Essentials of Palliative Care

Nalini Vadivelu • Alan David Kaye
Jack M. Berger

Editors

Essentials of Palliative Care

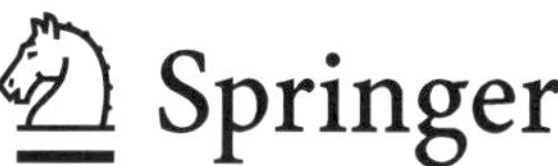 Springer

Editors
Nalini Vadivelu, MD
Department of Anesthesiology
Yale University School of Medicine
New Haven, CT, USA

Jack M. Berger, MS, MD, PhD
Department of Anesthesiology
Pain Medicine, and Critical Care
Keck School of Medicine of the
    University of Southern California
Los Angeles, CA, USA

Alan David Kaye, MD, PhD
Departments Anesthesiology
Louisiana State University School
    of Medicine,
New Orleans, LA, USA

ISBN 978-1-4614-5163-1   ISBN 978-1-4614-5164-8 (eBook)
DOI 10.1007/978-1-4614-5164-8
Springer New York Heidelberg Dordrecht London

Library of Congress Control Number: 2012951667

I wish to thank my parents, Major General Vadivelu and Gnanambigai Vadivelu, my husband, Thangamuthu Kodumudi, and my sons, Gopal and Vijay, for their steadfast support. I would also wish to thank my brother, Dr. Amarender Vadivelu, and sister, Suguna Vadivelu, for their inspiration, and my innumerable friends, colleagues, and students who encourage me to reach for heights higher than the day before.

–NV

I want to thank my wife, Dr. Kim Kaye, for her dedication and love over many decades; my brother, Dr. Adam Kaye, for a lifetime of friendship and support; and my mother-in-law, Dr. Patricia B. Sutker, for the thousands of loving and helpful things she has done for me over the past 25 years. Finally, I want to thank my mother, Florence Feldman, for inspiring me to be a doctor many years ago and for her love and support during my life.

–AK

I would like to thank my wife, Ethel, and my family for all their support, love, and understanding over the years of having to miss family functions because I became a doctor and my parents, Sol and Gertrude Berger, for all their support and encouragement to pursue my dreams. Special thanks to Angèle Ryan, MD, Jackie Carter, RN, MNS, and Janet Lucas, MSW, for teaching me about compassionate care and what it really means to be a doctor.

–JB

Foreword

When my mother turned 90 years old, she had moderately advanced Parkinson's disease, but no other major ailments. Her function was declining gradually, and she began to fall and become a bit forgetful. Her ability to live independently was waning. But her need for palliative care was clear and rapidly growing. It began with a general consideration of her medical goals—she did not want any big medical adventures, so resuscitation and intubation were easily taken off the table. But she still had a lot of things to enjoy in life, so she was willing to have her doctors try to fix easily treatable problems as long as she had a good chance of returning to an acceptable level of independence. But the ground rules of this approach were not clear, because her condition was fragile and her ability to live alone in her beloved house was becoming more and more difficult because of the ravages of her Parkinson's disease.

The next big event in her life was a fall where she sustained a broken hip. Surgically repairing the hip made sense given her goals (and the absence of good alternatives), but her recovery was complicated by pain, postoperative delirium, deconditioning, and worsening of her Parkinson's disease. The need for palliative care expertise to address the growing complexity of her symptoms and her condition was clearly growing, as her goals were now shifting more toward purely comfort-oriented approach. She had no definable terminal illness, so she did not qualify for a formal hospice program (even though that was the philosophy of treatment both she and we wanted), and no one could say with honesty that she was more likely than not to die in the next 6 months. With excellent palliation, she eventually made it to a rehabilitation program in a skilled nursing facility. Although her function improved modestly, she did not return to her former baseline. She hated living there, and her inability to safely walk without someone with her at all times was a real challenge to her sense of identity and personhood. Palliation now required multidimensional interventions that included orthopedic guidance, pain management, physical therapy, neurologic management of her Parkinson's disease, and psychological treatment of her grief.

My mother was adamant in her desire to return to her home, yet we as a family knew it was unsafe without 24-hour supervision, which she flatly refused. As we were struggling with next steps, she suddenly became jaundiced. Her doctor fortunately was skilled in palliative care and knowledgeable about hospice care. He helped us think through her limited options. My mother was painfully aware that her quality of life was waning rapidly, as was her ability to live independently, and that more medical intervention was the last thing she wanted unless it had a high likelihood of returning her to full independence. A biopsy or a biliary drainage procedure would not help her achieve these goals, and therefore would not be in her best interest. It was time to shift gears toward pure, noninvasive palliation, and a hospice referral was made without any biopsies or interventions. With her new found terminal illness, she now qualified for hospice medically as well as philosophically, and we began to think through where she would spend her final time. Although our extended family lived on the North Shore of Boston where my mother was living, she agreed to a move to Rochester to be near us so that we could help care for her over her final weeks or months. She put on my Red Sox cap for her final road trip, and my brother and I brought her to Rochester where she lived in a comfort care home for her final weeks. With the help of a skilled hospice team, we were able to keep her very comfortable. There were symptoms that required intensive management, including pruritis, pain, and delirium, but there were also wonder times of storytelling and family members coming together. She died very peacefully in our presence 3 weeks after her move to Rochester.

There ought not to be very much special or unique about this story, but in fact in the current environment it is probably the exception rather than the rule. Part of the reason it is exceptional is that many physicians do not have the knowledge and skill about palliative care and hospice that her physician and our family had. Such knowledge, skill, and advice is thoughtfully and accessibly presented in *Essentials of Palliative Care*, co-edited by three highly skilled and respected palliative care physicians, Drs. Vadivelu, Kaye, and Berger. The physicians caring for my mother were not specialists in palliative care or hospice, but they knew enough about palliative treatments to be able to help us think through a broad range of options at each clinical curve in the road. Although they did not always have all the palliative care treatment options at their fingertips, they knew how to find them and how to adapt the treatment plan to my mother's preferences and changing clinical circumstances. Many of the chapters in this book would have been relevant to my mother's care, including the chapters on pain management, on physical and occupational therapy, and psychological distress, as well as the chapter covering the transition to hospice. There are other chapters that provide guidance about vascular access, ostomy care, and palliative use of interventional radiology that might not be within the knowledge base of all clinicians, but would increase awareness of potential palliative options to address difficult symptom-related problems.

Not everyone providing palliative care needs to be a subspecialist (there is far too much work and too few fully trained and certified clinicians), but all clinicians who care for seriously ill patients should have solid basic palliative care skills both in terms of pain and symptom management, and in terms of helping patients negotiate the medical system in light of a full understanding of their patients' goals and clinical options. *Essentials of Palliative Care* should be a part of that toolkit, and we are indebted to Drs. Vadivelu, Kaye, Berger, and their other chapter authors for providing such an accessible, useful resource.

Rochester, NY, USA   Timothy E. Quill Rochester

Preface

Palliative Medicine has become a familiar term in recent years and is becoming established as a key component in modern health care, and many institutions promote Palliative Care teams. Although this is a term relatively new to many practitioners, palliative care was coined several decades ago by Dr. Balfour Mount, a Canadian physician. After training in Dame Cicely Saunders' St. Christopher's Hospice in London, he was so impressed that he was inspired to bring this type of care to mainstream curative medicine. As a result, he founded the Royal Victoria Hospital Palliative Care Service in 1974 and is credited with establishing the first in-patient palliative care unit in North America. Having emerged from the nurse driven hospice movement, the care of the dying has evolved to a formal hospice benefit and development of a recognized subspecialty.

This specialty of Hospice and Palliative Medicine (HPM) is dedicated to promoting quality end of life care to patients and families struggling with advanced disease. In recent years, palliative care has become increasingly common in the medical literature as well as in public media. Although the delivery of palliative care is influenced by the hospice model, the composition of a hospital-based palliative care team varies significantly from one institution to another, but fundamental roles are generally identified as the provision of physical, emotional, social, and spiritual comfort. The requirements for a "home" based palliative care team service is similar to those of the hospital-based service.

In developing an education program for symptom management and palliative care, physicians and other healthcare providers will need to learn how to make the difficult decisions with respect to recommending or initiating therapeutic interventions or recommending and discontinuing interventions. Examples of symptoms which would have to be considered can be grouped as follows:

- Pain of any etiology, tumor metastasis, spinal cord or nerve root compression, lymphedema, bowel obstruction, electrolyte abnormalities.
- Dehydration, malnutrition, anorexia–cachexia syndrome, radiation enteritis, diarrhea, nausea, vomiting.
- Asthenia, fatigue, weakness.

- Dyspnea, respiratory failure, respiratory tract infections, pleural effusions, lymphangitis carcinomatosis.
- Anemia, wound breakdown, ulcerations, decubitus ulcers, ostomies.
- Anxiety, confusion, sleep disorders, depression, sadness, anger.
- Hiccoughs, cough, bloating, belching, mucositis, foul body ordors, wheezing.

It is necessary to develop systems for evaluating the necessity or futility of intervening based upon an understanding of the pathophysiology of the above symptoms in the terminally ill patient. The costs both economic and psychosocial of intervening or not intervening or cessation of ongoing interventions must be better defined. Only through facing these difficult problems critically can we learn how best to deal with them.

The Physician

The American Board of Medical Specialties is a self-policing organization that sets standards and grants certification for medical practice beyond the minimum requirements for licensure. In a given field of medical practice, a physician seeks recognition for expertise. When Palliative Medicine became part of modern medical practice, the logical result was the pursuit of formal certification. As a result, the American Board of Hospice and Palliative Medicine was formed, an independent certifying organization.

From 1996 to 2006, the available certification for physicians practicing palliative medicine was through the independent American Board of Hospice and Palliative Medicine. This entity provided recognition of expertise for practitioners caring for the dying, while promoting the importance of the specialty and working toward transition to formal recognition by the American Board of Medical Specialties, the official body that is recognized by healthcare systems as the stamp of approval of medical specialties. Currently, there are ten co-sponsoring boards that offer subspecialty certification in Hospice and Palliative Medicine (HPM), including the American Boards of Anesthesiology, Emergency Medicine, Family Medicine, Internal Medicine, Obstetrics and Gynecology, Pediatrics, Physical Medicine and Rehabilitation, Psychiatry and Neurology, Radiology, and Surgery.

Competencies of subspecialist-level hospice and palliative medicine include skills in symptom management, relief of suffering and improving the quality of life for patients and families living with life-threatening illness, provision of assistance for patients and families coping with loss, and management of challenging problems associated with end-of-life care.

Nursing

The nursing profession has been in the forefront of the hospice movement and plays a pivotal role in modern palliative medicine. The National Board for Certification of Hospice and Palliative Nurses (NBCHPN), established in 1993, provides nursing certification for hospice and palliative medicine for several categories of nursing positions. The classifications of expertise include Advanced Certified Hospice and Palliative Nurse (ACHPN), Certified Hospice and Palliative Nurse (CHPN), Certified Hospice and Palliative Pediatric Nurse (CHPPN), Certified Hospice and Palliative Licensed Nurse (CHPLN), Certified Hospice and Palliative Nursing Assistant (CHPNA), Certified Hospice and Palliative Care Administrator (CHPCA). Each certification period is valid for 4 years and is renewable.

Advanced practice nursing certification is granted for nursing professionals who either hold a Clinical Nurse Specialist or Nurse Practitioner license, and have graduated from an accredited education program specializing in palliative care that includes a minimum of 500 hours of palliative care training, or have post master's graduate practice experience of 500 hours in providing palliative care in the year prior to examination. Successful completion of the examination establishes excellence in the area of clinical judgment, advocacy and ethics and systems thinking, professionalism and research, collaboration, facilitation of learning and communication, and cultural and spiritual competence.

For a registered nurse to test for CHPN status, the candidate must hold a valid registered nurse license. It is recommended that the individual also have at least 2 years of practice in end-of-life care prior to testing. Successful completion of the examination demonstrates ability in recognition of life-limiting conditions in adult patients, pain and symptom management, care of patient and family, education and advocacy, interdisciplinary/collaborative practice, and professional issues.

A nursing professional seeking certification for NBCHPN is required to hold a valid registered nurse license and is encouraged to have a minimum of 2 years experience in the care of terminally ill children. This encompasses the care of patients ranging in age from perinatal to young adulthood. As a result of certification, the pediatric nurse establishes competencies in recognition of life-threatening conditions in children, pain and symptom management, treatments and procedures, family centered care, education and advocacy, care at end of life, grief and bereavement, and professional issues.

The certification exam for licensed practical nurses (LPN) and licensed vocational nurses (LVN) has been offered since 2004. Successful candidates achieve the CHPLN credential, which is valid for 4 years. Candidates holding a valid LPN or LVN are eligible to take the exam. Two years experience in the hospice or palliative care setting is recommended. Clinical areas of expertise include various aspects of patient care such as end-stage disease process in adult patients, pain, symptom, and comfort management, treatments and procedures, care of patient, family, and other caregivers, patient and family education and advocacy, and interdisciplinary and collaborative practice issues.

Nursing assistants are eligible to test for the CHPNA credential if the candidate can provide documentation of 2000 practice hours under the supervision of a registered nurse in the previous 2 years. It is also recommended that the candidates have 2 years of experience specifically in the field of hospice or palliative care.

Examination for the CHPCA credential is offered for any individual with 2 years experience in an administrative role, verified by a supervisor, that involves hospice or palliative care. The NBCHPN administrator examination tests for competency in leadership, planning, operations, fiscal and human resource management, quality management, marketing, public relations, and ethics.

Social Work

The advanced certified hospice and palliative social worker (ACHP-SW) credential was added in 2009, adapted for the specialized skills and expertise of social work professionals who provide care in the hospice and palliative care setting . The eligibility requirements include a master's degree in social work from an accredited university, 20 or more continuing education credits specific to hospice and palliative care, documentation of at least 2 years of supervised social work experience in hospice or palliative care setting, and a current license to practice as a professional social worker.

Program Certification

With the ambitious credentialing process for all members of the palliative care team, it is logical to expect progression to program certification. The Joint Commission on Accreditation of Healthcare Organizations has developed an Advanced Certification Program for Palliative Care. Expertise and commitment of dedicated individuals representing the credentialed disciplines is greatly enhanced in the setting of institutional support. Standards set forth by the Joint Commission certification program emphasize this need to consign resources and support for palliative care teams. Eligibility requirements for palliative care program certification include: be a joint commission accredited hospital or facility, have full time coverage for palliative care services, have served a minimum of ten patients and have at least one active patient at the time of the initial joint commission review, provide care based on clinical practice guidelines and/or evidence-based practice, have control in the clinical management of patients and coordination of care, follow an organized approach supported by an interdisciplinary team of health professionals, and use performance measurement to improve its performance over time.

These standards are based on The National Consensus Project's Clinical Practice Guidelines for Quality Palliative Care and the National Quality Forum's National Framework and Preferred Practices for Palliative and Hospice Care Quality.

The common goals and standards of all the credentialing disciplines and organizations reflect the scope and complexity of palliative care. All entities strive for complete care of the dying patient and family, including the physical, spiritual, emotional, cultural, legal, and ethical components treatments. Features that are shared by all programs stress the importance of the interdisciplinary approach for alleviation of suffering, care in multiple settings, education, quality improvement, and attention to family and caregivers.

The monumental efforts that have led to the entry of palliative care into the mainstream of medical practice provide a sound foundation for individual institutions to incorporate this practice into the network of customary hospital services . Although the number of institutions that provide a palliative care team continues to grow, there is a lack of standardization regarding the composition and role of such a team. There is opportunity for institutions to support the excellence and standards of specialized professionals, and offer customized service that is focused on the unique patient populations that they serve. Each hospital has tools available developing its own unique approach for delivery of palliative care.

Education, of course, should be a major component of any symptom management and palliative care program. Mark Lema, MD, PhD commented in the ASA Newsletter, July 1998, that "The AMA is concerned that physician assisted suicide is a symptom of a much bigger problem, that physicians are not prepared to properly care for dying patients" [6]. Changing one's focus from cure to comfort care is not in the traditional medical curriculum or philosophy. Attendings, fellows, residents, interns, and medical students as well as nursing staff and all other ancillary personnel of the team have to be taught this reorientated mind-set. How to approach the patient and/or significant others with the diagnosis of terminal illness, the presentation of options for end-of-life care, the emphasis that palliative care does not mean "nothing else can be done," or that no care will be offered, but rather that the goal of therapy will be comfort and dignity is something that must be taught and practiced. How one obtains a "true informed consent" for do not resuscitate (DNR), and how one approaches the completion of an advanced directive needs to be taught and needs to be learned.

In summary, true palliative care involves a paradigm shift. A patient used to receive a diagnosis of a life-threatening disease and a treatment plan was laid out with little attention paid to the consequences of the treatment or what will be done if the treatment fails to arrest the disease. And it was only in the last few days or weeks of life that a patient was offered comfort care measures. Today, as compassionate healthcare providers it is incumbent upon us to introduce comfort care early in the process. Comfort measures (palliative care) will intensify as curative measures are exhausted. Thus, the needs of the patient and his/her family can be met at all stages of the disease process. We hope that our book, *Essentials of Palliative Care*, is useful for clinicians of all disciplines as we move forward in this ever changing and complex world.

New Haven, CT, USA
New Orleans, LA, USA
Los Angeles, CA, USA Nalini Vadivelu
Alan David Kaye
Jack M. Berger

References

1. Portenoy RK, Lupu DE, Arnold RM, Cordes A, Storey P. Formal ABMS and ACGME recognition of hospice and palliative medicine expected in 2006. J Palliat Med. 2006;9(1):21–3.
2. Berzoff J, Lucas G, Deluca D, Gerbino S, Browning D, Foster Z, Chatchkes E. Clinical social work education in palliative and end-of-life care: relational approaches for advanced practitioners. J Soc Work End Life Palliat Care. 2006;2(2):45–63.
3. Von Gunten CF. Set an example. J Palliat Med. 2009;12(5):409.
4. Weissman DE, Meier DE. Identifying patients in need of a palliative care assessment in the hospital setting, a consensus report from the Center to Advance Palliative Care. J Palliat Med. 2011;14(1):17–22.
5. Weissman DE, Meier DE. Operational features for hospital palliative care programs: consensus recommendations. J Palliat Med. 2008;11(9):1189–94.
6. Lema M. Comments in the ASA Newsletter, July 1998.

Contents

1 Introduction and Education... 1
Angèle Ryan and Jack M. Berger

2 Multidisciplinary Approach and Coordination of Care..................... 7
Sukanya Mitra and Nalini Vadivelu

**3 Psychological Distress and Psychiatric Comorbidities
in Palliative Care**... 23
Raphael J. Leo and Maria Theresa Mariano

4 Hospice for the Terminally Ill and End-of-Life Care 49
Jamie Capasso, Robert Byron Kim, and Danielle Perret

5 Communication in Palliative Care 73
Dominique Anwar, Sean Ransom, and Roy S. Weiner

6 Guidance with Complex Treatment Choices..................................... 89
Sukanya Mitra and Nalini Vadivelu

7 Symptom Management.. 107
Angèle Ryan

8 Nutrition in Palliative Care... 137
M. Khurram Ghori and Susan Dabu-Bondoc

9 Nursing Perspective and Considerations 163
Ena M. Williams and Tong Ying Ge

10 Physical and Occupational Therapy in Palliative Care..................... 177
Kais Alsharif and Justin Hata

11 Social Work in Palliative Care... 189
Janet Lucas, Bill Mejia, and Anne Riffenburgh

12 The Healthcare System: More Questions than Answers.................... 209
Jackie D.D. Carter

**13 Vascular Access: Ostomies and Drains Care
in Palliative Medicine** 217
Patricia L. Devaney

14 Drug Formulary 229
Angèle Ryan

15 Interventional Radiology in Palliative Care 253
Oliver Hulson, Neal Larkman, and S. Kunnumpurath

16 Stroke, Epilepsy, and Neurological Diseases 279
María Gudín

17 Interventional Techniques in Palliative Care 299
Rinoo V. Shah, Alan David Kaye,
Christopher K. Merritt, and Lien B. Tran

18 Headache in Palliative Care 315
Nicholas Connolly, Matthew Peña, and Tara M. Sheridan

**19 Endoscopic Therapies for Palliation of Gastrointestinal
Malignancies** 349
Henry C. Ho and Uzma D. Siddiqui

20 The Role of Palliative Care in Cardiothoracic Surgery 369
Amit Banerjee

21 Management of Advanced Heart Failure Patients 375
Dominique Anwar and Asif Anwar

22 Palliative Care in Cardiac Electrophysiology 385
Eric Grubman

23 Palliation in Respiratory Disease 395
David R. Meek, Martin D. Knolle, and Thomas B. Pulimood

24 Palliative Care in Critical Care Units 417
Rita Agarwala, Ben Singer, and Sreekumar Kunnumpurath

25 Pediatric Palliative Care 441
Shu-Ming Wang, Paul B. Yost, and Leonard Sender

26 New Pain Management Vistas in Palliative Care 457
Christopher K. Merritt, Lien B. Tran, Rinoo V. Shah,
and Alan David Kaye

27 Ethics in Palliative and End-of-Life Care 483
Jack M. Berger

**28 Physician Coding, Billing, and Reimbursement
for Palliative Care** 501
Rene R. Rigal

Index 505

Contributors

Rita Agarwala, B.M., B.Sc. Department of Anesthetics, Epsom and St Helier University Hospitals NHS Trust, Carshalton, Surrey, UK

Kais Alsharif, M.D. Department of Anesthesiology and Perioperative Care, University of California, Irvine School of Medicine, Irvine, CA, USA

Asif Anwar, M.D. Heart and Vascular Institute, Department of Medicine, Tulane University School of Medicine, New Orleans, LA, USA

Dominique Anwar, M.D. Section of General Internal Medicine and Geriatrics, Tulane University School of Medicine, New Orleans, LA, USA

Amit Banerjee, M.S., M.Ch. Department of Cardiothoracic Surgery, Maulana Azad Medical College, New Delhi, India

Govind Ballabh Pant Hospital, University of Delhi, New Delhi, India

Jack M. Berger, M.S., M.D., Ph.D. Department of Anesthesiology, Keck School of Medicine, University of Southern California, Los Angeles, CA, USA

Jamie Capasso, D.O. Department of Medicine, University of California, Irvine School of Medicine, Irvine, CA, USA

Jackie D.D. Carter, R.N., M.S.N., C.N.S. Department of Nursing, LAC+USC Medical Center, Los Angeles, CA, USA

Nicholas Connolly, M.D. Department of Anesthesiology, Naval Medical Center San Diego, San Diego, CA, USA

Susan Dabu-Bondoc, M.D. Department of Anesthesiology, Yale University School of Medicine, New Haven, CT, USA

Patricia L. Devaney, R.N., B.S., M.S. Department of Diagnostic Radiology, Yale-New Haven Hospital, New Haven, CT, USA

Tong Ying Ge, R.N., M.S.N. (Master Degree of Nursing) Pain Advanced practice nurse, Sir Run Run Shaw Hospital, Hangzhou, China

M. Khurram Ghori, M.D. Department of Anesthesiology, Yale University School of Medicine, New Haven, CT, USA

Eric Grubman, M.D. Department of Internal Medicine, Yale University School of Medicine, New Haven, CT, USA

María Gudín, Ph.D. Neurology Department, Ciudad Real General University Hospital, Ciudad Real, Castilla–La Mancha, Spain

Justin Hata, M.D. Department of Anesthesiology and Perioperative Care, University of California, Irvine School of Medicine, Irvine, CA, USA

Henry C. Ho, M.D. Section of Digestive Diseases, Department of Internal Medicine, Yale University School of Medicine, New Haven, CT, USA

Oliver Hulson, M.B.Ch.B. (Hons.) Leeds and Bradford Radiology Training Scheme, Leeds General Infirmary, Leeds, UK

Alan David Kaye, M.D., Ph.D. Department of Anesthesiology, Louisiana State University School of Medicine, New Orleans, LA, USA

Robert Byron Kim, M.D. Department of Anesthesiology & Perioperative Care, University of California, Irvine School of Medicine, Irvine, CA, USA

Martin D. Knolle, M.B., B.Chir., M.R.C.P. Department of Respiratory Medicine, Lister Hospital, Stevenage, UK

Sreekumar Kunnumpurath, M.B.B.S., M.D. Department of Anaesthetics, Epsom and St Helier University Hospitals NHS Trust, Carshalton, Surrey, UK

Neal Larkman, M.B.B.S. M.P.H., Leeds and Bradford Radiology Training Scheme, Leeds General Infirmary, Leeds, UK

Raphael J. Leo, M.A., M.D. Department of Psychiatry, School of Medicine and Biomedical Sciences, State University of New York, Buffalo, NY, USA

Janet Lucas, L.C.S.W., B.S., M.S.W. Family Practice Residency Program, Glendale Adventist Medical Center, Glendale, CA, USA

Maria Theresa Mariano, M.D. Department of Psychiatry, School of Medicine and Biomedical Sciences, State University of New York, Buffalo, NY, USA

David R. Meek, M.R.C.P. Department of Respiratory and General Internal Medicine, West Suffolk Hospital, University of Cambridge Teaching Hospital, Bury St Edmunds, Suffolk, UK

Bill Mejia, L.C.S.W., B.S., M.S.W. Palliate Care Consult Service, Huntington Hospital, Pasadena, CA, USA

Christopher K. Merritt, M.D. Department of Anesthesiology, Louisiana State University School of Medicine, New Orleans, LA, USA

Sukanya Mitra, M.D. Department of Anaesthesia and Intensive Care, Government Medical College and Hospital, Chandigarh, India

Matthew Peña, M.D. Department of Anesthesiology, Naval Medical Center San Diego, San Diego, CA, USA

Danielle Perret, M.D. Department of Anesthesiology & Perioperative Care, University of California, Irvine School of Medicine, Irvine, CA, USA

Thomas B. Pulimood, M.B.B.S., F.R.C.P. Department of Respiratory and General Internal Medicine, West Suffolk Hospital, University of Cambridge Teaching Hospital, Bury St Edmunds, Suffolk, UK

Sean Ransom, Ph.D. Department of Psychiatry and Behavioral Sciences, Tulane University School of Medicine, New Orleans, LA, USA

Anne Riffenburgh, L.C.S.W., B.S., M.S.W. Huntington Cancer Center, Huntington Hospital, Pasadena, CA, USA

Rene R. Rigal, M.D. Pain Management Center, Divine Providence Hospital, Williamsport, PA, USA

Angèle Ryan, M.D. Department of Anesthesiology, Keck School of Medicine, University of Southern California, Los Angeles, CA, USA

Leonard Sender, M.D. Department of Medicine, University of California, Irvine School of Medicine, Irvine, CA, USA

Rinoo V. Shah, M.D., M.B.A. Department of Anesthesiology, Guthrie Clinic-Big Flats, Horseheads, NY, USA

Tara M. Sheridan, M.D. Department of Anesthesiology, Naval Medical Center San Diego, Bethesda, MD, USA

Uzma D. Siddiqui, M.D. Department of Medicine, University of Chicago Pritzker School of Medicine, Chicago, IL, USA

Ben Singer, M.B.B.S., F.R.C.A. Department of Anaesthetics, Epsom and St Helier University Hospitals NHS Trust, Carshalton, Surrey, UK

Lien B. Tran, M.D. Department of Anesthesiology, Louisiana State University School of Medicine, New Orleans, LA, USA

Nalini Vadivelu, M.D. Department of Anesthesiology, Yale University School of Medicine, New Haven, CT, USA

Shu-Ming Wang, M.D. Department of Anesthesiology and Perioperative Care, University of California, Irvine School of Medicine, Irvine, CA, USA

Roy S. Weiner, M.D. Tulane Cancer Center, Tulane University School of Medicine, New Orleans, LA, USA

Ena M. Williams, R.N., M.S.M., M.B.A. Department of Perioperative Services, Yale-New Haven Hospital, New Haven, CT, USA

Paul B. Yost, M.D., F.A.A.P. Department of Anesthesiology, St. Joseph's of Orange, Orange, CA, USA

Chapter 1
Introduction and Education

Angèle Ryan and Jack M. Berger

Palliative Medicine has become a familiar term in recent years and is becoming established as a key component in modern health care, and many institutions promote Palliative Care teams. Although this is a term relatively new to many practitioners, palliative care was coined several decades ago by Dr. Balfour Mount, a Canadian physician. After training in Dame Cicely Saunders' St. Christopher's Hospice in London, he was so impressed that he was inspired to bring this type of care to mainstream curative medicine. As a result, he founded the Royal Victoria Hospital Palliative Care Service in 1974 and is credited with establishing the first in-patient palliative care unit in North America. Having emerged from the nurse driven hospice movement, the care of the dying has evolved to a formal hospice benefit and development of a recognized subspecialty.

This specialty of Hospice and Palliative Medicine (HPM) is dedicated to the promotion of quality end of life care to patients and to families struggling with advanced disease. In recent years, palliative care has become increasingly common in the medical literature as well as in the public media. Although the delivery of palliative care is influenced by the hospice model, the composition of a hospital-based palliative care team varies significantly from one institution to another, but fundamental roles are generally identified for the provision of physical, emotional, social, and spiritual comfort. The requirements for a "home" based palliative care team service are similar to those of the hospital-based service.

In developing an educational program for symptom management and palliative care, physicians and other healthcare providers need to learn how to make difficult decisions with respect to recommending or initiating therapeutic interventions or recommending and discontinuing interventions. Examples of symptoms which have to be considered can be grouped as follows:

A. Ryan, M.D. (✉) • J.M. Berger, M.S., M.D., Ph.D.
Department of Anesthesiology, Keck School of Medicine, University of Southern California, Los Angeles, CA, USA
e-mail: angel@ix.netcom.com; jmberger@usc.edu

N. Vadivelu et al. (eds.), *Essentials of Palliative Care*,
DOI 10.1007/978-1-4614-5164-8_1,
© Springer Science+Business Media New York 2013

- Pain of any etiology, tumor metastasis, spinal cord or nerve root compression, lymphedema, bowel obstruction, electrolyte abnormalities.
- Dehydration, malnutrition, anorexia–cachexia syndrome, radiation enteritis, diarrhea, nausea, vomiting.
- Asthenia, fatigue, weakness.
- Dyspnea, respiratory failure, respiratory tract infections, pleural effusions, lymphangitis carcinomatosis.
- Anemia, wound breakdown, ulcerations, decubitus ulcers, ostomies.
- Anxiety, confusion, sleep disorders, depression, sadness, anger.
- Hiccoughs, cough, bloating, belching, mucositis, foul body odors, wheezing.

It is necessary to develop systems for evaluating the necessity or futility of intervening based upon an understanding of the pathophysiology of the above symptoms in the face of the terminally ill patient. The costs both economic and psychosocial of intervening or not intervening or cessation of ongoing interventions must be better defined. Only through facing these difficult problems critically can we learn how best to deal with them.

The Physician

The American Board of Medical Specialties is a self-policing organization that sets standards and grants certification for medical practice beyond the minimum requirements for licensure. In a given field of medical practice, a physician seeks recognition for expertise. When Palliative Medicine became part of modern medical practice, the logical result was the pursuit of formal certification. As a result, the American Board of Hospice and Palliative Medicine was formed, an independent certifying organization.

From 1996 to 2006, the available certification for physicians practicing palliative medicine was through the independent American Board of Hospice and Palliative Medicine. This entity provides recognition of expertise for practitioners caring for the dying, while promoting the importance of the specialty and working toward transition to formal recognition by the American Board of Medical Specialties, the official body that is recognized by healthcare systems as the stamp of approval of medical specialties [1]. Currently, there are ten cosponsoring boards that offer subspecialty certification in Hospice and Palliative Medicine (HPM), including the American Boards of Anesthesiology, Emergency Medicine, Family Medicine, Internal Medicine, Obstetrics and Gynecology, Pediatrics, Physical Medicine and Rehabilitation, Psychiatry and Neurology, Radiology, and Surgery.

Competencies of subspecialist-level hospice and palliative medicine include skills in symptom management, relief of suffering and improving the quality of life for patients and families living with life-threatening illness, provision of assistance for patients and families coping with loss, and management of challenging problems associated with end-of-life care.

Nursing

The nursing profession has been at the forefront of the hospice movement and plays a pivotal role in modern palliative medicine. The National Board for Certification of Hospice and Palliative Nurses (NBCHPN), established in 1993, provides nursing certification for hospice and palliative medicine for several categories of nursing positions. The classifications of expertise include: Advanced Certified Hospice and Palliative Nurse (ACHPN), Certified Hospice and Palliative Nurse (CHPN), Certified Hospice and Palliative Pediatric Nurse (CHPPN), Certified Hospice and Palliative Licensed Nurse (CHPLN), Certified Hospice and Palliative Nursing Assistant (CHPNA), and Certified Hospice and Palliative Care Administrator (CHPCA). Each certification period is valid for 4 years and is renewable.

Advanced practice nursing certification is granted for nursing professionals who hold a Clinical Nurse Specialist or Nurse Practitioner license and have graduated from an accredited education program specializing in palliative care. The program must include a minimum of 500 hours of palliative care training or have post master's graduate practice experience of 500 hours in providing palliative care in the year prior to examination. Successful completion of the examination establishes excellence in the area of clinical judgment, advocacy and ethics and systems thinking, professionalism and research, collaboration, facilitation of learning and communication, and cultural and spiritual competence.

The eligibility requirements for a registered nurse to test for CHPN status, the candidate must hold a valid registered nurse license. It is recommended that the individual also have at least 2 years of practice in end-of-life care prior to testing. Successful completion of the examination demonstrates abilities in recognition of life-limiting conditions in adult patients, pain and symptom management, care of patient and family, education and advocacy, interdisciplinary/collaborative practice, and professional issues.

A nursing professional seeking certification for NBCHPN is required to hold a valid registered nurse license and is encouraged to have a minimum of 2 years experience in the care of terminally ill children. This encompasses the care of patients ranging in age from prenatal to young adulthood. As a result of certification, the pediatric nurse establishes competencies in recognition of life-threatening conditions in children, pain and symptom management, treatments and procedures, family centered care, education and advocacy, care at end of life, grief and bereavement, and professional issues.

The certification exam for licensed practical nurses (LPN) and licensed vocational nurses (LVN) has been offered since 2004. Successful candidates achieve the CHPLN credential, which is valid for 4 years. Candidates holding a valid LPN or LVN are eligible to take the exam. Two years experience in the hospice or palliative care setting is recommended. Clinical areas of expertise include: various aspects of patient care, such as end-stage disease process in adult patients, pain, symptom, and comfort management, treatments and procedures, care of patient, family, and other caregivers, patient and family education and advocacy, and interdisciplinary and collaborative practice issues.

Nursing assistants are eligible to test for the CHPNA credential if the candidate can provide documentation of 2000 practice hours under the supervision of a registered nurse in the previous 2 years. It is also recommended that the candidates have 2 years of experience specifically in the field of hospice or palliative care.

Examination for the CHPCA credential is offered for any individual with 2 years experience in an administrative role, verified by a supervisor which involves hospice or palliative care. The NBCHPN administrator examination tests for competency in leadership, planning, operations, fiscal and human resource management, quality management, marketing, public relations, and ethics.

Social Work

The advanced certified hospice and palliative social worker (ACHP-SW) credential was added in 2009. It was adapted for the specialized skills and expertise of social work professionals who provide care in the hospice and palliative care setting [2]. The eligibility requirements include a master's degree in social work from an accredited university, 20 or more continuing education credits specific to hospice and palliative care, documentation of at least 2 years of supervised social work experience in hospice or palliative care setting, and current license to practice as a professional social worker.

Program Certification

With the ambitious credentialing process for all members of the palliative care team, it is logical to expect progression to program certification. The Joint Commission on Accreditation of Healthcare Organizations has developed an Advanced Certification Program for Palliative Care. Expertise and commitment of dedicated individuals representing the credentialed disciplines is greatly enhanced in the setting of institutional support. Standards set forth by the Joint Commission certification program emphasize this need to consign resources and support for palliative care teams.

Eligibility requirements for palliative care program certification include joint commission accredited hospital or facility, full-time coverage for palliative care services, have served a minimum of ten patients and have at least one active patient at the time of the initial joint commission review, provide care based on clinical practice guidelines and/or evidence-based practice, have control in the clinical management of patients and coordination of care, follow an organized approach supported by an interdisciplinary team of health professionals, and use performance measurement to improve its performance over time. These standards are based on The National Consensus Project's Clinical Practice Guidelines for Quality Palliative

Care and the National Quality Forum's National Framework and Preferred Practices for Palliative and Hospice Care Quality.

The common goals and standards of all the credentialing disciplines and organizations reflect the scope and complexity of palliative care. All entities strive for complete care of the dying patient and family, including the physical, spiritual, emotional, cultural, legal, and ethical components treatments. Features that are shared by all programs stress the importance of the interdisciplinary approach for alleviation of suffering, care in multiple settings, education, quality improvement, attention to family and caregivers.

The monumental efforts that have led to the entry of palliative care into the mainstream of medical practice provide a sound foundation for individual institutions to incorporate this practice into the network of customary hospital services [3]. Although the number of institutions that provide a palliative care team continues to grow, there is a lack of standardization regarding the composition and role of such a team. There is opportunity for institutions to support the excellence and standards of specialized professionals, and offer customized service that is focused on the unique patient populations that they serve [4, 5]. Each hospital has tools available for development of its own unique approach for delivery of palliative care.

Education of course should be a major component of any symptom management and palliative care program. Mark Lema M.D., Ph.D. commented in the American Society of Anesthesiologists Newsletter, July 1998, that "The American Medical Association is concerned that physician assisted suicide is a symptom of a much bigger problem, that physicians are not prepared to properly care for dying patients" [6].

Changing one's focus from cure to comfort care is not in the traditional medical curriculum or philosophy. Attendings, fellows, residents, interns, and medical students as well as nursing staff and all other ancillary personnel of the team have to be taught this reorientation of mind-set. How to approach the patient and/or significant others with the diagnosis of terminal illness, the presentation of options for end of life care, the emphasis that palliative care does not mean "nothing else can be done," or that no care will be offered, but rather that the goal of therapy will be comfort and dignity is something that must be taught and practiced. How one obtains a "true informed consent" for do not resuscitate (DNR), and how one approaches the completion of an advanced directive needs to be taught and needs to be learned.

In summary, true palliative care involves a paradigm shift. A patient used to receive a diagnosis of a life-threatening disease and a treatment plan was laid out with little attention paid to the consequences of the treatment or what will be done if the treatment fails to arrest the disease. And it was only in the last few days or weeks of life that a patient was offered comfort care measures. Today, as compassionate healthcare providers it is incumbent upon us to introduce comfort care early in the process. Comfort measures (palliative care) will intensify as curative measures are exhausted. Thus, the needs of the patient and his/her family can be met at all stages of the disease process.

References

1. Portenoy RK, Lupu DE, Arnold RM, Cordes A, Storey P. Formal ABMS and ACGME recognition of hospice and palliative medicine expected in 2006. J Palliat Med. 2006;9(1):21–3.
2. Berzoff J, Lucas G, Deluca D, Gerbino S, Browning D, Foster Z, Chatchkes E. Clinical social work education in palliative and end-of-life care: relational approaches for advanced practitioners. J Soc Work End Life Palliat Care. 2006;2(2):45–63.
3. Von Gunten CF. Set an example. J Palliat Med. 2009;12(5):409.
4. Weissman DE, Meier DE. Identifying patients in need of a palliative care assessment in the hospital setting, a consensus report from the Center to Advance Palliative Care. J Palliat Med. 2011;14(1):17–22.
5. Weissman DE, Meier DE. Operational features for hospital palliative care programs: consensus recommendations. J Palliat Med. 2008;11(9):1189–94.
6. Lema M. Comments in the ASA Newsletter, July 1998.

Chapter 2
Multidisciplinary Approach and Coordination of Care

Sukanya Mitra and Nalini Vadivelu

Introduction and Basic Concepts

On September 1, 2011, The Joint Commission (formerly the Joint Commission on Accreditation of Healthcare Organizations) announced the Advanced Certification Program for Palliative Care, "designed to recognize hospital inpatient programs that demonstrate exceptional patient and family-centered care in order to optimize the quality of life for patients with serious illness" [1]. This development represents the latest important milestone marked on a long and arduous journey that began in the hospice movement in the 1960s and then the related palliative care movement in the 1980s.

The word "palliative" or "palliation" is derived from Latin "palliare," which means "to cloak," or in other words, to mask, to cover up, or to mitigate. Traditional medicine has generally been curative, i.e., focused on cure of the underlying cause of a disease. Symptom removal (or "symptomatic treatment") has often been perceived as incomplete and facile. In a similar vein, traditional medicine has usually regarded issues such as distress reduction and improvement in quality of life as secondary to the primary aim of treating the actual disease. Understandably, such an approach immediately faces an obvious roadblock when dealing with diseases that are remotely curable or incurable (e.g., some cancers, cancers with widespread metastasis, advanced HIV disease, some neurological, renal, and pulmonary diseases, etc.). In these unfortunate progressive and life-threatening illnesses, where

S. Mitra, M.D. (✉)
Department of Anaesthesia and Intensive Care,
Government Medical College and Hospital,
Chandigarh, India
e-mail: Drsmitra12@yahoo.com

N. Vadivelu, M.D.
Department of Anesthesiology,
Yale University School of Medicine,
New Haven, CT, USA

N. Vadivelu et al. (eds.), *Essentials of Palliative Care*,
DOI 10.1007/978-1-4614-5164-8_2,
© Springer Science+Business Media New York 2013

the prospect of a "cure" is largely nonexistent, one is forced to "shift gear" and adopt a modified perspective. The focus then changes to one of symptom reduction, distress management, and eventually, improving the quality of life under the circumstances. This, in essence, is the palliative care approach.

The World Health Organization (WHO) has defined palliative care as:

> Palliative care is an approach that improves the quality of life of patients and their families facing the problems associated with life-threatening illness, through the prevention and relief of suffering by means of early identification and impeccable assessment and treatment of pain and other problems, physical, psychosocial and spiritual [2].

It goes on further to clarify that palliative care:

- Provides relief from pain and other distressing symptoms.
- Affirms life and regards dying as a normal process.
- Intends neither to hasten nor postpone death.
- Integrates the psychological and spiritual aspects of patient care.
- Offers a support system to help patients live as actively as possible until death.
- Offers a support system to help the family cope during the patient's illness and in their own bereavement.
- Uses a team approach to address the needs of patients and their families, including bereavement counseling, if indicated.
- Will enhance quality of life, and may also positively influence the course of illness.
- Is applicable early in the course of illness, in conjunction with other therapies that are intended to prolong life, such as chemotherapy or radiation therapy, and includes those investigations needed to better understand and manage distressing clinical complications [2].

Similar definitions of palliative care are found elsewhere. For example, The National Consensus Project (NCP) has given a comprehensive definition and characterization of palliative care as follows:

> The goal of palliative care is to prevent and relieve suffering and to support the best possible quality of life for patients and their families, regardless of the stage of the disease or the need for other therapies. Palliative care is both a philosophy of care and an organized, highly structured system for delivering care. Palliative care expands traditional disease-model medical treatments to include the goals of enhancing quality of life for patient and family, optimizing function, helping with decision making, and providing opportunities for personal growth. As such, it can be delivered concurrently with life-prolonging care or as the main focus of care. Palliative care is operationalized through effective management of pain and other distressing symptoms, while incorporating psychosocial and spiritual care with consideration of patient/family needs, preferences, values, beliefs, and culture. Evaluation and treatment should be comprehensive and patient-centered with a focus on the central role of the family unit in decision making. Palliative care affirms life by supporting the patient and family's goals for the future, including their hopes for cure or life-prolongation, as well as their hopes for peace and dignity throughout the course of illness, the dying process, and death. Palliative care aims to guide and assist the patient and family in making decisions that enable them to work toward their goals during whatever time they have remaining. Comprehensive palliative care services often require the expertise of various

providers to adequately assess and treat the complex needs of seriously ill patients and their families. Leadership, collaboration, coordination, and communication are key elements for effective integration of these disciplines and services [3].

Finally, the National Quality Forum (NQF) has provided this rather concise definition:

Palliative care refers to patient- and family-centered care that optimizes quality of life by anticipating, preventing, and treating suffering. Palliative care throughout the continuum of illness involves addressing physical, intellectual, emotional, social, and spiritual needs and facilitating patient autonomy, access to information, and choice [4].

The NCP and the NQF both espoused eight domains of palliative care as follows:

1. Structure and processes of care
2. Physical aspects of care
3. Psychosocial and psychiatric aspects of care
4. Social aspects of care
5. Spiritual, religious, and existential aspects of care
6. Cultural aspects of care
7. Care of the imminently dying patient
8. Ethical and legal aspects of care

Multidisciplinary Approach in Palliative Care

From all the above definitions and characterizations of palliative care, one key element of palliative care that stands out is the element of *multidisciplinary (also termed interdisciplinary; but see later) approach*. All the definitions either directly or indirectly include this element as a defining component of palliative care. The basic logic behind this approach is simple: the needs to be addressed in palliative care are diverse, complex, multidimensional, and dynamic. These needs transgress the narrow bounds of disease-governed dimensions (e.g., metastasis, CD4 cell counts) and extend to several symptom and syndromal domains (e.g., pain, dyspnea, delirium, depression, nausea, weight loss, and many others). More importantly, as repeatedly emphasized in all the definitions of palliative care, these needs transverse multiple overlapping dimensions: physical, emotional, intellectual, familial and other interpersonal, financial and other practical, social and cultural, and, finally, spiritual or existential. It naturally follows that so many aspects of palliative care (see the domains of care mentioned by both NCP and NQF) cannot be addressed by one person or even one team from a particular discipline. Hence the essential need for a multidisciplinary approach in palliative care. The NCP, for example, has explicitly stated this as the fifth of their 11 "key elements of palliative care":

Interdisciplinary team: Palliative care presupposes indications for, and provision of, inter-disciplinary team evaluation and treatment in selected cases. The palliative-care team must be skilled in care of the patient population to be served. Palliative-care teams may be expanded to include a range of professionals based on the services needed. They include a core group of professionals from medicine, nursing and social work, and may include some combination of volunteer coordinators, bereavement coordinators, chaplains, psychologists, pharmacists, nursing assistants and home attendants, dietitians, speech and language pathologists, physical, occupational, art, play, music, and child-life therapists, case managers, and trained volunteers [3].

As an aside, it is to be noted that although the terms multidisciplinary and interdisciplinary are used interchangeably in this chapter, these two are not exactly synonymous. Both the terms refer to inputs from different disciplines regarding individual patient care. In multidisciplinary model, however, each member of a particular discipline provides an expert consultation in his or her area of expertise, clearly maintains one's own disciplinary identity, and works in relative isolation where team membership, while important, is secondary. There is usually a clearly defined hierarchy in the multidisciplinary team. The identified "leader" of the multidisciplinary team (MDT) integrates the inputs from different disciplines and takes the final decision. In interdisciplinary model, however, the approach is more of sharing and integration from the beginning, less clear role distinction and hierarchy, and leadership is task dependent rather than hierarchy dependent. Also, the patient is kept at the center of an interdisciplinary approach and he or she takes an active part in the consultative and decision-making process [5, 6]. Many of the current documents (NCP, NQF) use the term interdisciplinary rather than multidisciplinary. Research literature and general clinical practice, however, maintain the term multidisciplinary. Further, the differences between these two terms are subtle and graded. In keeping with the title of this chapter, the term multidisciplinary will be consistently used here.

Models of Palliative Care and Multidisciplinary Approach

Palliative care can be provided at various levels. Because the current expanded concept of palliative care encompasses this care of the patient to start ideally right from the diagnosis of a potentially life-threatening illness, the first level of palliative care can start at the primary care level itself. Depending upon the stage of progression of disease, its complications and newly emergent needs of the patient and the family, the level of such care then moves through secondary care and finally specialist tertiary care. Understandably, the composition and activities (structure and process) of the multidisciplinary team will also vary according to these levels of care.

There are different models of palliative care depending upon the different levels. These may be:

(a) Outpatient Palliative Care Programs—these occur in ambulatory care settings to provide continuity of care for patients with serious or life-threatening illnesses.
(b) Community Palliative Care Programs—these occur in communities as consultative teams who collaborate with hospices or home health agencies to support seriously ill patients who have not yet accessed hospice.

(c) Institutional Palliative Care Programs—these are institutional-based programs in the hospital or nursing home to serve patients with life-threatening or life-limiting illnesses. They occur in hospital settings (academic, community, rehabilitation) and skilled nursing facilities. These provide services to patients anywhere along the disease continuum between initial diagnosis and death.

(d) Hospice Care—this is a well-established program to provide patients with a prognosis of 6 months or less. As delineated within the Medicare Hospice Benefit, these services can be provided in the home, nursing home, residential facility, or on an inpatient unit.

Role Played by the Multidisciplinary Team in Palliative Care

The MDT plays an essential role in virtually every stage of the palliative care process, starting from the comprehensive assessment of the patient in the beginning till the final days of end-of-life care.

Under the first domain of palliative care (structure and processes of care), the very first guideline (1.1) of NCP stresses this fact: The timely plan of care is based on a comprehensive interdisciplinary assessment of the patient and family. It elaborates that "Assessment includes documentation of disease status, including diagnoses and prognosis; comorbid medical and psychiatric disorders; physical and psychological symptoms; functional status; social, cultural, spiritual, and advance care planning concerns and preferences, including appropriateness of referral to hospice."

The guideline 1.2 (care plan) too emphasizes the role of the MDT: "The interdisciplinary team coordinates and shares the information, provides support for decision making, develops and carries out the care plan, and communicates the palliative care plan to patient and family, to all involved health professionals, and to the responsible providers when patients transfer to different care settings."

Guideline 1.3 most clearly espouses the role of the MDT in palliative care and is worth quoting in full:

> **Guideline 1.3** An interdisciplinary team provides services to the patient and family consistent with the care plan. In addition to nursing, medicine, and social work, other therapeutic disciplines with important assessment of patients and families include physical therapists, occupational therapists, speech and language pathologists, nutritionists, psychologists, chaplains, and nursing assistants. For pediatrics, this should include child-life specialists. Complementary and alternative therapies may be included.

Criteria:

- Specialist-level palliative care is delivered by an interdisciplinary team.
- The team includes palliative care professionals with the appropriate patient-population-specific education, credentialing, and experience and the ability to meet the physical, psychological, social, and spiritual needs of both patient

and family. Of particular importance is hiring physicians, nurses, and social workers "appropriately trained" and ultimately certified in hospice and palliative care. Education should include a fundamental understanding of the domains of palliative care and the goals of the Medicare Hospice Benefit, in addition to pain, symptoms, grief, bereavement, and communication. Ideally this occurs in preceptorships, fellowships, or in baccalaureate and graduate specific programs. Continuing education is an essential for professionals currently in practice.

- The interdisciplinary palliative care team involved in the care of children, either as patients or as the children of adult patients, has expertise in the delivery of services for such children.
- The patient and family have access to palliative care expertise and staff 24 hours a day, seven days a week. Respite services are available for the families and caregivers of children or adults with life-threatening illnesses.
- The interdisciplinary team communicates regularly (at least weekly or more often as required by the clinical situation) to plan, review, and evaluate the care plan, with input from both the patient and family.
- The team meets regularly to discuss provision of quality care, including staffing, policies, and clinical practices.
- Team leadership has appropriate training, qualifications, and experience.
- Policies for prioritizing and responding to referrals in a timely manner are documented [3].

Specific instances of the roles of the MDT in other domains of palliative care are mentioned as well. For example, under domain 2 (Physical aspects of care), Guideline 2.1 mentions as its first criterion: "The interdisciplinary team includes professionals with specialist-level skill in symptom control for all types of life-threatening illnesses, including physicians, nurses, social workers, rehabilitation specialists, physical therapists, occupational therapists, speech and language pathologists, psychologists, child-life specialists (and other appropriate therapists for children), and chaplains" [3]. Similarly, under domain 3 (Psychological and psychiatric aspects of care), Guideline 3.1 mentions as its first criterion: "The interdisciplinary team includes professionals with patient-specific skills and training in the psychological consequences and psychiatric comorbidities of serious illness for both patient and family, including depression, anxiety, delirium, and cognitive impairment" [3]. Under the same domain, the first criterion of Guideline 3.2 mentions: "The interdisciplinary team includes professionals with patient-population-appropriate education and skill in the care of patients, families, and care staff experiencing loss, grief, and bereavement" [3].

Domain 4 (Social aspects of care) again heavily stresses the role of the MDT in case assessment and care plan formulation, and is quoted below:

Guideline 4.1 Comprehensive interdisciplinary assessment identifies the social needs of patients and their families, and a care plan is developed to respond to these needs as effectively as possible.

Criteria:

- The interdisciplinary team includes professionals with patient-population-specific skills in the assessment and management of social and practical needs during a life-threatening or chronic debilitating illness
- It is essential that practitioners skilled in the assessment and management of the developmental needs of children are available for pediatric patients and the children of adult patients, as appropriate.
- A comprehensive interdisciplinary social assessment is completed and documented to include: family structure and geographic location; relationships; lines of communication; existing social and cultural networks; perceived social support; medical decision making; work and school settings; finances; sexuality; intimacy; living arrangements; caregiver availability; access to transportation; access to prescription and over-the-counter medicines and nutritional products; access to needed equipment; community resources, including school and work settings; and legal issues
- Routine patient and family meetings are conducted with appropriate members of the interdisciplinary team to assess understanding and address questions; provide information and help with decision making, discuss goals of care and advance care planning; determine wishes, preferences, hopes and fears; provide emotional and social support; and enhance communication.
- The social care plan is formulated from a comprehensive social and cultural assessment and reassessment and reflects and documents values, goals, and preferences as set by the patient and family over time. Interventions are planned to minimize the adverse impact of caregiving on the family and to promote caregiver and family goals and well-being.
- Referrals to appropriate services are made that meet identified social needs and promote access to care, help in the home, school or work, transportation, rehabilitation, medications, counseling, community resources, and equipment [3].

Indeed, the roles of the MDT have been mentioned for all the other domains of palliative care (Spiritual, religious, and existential aspects of care; Cultural aspects of care; Care of the imminently dying patient; Ethical and legal aspects of care). It is especially worthwhile to note that the MDT has an important role to play after death of the patient as well: ("**Guideline 7.3** A post-death bereavement plan is activated. An interdisciplinary team member is assigned to the family in the post-death period to help with religious practices, funeral arrangements, and burial planning" [3]).

The NQF too echoes this general emphasis as reflected in many of its "Preferred Practices" starting, for example, from its Preferred Practice number 1: "Provide palliative and hospice care by an interdisciplinary team of skilled palliative care professionals, including, for example, physicians, nurses, social workers, pharmacists, spiritual care counselors, and others who collaborate with primary healthcare professional(s)" [4].

Advantages and Effectiveness and of MDT Approach

The most obvious advantage of MDT is that more heads put together may work better than one head. In other words, MDT approach may generate new options and yield creative solutions to complex and multidimensional problems. The other advantages include:

- Decrease the time from presentation to treatment.
- Decrease fragmentation, with better communication, decreased errors and duplicate tests, and clarified treatment plan.
- Decrease variability between physicians, ensuring application of good clinical practice.
- Increase patient satisfaction through fewer visits and consistent communication.
- Enable doctors to focus on multiple aspects of a patient's care (socio-emotional, nutrition, etc).
- Decrease medico-legal risk.
- Improve quality of life.
- Foster the setting wherein complex treatment plans can be created and sustained.
- Increase enrollment in research studies.
- Improve the education and support of family members.
- Provide a marketable service for an institution.
- Create a unique experience for graduate medical education.
- Decrease the number of procedures needed to make a diagnosis.
- Align programs.
- Improve survival [7].

The benefits of MDT approach, supported by data, include: increased patient satisfaction; enhanced quality of life; increased accuracy of care; decreased time to treatment; decreased variability of care; and even some data to show a modest increase in survival in cancer patients [7–13]. There is, however, a need to conduct more methodologically rigorous controlled trials in this area [14].

Barriers and Challenges

Theoretically and conceptually, the MDT approach lies at the heart of the palliative care. However, there are a number of practical challenges in setting up and running a successful MDT [15–17]. Like any other program, setting up a MDT in a busy and resource-competitive hospital can be a daunting task. It requires, among other things, political will and administrative support, institutional back-up, adequate and sustainable funding, identifying specific team members and securing professional support from the identified team members in terms of time, effort, and commitment. All these can prove quite an uphill task!

After these barriers have been overcome, other issues remain. These involve practical logistic issues such as the format, location, frequency, duration, and order of prioritization of the MDT meetings. During the meetings, certain professionals may view it as a duplication of their efforts (and hence waste of their time, especially if there is no reimbursement for the same) because of repetition of parts of information from different sources. On the other hand, at times, professionals from widely diverse disciplines (neurosurgeon, radiation oncologist, nursing staff, psychologist, social worker, counselor, chaplain) speak different "languages" and may find it difficult understanding one another's perspectives and priorities. Communication barriers may ensue, which may further complicate matters and perhaps foster a sense of alienation and futility. Leadership issues may arise, either directly or covertly. Finally, the sheer arrangement of such meetings can prove an arduous task given the busy schedules and prior commitments of the individual members of the MDT.

Even when a MDT is put in place and has been running its services for a while, barriers and challenges continue to haunt these services. As recently found in a survey conducted in Australia, these barriers are of six thematic types [17]:

1. Confusion about the roles and responsibilities of the different members of the MDT involved in care (e.g., perceived lack of recognition of the identified care coordinator as a professional in her own right, role tensions between the primary care providers and MDT members, confusion in the patient's mind as to what a "care coordinator" means and who is that—the primary referring doctor, the surgeon, the oncologist(s), or the named care coordinator, etc.)
2. Problems in implementing comprehensive multidisciplinary team meetings (e.g., time constraints, lack of support for meetings, logistical issues in trying to get all members of the MDT together at the onetime, large geographical distances between team members, staff shortages in key disciplines such as oncology, alack of administrative support for these meetings and dominant personalities limiting open discussion
3. Transitioning of care: "Falling through the cracks" (e.g., lack of communication and effective referral between these centers, particularly from large urban centers of expertise back to the local services from which patients sought support, lack of communication and coordination between the public and private sectors)
4. Inadequate communication between specialist and primary care (inconsistent, delayed and incomplete communication among the health care team, particularly between family physicians and specialists which inhibited the delivery of coordinated patient care)
5. Inequitable access to health services (rural or regional disadvantages, public/ private care differences)
6. Managing scarce resources and personnel (in terms of primary care physicians, specialists, care coordinators, and other members of the MDT)

Coordination of Care

Many of these barriers and challenges may be overcome by an effective and continuous coordination of care. Coordination of care, in fact, is one of the central tenets of the MDT approach. Coordination of care is vitally important:

(a) For the patient: for ensuring proper continuity of care of the individual patient through different stages of the disease and emergent needs
(b) For the MDT: for ensuring its smooth operation and overcoming many of the barriers mentioned above
(c) For the healthcare system: for enhancing its efficiency and minimizing fragmentation of the system involved in palliative care as a whole

Lack of coordinated care can lead to fragmented care, patients getting "lost" in the system and failing to access appropriate services, as well as more unplanned health utilization [17]. On the other hand, a proper system of care coordination has multiple benefits, both over short and long term.

Coordination of palliative care can:

- Improve patient outcomes (when patients receive the appropriate care at the right time)
- Improve use of recommended treatments, including increased referral to appropriate services and patient compliance (when system processes are known and used)
- Improve communication between providers (when reliable and trusting relationships are built over time)
- Streamline services, decrease duplication, and reduce costs (when processes and communication are efficient and monitored or reviewed over time) [18, 19]

Care coordination is a comprehensive approach to achieving continuity of care for patients.

This approach aims to ensure that care is delivered in a logical, connected, and timely manner so that the medical and personal needs of patients are met.

Coordinated care is an important part of management for all patients who require a variety of treatments and care, particularly when care is provided over time and between settings. This is often the case for people with chronic and progressive diseases in need of palliative care.

Effective care coordination provides the necessary interface between patients and healthcare providers, between the providers themselves, between the providers and the healthcare system, and, importantly, between different healthcare settings as the patient "transitions" from the primary care to various levels of specialist care during the phases of the illness, in order to prevent the patient "falling through the cracks." For cancer patients, for example, it is well known that the treatment journey is complex and challenging. It is not uncommon for these patients to be seen by many health professionals within and across multiple health services and across different health sectors including public, private, and community health in both metropolitan and rural regions.

The Victorian Government Department of Human Services, Melbourne, Victoria, Australia, in their important document "Linking cancer care: A guide for implementing coordinated cancer care" has identified the following as the key principles of care coordination in the context of cancer care (which are easily applicable for palliative care in general) [19]:

- Patients, their families and carers affected by cancer are at the center of care
- Care coordination initiatives should take into consideration the continuum of care including the various health sectors involved in delivering care across tumor streams
- Care coordination initiatives should take into consideration rural/regional and metropolitan contexts of care
- Enhancing continuity of care across the health sector requires a whole-of-system response, that is, initiatives developed to address continuity of care need to occur across a number of key levels—that of the health system, health service, team, and individual
- Improving care coordination is the responsibility of all health professionals involved in the care of individual patients and should therefore be considered in their practice

Conclusion

Palliative care aims to reduce distress, enhance functioning, and improve the quality of life of people and their families facing life-threatening diseases, rather than directly aiming at cure or disease modification. Palliative care should start early and alongside disease-modifying treatment, and become the predominant mode of care with more advanced stages of disease, finally ending in bereavement care. Palliative care thus is a continuum. During this continuum, palliative care addresses the multiple domains of needs and concerns of the patient and the family—physical, psychological, social, and spiritual. These needs cannot be addressed by one single person or agency without causing fragmentation of care. Hence a multidisciplinary approach is the backbone of palliative care. In this approach, inputs are obtained and integrated from multiple sources depending upon, among other factors, stage of disease progression, pain and other symptoms, patient's and family's psychological state, social and practical requirements, and available resources. The doctors (both primary care and specialists), nursing staff, social worker, and many others involved in the multifaceted care of the patient form the multidisciplinary team, which provides this care in a coordinated manner so as to provide continuity of care. There are many obvious advantages of the multidisciplinary approach, and its efficacy has been demonstrated convincingly in increasing satisfaction of the patient and family, improving quality of life, and even a modest increase in survival for some patients. However, the multidisciplinary approach has its own barriers and challenges. Some of these can be at least partly overcome with an effective coordination of care between different locations (primary, secondary), personnel (both between the patient and the healthcare providers, and between different categories of the providers themselves), and time points of care. With proper coordination of care, people living with life-threatening diseases can look forward to receiving palliative care.

References

1. jointcommission.org. Washington, DC: The Joint Commission. Advanced certification for palliative care programs. http://www.jointcommission.org/certification/palliative_care.aspx. Updated 24 Oct 2011; cited 25 Oct 2011.
2. who.int. Geneva, Switzerland: World Health Organization. WHO definition of palliative care. http://www.who.int/cancer/palliative/definition/en/. Updated 24 Oct 2011; cited 25 Oct 2011.
3. National Consensus Project for Palliative Care. Clinical practice guidelines for quality palliative care. 2nd ed. Pittsburgh: National Consensus Project for Palliative Care; 2009.
4. National Quality Forum. A national framework and preferred practices for palliative and hospice care quality. Washington, DC: National Quality Forum; 2006.
5. Crawford GB, Price SD. Team working: palliative care as a model of interdisciplinary practice. Med J Aust. 2003;179:S32–4.
6. Jessup RL. Interdisciplinary versus multidisciplinary care teams: do we understand the difference? Aust Health Rev. 2007;31:330–1.
7. Horvath LE, Yordan E, Malhotra D, Leyva I, Bortel K, Schalk D, et al. Multidisciplinary care in the oncology setting: historical perspective and data from lung and gynecology multidisciplinary clinics. J Oncol Pract. 2010;6:e21–6.
8. Rummans TA, Clark MM, Sloan JA, et al. Impacting quality of life for patientswith advanced cancer with a structured multidisciplinary intervention: a randomized controlled trial. J Clin Oncol. 2006;24:635–42.
9. Walker MS, Ristvedt SL, Haughey BH, et al. Patient care in multidisciplinary cancer clinics: does attention to psychosocial needs predict patient satisfaction? Psychooncology. 2003;12:291–300.
10. Newman EA, Guest AB, Helvie MA, et al. Changes in surgical management resulting from case review at a breast cancer multidisciplinary tumor board. Cancer. 2006;107:2346–51.
11. Bakitas M, Lyons KD, Hegel MT, et al. Effects of a palliative care intervention on clinical outcomes in patients with advanced cancer: the Project ENABLE II randomized controlled trial. JAMA. 2009;302:741–9.
12. Temel JS, Greer JA, Muzikansky A, et al. Early palliative care for patientswith metastatic non-small-cell lung cancer. N Engl J Med. 2010;363:733–42.
13. Meier DE, Brawley OW. Palliative care and the quality of life. J Clin Oncol. 2011;29:2750–2.
14. Carey M, Sanson-Fisher R, Lotfi-Jam K, Schofield P, Aranda S. Multidisciplinary care in cancer: do the current research outputs help? Eur J Cancer Care. 2010;19:434–41.
15. Hammond DB. Multidisciplinary cancer care in a hospital setting: challenges and rewards. J Oncol Pract. 2010;6:281–3.
16. Look Hong NJ, Gagliardi AR, Bronskill SE, Paszat LF, Wright FC. Multidisciplinary cancer conferences: exploring obstacles and facilitators to their implementation. J Oncol Pract. 2010;6:61–8.
17. Walsh J, Harrison JD, Young JM, Butow PN, Solomon MJ, Masya L. What are the current barriers to effective cancer care coordination? A qualitative study. BMC Health Serv Res. 2010;10:132.
18. Morrison RS, Meier DE. Palliative care. N Engl J Med. 2004;350:2582–90.
19. Victorian Government Department of Human Services. Linking cancer care: a guide for implementing coordinated cancer care. Melbourne: Victorian Government Department of Human Services; 2007.

Review Questions

1. According to the World Health Organization definition of palliative care, the essential aim of palliative care is to:

    (a) Correct the underlying metabolic derangements in life-threatening disease
    (b) Focus on disease modification
    (c) Improve the quality of life
    (d) Provide symptomatic and psychosocial support exclusively for the patient

2. Palliative care is:

    (a) Disease centered
    (b) Patient centered
    (c) Family centered
    (d) Patient- and family centered

3. The needs addressed by palliative care does *not* include:

    (a) Spiritual
    (b) Curative
    (c) Psychosocial
    (d) Physical

4. The number of domains of palliative care endorsed by both National Consensus Project (NCP) and National Quality Forum (NQF) is:

    (a) 4
    (b) 6
    (c) 8
    (d) 10

5. According to NCP Clinical Practice Guidelines 2009, the core group in an interdisciplinary (multidisciplinary) palliative care team should have professionals from all the following disciplines *except*:

    (a) Psychology
    (b) Social work
    (c) Nursing
    (d) Medicine

6. According to expanded model and scope of palliative care, such care can start at the level of :

    (a) Primary care
    (b) Secondary care
    (c) Tertiary care
    (d) Any of the above levels

7. The following statement is true regarding research-evidenced benefits of a multidisciplinary team (MDT) in palliative care:

    (a) Modest increase in survival of certain cancer patients
    (b No effect on patient satisfaction
    (c) No effect on quality of life
    (d) Time delay in reaching consensus opinions

8. Coordination of care is important for:

    (a) The patient
    (b) The MDT
    (c) The healthcare system
    (d) All of the above

9. For patients in palliative care, the overall aim of coordination of care is to provide:

    (a) Consultations from various doctors
    (b) Arrangement of MDT meetings
    (c) Continuity of care over time and across settings
    (d) Bereavement counseling

10. The Advanced Certification Program for Palliative Care announced by the Joint Commission is designed for the following type of palliative care program (as of September 2011):

    (a) Outpatient based
    (b) Inpatient based
    (c) Community based
    (d) Hospice based

Answers

1. (c)
2. (d)
3. (b)
4. (c)
5. (a)
6. (d)
7. (a)
8. (d)
9. (c)
10. (b)

Chapter 3
Psychological Distress and Psychiatric Comorbidities in Palliative Care

Raphael J. Leo and Maria Theresa Mariano

Introduction

Palliative care medicine has expanded awareness of, and the refinement of treatment efforts directed at, alleviating physical symptoms of patients with terminal conditions. Over the years, medical and psychological discourse on end-of-life care has increasingly drawn attention to many of the distinct psychosocial challenges that patients confront, emphasizing the importance of integrating the physical and psychological aspects of care essential to improving quality of life. Addressing the multiplicity of psychological issues faced by patients can be daunting, especially when considered in the context of the limited time available before death ensues. This chapter highlights the psychological needs of the terminal patient. An emphasis will be placed on subsyndromal, but nonetheless distressing, psychological states, as well as the assessment and management of psychiatric disorders frequently encountered within the context of palliative care. Although much of the data come from studies of patients with terminal cancer, many of the principles outlined herein are likely to apply to a broad spectrum of patients requiring end-of-life care.

Psychosocial Demands at the End of Life

Having a terminal prognosis alters, and often disrupts, one's view of the world, one's self and the future. Several, perhaps all, aspects of one's life may be suspended because of prevailing physical needs, e.g., one's life may become centered on pain and/or other physical symptoms and the securing of basic bodily needs.

R.J. Leo, M.A., M.D. (✉) • M.T. Mariano, M.D.
Department of Psychiatry, School of Medicine and Biomedical Sciences,
State University of New York,
Buffalo, NY, USA
e-mail: rleomd@aol.com

N. Vadivelu et al. (eds.), *Essentials of Palliative Care*,
DOI 10.1007/978-1-4614-5164-8_3,
© Springer Science+Business Media New York 2013

The patient may be thrust into positions of marked dependency on others. Progressive physical deconditioning may interfere with one's capacity to engage in customary activities and interests, and may restrict access to customary social support networks. There may be limited emotional reserve to invest in others or to maintain relationships. The patient may experience a loss of hope for goals and aspirations. Concerns may arise about one's transcendence and generativity, i.e., leaving a legacy, and how one is remembered by those who are left behind.

Any of these factors, in isolation or combined, can trigger, and amplify, psychological reactions that present significant sources of distress and suffering for the terminal patient as well as caregivers. Acknowledgement of the finite nature of one's future requires coping with grief and highlights one's concerns about life meaning. These issues will be briefly discussed below.

Grief, Life Meaning, and Spiritual Distress

Grief is the emotional and psychological reaction to a loss, not necessarily limited to death. Many patients with medical illness, especially those confronting terminal illness, suffer grief reactions related to losses arising from the illness, e.g., loss of a sense of future, self-image, self-esteem and self-efficacy, and material losses. The process of mourning allows for the expression of loss, facilitates acceptance of prevailing life circumstances, and enables the individual to begin to channel energy into maintaining relationships, resolving interpersonal conflicts, and managing the challenges faced as death approaches [1].

For family and loved ones too, there can be sadness in anticipation of the impending death. Anticipatory grief, therefore, has the potential for drawing families and loved ones closer to the patient, as well as to one another. Effective and open communication during this time between the patient and loved ones, engendered by exchanging gratitude, story-telling and reminiscing, and celebrating the life and contributions of the dying person, may facilitate the mourning process, providing opportunities for "saying goodbye" and sharing in the completion of "unfinished business" [1, 2].

Symptoms of grief include profound sadness, which can sometimes be expressed as a focus on physical symptoms, withdrawal from others, and even fleeting thoughts of despair. However, there can be variability in mood during mourning that serves to distinguish it from depression [3]. Impediments to mourning can arise from denial, avoidance of the inevitability of death, and unaddressed anger, triggering persisting, i.e., less variability in, symptoms. Persistent and unremitting dysphoria, hopelessness, helplessness, preoccupations with guilt and/or worthlessness, anhedonia, and death preoccupation, by contrast, may signal an underlying depressive disorder, and should not be dismissed as an expected grief-related reaction. If present, these symptoms should prompt efforts to secure treatment.

Dying patients may experience existential distress, i.e., despair engendered by threats to one's perception of the meaningfulness of life and a sense of disconnection from one's sense of purpose. Such distress can present with an admixture of emotional and psychological reactions including fear, shock, anger, vulnerability, uncertainty, isolation, hopelessness, and desires for hastening death. Having an opportunity to express concerns related to the meaningfulness of one's life and to pursue goals and responsibilities towards others may assist patients to alter their attitudes and begin to view their lives as worthwhile despite the severe illness.

Closely related to existential distress is a perceived disruption from one's spirituality. For some persons, the experience of spirituality will guide one's ability to derive meaning from life experiences, e.g., lending a framework within which to understand suffering and impart a means for understanding existential issues and one's imminent death [4].

Research has demonstrated that spirituality can serve to buffer against depression [5, 6] and hopelessness [7, 8], and fosters coping [6, 9]. Thus, spirituality and one's ability to cultivate and sustain life meaning and purpose may be particularly predictive of psychological well-being and quality of life among patients with terminal illness [10]. However, facing a life-threatening illness can pose challenges to one's spiritual framework, e.g., causing one to question fundamental belief systems such as beliefs in the afterlife, or to face issues related to the meaningfulness of one's life and existential issues, and thereby trigger distress [11].

A broad range of psychological and emotional reactions are therefore possible in the context of terminal illness. The challenge for treatment providers is to effectively identify those patients for whom such emotional and psychological reactions constitute pathologic states warranting treatment measures and referral to other sources of support, e.g., pastoral and/or mental health services.

Patient–Provider Communication: When Is Distress Pathological?

It is common for terminal patients to experience transient feelings of sadness, apprehension, worry (e.g., about aspects of the illness or treatment), or manifest preoccupations with life meaning, futility or pessimism often contingent upon, and in response to, clinical developments. Patients may, nonetheless, successfully navigate the adaptational challenges posed at advanced stages of illness without significant and enduring suffering and distress, depending upon whether they have psychological resources (influenced by intrinsic emotional reserves, cognitive attributions, and problem-solving strategies) [12]. The meanings ascribed to, and expectations related to, the illness, the beliefs and assumptions one has about one's life and self-perceptions, one's coping strategies, and the perception one has about his/her competence with which to manage the illness can be significant determinants influencing the extent to which distress is experienced [13–16]. Distress incurred by ineffective coping strategies and beliefs about the illness or its effects can, however, be buffered by strong and supportive relationships, e.g., the accessibility of physical, psychological, spiritual, and emotional support from family, friends, caregivers, and treatment providers. For example, the degree to which family and other social supports are perceived as accessible and supportive can influence the extent to which psychological distress is experienced [17].

However, in some circumstances, the distress incurred may be overwhelming, leading to impairments in adaptation. Thus, for example, an individual perceiving the illness as uncontrollable and unpredictable and perceiving minimal social support is likely to experience significant distress as compared with another who is apt to appraise herself as capable of exerting control over at least some aspects of the illness or her life and/or perceiving greater social support.

Given the magnitude of psychological issues encountered in the advanced stages of illness, competence in the skills in providing grief/bereavement and spiritual support are critical and central components for the palliative care team [18]. The relationship with primary medical caregiver(s) may be the safest and the main source of support for exploration of psychological distress. Ongoing clinician–patient communication is essential to the assessment of the patient's psychological well-being. Being aware of the critical psychological tasks encountered at the end of life can influence the tenor of care offered by palliative care providers, potentially humanizing it and infusing it with a respect for the patient. Patients may find openness to discussions about matters pertaining to loss, grief, life meaning, and spirituality to be reassuring, conveying that such deeply personal experiences are esteemed and respected, and that their values will be honored in the context of the patient–clinician relationship. Typically, approaches that are advocated involve making time to foster a connection with the patient, respecting the unique aspects of the individual's experiences and spirituality, enabling the sharing of the patient's perspectives and conveying that s/he is heard [19]. Furthermore, ongoing communication between treatment provider and patient may unveil signs that psychological distress related to grief, existential matters, and spirituality are incapacitating, burdensome, and/or may be harbingers of more significant psychiatric disturbance that warrant treatment.

It is often difficult to determine when one's emotional and psychological reactions constitute appropriate and expected responses to life-altering experiences and when the patient's reactions signal a clinicopathological state; the benchmark for making this determination is defined in terms of the duration, flexibility, and consequences of symptoms. Thus, when negative emotions persist and/or when problematic cognitive appraisals remain inflexible, and thereby significantly disrupt functioning, hinder treatment, or impede one's capacity to take in pleasure or comfort, these psychological reactions are thought to reflect more of a pathological state. Under such circumstances, having access to psychiatrists, other mental health practitioners and pastoral care services can be particularly helpful, serving to bolster psychological and physical well-being, and foster life meaning.

Unfortunately, recognition of psychological distress and comorbid psychiatric conditions often goes unrecognized by palliative care clinicians [20–22]. Common impediments to open communication about the patient's emotional/psychological needs in palliative care are summarized in Table 3.1. For example, very brief clinical encounters, embarrassment, and the perception that one's care providers would be disinterested in such matters may prevent patients from disclosing information about their level of emotional distress. On the other hand, clinicians often are prone

Table 3.1 Patient–clinician factors impeding communication about psychological distress

Patient-related factors	Clinician-related factors
Embarrassment precluding open discussion about psychological distress	The perception that it is not one's role to address psychosocial concerns
Stigma associated with being labeled with a psychological disorder	Insufficient skills or training to address psychosocial concerns
Perception that doctors are too busy or disinterested	Clinician discomfort with emotionally-laden topics
Believing that psychological distress is expected	Lack of awareness of psychological stressors confronting patients at end of life
A tendency to somatize as a means of conveying psychological distress instead of directly expressing distress openly	Misattributions that emotional distress is expected and "normal" response to confronting terminal illness
	Greater weight given to physical ailments rather than psychological distress
	Under-recognition of psychiatric comorbidities potentially affecting patients at end-of-life

[23–25]

to prioritize medical diagnostic and treatment concerns and overlook emotional distress [23, 24]. This tendency may be fueled by the assumptions that dysphoria and depression are understandable reactions to being afflicted with an unremitting and terminal condition. In addition, clinicians may be reluctant to explore emotionally-laden issues with their patients because they fear that such discussion will be insulting or stigmatizing. However, failure to explore the presence of clinically significant emotional distress may leave potentially treatable conditions unidentified and unaddressed, further compromising quality of life in advanced stages of illness.

To bypass some of these impediments, palliative care practice guidelines strongly advocate for constant monitoring for, and use of screening assessments to assist in the identification of, psychological distress [18]. Although the utility of many of these screening instruments, e.g., the Distress Thermometer [26], the Functional Assessment of Chronic Illness Therapy Spiritual Well-Being Scale [10], among others, have not been empirically established [27], their use facilitates dialogue and can be the basis for the exploration of treatment options that can be potentially implemented to enhance patient comfort.

Psychiatric Disorders Encountered in the Palliative Care Setting

There is an extensive epidemiological literature that supports the high prevalence of primary psychiatric disorders among persons in the terminal phases of illness (e.g., [28, 29]). Several meta-analyses and systematic reviews of the literature revealed that adjustment disorders, depression, anxiety disorders, and delirium are among the most common psychiatric conditions encountered in palliative care settings [30–34]. (More specific features of each of these conditions and their management are discussed in the next section.)

It is noteworthy that prevalence estimates of psychiatric disorders vary across studies included in the aforementioned reviews depending upon the assessment methodologies employed, sampling heterogeneity and selection bias, and the ranges of symptoms upon which diagnoses were based. Thus, the types of assessments employed, e.g., clinical diagnostic interview versus self-rated questionnaire, can account for some of the variability in prevalence rates observed [35, 36]. Brief rating instruments customarily applied to, and standardized based upon, non-terminal patients may not be appropriate for terminal patients and thus results reported by investigations based on such self-report measures should be interpreted with caution [37]. Additionally, selection bias may have had a bearing on outcomes, e.g., severely ill patients who may ostensibly have comparatively high rates of psychiatric illness, may have been excluded from such investigations due to poor health limiting participation in assessments [38]. Lastly, the inclusiveness, or exclusiveness, in the range of symptoms upon which the diagnosis of various psychiatric disorders was based may have been inconsistent across studies influencing the reported prevalence rates. For example, many symptoms, e.g., sleep disturbances, fatigue, or anorexia, occurring as a direct result of medical illness may mimic neurovegetative symptoms of major mood and anxiety disorders. Reliance on these symptoms may yield false positives, and therefore, inflate reported rates of psychiatric comorbidities. On the other hand, studies utilizing stringent criteria, i.e., excluding symptoms with ambiguous etiologies, may have potentially led to missed cases and lower reported prevalence rates.

Despite the aforementioned methodological issues in the extant literature, it nonetheless appears that palliative care practitioners should prudently and judiciously consider an extensive array of psychiatric comorbidities among terminal patients and that psychiatric treatment be secured whenever appropriate. Generally, a multimodal approach to treatment, i.e., employing psychotherapeutic and psychopharmacologic interventions, may be necessary. Although it is not feasible to provide an exhaustive overview of available psychotherapeutic approaches useful in palliative care here, the reader should recognize that there are several approaches available. A summary of the possible uses of various psychotherapeutic and pharmacologic treatment approaches employed in palliative care settings is provided in Tables 3.2 and 3.3, respectively. Briefly, the goals of treatment include alleviation of subjectively perceived distress, facilitating comfort and hope, and, in as much as it is feasible given the severity of prevailing medical conditions, improvement of symptoms and the patient's functional capabilities. The implementation of psychotherapeutic interventions outlined herein can also be useful in assisting patients contending with subsyndromal psychological distress related to existential distress, grief, etc. The selection of a particular modality or combination of modalities would depend on the particular patient's needs, the commitment to pursue psychotherapy and the training/skills of the psychiatrist, and other available mental health practitioners, enlisted in the care of the terminal patient.

Table 3.2 Psychotherapeutic interventions that may be useful in addressing psychological distress and psychiatric comorbidities in the palliative care setting

Modality	Technique	Uses
Supportive psychotherapy	Active listening, problem-solving strategies; allowing the expression of distressing emotions; enhance availability and accessibility of social support networks	Reduce distressing emotions; expression of emotions in a safe environment; enhance focused problem-solving; enhancement of social supports to sustain patient through difficulties
Cognitive-behavioral therapy	Collaborative process identifying cognitive appraisals; cognitive restructuring and coping skills training	Reduce depression and anxiety; reduce problematic cognitive styles and faulty attributions; develop effective coping strategies
Interpersonal psychotherapy	Role-playing, analysis of and modification of problematic communication patterns	Address role transitions due to illness, relationship difficulties, and interpersonal conflicts
Existential therapy	Life narrative and life review, i.e., identifying and highlighting one's significant life experiences and achievements	Fostering a sense of meaningfulness; placing current experiences within the context of coping with illness
Grief therapy	Exploration of perceived losses, facilitating mourning, encouraging restoration of function and delineation of remaining goals, re-engagement with others	Fostering mourning, acceptance; fostering a sense of meaningfulness; and leaving a legacy/generativity
Dignity-preserving therapy	Preserving self-care and customary roles; ensuring appropriate privacy boundaries, preserving autonomy and control in life matters and decision-making whenever feasible	Maintaining pride, and sense of self-efficacy and autonomy; reducing perceived burden to others
Relaxation training	Deep breathing exercises; progressive muscle relaxation; guided imagery	Relaxation; distraction from physical discomfort, e.g., pain; fosters a sense of mastery and empowerment
Self-hypnosis	Focused attention and dissociation is directed at alleviating physical discomfort and anxiety/distress	Relaxation; distraction; pain relief

[38–40]

A few caveats are worth noting, however. First, recommendations for many of the treatment approaches delineated in the section below are not based upon a solid foundation of empirical work. For some of these, the proposed benefit is extrapolated from studies demonstrating the benefits obtained from employing these

Table 3.3 Uses of various classes of psychopharmacologic agents in palliative care

Antidepressants	Neuroleptics
Depression	Antiemetic
Anxiety	Delirium
Co-analgesic agents in pain	Psychosis
	Severe agitation/violent behavior

Benzodiazepines	Psychostimulants
Anxiety	Depressive disorders
Insomnia	Opioid-induced sedation
Neuroleptic-induced akathisia	Fatigue
Alcohol withdrawal	Narcolepsy
Muscle spasm	
Conscious sedation	

[12, 28, 40, 41]

interventions in nonterminal patients. There are limited prospective, randomized trials or systematic meta-analytic reviews to draw upon to guide or direct selection of optimal treatment strategies in the palliative care setting. Often, the evidence for the utility of many of the psychotherapeutic and psychopharmacologic approaches discussed herein has largely been anecdotal, or based upon few randomized controlled trials or investigations employing small sample sizes. Additionally, there has been little investigation comparing the efficacy of one approach versus another, or determining the efficacy of combined endeavors versus those administered in isolation. It is imperative, however, to point out that the dearth of empirical research does not constitute evidence of a lack of efficacy in these conditions [42, 43].

Second, the logistics of some of the treatment approaches outlined herein can sometimes be impractical. Prognostic factors, e.g., life expectancy and the time frame available for treatment, are significant determinants influencing selection of the types of psychopharmacologic and psychotherapeutic measures undertaken. The terminal patient expected to live several months may be able to afford the time it takes to undergo certain psychotherapeutic modalities and/or the time requirements to appreciate the clinical efficacy of certain psychopharmacologic interventions, e.g., antidepressant effects. By contrast, patients with extremely restricted life expectancies, e.g., a few weeks, may not be able to yield much benefit from such interventions, requiring more expedient palliative measures to allay distress and provide comfort. In addition, the limited stamina of the patient and/or diminished cognitive acuity may impede the ability to successfully engage a patient in psychotherapy. Under such circumstances, there may be a need to rely predominantly on psychopharmacologic approaches instead.

Adjustment Disorders

The literature has suggested high, albeit variable, prevalence rates for adjustment disorders among patients in palliative care settings, ranging from 10 to 22% [32]. Risk factors associated with the development of adjustment disorders have been suggested to include physical limitations, problems related to social supports, and existential issues [44].

As a cluster, adjustment disorders refer to subthreshold conditions, possessing features of other conditions, e.g., anxiety and depression. According to the Diagnostic and Statistical Manual of Mental Disorders (DSM), the diagnosis rests on an assessment of one's emotional and behavioral responses to a stressor, and determining whether those responses appear to be in excess of normative standards, i.e., what would be expected by most persons facing comparable circumstances [45]. The potential pitfall to this diagnostic scheme is that it is subjective. Often, it is unclear how one knows what the normative response to a stressor might be; this issue is likely to become particularly onerous given the complexities of the stressors confronting patients at the end of life. The parameters for what constitutes maladaptive responses to stress can vary depending on one's gender, as well as societal and cultural influences further obscuring diagnosis. Unfortunately, adjustment disorders, unlike depressive and anxiety disorders, possess indefinite symptoms and lack an objective checklist of diagnostic criteria upon which to rely.

The confusion around diagnosis of adjustment disorders is paralleled by the numerous attempts within the literature to characterize psychological and emotional distress among palliative care patients, encapsulated in terms such as emotional suffering [46, 47], psychological distress [48], existential distress [49], and demoralization [50, 51]. Many of these terms reflect unpleasant and aversive emotions and behaviors, possessing features overlapping with, although not quite meeting, diagnostic criteria for major mood or anxiety disorders as outlined in DSM phenomenology. For example, demoralization has been described as a state encompassing isolation, hopelessness, dysphoria, apprehension, and an inability to cope [52]. It would be an oversimplification to merely suggest that demoralization, or any of the other aforementioned terms, be cast under the general rubric of adjustment disorders. It is plausible that the distress encapsulated by some of these terms might exist along a continuum, ranging from normal or appropriate responses to the challenges faced at the end of life to more extreme forms representing adjustment disorders and perhaps a more pernicious depressive or anxiety disorder [51]. However, as alluded to previously, distinguishing between a normal variant and psychiatric disorder can be difficult. When distress diminishes one's capacity for pleasure or to maintain connections with others or detracts from one's sense of meaning, clinicians ought to consider the possibility of an underlying psychiatric disorder [26].

Because of a lack of operationalized diagnostic criteria, there are no screening instruments that can be implemented to unearth the presence of adjustment disorders. Other screening instruments, e.g., the Distress Thermometer among others, may be considered surrogate assessments of subjective distress that can be incorporated routinely to unveil whether a condition exists that may be responsive to treatment [26].

Treatment approaches for adjustment disorders primarily rest upon psychotherapeutic measures that foster coping, reduce the impact of stress, and enhance social support systems to bolster and sustain the patient so as to enhance adaptation (see Table 3.2). Essentially, the goals of psychotherapy include the provision of a nurturing environment and support, cultivation of patient empowerment over psychological distress, the fostering of problem-solving and coping strategies with which to effectively deal with adversity, and to mitigate psychological distress that can potentially exacerbate, perpetuate, or maintain physical discomfort, e.g., pain.

In some cases, short-term courses of pharmacotherapy may be indicated to mitigate distress. For example, anxiolytics and sedative-hypnotics may be useful in reducing the impact of incapacitating symptoms that otherwise compromise functioning and impede one's ability to participate in short-term psychotherapy.

Depression

The experience of sadness is a natural and expected reaction to the multiple adversities encountered when one is confronted with advanced stages of illness, e.g., alteration of one's life trajectory, changes in body image, disability and dependency, etc. The inability to mourn loss or adapt to new challenges may manifest with signs and symptoms of clinical depression. Individuals who possess a prior history of depression, a family history of depression, or who have limited social supports may be more likely to develop clinical depression in the context of medical illnesses [53, 54]. Among patients with cancer, the severity of cancer-related symptoms and decrements in functioning that they produce may be factors predisposing patients to depression [55]. Prevalence rates of depression among patients in palliative care settings are substantially higher than those in the general population; a recent meta-analysis reported prevalence rates ranging from 13 to 20% [32].

Symptoms of depression can manifest with psychological symptoms, i.e., pervasive sadness, loss of interests in customarily pleasurable activities, preoccupations with guilt, worthlessness, death, dying and/or suicide, social withdrawal, indecisiveness and concentration deficits, as well as vegetative symptoms, i.e., appetite changes, sleep disturbances [45]. Depression is a significant cause of suffering and distress, resulting in the intensification and perpetuation of significant physical symptoms, e.g., pain and fatigue, and is associated with increased mortality among patients with cancer [7, 24, 56–61].

Depression can play a pivotal role in the expressed desires of patients for hastened death. Although fleeting thoughts of a desire to hasten death are relatively commonly encountered among terminal patients [62, 63], those patients with persisting desires for hastened death were most apt to be clinically depressed. Conversely, depressed terminally ill cancer patients were more likely than those who were not to endorse a desire for hastened death [7]. However, one should be aware that a desire for hastened death is not invariably associated with depression [64], for some, such passive desires for hastened death may be linked with inadequate pain treatment and other physical symptoms, and that, once appropriately managed, such desires for death may abate [65, 66].

Transient and intermittent suicidal ideas are reportedly experienced by patients with advanced phases of illness [67], however, persistent suicidal ideation is likely to signal severe psychiatric illness, including depression, adjustment disorder, or delirium [68, 69]. Vulnerability to enduring suicidal ideation is related to inadequately treated pain, the perception that one is helpless or that one is inefficacious in exerting control over aspects of one's illness/life [70, 71]. Hopelessness is a significant predictor of completed suicide in the general population [72, 73] and is a clinical predictor of suicidal ideation among the terminally ill [57]. Sensitive inquiry into the patient's harboring of suicidal ideas, intent, and/or plans is imperative so as to effectively develop, in conjunction with psychiatric consultation, appropriate measures to ensure the patient's safety, mitigate risk, and more effectively manage pain, mood disorders, and/or delirium.

According to the DSM, the diagnosis of a depressive disorder is restricted to situations in which patients manifest prototypic signs and symptoms that would not otherwise be accounted for by another medical/psychiatric condition or their treatment [45]. As alluded to previously, this exclusionary approach to assessment can present a diagnostic dilemma particularly in the palliative care setting. Uncertainties may arise as to whether symptoms that are commonly included among the diagnostic criteria for depression should be excluded if these can be otherwise ascribed to the medical illness. Thus, for example, many symptoms of medical illnesses, e.g., fatigue, anorexia, diminished concentration, and sleep disturbances, among others, can resemble the somatic symptoms of depression. Similarly, reductions in endurance and physical deconditioning can compromise one's capacity for engaging in pleasurable activities, resembling anhedonia. Exclusion of such symptoms when evaluating patients may reduce ambiguities, but conversely, potentially incurs the risk of missing a potentially treatable depressive disorder.

It is generally agreed that screening methods for depression should be accurate and easily administered, so as to facilitate development of timely and effective treatment approaches and resource planning, e.g., psychological and/or psychiatric referral. The Center for Epidemiologic Studies Depression Scale (CES-D) [74], the Hospital Anxiety and Depression Scale (HADS) [75], and the Beck-Depression Inventory-II (BDI-II) [76] have been demonstrated to be effective depression screening instruments employed among the medically ill. Part of the confusion surrounding the use of these measures has to do with decisions regarding the selection of appropriate cutoff scores. Certainly, if the intent is to avoid missing patients with depression who could, therefore, benefit from treatment, less stringent cutoff scores should be employed. The HADS is perhaps the most frequently used screening instrument employed in palliative care settings, partly attributable to its brevity and ease of administration and the fact that it places less emphasis on somatic symptoms [77, 78]. However, controversy attends whether the HADS is a particularly useful measure, i.e., having demonstrated unacceptably low sensitivity and specificity values [79]. Recently, there has been increased interest in the use of a single item screen asking the question "Are you depressed?" [80]. Although there has been some evidence to suggest the utility of straightforward inquiry in medical settings, the low sensitivity and specificity values of affirmative replies in assessing major depression in palliative care settings raise questions about their utility [81]. Regardless of the screening instrument employed, diagnosis requires a thorough clinical interview based upon clinical criteria as specified in the DSM; when uncertainties arise, consultation with mental health providers may clarify diagnosis and guide treatment approaches [82].

In evaluating a terminal patient with symptoms of depression, it is essential to consider the full range of potential causes as these may have implications for how treatment is contoured. It would be presumptuous to assume that depression is ascribable to the patient's reactions to having a terminal diagnosis, to a primary (functional) depressive disorder, or to the social sequelae of grave illness, e.g., isolation from customary supports. Thus, medical conditions (hypothyroidism and other metabolic abnormalities, HIV, cerebral metastasis, etc.) and medication use (corticosteroids, several chemotherapeutic agents, narcotics, anticonvulsants, antibiotics, digitalis, beta adrenergic blockers, among others) may need to be considered among the possibilities to unearth potential causes of depression [40]. It should be noted that for a particular patient, multiple factors can contribute to or exacerbate depression symptoms concurrently and that these factors can often have reciprocal influences. For example, chemotherapy may have direct depressogenic effects while concomitantly triggering marked dysphoria related to changes in body image. Therefore, consideration of multiple factors can inform treatment approaches that are individualized to the unique needs of the patient. In some cases, addressing remediable medical illnesses and/or modifications in medication selection or doses whenever possible or reasonable, may be helpful, and possibly sufficient, measures undertaken to mitigate depressive symptoms.

As a general class, antidepressants have established efficacy in the management of major depression in the context of palliative care [83]. Among the various classes of antidepressants available, tricyclic antidepressants (TCAs), serotonin-selective reuptake inhibitors (SSRIs), and mirtazapine have demonstrated clinical efficacy as compared to placebo conditions [84]. Although, the clinical benefits of TCAs may be apparent sooner than those acquired from SSRIs, the extant literature has not demonstrated greater efficacy of any particular antidepressant class over another [82, 85]. Evaluation of the utility of alternate antidepressant classes, e.g., serotonin–norepinephrine reuptake inhibitors (SNRIs) and bupropion has not been extensively investigated in the palliative care setting.

Selection of an antidepressant is predicated on several factors, i.e., the side effect profile of the drug, drug tolerability, safety concerns in light of prevailing medical conditions, and a history of the patient's personal or familial successful use of a particular agent or class of agent. For example, so as to minimize the encumbrance of, and potential risks associated with, polypharmacy, it may be prudent to select an agent which has demonstrated efficacy in addressing two or more conditions concurrently, e.g., depression and pain,. In such circumstances, use of a TCA or perhaps an SNRI, may be preferable. The side effects of a particular medication might be used to the patient's advantage as well. Thus, individuals experiencing insomnia and/or diminished appetite as part of their symptom complex may benefit from agents that can simultaneously yield these benefits, e.g., mirtazapine or TCAs; whereas persons who experience marked and incapacitating fatigue may benefit from the addition of antidepressants with less sedating side effects, e.g., an SNRI or bupropion.

Similarly, the adverse effects of antidepressants can be prohibitive and intolerable for some patients, and/or the use of selected agents may be contraindicated in light of the patient's comorbid medical conditions. For example, the anticholinergic side effects of TCAs can predispose medically compromised individuals toward development of a delirium, limiting their utility. Interestingly, although the potential for adverse effects of TCAs can render them poorly tolerable by palliative patients, drop-out rates for patients treated with TCAs did not differ significantly from those of other agents, i.e., SSRIs [84]. Furthermore, use of TCAs is contraindicated in patients with closed-angle glaucoma, recent myocardial infarction, cardiac arrhythmias, poorly controlled seizures, or severe benign prostatic hypertrophy.

It is noteworthy however, that it may take 2–4 weeks (and perhaps longer durations) at optimal doses before benefits of the antidepressants can be appreciated. As such, the delayed response to achieve antidepressant efficacy may prove to be a limiting factor for patients with short life expectancies. Use of psychostimulants, e.g., methylphenidate or dextroamphetamine, has been advocated as alternatives for rapid treatment of depression in the palliative care setting [86]. These agents may offer an advantage of producing stimulating effects, e.g., potentially reducing opioid-induced sedation [87, 88]. However, the utility of psychostimulants in palliative care settings is uncertain; a recent review indicated that there was insufficient empirical evidence to recommend the use of psychostimulants for the treatment of depression [89].

Psychotherapeutic interventions, e.g., supportive therapy or cognitive-behavioral therapy, may be helpful in mitigating symptoms of depression as long as there is reasonable life expectancy to make such interventions worthwhile. Additionally, the feasibility of psychotherapeutic interventions will be contingent upon the patient's cognitive capabilities and motivation. A recent meta-analysis, based on very few randomized controlled trials, suggested that psychotherapy, and supportive psychotherapy in particular, is effective in mitigating depression among patients with advanced cancer [39]; it is important to note that empirical investigations addressing the effectiveness and utility of such psychotherapeutic interventions are limited, thereby making it impossible to make definitive statements about their utility in palliative care settings [90].

Anxiety

Symptoms of anxiety are commonly encountered in the terminal phases of illness, particularly as one confronts the stark reality of the limitations of treatment and a limited life expectancy. Anxiety can manifest in a variety of forms, including symptoms of apprehension, restlessness, jitteriness, hypervigilance, distractibility, tachycardia and palpitations, dyspnea, and numbness [91–93]. In addition, patients may experience distressing rumination and worry [40]; a sense of foreboding can predispose one to catastrophizing and a preoccupation with the inevitability of harm/threat which can strain the patient–physician relationship and thereby undermine treatment [94]. Although many of the aforementioned symptoms can mimic those of an underlying medical conditions, consideration of, and formal assessment for, the presence of a treatable anxiety disorder should be considered.

Estimates suggest that anxiety disorders are relatively common among terminally ill patients [35], reportedly ranging between 7 and 13% [32]. Frequently, anxiety can coexist with other psychiatric conditions, including depression [30, 95]. Commonly encountered anxiety disorders include panic disorder, post-traumatic stress disorder, and generalized anxiety disorder [30, 94]. Anxiety disorders can incur significant functional deficits among afflicted patients [96]; greater impediments to functioning are likely to be encountered when anxiety and depression coexist [95].

Screening for anxiety can be accomplished with instruments such as the State Trait Anxiety Inventory (STAI) [97] and the HADS. The STAI was not developed specifically for medically ill patients, and due to its length, may be cumbersome for use in palliative care settings [26, 27]. The HADS is perhaps more commonly used, owing to its brevity and because it simultaneously screens for depression, despite some of the previously mentioned concerns about its sensitivity and specificity [78, 79]. As noted previously, it serves as an effective screening instrument, but should not be employed for diagnostic purposes [78]; ultimately, diagnosis of an anxiety disorder would depend upon a thoroughly conducted clinical interview based upon DSM diagnostic criteria.

As with depression, in evaluating a terminal patient with symptoms of anxiety, it is essential to consider whether other factors, apart from a functional anxiety disorder, may be precipitating or exacerbating the symptoms. Thus, medical conditions (e.g., hypoxia arising from chronic obstructive pulmonary disease, pulmonary edema, congestive heart failure, lung cancer; endocrine disturbances such as hyperthyroidism, hyperparathyroidism, carcinoid, pheochromocytoma; cardiac disease such as myocardial infarction, congestive heart failure, arrhythmia; electrolyte disturbances, e.g., hypocalcemia, hypomagnesemia) and adverse effects of medication (e.g., bronchodilators, β-adrenergic receptor stimulants, corticosteroids, antiemetics, i.e., metoclopramide and prochlorperazine, antipsychotic-induced akathisia, and serotonin syndrome) ought to be given consideration, as these may have treatment implications. Addressing these potential precipitating/exacerbating factors, if possible, may well mitigate anxiety symptoms.

The treatment of comorbid anxiety can serve to reduce somatic preoccupation and improve patient comfort, and therefore is a necessary component of comprehensive palliative care. Benzodiazepines are effective for the rapid amelioration of anxiety symptoms, e.g., apprehension, agitation, and restlessness, which are commonly encountered in terminal phases of illness [28, 40, 98, 99]. Several factors need to be considered when making medication selections. For example, agents with long half-lives, e.g., diazepam or clonazepam, may offer the advantage of more sustained anxiolytic effects over those which are short-acting, e.g., lorazepam or alprazolam, and thereby necessitate less frequent dosing. Abrupt discontinuation of long-acting agents will precipitate less severe withdrawal phenomena as compared with that associated with short-acting agents. On the other hand, side effects, e.g., excess sedation, memory impairments, and confusion, can be more troublesome and enduring with long acting as compared with short-acting agents [99]. Adverse effects associated with toxic accumulation of benzodiazepines can become especially problematic in patients with significant hepatic dysfunction, necessitating that benzodiazepine selection be restricted to lorazepam, oxazepam, or temazepam instead. The routes of administration may influence selection of specific agents. For example, only lorazepam and midazolam are rapidly and reliably absorbed following intramuscular administration, while diazepam can be effectively absorbed through rectal administration and alprazolam from sublingual administration. Although there is a risk of abuse encountered with administration of benzodiazepines, this is rarely a concern in palliative care settings.

The use of benzodiazepines may be precluded because of the potential for adverse effects, e.g., for patients with significant respiratory compromise or obstructive sleep apnea, or those persons for whom excess sedation can be particularly incapacitating or undesirable. It may be possible to employ alternate agents under such circumstances. For example, buspirone or antidepressants with anxiolytic properties, e.g., SSRIs or SNRIs, may be considered, however, as alluded to previously the time course required to achieve sufficient therapeutic benefits may be a limiting factor. Antipsychotics may be considered as possible alternatives, e.g., olanzapine or quetiapine [99]. Opioids, although intended for analgesic use, can offer relief from perceived dyspnea and anxiety as well, particularly in the late stages as death becomes imminent [100].

Interventions such as relaxation training and deep breathing exercises may be expedient measures to employ to mitigate periods of marked apprehension and distress. Effective use of such self-soothing strategies may also foster the patient's sense of self-empowerment in being able to control and modulate periods of distress. Although other strategies, e.g., Cognitive-Behavioral Therapy and supportive psychotherapy, have also been advocated in the treatment of anxiety, the utility and efficacy of such formalized interventions in the palliative care setting has not been extensively established in empirical work. One meta-analysis, based upon few randomized controlled trials, demonstrated only a marginal benefit from psychotherapy in mitigating anxiety among patients with incurable cancer [39].

Delirium

The presence of delirium can be a significant source of distress among patients in the advanced phases of illness, interfering with functioning, adaptation, and communication with others. Estimates suggest that the prevalence of delirium can be astonishingly high, as much as 80%, among terminal patients in the weeks before death [101].

The symptoms of delirium manifest with an inability or reduced ability to maintain attention, fluctuation of consciousness, disorientation, and sudden and dramatic memory impairments. Patients may experience distressing perceptual disturbances, i.e., misperceptions of their surroundings and hallucinations (usually visual). The patient is unlikely to perceive events in the environment accurately, e.g., may be incapable of understanding what is said to, or done for, them and may have impairments in communicating effectively with others. Because of these experiences, patients may display fear, sadness, defensive and aggressive behaviors overtly. Family members and caregivers may find the cognitive and behavioral aberrations alarming and the impediments to providing care overtaxing.

Because of its pervasiveness, and the distress it produces for the patient and caregivers alike, it is essential that clinicians be vigilant for delirium. The symptoms can be variable, often changing over time, contributing to misidentification, e.g., it can sometimes be difficult to distinguish from dementia, mood disturbances, anxiety, and psychosis e.g., [102]. Instruments available to assist in the identification of delirium in palliative care settings include the Confusion Assessment Method (CAM) [103] and the Memorial Delirium Assessment Scale (MDAS) [104], among others. The use of screening instruments, when combined with appropriate physical and cognitive examination along with laboratory investigations, can be useful for diagnostic purposes and quantification of the severity of symptoms [26]. The CAM is a simple, observer-based rating scale, useful for case finding, originally intended for use by nonpsychiatric clinicians to assess patients in hospital settings. Its validity for use in palliative care settings has only recently been investigated but not yet established [31, 105]. Although the CAM has been demonstrated to be reliable, its sensitivity varies as a function of the skills of the individual completing the assessment [106]. In one study conducted within a palliative care setting, the sensitivity of the CAM when completed by nonphysicians was markedly enhanced when formal instruction was provided to assist raters in detection of clinical signs of delirium [105]. Because of these limitations, the CAM is primarily recommended for use as a screening as opposed to a diagnostic instrument, formal neurocognitive assessment is still necessary to enhance detection and to avoid missing subtle or atypical presentations of delirium [107]. The MDAS, by contrast, has been developed for use in palliative care populations, e.g., hospitalized patients with advanced cancer and AIDS. One of the shortcomings of the MDAS is that it does not incorporate an assessment of the time course over which symptoms manifest and the degree to which the symptoms fluctuate over time, critics argue that without these features, it is sometimes difficult to distinguish features of delirium from other conditions with which some features may overlap, e.g., dementia. The MDAS is easy to complete, has good sensitivity ratings, and when administered repeatedly, can provide an indicator of the effectiveness of treatment interventions [104, 108].

Standard recommendations to the management of delirium include a tripartite approach involving a search for the etiology, correction of the underlying cause(s), and management of distressing symptoms associated with the altered mental state [109]. Several points of interest are worth noting about this approach. It has long been established that there are multiple causes for delirium including infection, metabolic and electrolyte abnormalities, nutritional deficits, brain tumors/metastasis, hypoxia, seizure, paraneoplastic syndrome, as well as medication use [101, 110]. Although identification and remediation of the pathology underlying delirium is ideal, there are several limiting factors encountered in palliative care settings. First, the extant literature suggests that it is often difficult to clearly establish a

Table 3.4 Medications with the potential for causing delirium

Anticholinergics, e.g., antihistamines, antispasmodics, atropine
Anti-inflammatory, e.g., corticosteroids
Antineoplastics, e.g., vincristine, vinblastine, asparaginase
Antimicrobials, e.g., acyclovir, aminoglycosides, vancomycin
Anticonvulsants, e.g., phenytoin, valproate
Antiemetics, e.g., metoclopramide
Analgesics, e.g., opioids (especially meperidine)
Cardiac medications, e.g., antiarrhythmics, beta-blockers, digitalis
Psychoactive medications, e.g., tricyclic antidepressants, lithium, antipsychotics
Sedative-hypnotics, e.g., barbiturates, benzodiazepines
Sympathomimetics, e.g., methylphenidate, ephedrine, phenylephrine, theophylline

[31, 109, 114]

specific cause for the delirium among patients with advanced diseases [41, 111]. For example, there may be restrictions on pursuing extensive investigative studies and diagnostic procedures for terminal patients because of concerns that these procedures can be invasive, burdensome, or incur discomfort. Second, the causes are often multifactorial [112, 113], however, determining which factors constitute essential causes of the delirium as opposed to those which are facilitating factors, and not necessarily directly related to the delirium, can be difficult. Third, even when causes are unveiled, treatment may not be possible due to the irreversibility of the underlying condition, e.g., brain metastasis.

However, the clinician should be aware that there are many causes of delirium that can, nonetheless, be reversible and easily remediated. The most common reversible medical causes of delirium include dehydration, electrolyte disturbances, e.g., hypercalcemia, and certain infections, e.g., urinary tract infections [101, 113]. Additionally, adverse effects of prescribed medication are capable of producing alterations in cognitive status; several medication classes that are commonly implicated in causing/exacerbating delirium are listed in Table 3.4. Consideration must be given to the possibility of addressing delirium by modifying the patient's medication regimen, e.g., by means of dose reduction or substitution of an alternative agent [31]. Unfortunately, in the last days of life, delirium can remain refractory to corrective measures, perhaps attributable to general organ failure [101].

Several medications can be used to address the symptoms associated with delirium. Antipsychotic medications are frequently invoked for the management of the psychomotoric restlessness, distress, and confusion encountered in delirium. Evidence for the efficacy of antipsychotics in the treatment of delirium has largely been anecdotal (based upon case reports and case series). Although conventional agents, e.g., haloperidol, have been frequently employed because of ease of use (parenterally, intramuscularly, subcutaneously, and orally), there are potential risks associated with their use. For example, extrapyramidal side effects, e.g., parkinsonism and akathisia, may, in turn, become particularly distressing to patients, precluding their use in patients with certain comorbid conditions, e.g., Parkinson's disease and Lewy-body dementia. Because of concerns that delirium may be related to disruptions in central nervous system cholinergic transmission, highly anticholinergic agents may be best avoided as these can potentially exacerbate delirium. More recently, atypical antipsychotics, e.g., risperidone or olanzapine, have been employed as alternatives [115, 116]. However, very few randomized controlled trials have thus far been conducted, thereby limiting the ability to make definitive statements about the efficacy of the atypical antipsychotics in the management of delirium in terminal disease [114, 116, 117]. In severe forms of delirium refractory to antipsychotic use, sedation with agents such as midazolam or propofol may be useful to mitigate distress and induce marked sedation [118–120]. However, these agents, by virtue of their central nervous system effects, can significantly interfere with processing of sensory information, impede memory formation and thereby, contribute to further cognitive decline [109].

Lastly, there are several environmental and psychosocial interventions that can be helpful in mitigating patient and caregiver distress. It is imperative that the risks of inadvertent harm be reduced by ensuring that the environment is safe. Patients may be calmed by reducing unnecessary stimulation, e.g., noise and light, and by having familiar objects, e.g., photographs and personal mementos, and familiar persons around them. Afflicted patients may require frequent redirection, it is imperative to invoke simple, clear directives, and to gently redirect the patient with soft vocal tones and physical contact. Education of family members may help to mitigate caregiver distress. They may need to be advised not to overinterpret erratic behaviors, gestures, and grimacing and to avoid personalizing hostile, resistive, or aggressive behaviors; education can demystify such aberrant behaviors when caregivers are informed that such behaviors are likely to instead reflect disturbances in processing/integration of information and coordination of goal-directed behaviors [109, 121]. Transition to a higher level care, e.g., acute settings or hospices, may be required if appropriate safety measures cannot be implemented in the home or if the burdens to caregivers exceed what they can reasonably provide to the patient.

Conclusions

The approach of palliative care medicine is embedded in the perspective that treatment efforts, albeit noncurative, should be directed at reduction of suffering and improving well-being. Palliative care guidelines recognize the indispensable psychological, existential, and social domains to the comprehensive management of patients in the terminal phases of illness. A multimodal approach, i.e., employing psychotherapeutic and psychopharmacologic treatments, may therefore be necessary to address psychological distress, e.g., grief, spiritual distress, and existential concerns, along with psychiatric complications, e.g., adjustment disorder, depression, anxiety, and delirium that significantly impact quality of life. Care of the patient can be greatly enriched when mental health specialists are enlisted in the assessment and treatment of the terminal patient, working in a coordinated fashion with palliative care physicians, nurses, caregivers, and family members. Although advances have been made in identifying the psychiatric comorbidities and subthreshold psychological states that impact the terminal patient, further investigation is required to inform evidence-based treatment guidelines as well as to determine which treatment approaches are most practical and under what circumstances and for whom such interventions prove to be most effective.

References

1. Worden JW. Grief counseling and grief therapy – a handbook for the mental health practitioner. 4th ed. New York: Springer; 2009.
2. Meares RA. On saying goodbye before death. JAMA. 1981;246(11):1227–9.
3. Periyakoil VS, Kraemer HC, Noda A, Moos R, Hallenbeck J, Webster M, Yesavage JA. The development and initial validation of the Terminally Ill Grief or Depression Scale (TIGDS). Int J Methods Psychiatr Res. 2005;14(4):202–12.
4. Larson DB, Swyers JP, McCullough ME. Scientific research on spirituality and health. Rockville, MD: National Institute for Healthcare Research; 1997.
5. Koenig HG, Cohen HJ, Blazer DG, Pieper C, Meador KG, Shelp F, Goli V, DiPasquale B. Religious coping and depression among elderly, hospitalized medically ill men. Am J Psychiatry. 1992;149:1693–700.
6. Nelson CJ, Rosenfeld B, Breitbart W, Galietta M. Spirituality, religion, and depression in the terminally ill. Psychosomatics. 2002;43:213–20.
7. Breitbart W, Rosenfeld B, Pessin H, Kaim M, Funesti-Esch J, Galietta M, Nelson CJ, Brescia R. Depression, hopelessness, and desire for hastened death in terminally ill patients with cancer. JAMA. 2000;284:2907–11.
8. McClain CS, Rosenfeld B, Breitbart W. Effect of spiritual well-being on end-of-life despair in terminally-ill cancer patients. Lancet. 2003;361:1603–7.
9. Baider L, Russak SM, Perry S, Kash K, Gronert M, Fox B, Holland J, Kaplan-Denour A. The role of religious and spiritual beliefs in coping with malignant melanoma: an Israeli sample. Psychooncology. 1999;8(1):27–35.
10. Peterman AH, Fitchett G, Brady MJ, Hernandez L, Cella D. Measuring spiritual well-being in people with cancer: the functional assessment of chronic illness therapy-spiritual well-being scale (FACIT-Sp). Ann Behav Med. 2002;24(1):49–58.
11. Holland J. Psychosocial distress in the patient with cancer. Standards of care and treatment guidelines. Oncology. 2000;15(4 Suppl 2):19–24.
12. Block SD. Psychological issues in end-of-life care. J Palliat Med. 2006;9(3):751–72.
13. Greer S, Watson M. Mental adjustment to cancer: its measurement and prognostic importance. Cancer Surv. 1987;6(3):439–53.
14. Lazarus RS, Folkman S. Stress, appraisal and coping. New York: Springer; 1984.
15. Park CL, Folkman S. Meaning in the context of stress and coping. Rev Gen Psychol. 1997;1:115–44.
16. Parkes CM. What becomes of redundant world models? A contribution to the study of adaptation to change. Br J Med Psychol. 1975;48:131–7.
17. Baider L, Ever-Hadani P, Goldzweig G, Wygoda MR, Peretz T. Is perceived family support a relevant variable in psychological distress? A sample of prostate and breast cancer couples. J Psychosom Res. 2003;55:453–60.
18. National Consensus Project for Quality Palliative Care Consortium. National consensus project for quality palliative care: clinical practice guidelines for quality palliative care, executive summary. J Palliat Med. 2004;7(5):611–27.
19. Edwards A, Pang N, Shiu V, Chan C. The understanding of spirituality and the potential role of spiritual care in end-of-life and palliative care: a meta-study of qualitative research. Palliat Med. 2010;24(8):753–70.

20. Fallowfield L, Ratcliffe D, Jenkins V, Saul J. Psychiatric morbidity and its recognition by doctors in patients with cancer. Br J Cancer. 2001;84(8):1011–5.
21. McDonald MV, Passik SD, Dugan W, Rosenfeld B, Theobald DE, Edgerton S. Nurses' recognition of depression in their patients with cancer. Oncol Nurs Forum. 1999;26(3):593–9.
22. Passik SD, Dugan W, McDonald MV, Rosenfeld B, Theobald DE, Edgerton S. Oncologists' recognition of depression in their patients with cancer. J Clin Oncol. 1998;16(4):1594–600.
23. Maguire P, Pitceathly C. Improving the psychological care of cancer patients and their relatives – the role of specialist nurses. J Psychosom Res. 2003;55:469–74.
24. Leo RJ. Clinical manual of pain management in psychiatry. Washington, DC: American Psychiatric Press; 2007.
25. Ryan H, Schofield P, Cockburn J, Butow P, Tattersall M, Turner J, Girgis A, Bandaranayake D, Bowman D. How to recognize and manage psychological distress in cancer patients. Eur J Cancer Care. 2005;14:7–15.
26. Kelly B, McClement S, Chochinov HM. Measurement of psychological distress in palliative care. Palliat Med. 2006;20:779–89.
27. Carlson LE, Bultz BD. Cancer distress screening – needs, models, and methods. J Psychosom Res. 2003;55:403–9.
28. Breitbart W, Bruera E, Chochinov H, Lynch M. Neuropsychiatric syndromes and psychological symptoms in patients with advanced cancer. J Pain Symptom Manage. 1995;10(2):131–41.
29. Minagawa H, Uchitomi Y, Yamawaki S, Ishitani K. Psychiatric morbidity in terminally ill cancer patients. A prospective study. Cancer. 1996;78(5):1131–7.
30. Kadan-Lottick NS, Vanderwerker LC, Block SD, Zhang B, Prigerson HG. Psychiatric disorders and mental health service use in patients with advanced cancer: a report from the coping with cancer study. Cancer. 2005;104(12):2872–81.
31. Leonard M, Agar M, Mason C, Lawlor P. Delirium issues in palliative care settings. J Psychosom Res. 2008;65:289–98.
32. Mitchell AJ, Chan M, Bhatti H, Halton M, Grassi L, Johansen C, Meader N. Prevalence of depression, anxiety, and adjustment disorder in oncological, haematological, and palliative-care settings: a meta-analysis of 94 interview-based studies. Lancet Oncol. 2011;12:160–74.
33. Stark DP, House A. Anxiety in cancer patients. Br J Cancer. 2000;83:1261–7.
34. van't Spijker A, Trijsburg RW, Duivenvoorden HJ. Psychological sequelae of cancer diagnosis: a meta-analytical review of 58 studies after 1980. Psychosom Med. 1997;59:280–93.
35. Stark D, Kiely M, Smith A, Velikova G, House A, Selby P. Anxiety disorders in cancer patients: their nature, associations and relation to quality of life. J Clin Oncol. 2002;20(14):3137–48.
36. Wasteson E, Brenne E, Higginson IJ, Hotopf M, Lloyd-Williams M, Kaasa S, Loge JH. Depression assessment and classification in palliative cancer patients: a systematic literature review. Palliat Med. 2009;23(8):739–53.
37. Hopwood P, Stephens RJ. Depression in patients with lung cancer: prevalence and risk factors derived from quality-of-life data. J Clin Oncol. 2000;18:893–903.
38. Sellick SM, Crooks DL. Depression and cancer: an appraisal of the literature for prevalence, detection, and practice guideline development for psychological interventions. Psychooncology. 1999;8(4):315–33.
39. Akechi T, Okuyama T, Onishi J, Morita T, Furukawa TA. Psychotherapy for depression among incurable cancer patients (Review). Cochrane Database Syst Rev. 2010;(11):CD005537. doi:10.1002/14651858.
40. Miller K, Massie MJ. Depression and anxiety. Cancer J. 2006;12:388–97.
41. Stiefel F, Fainsinger R, Bruera E. Acute confusional states in patients with advanced cancer. J Pain Symptom Manage. 1992;7:94–8.
42. Kutner JS. Applying the evidence base to terminal care. J Palliat Med. 2005;8(5):1040–1.
43. Plonk WM, Arnold RM. Terminal care: the last weeks of life. J Palliat Med. 2005;8(5):1042–54.
44. Akechi T, Okuyama T, Sugawara Y, Nakano T, Shima Y, Uchitomi Y. Major depression, adjustment disorders, and post-traumatic stress disorder in terminally ill cancer patients: associated and predictive factors. J Clin Oncol. 2004;22(10):1957–65.

45. American Psychiatric Association. Diagnostic and statistical manual of mental disorders. 4th ed. Washington, DC: American Psychiatric Association; 2000. Text revision.
46. Cassel EJ. The nature of suffering and the goals of medicine. N Engl J Med. 1982;306(11):639–45.
47. Cherny NI, Coyle N, Foley KM. Suffering in the advanced cancer patient: a definition and taxonomy. J Palliat Care. 1994;10:57–70.
48. Ridner SH. Psychological distress: concept analysis. J Adv Nurs. 2004;45(5):536–45.
49. Kearny M, Mount B. Spiritual care of the dying patient. In: Chochinov HM, Breitbart W, editors. Handbook of psychiatry in palliative medicine. New York: Oxford University Press; 2000. p. 357–73.
50. Kissane DW, Clarke DM, Street AF. Demoralization syndrome: a relevant psychiatric diagnosis for palliative care. J Palliat Care. 2001;17:12–21.
51. Kissane DW, Wein S, Love A, Lee XQ, Kee PL, Clarke DM. The demoralization scale: a report of its development and preliminary validation. J Palliat Care. 2004;20(4):269–76.
52. Clarke DM, Kissane DW, Trauer T, Smith GC. Demoralization, anhedonia and grief in patients with severe physical illness. World Psychiatry. 2005;4(2):96–105.
53. Cavanaugh S, Clark DC, Gibbons RD. Diagnosing depression in the hospitalized medically ill. Psychosomatics. 1983;24:809–15.
54. Craven JL, Rodin GM, Johnson L, Kennedy SH. The diagnosis of major depression in renal dialysis patients. Psychosom Med. 1987;49(5):482–92.
55. Kurtz ME, Kurtz JC, Stommel M, Given CW, Given B. Predictors of depressive symptomatology of geriatric patients with lung cancer – a longitudinal analysis. Psychooncology. 2002;11:12–22.
56. Breitbart W, Rosenfeld BD, Passik SD. Interest in physician-assisted suicide among ambulatory HIV-infected patients. Am J Psychiatry. 1996;153(2):238–42.
57. Chochinov HM, Wilson KG, Enns M, Lander S. Depression, hopelessness, and suicidal ideation in the terminally ill. Psychosomatics. 1998;39:366–70.
58. Onitilo AA, Nietert PJ, Egede LE. Effect of depression on all-cause mortality in adults with cancer and differential effects by cancer site. Gen Hosp Psychiatry. 2006;28:396–402.
59. Pinquart M, Duberstein PR. Depression and cancer mortality: a meta-analysis. Psychol Med. 2010;40:1797–810.
60. Satin JR, Linden W, Phillips MJ. Depression as a predictor of disease progression and mortality in cancer patients – a meta-analysis. Cancer. 2009;115:5349–61.
61. Watson M, Haviland JS, Greer S, Davidson J, Bliss JM. Influence of psychological response on survival in breast cancer: a population-based cohort study. Lancet. 1999;354:1331–6.
62. Chochinov HM, Wilson KG, Enns M, Mowchun N, Lander S, Levitt M, Clinch JJ. Desire for death in the terminally ill. Am J Psychiatry. 1995;152(8):1185–91.
63. Chochinov HM, Tataryn D, Clinch JJ, Dudgeon D. Will to live in the terminally ill. Lancet. 1999;354:816–9.
64. Jones JM, Huggins MA, Rydall AC, Rodin GM. Symptomatic distress, hopelessness, and the desire for hastened death in hospitalized cancer patients. J Psychosom Res. 2003;55:411–8.
65. Mystakidou K, Parpa E, Katsouda E, Galanos A, Vlahos L. Pain and desire for hastened death in terminally ill cancer patients. Cancer Nurs. 2005;28(4):318–24.
66. Mystakidou K, Parpa E, Katsouda E, Galanos A, Vlahos L. The role of physical and psychological symptoms in desire for death: a study of terminally ill cancer patients. Psychooncology. 2006;15:355–60.
67. Brown JH, Henteleff P, Barakat S, Rowe CJ. Is it normal for terminally ill patients to desire death? Am J Psychiatry. 1986;143:208–11.
68. Breitbart W. Suicide in cancer patients. Oncology. 1987;1:49–55.
69. Breitbart W. Identifying patients at risk for, and treatment of major psychiatric complications of cancer. Support Care Cancer. 1995;3(1):45–60.
70. Bolund C. Suicide and cancer: II. Medical and care factors in suicides by cancer patients in Sweden, 1973–1976. J Psychosoc Oncol. 1985;3(1):31–52.

71. Filiberti A, Ripamonti C, Totis A, Ventafridda V, De Conno F, Contiero P, Tamburini M. Characteristics of terminal cancer patients who committed suicide during a home palliative care program. J Pain Symptom Manage. 2001;22(1):544–53.
72. Beck AT, Steer RA, Kovacs M, Garrison B. Hopelessness and eventual suicide: a ten-year prospective study of patients hospitalized with suicidal ideation. Am J Psychiatry. 1985;142:559–63.
73. Cooper-Patrick L, Crum RM, Ford DE. Identifying suicidal ideation in general medical patients. JAMA. 1994;272:1757–62.
74. Radloff LS. The CES-D Scale: a self-report depression scale for research in the general population. Appl Psychol Meas. 1977;3:385–401.
75. Zigmond AS, Snaith RP. The Hospital Anxiety and Depression Scale. Acta Psychiatr Scand. 1983;67:361–70.
76. Beck AT, Steer RA, Brown GK. Manual for the Beck Depression Inventory-II. San Antonio, TX: Psychological Corporation; 1996.
77. Hotopf M, Chidgey J, Addington-Hall J, Ly KL. Depression in advanced disease: a systematic review Part 1. Prevalence and case finding. Palliat Med. 2002;16:81–97.
78. Mitchell AJ, Meader N, Symonds P. Diagnostic validity of the Hospital Anxiety and Depression Scale (HADS) in cancer and palliative settings: a meta-analysis. J Affect Disord. 2010;126(3):335–48.
79. Lloyd-Williams M, Friedman T, Rudd N. An analysis of the validity of the Hospital Anxiety and Depression Scale as a screening tool in patients with advanced metastatic cancer. J Pain Symptom Manage. 2001;22:990–6.
80. Chochinov HM, Wilson KG, Enns M, Lander S. "Are you depressed?" Screening for depression in the terminally ill. Am J Psychiatry. 1997;154:674–6.
81. Lloyd-Williams M, Spiller J, Ward J. Which depression screening tools should be used in palliative care? Palliat Med. 2003;17:40–3.
82. Rayner L, Price A, Hotopf M, Higginson IJ. The development of evidence-based European guidelines on the management of depression in palliative cancer care. Eur J Cancer. 2011;47:702–12.
83. Massie MJ, Popkin MK. Depressive disorders. In: Holland JC, Rowland JH, editors. Psycho-oncology. New York: Oxford University Press; 1998. p. 518–40.
84. Rayner L, Price A, Evans A, Valsraj K, Hotopf M, Higginson IJ. Antidepressants for the treatment of depression in palliative care: systematic review and meta-analysis. Palliat Med. 2011;25(1):36–51.
85. Ly KL, Chidgey J, Addington-Hall J, Hotopf M. Depression in palliative care: a systematic review. Part 2. Treatment. Palliat Med. 2002;16:279–84.
86. Orr K, Taylor D. Psychostimulants in the treatment of depression. CNS Drugs. 2007;21(3): 239–57.
87. Bruera E, Chadwick S, Brenneis C, Hanson J, MacDonald RN. Methylphenidate associated with narcotics for the treatment of cancer pain. Cancer Treat Rep. 1987;71(1):67–70.
88. Reissig JE, Rybarczyk AM. Pharmacologic treatment of opioid-induced sedation in chronic pain. Ann Pharmacother. 2005;39(4):727–31.
89. Candy B, Jones L, Williams R, Tookman A, King M. Psychostimulants for depression. Cochrane Database Syst Rev. 2008;(2):CD006722.
90. Massie MJ, Holland JC, Straker N. Psychotherapeutic interventions. In: Holland JC, Rowland JH, editors. Handbook of psycho-oncology: psychological care of the patient with cancer. New York: Oxford University Press; 1989. p. 455–69.
91. Breitbart W, Jacobsen PB. Psychiatric symptom management in terminal care. Clin Geriatr Med. 1996;12:329–47.
92. Noyes R, Holt CS, Massie MJ. Anxiety disorders. In: Holland JC, editor. Psycho-oncology. New York: Oxford University Press; 1998. p. 548–63.
93. Roth AJ, Breitbart W. Psychiatric emergencies in terminally ill cancer patients. Hematol Oncol Clin North Am. 1996;10(1):235–59.
94. Spencer R, Nilsson M, Wright A, Pirl W, Prigerson H. Anxiety disorders in advanced cancer patients correlates and predictors of end-of-life outcomes. Cancer. 2010;116:1810–9.

95. Wilson KG, Chochinov HM, Skirko MG, Allard P, Chary S, Gagnon PR, Macmillan K, De Luca M, O'Shea F, Kuhl D, Fainsinger RL, Clinch JJ. Depression and anxiety disorders in palliative cancer care. J Pain Symptom Manage. 2007;33(2):118–29.
96. Skarstein J, Aass N, Fossa SD, Skovlund E, Dahl AA. Anxiety and depression in cancer patients: relation between the Hospital Anxiety and Depression Scale and the European Organization for Research and Treatment of Cancer Core Quality of Life Questionnaire. J Psychosom Res. 2000;49:27–34.
97. Speilberger CD. Manual for the State-Trait Anxiety Inventory: STAI (Form Y). Palo Alto, CA: Consulting Psychologists Press; 1983.
98. Henderson M, MacGregor E, Sykes N, Hotopf M. The use of benzodiazepines in palliative care. Palliat Med. 2006;20:407–12.
99. Roth AJ, Massie MJ. Anxiety and its management in advanced cancer. Curr Opin Support Palliat Care. 2007;1:50–6.
100. Portenoy RK, Foley KM. Management of cancer pain. In: Holland JC, Rowland JH, editors. Handbook of psychooncology: psychological care of the patient with cancer. New York: Oxford University Press; 1989. p. 369–82.
101. Lawlor PG, Gagnon B, Mancini IL, Pereira JL, Hanson J, Suarez-Almazor ME, Bruera ED. Occurrence, causes, and outcome of delirium in patients with advanced cancer – a prospective study. Arch Intern Med. 2000;160:786–94.
102. Ostgathe C, Gaertner J, Voltz R. Cognitive failure in end of life. Curr Opin Support Palliat Care. 2008;2:187–91.
103. Inouye SK, van Dyck CH, Alessi CA, Balkin S, Siegal AP, Horwitz RI. Clarifying confusion: the confusion assessment method. Ann Intern Med. 1990;113:941–8.
104. Breitbart W, Rosenfeld B, Roth A, Smith MJ, Cohen K, Passik S. The memorial delirium assessment scale. J Pain Symptom Manage. 1997;13:128–37.
105. Ryan K, Leonard M, Guerin S, Donnelly S, Conroy M, Meagher D. Validation of the confusion assessment method in the palliative care setting. Palliat Med. 2009;23:40–5.
106. Rolfson DB, McElhaney JE, Jhangri GS, Rockwood K. Validity of the confusion assessment method in detecting post-operative delirium in the elderly. Int Psychogeriatr. 1999;11(4):431–8.
107. Wei LA, Fearing MA, Sternberg EJ, Inouye SK. The confusion assessment method (CAM): a systematic review of current usage. J Am Geriatr Soc. 2008;56(5):823–30.
108. Lawlor PG, Nekolaichuk C, Gagnon B, Mancini IL, Pereira JL, Bruera ED. Clinical utility, factor analysis, and further validation of the memorial delirium assessment scale in patients with advanced cancer: assessing delirium in advanced cancer. Cancer. 2000;88:2859–67.
109. Centeno C, Sanz A, Bruera E. Delirium in advanced cancer patients. Palliat Med. 2004;18:184–94.
110. Jackson KC, Lipman AG. Delirium in palliative care patients. J Pharm Care Pain Symptom Control. 1999;7(4):59–70.
111. Bruera E, Miller J, McCallion J, Macmillan K, Krefting L, Hanson J. Cognitive failure in patients with terminal cancer: a prospective study. J Pain Symptom Manage. 1992;7(4):192–5.
112. Casarett DJ, Inouye SK. Diagnosis and management of delirium near the end of life. Ann Intern Med. 2001;135:32–40.
113. Morita T, Tei Y, Tsunoda J, Inoue S, Chihara S. Underlying pathologies and their associations with clinical features in terminal delirium of cancer patients. J Pain Symptom Manage. 2001;22(6):997–1006.
114. Gagnon PR. Treatment of delirium in supportive and palliative care. Curr Opin Support Palliat Care. 2008;2:60–6.
115. Breitbart W, Tremblay A, Gibson C. An open trial of olanzapine for the treatment of delirium in hospitalized cancer patients. Psychosomatics. 2002;43:175–82.
116. Jackson KC, Lipman AG. Drug therapy for delirium in terminally ill adult patients (Review). Cochrane Database Syst Rev. 2009;(4):CD004770.
117. Lonergan E, Britton AM, Luxenberg J, Wyller T. Antipsychotics for delirium. Cochrane Database of Systematic Reviews. (2):CD005594, 2007.

118. Bottomley DM, Hanks GW. Subcutaneous midazolam infusion in palliative care. J Pain Symptom Manage. 1990;5(4):259–61.
119. Fainsinger R, Miller MJ, Bruera E, Hanson J, Maceachern T. Symptom control during the last week of life on a palliative care unit. J Palliat Care. 1991;7(1):5–11.
120. Mercadante S, De Conno F, Ripamonti C. Propofol in terminal care. J Pain Symptom Manage. 1995;10:639–42.
121. Bruera E, Bush SH, Willey J, Paraskevopoulos T, Li Z, Palmer JL, Cohen MZ, Sivesind D, Elsayem A. Impact of delirium and recall on the level of distress in patients with advanced cancer and their family caregivers. Cancer. 2009;115(9):2004–12.

Review Questions

1. Which of the following is the most common psychiatric disorder encountered in palliative care settings?

   (a) Adjustment disorder
   (b) Depression
   (c) Anxiety disorder
   (d) Delirium

2. What is the primary treatment for adjustment disorders in the palliative care setting?

   (a) Anxiolytics
   (b) Sedatives
   (c) Psychotherapy
   (d) Hypnotics

3. Psychostimulants may be a reasonable consideration for the treatment of a terminal cancer patient who is experiencing which of the following?

   (a) Generalized worry and apprehension, with episodic dyspnea and perceived palpitations
   (b) Depressive symptoms and incapacitating opioid-induced sedation
   (c) Depressive symptoms including insomnia, anorexia, and irritability
   (d) Alcohol withdrawal

4. Which of the following is the best assessment for diagnosis of an anxiety disorder in palliative care settings?

   (a) Clinical interview based on DSM criteria
   (b) Hospital Anxiety and Depression Scale
   (c) State Trait Anxiety Scale
   (d) Distress Thermometer

5. Each of the following factors is likely to bode favorably in terms of adapting to the challenges faced at the end-of-life *except*:

   (a) Having a spiritual framework
   (b) The perception that one has an accessible social support network
   (c) Believing that one's illness and clinical course is uncontrollable and unpredictable
   (d) The perception that one has a repertoire of skills with which to manage stressors

Answers

1. Answer: (d). As high as 80% of terminally ill patients can experience delirium, especially in the weeks before death. Depression and adjustment disorders have a prevalence range of 13–22%, and 10–22%, respectively. Anxiety disorder is the fourth most common psychiatric comorbidity ranging from 7 to 13%.
2. Answer: (c). Psychotherapy is the primary treatment for adjustment disorders. Anxiolytics, sedatives-hypnotics can be used as an adjunct for patients who experience incapacitating symptoms that can impede their ability to participate in psychotherapy.
3. Answer: (b). Although there is insufficient evidence to recommend the use of psychostimulants in palliative care settings, these agents have been advocated for the rapid improvement of depressive symptoms. In addition, psychostimulants offer the potential benefit of reducing incapacitating opioid-induced sedation. The potential adverse effects, e.g., insomnia, anorexia, and heightened anxiety, would preclude their use in patients experiencing many of these symptoms. Psychostimulants would not be indicated for the treatment of alcohol withdrawal.
4. Answer: (a). The Hospital Anxiety and Depression Scale, State Trait Anxiety Scale, and Distress Thermometer are screening instruments. However, a clinical interview based on DSM criteria is the gold standard in diagnosing anxiety disorders in the palliative care setting.
5. Answer: (c). Terminal patients can successfully navigate the adaptational challenges posed in the advanced phases of illness. Among the factors listed here, inflexible and maladaptive beliefs, i.e., perceiving that one's illness is uncontrollable and unpredictable, may bode poorly with regard to managing psychological distress.

Chapter 4
Hospice for the Terminally Ill and End-of-Life Care

Jamie Capasso, Robert Byron Kim, and Danielle Perret

Introduction

Some healthcare professionals are privileged with the opportunity to care for patients at or near the end of their lives. This is an important and vital service that can make a significant and lasting difference in the lives of patients and their families. Patients nearing death have unique needs that frequently are more complex or urgent than patients with transient or chronic disease, and therefore require specialized care.

Most patients cared for during the terminal portion of their life are a challenge for clinicians, and those that are best prepared for this challenge have knowledge in several areas. These include advanced pain and symptom management, knowing how and when to enlist the assistance of programs such as hospice or home care, how to customize treatment plans in accordance with the patient's changing clinical status, and being familiar with the natural progression of signs and symptoms in the actively dying patient.

J. Capasso, D.O. (✉)
Department of Medicine, University of California,
Irvine School of Medicine, Irvine, CA, USA
e-mail: jcapasso@uci.edu

R.B. Kim, M.D. • D. Perret, M.D.
Department of Anesthesiology & Perioperative Care,
University of California, Irvine School of Medicine,
Irvine, CA, USA

N. Vadivelu et al. (eds.), *Essentials of Palliative Care*,
DOI 10.1007/978-1-4614-5164-8_4,
© Springer Science+Business Media New York 2013

The Beginnings of Hospice: A Historic Perspective

St. Christopher's Hospice, widely regarded as one of the most important founding hospice institutions, was founded in 1967 by Dr. Cicely Saunders. Located in London, it was founded to help address the changing climate of death and dying. As medicine advanced, more treatments were available to end stage patients. Consequently, more patients were dying in hospitals rather than in their own homes, as had been the case for hundreds of years.

Patients were living longer with "terminal" diagnoses due to new medical innovations but progress in pain and symptom control unfortunately lagged behind. This lag left a critical need for new methods of caring for dying patients [1, 2].

In the early 1960s, Dr. Saunders spoke at Yale University about her vision for comprehensive, comfortable, and dignified end-of-life care for patients and support for their families. The dean of nursing, Florence Weld, who attended this event, later said that the encounter changed the direction of her life. She decided to leave Yale to learn more about Dr. Saunders' vision and to train at St. Christopher's in London. Upon her return in 1974, she established Connecticut Hospice in Branford, Connecticut [3].

Over the next several years, the hospice movement gained momentum, and by 1980 there were 138 hospice programs in the USA The hospice Medicare benefit was established in 1982, and although initially opposed by many, it allowed for widespread expansion of hospice with increased availability to patients. Today, there are over 4,700 hospice organizations in the USA. This exponential growth has led to hospice evolving from a relatively insignificant part of the US health care system to the fastest growing component of Medicare spending. The National Hospice and Palliative Care Organization estimates that the number of patients served in 2007 was 1.4 million [4].

Hospice Defined

In the US, hospice is the predominant model of care for the diverse group of patients with life-limiting illness or injury. It is centered on the philosophy that all individuals should have the ability to die with comfort, dignity, and on their own terms. It consists of a team-oriented approach to medical care, pain and symptom management, and emotional and spiritual support for both patient and the family unit. This care is provided by an interdisciplinary team consisting of experts in their specific component of patient care (see Table 4.1). The team consists of a physician, nurse, social worker, chaplain, home health aide, and volunteers, all with specialized training in hospice. Additionally, a physical, speech, occupational, massage, or music therapist may be available to address specific needs if necessary. The team members meet frequently as a group with the goal of creating a cohesive, inclusive care plan [5].

Table 4.1 Interdisciplinary team members

Hospice medical director	• Leads the interdisciplinary team in developing the plan of care • Provides consultation to other physicians regarding hospice care • Certifies patient for hospice eligibility
Hospice physician	• May serve as primary care physician (PCP) or consultant managing patient's pain and symptoms after enrollment in hospice • Assesses patient needs, manages and prescribes treatments • Co-certifies patient for hospice eligibility
Registered nurse	• Assesses patient and family needs • Ensures patient has adequate pain and symptom control • Coordinates team visits • Ensures plan of care is successfully implemented
Social worker	• Assesses patient and family emotional, social, financial, and spiritual needs • Provides bereavement support • Provides direct counseling or referral to appropriate community agencies
Chaplain	• Assesses patient and family spiritual needs • Assists with memorial preparations • Provides counseling and bereavement support
Therapist	• Provides physical, occupational, speech, massage, or music therapy, if necessary
Volunteers	• Provides needed nonmedical services such as life review, letter writing, and respite care • Provides support and companionship to patient and family
Home health aid	• Provides direct personal care to the patient • Provides comfort measures and reports issues to be addressed to the registered nurse

Hospice Benefits and Coverage

Medicare regulations require hospice to cover medications and interventions that provide comfort related to the terminal diagnosis. This coverage includes durable medical equipment such as a hospital bed, commode, and oxygen, medications for symptoms such as pain, dyspnea, depression, and anxiety, as well as the professional services of the interdisciplinary team. Medicare hospice benefit requires the hospice to provide a minimum of 13 months of bereavement care to the family after the patient's death. Hospice also provides around the clock emergency services for symptom management. The benefit does not cover custodial services—care that can be provided by a family member or nonlicensed caregiver—such as cooking and cleaning. Hospice also does not cover services related to nonhospice conditions, whether they are preexisting such as diabetes or hypertension, or are acute new conditions such as nonpathological fractures [5].

Levels of Care

Hospice has several levels of care available. The most commonly employed level of care is routine home care. It is provided at the patient's residence and is flexible to ensure a level of support that is tailored to the individual patient and family. These weekly visits from the various team members include 2–3 nursing visits, 1–2 bath aide visits, and social work, chaplain, and volunteer visits commensurate with patient need, up to several times a week. There is an initial physician visit near the time of enrollment, as needed for issues that require physician attention thereafter, and at least one face-to-face encounter before each recertification.

Hospice also offers an inpatient option in appropriate circumstances. General inpatient care (GIP) is given either in a dedicated hospice facility or nursing facility for those patients with problems or issues that cannot be adequately controlled in a home setting. It is used only for short, defined periods of time, typically only a few days, until the problem is controlled. The problems are usually pain or poorly controlled symptoms that require more than once a day nursing intervention or medication adjustment. This level of care would also be appropriate for patients whose home support is disrupted to the point where they would otherwise require hospital admission. Respite care is also available for up to 5-day intervals. The patient is placed in a facility in order to provide a break for the caregiver(s) that may be experiencing "burn out" [6].

Another option for some patients is continuous care. With this level of care a patient receives nursing care in the home for 8–24 h a day. Continuous care is furnished only during brief periods of crisis for problems or issues that cannot be managed at home with routine care. Like GIP, it is intended only for short-term use of a few days with the target goal of control of the particular problem.

Hospice Funding and Eligibility

The majority of hospice services in the USA are paid for through the Medicare Hospice Benefit or its Medicaid counterpart. Most hospice organizations use the Medicare criteria for qualification, which are based on the guidelines of the National Hospice and Palliative Care Organization (NHPCO).

Medicare requires that two physicians certify that if the patient's condition follows the natural course of its disease, the patient has reasonable likelihood of living 6 months or less. "Reasonable likelihood" means that the majority of patients in the same condition will die within 6 months—in other words, 51% of patients in

Table 4.2 Summary of Medicare guidelines

General debility/
failure to thrive
	Progression:
	1. Documented progression of a primary disease, documented serially
	2. Multiple emergency room visits or hospitalizations over the last 6 months
	3. Homebound patients with decline in function:
	  • Recent decline in function, distinguished from those with reduced baseline functioning. Documented using either:
	    (a) Karnofsky Performance status of ≤50% [10, 11]
	    (b) Dependence in at least 3/6 activities of daily living (ADLs)
	  • Recent decreased nutritional status:
	    (a) Unintentional, progressive weight loss of 10% < over 6 months
	    (b) Serum albumin < 2.5 g/dl
		Condition must be "life limiting" but need not be a single or specific disease state
		Patient and family have elected that goals of treatment consist of comfort rather than cure

Cardiac disease	1. Symptoms of heart failure at rest (New York Heart Association class IV) 2. Symptoms of heart failure despite "optimal treatment" with vasodilators and diuretics. *If not on these agents, there should be a medical reason for foregoing these drugs, such as hypotension* [12]	1. Ejection fraction <20% 2. Symptomatic, treatment-resistant supraventricular or ventricular tachycardia 3. History of cardiac arrest 4. History of unexplained syncope 5. Cardiogenic brain embolism 6. Concomitant HIV disease
Pulmonary disease	1. Disabling dyspnea at rest, despite optimal treatment, that results in markedly reduced functional activity 2. Function is frequently exacerbated with chronic cough or fatigue 3. Evidence of progressive disease: increasingly frequent medical attention for pulmonary infections or failure 4. Presence of cor pulmonale or right heart failure. *This should be due to pulmonary disease, not left heart failure or valve disease. May be documented with: Echocardiogram, EKG, CXR, or physical signs of right heart failure* [13]	1. FEV_1 < 30% of predicted (postbronchodilator) 2. Decrease in FEV_1 on serial testing of greater than 40 ml/year 3. Hypoxemia on oxygen: pO_2 < 55 mmHg 4. O_2 saturation < 88% on oxygen 5. Hypercapnia: pCO_2 > 50 mmHg 6. Weight loss of >10% body weight/6 months 7. Resting tachycardia > 100 bpm

(continued)

Table 4.2 (continued)

Dementia	1. Patient should be at or beyond stage 7 on the Functional Assessment Staging Scale (FAST): (a) Unable to ambulate without assistance (b) Unable to dress without assistance (c) Unable to bathe properly (d) Urinary and fecal incontinence; occasional or increasing in frequency (e) Limited communication—6 words or less per day 2. Difficulty eating, or refusal to eat causing inadequate fluid/calorie intake [9]	1. Patients receiving tube feedings should have documented weight loss of greater than 10% of body weight over 6 months 2. Serum albumin<2.5 g/dl
HIV/AIDS	1. CD4+ count<25 cells/ml, as measured during a period where the patient is relatively free of acute disease 2. Patients with a persistent HIV RNA (viral load) of >100,000 copies/ml 3. Patients with lower viral loads, if they: (a) Elect not to use antiretrovirals (b) Have a declining functional status (c) Are experiencing persistent diarrhea for at least a year, regardless of etiology or have a persistently low albumin (<2.5 g/dl) (d) Are aged >50 years or have severe heart failure Important to consult with HIV specialist regarding complex HIV cases, as mortality is highly variable due to new and changing therapies, as well as individual tolerance to treatment	The following HIV-related diseases are associated with <6 months prognosis: (a) CNS lymphoma (b) Progressive multifocal leukoencephalopathy (c) Cryptosporidiosis (d) Wasting (loss of 1/3 lean body mass) (e) Mycobacterium avium complex (MAC) bacteremia, untreated (f) Treatment-refractory visceral Kaposi's sarcoma (g) Renal failure without hemodialysis (h) Advanced AIDS dementia complex (i) Toxoplasmosis

(continued)

Table 4.2 (continued)

| Liver disease | The following factors correlate with shortened prognosis with additive effects:
1. Both serum albumin <2.5 and prolonged PTT more than 5 s over control
2. Ascites; refractory to sodium restriction/diuretics or due to patient noncompliance
 (a) Spontaneous bacterial peritonitis
 (b) Hepatorenal syndrome
3. Hepatic encephalopathy, as evidenced by:
 (a) somnolence, obtundation, emotional lability
 (b) flapping tremor/asterixis
4. Recurrent variceal bleeding despite treatments such as transjugular intrahepatic portosystemic shunt (TIPS), sclerotherapy/band ligation, or oral beta blockers [14] | Prognosis worsens with the addition of:
1. Progressive malnutrition
2. Muscle wasting, reduced strength/endurance
3. Continued active alcoholism
4. Hepatocellular carcinoma
5. HBsAg positivity |
| Renal disease | Critical renal failure defined:
Creatinine clearance < 10 cc/min (<15 for diabetics) and
Serum creatinine > 8 mg/dl (>6 for diabetics)
Clinical signs and syndromes associated with renal failure:
1. Uremia: confusion, obtundation, nausea/vomiting, pruritus, restlessness
2. Oliguria (<400 cc urine/day)
3. Persistent serum K > 7.0, unresponsive to medical management
4. Uremic pericarditis
5. Hepatorenal syndrome
6. Intractable fluid overload [15, 16] | Clinical manifestations:
1. Confusion, obtundation
2. Intractable nausea/vomiting
3. Generalized pruritus
4. Restless legs
In hospitalized patients, increased mortality is seen with:
1. Mechanical ventilation
2. Chronic lung disease
3. Advanced cardiac disease
4. Advanced liver disease
5. Sepsis
6. Immunosuppression/AIDS
7. Albumin < 3.5 g/dl
8. Cachexia
9. Age > 75
10. Disseminated intravascular coagulation (DIC)
11. Gastrointestinal bleeding |

(continued)

Table 4.2 (continued)

| Stroke and coma | Patients who do not die in the acute hospitalization tend to stabilize with supportive care only. Those with continuous decline have a poorer prognosis
During the acute phase (immediately following CVA) any of the following predict early mortality:
1. Coma/persistent vegetative state > 3 days
2. In anoxic CVA, coma, obtundation with myoclonus > 3 days
3. Comatose patients with 4/5 of the following have a 97% 2 month mortality:
  (a) Abnormal brain stem response
  (b) Absent verbal response
  (c) Absent withdrawal to pain
  (d) Creatinine > 1.5 mg/dl
  (e) Age > 70 | Computed tomography (CT) findings that indicate poor prognosis or minimal recovery:
For hemorrhagic stroke:
  (a) Large volume hemorrhage (>20 ml infra- and >50 ml supratentorial)
  (b) Ventricular extension of hemorrhage
  (c) >30% surface area involvement
  (d) Midline shift >1.5 cm
  (e) Obstructive hydrocephalus without ventriculo-peritoneal (VP) shunt
For thrombotic/embolic stroke:
  (a) Large anterior infarcts with both cortical and subcortical involvement
  (b) Large bi-hemispheric infarcts
  (c) Basilar artery occlusion
  (d) Bilateral vertebral artery occlusion |
| ALS | Best to be educated on the natural history of amyotrophic lateral sclerosis (ALS):
1. It progresses linearly with a fairly constant rate of decline, but this rate can vary greatly from patient to patient. Thus, it is important to know the history of the rate of progression to prognosticate
2. Neurology involvement within 3 months of hospice assessment is recommended for assistance | Important factors that imply decreased survival:
1. Rapidly progressing muscle weakness, bulbar function (swallowing, chewing, speaking)
Patient should develop the majority of their disability within the last year
2. Critically impaired ventilatory capacity:
FVC < 30%, significant dyspnea at rest, O_2 requiring, declines tracheostomy/intubation
3. Critical nutritional impairment, declining artificial nutrition
Continued weight loss, dehydration |

the same condition will die within 6 months. This is a somewhat outdated notion, as even experienced hospice physicians have traditionally been unable to prognosticate accurately, resulting in late hospice referral and decreasing lengths of stay. Although physicians are compelled to utilize the hospice criteria for patient eligibility, the resulting delay in referral can deprive patients from receiving the full spectrum of hospice services. In 2008, the average hospice length of stay was 83 days, less than half of the 6-month criterion [7].

The first hospice benefit period is 90 days, and if a patient continues to decline, he or she may be recertified for an additional 90 days, and then for an indefinite number of 60-day benefit periods. These may be renewed as long as the patient continues to decline [8].

Medicare uses the NHPCO criteria for several noncancer designated diagnoses and specific guidelines for prognosticating in each condition (see Table 4.2). The NHPCO uses evidence-based data from clinical experience and research in an effort to provide these prognosticating guidelines. Unfortunately, despite these efforts, the tools available to physicians for determining the appropriate point for hospice referral are often cumbersome and ineffective. Some of the most widely utilized prognostication guides include the modified Functional Assessment Staging (FAST) tool for dementia [9], the Karnofsky Performance Status Scale for general debility [10, 11], The Seattle Heart Failure Model for heart disease [12], and the Model for End Stage Liver Disease (MELD) for liver failure [13].

As in any end-stage disease, optimum life-prolonging therapy should have been exhausted or refused by the patient prior to consideration for hospice.

In dementia, stroke/coma, and amyotrophic lateral sclerosis (ALS), common comorbid medical conditions additively portend a worsened prognosis. These include: aspiration pneumonia, upper urinary tract infection (UTI)/pyelonephritis, septicemia, multiple decubitus ulcers (stage 3–4), and recurrent fever after antibiotics [9].

Hospice Alternatives

Depending on the needs of the individual patient, various alternatives to traditional hospice are available. To address basic medical needs, traditional regular home nursing services are available for patients that may not need palliation or have a life-threatening illness. These services may include medication or blood pressure monitoring and patient education, and are typically available weekly.

Home palliative care is more comprehensive and can provide all the services of traditional regular home health care plus providing skilled nursing care for pain or symptom management. It therefore can provide a longer duration of home care for the patient than traditional regular home health care as long as the patient has pain or symptoms to be managed. It is more appropriate for patients who are not yet ready for hospice. Home palliative care is less comprehensive than hospice and lacks the interdisciplinary care of the hospice team, but its advantage over hospice is that this care can be provided simultaneously with curative treatments in seriously ill patients.

The most comprehensive alternative option is open access hospice. This new phenomenon acts as a "bridge" from curative to comfort care. A small number of larger hospices (serving 400 or more patients) are able to offer potentially life-extending interventions to their patients simultaneously with hospice care. These interventions may include TPN, chemotherapy, and radiation. These hospices are able to offset the costs of these treatments from the increased revenue that comes from enrolling more patients earlier in the course of the disease [17].

The Terminal Phase

While caring for someone with a terminal illness, the terminal phase of the illness can be one of the most challenging times. The terminal phase of an illness is defined as the time when a person's disease process is incurable and their health deteriorates to the point where he or she is not expected to live more than a few days, weeks, or months. The goal at this point is mainly supportive: to ensure the most comfort for the patient and the people providing care. Other goals at this point include symptom management, emotional and spiritual support, assistance with personal care, transportation assistance, and improving communication with health care providers [18]. Although these goals are not unique to the terminal phase, there is now an urgency to address these goals in a limited time.

Functional Decline

As with any of the challenges during the terminal phase, the functional decline can be met with increased burden of illness and diminished functional capacity for activities of daily living (ADL). The earliest way to assess this clinically is a sudden decline in the functional status that often signals shortened survival and acts as a sentinel event that can be readily seen [19]. This decline before death differs by age and with the chronically ill; it is the medical condition that influences the pattern of functional disability [20, 21]. For example, patients with cancer tend to show a steady decline in ADLs in the 6 months prior to death, while patients with noncancerous illnesses tend to show a more variable course of decline [19, 22]. Although in the USA, only 23% die from cancer [20, 23], a significant number of patients die from acute complications of an otherwise chronic condition. End-of-life care should also serve those who become increasingly frail, even without immediately life-threatening illness [20, 24].

It may be advantageous to have assessments done by occupational and physical therapists to help determine the degree of assistance required and if there is any durable medical equipment (DME) that may assist with remaining functional capacity. Occupational and physical therapists can have a significant impact on the quality of life of terminally ill patients. While rehabilitation is often overlooked in the critical care setting, occupational and physical therapists work with critically ill patients to create realistic and meaningful goals for improving comfort, mobility, socialization skills, and ability to care for oneself regardless of disease state and medical status [25].

Reduced Oral Intake

Although oral administration of medication is generally preferable, a parenteral route is often advisable in many circumstances during the progression of a terminal illness. Not only are there problems of medication administration with reduced oral intake, but also there are implications for food/fluid intake. Disease processes like cancer have a profound impact on patients' metabolism. Proteolysis and lipolysis are accelerated while muscle protein synthesis is depressed, resulting in a loss of lean body mass and fat tissue. Despite hypermetabolism and weight loss (exacerbated by stress, pain, infection, and surgical procedures), patients' food intake is usually not increased leading to further wasting [26].

Starvation and dehydration are not caused by lack of intake but by the disease process itself. Providing or even forcing food and fluids will not prolong or enhance life and may be a burden or detrimental. A healthy individual has an anabolic metabolism, which can use nutrients to build and repair tissue. However, during the dying process, the body shifts from an anabolic to a catabolic state. It is this catabolic condition that leads to starvation and dehydration. This shift is a natural part of the dying process and occurs whether or not food and fluids are provided. Furthermore, there is a possibility of additional problems due to complications of central line infections and metabolic derangement associated with total parenteral nutrition (TPN). Even tube feeding is not without risks, which include dislodgement, infection, discomfort, and aspiration [27].

It is often not realized that starvation produces a euphoric state that increases comfort. As the body uses fat as the main energy source and ketones build up, the resulting ketonemia causes euphoria. Even small amounts of feeding can prevent ketonemia and prolong the sensation of hunger. The most common complaint patients have when withholding food or fluids is a dry mouth; therefore, good mouth care can alleviate most discomfort and provide an outlet for the caregiver to still nurture [27].

Alternative Routes of Medication Administration

Pharmacologic symptom management can improve the quality of life of patients with a severe life-limiting illness. Although pharmacotherapy is only one component of end-of-life care, ensuring timely access to needed medication is a fundamental component of effective palliative care with increasing importance as death approaches [28]. The loss of an oral intake route is a possibility that can occur at any time; therefore, the need for effective alternate route for administering medication may become more urgent due to the inability to swallow, dyspnea due to pneumonia, and/or agitation due to end-of-life delirium. Additionally, since parenteral medications may not be available emergently, medications delivered via alternate routes should be made accessible for immediate administration [29].

Transdermal Route

Transdermal fentanyl is an effective and well-tolerated pharmacotherapy for cancer pain patients. It should not be used in opioid-naïve patients and watching for drug accumulation is required when doses are increased [30, 31]. However, clinicians need to be cognizant that the US/UK manufacturer's recommendations for equianalgesic dosing of transdermal fentanyl may result in initial doses that produce subtherapeutic levels and unrelieved pain in some patients [31, 32].

Transdermal buprenorphine is now being prescribed in the US, but was initially used in Europe and Australia for chronic and cancer pain management. Buprenorphine's mixed agonist/antagonist activity, dosage ceiling, and high affinity to the opiate receptor limit its use to those patients who do not already require large daily doses of opioids. Thus, buprenorphine may not be an appropriate medication for some patients with advanced unremitting cancer pain [31, 33].

Transdermal scopolamine is effective for severe drug-resistant nausea and vomiting in advanced cancer. It is most appropriate for vestibular causes of nausea and vomiting precipitated or exacerbated by head or body movement, with or without dizziness [34].

Most topical nonsteroidal anti-inflammatory drugs (NSAIDs), such as diclofenac, have shown improved safety and tolerability compared with oral NSAIDs. Topical salicylates and capsaicin are available in the US without a prescription, but neither has shown substantial efficacy in clinical trials, and both have potential to cause serious adverse reactions. Accidental poisonings have been reported with salicylates, and concerns exist that capsaicin-induced nerve desensitization may not be fully reversible and that its autonomic nerve effects may increase the risk of skin ulcers in diabetic patients [35].

Good adhesion of the patch to the skin is essential for maximum efficacy; therefore, patients must be instructed on the proper technique for patch application. Hair on the skin should be clipped, not shaved, in order to avoid abrasions where the patch is to be applied. This skin should be clean, dry, and undamaged. After removal of the plastic backing, the patch should be held firmly in place for about 30 s. A finger should be run around the edge of the patch to ensure that adhesion has occurred around all edges. The top of the patch should be rubbed for approximately 3 min. Patients should also be instructed to rotate sites when changing patches in order to minimize changes in serum levels due to build up of subcutaneous depots and to minimize skin irritation [31, 36].

Subcutaneous Route

Fluids can be administered as subcutaneous rehydration using NaCl 0.9%, combined solutions of glucose 5%/NaCl 0.9%, and NaCl 0.45%. Site of injection is primarily in the thighs, back, or arms at a maximum of 2 l/day [37].

A wide variety of medications can be given subcutaneously; these include analgesics (morphine, hydromorphone, sufentanil, methadone, fentanyl, and ketorolac), corticosteroids (dexamethasone), diuretics (furosemide), barbituates (phenobarbital), anticholinergic agents (glycopyrrolate and scopolamine), antiemetics (ondansetron and metoclopramide), neuroleptics (haldoperidol, levomepromazine), and benzodiazepines (clonazepam and midazolam). Many of these medications are off-label for subcutaneous use, but are recommended for use in palliative care [37].

Transmucosal Route

An intranasal, sublingual, or buccal route of fentanyl administration is a treatment option for breakthrough cancer pain (BTCP). Transmucosal fentanyl is an attractive and convenient treatment modality in opioid-tolerant patients due to its quick onset and short duration of action, noninvasive administration route, high bioavailability, and avoidance of a hepatic first-pass effect. Few clinical trials have been conducted with intranasal fentanyl, but all have confirmed its usefulness and acceptability in BTCP treatment. It may be used in opioid-tolerant patients without nasal pathologies [38]. Oral transmucosal fentanyl citrate (Actiq and Cephalon) is specifically developed and approved for the management of breakthrough pain in cancer patients and it has the potential to be a useful tool for clinicians [39].

Other medications can be used transmucosally, such as Lorazepam, Ketorolac, Insulin, or Ketamine. The general rule is to start with the recommended IV dose and titrate to desired response. As a safety factor, the bioavailability of the transmucosal route will not exceed the intravenous route as absorption is only 35–70% [40–43].

Rectal Route

In some circumstances, it is impractical or even impossible (during nausea/emesis, convulsions, uncooperative patients, and before surgery) to give medications in the methods listed above. In these cases, the rectal route may represent a practical alternative. Rectal administration is now well accepted for delivering, for example, anticonvulsants, non-narcotic and narcotic analgesics, theophylline, antiemetics, and antibacterial agents. The rate and extent of rectal drug absorption are often lower than with oral absorption, possibly an inherent factor owing to the relatively small surface area available for drug uptake [44].

Specific Symptom Management

The prediction of impending death remains an imprecise science, but studies have shown several common terminal signs and symptoms. Clinicians and family members need to be aware of and be prepared to address specific symptoms during the final few days without delay. These include symptoms of breathlessness, accumulation of respiratory tract secretions (death rattle), and terminal delirium.

Death Rattle

The accumulation of respiratory tract secretions (ARTS) prior to death, which leads to gurgling respirations, is presumably caused by a decreased gag and clearing reflex. This "death rattle" occurs in 25–50% of dying patients, more commonly in men, and in patients with brain and lung cancers, and predicts most (76% in one study) will die within 48 h [45, 46]. Nonpharmacologic interventions such as stopping parenteral fluids, repositioning, and postural drainage are frequently suggested but have not been studied specifically. Oropharyngeal suctioning is considered generally ineffective for this condition and may cause discomfort for both the patient and patient's family [45, 46].

A majority (50–80%) of patients respond to treatment with antimuscarinics [45, 47]. Subcutaneous scopolamine (hyoscine hydrobromide) is immediately more effective, in studies, than subcutaneous glycopyrrolate, but glycopyrrolate has a longer duration of action. Since glycopyrrolate is a quaternary amine, it has the advantage of not crossing the blood–brain barrier. Therefore, unlike scopolamine, it is less likely to cause sedation or delirium [45, 48].

Terminal Agitated Delirium

Delirium is characterized by fluctuating disturbances in consciousness, cognition, and perception, which occur in up to 83% of patients near the end of life [45, 49]. Terminal delirium is often associated with signs of decreased perfusion, which is commonly divided into three types: hyperactive (with restlessness, agitation, or hallucinations), hypoactive (with somnolence), and mixed (with alternating features of both) [45, 50]. Terminal delerium is thought to be multifactorial in etiology and often is confused with sedation, dementia, or near-death awareness. Frequent symptoms, including both the psychomotor and cognitive symptoms of hyperactive delirium, can be enormously upsetting for families because they remain a lasting image after a patient's death [45, 51].

The moaning, groaning, and grimacing that often accompany delirium may also be misunderstood as physical pain [45, 47]. Many experts feel that terminal delirium may be precipitated *not* by the pain medication itself, but rather by poor pain control [45, 52], and that uncontrollable pain rarely develops near death if it has not previously been a problem [45, 53]. While reversible factors such as psychoactive medications, metabolic disarray, or infection may be identified in up to half of cases, terminal delirium management typically focuses on symptom control with medications [45, 53]. Benzodiazepines like Midazolam or Lorazepam can be used with good success, but may result in disinhibition and increased restlessness [45, 46]. Haloperidol was demonstrated to be superior when compared to Lorazepam in a small randomized controlled trial in delirium patients with AIDS [45, 54]. Other antipsychotics (e.g., levomepromazine) have shown benefit in treating delirium with dementia, but it is unclear how these results translate to the treatment of actively dying patients [45, 55].

Normal Physiology of Death and Dying, Progression, and Time of Symptoms

Several clinical features have been identified as indicators of death within days, but evidence for the reliability of these signs is limited. Evidence does show that physicians consistently overestimate patient survival, and those most familiar with the patient are often the least accurate [45, 56]. One observational study looking at terminally ill patients with cancer noted that patients, on average, developed respirations with mandibular movement at 8 h, acrocyanosis at 5 h, and radial pulselessness at 3 h before death but there was wide individual variation, with most patients developing these symptoms less than 2.5 h before they died. Decreased consciousness was identified in 84% at 24 h and 92% at 6 h prior to death [45, 57]. Development of a death rattle is predictive of death within 48 h but typically occurs in less than half of patients [45, 58]. Except for symptoms of drowsiness, fatigue, and confusion; symptoms in patients with cancer followed at home tended to improve in the last days of life [45, 59]. According to some expert opinions, other signs of impending death include becoming bedbound, irregular breathing, tolerating sips of fluid only, and cool or mottled extremities [45, 60]. Distressing physical symptoms are common at the end of life. The SUPPORT study showed that during the last 3 days of life, 80% of dying hospitalized patients suffered severe fatigue, 50% severe dyspnea, and 40% severe pain [45, 61]. Common symptoms reported by families during final week of life were fatigue, dyspnea, and dry mouth, while the most distressing were fatigue, dyspnea, and pain [45, 62]. Anorexia, anxiety, constipation, nausea/vomiting, incontinence, pressure sores, and insomnia have also been identified as particularly distressing in certain patients [45, 63].

Conclusion

The discomfort of dying patients is substantial and hospice represents a unique interdisciplinary team-based approach to the management of the many symptoms that burden patients at the end of life. Guidelines for hospice vary by terminal illness and disease; despite guidelines physicians typically refer patients to hospice care late. Earlier referrals, when patients with terminal illness reasonably have 6 months or less to live, will maximize the resources that hospice can offer. As terminal illness progresses, the urgency of symptom management becomes more impressive. Functional decline and reduced oral intake are common. The hospice provider should be well versed in employing other routes of medication administration for analgesia and for management of terminal symptoms. In the final stages of life, symptoms of breathlessness, accumulation of respiratory tract secretions (death rattle), and delirium may be present and typically signal impending death. Being familiar with the natural progression of signs and symptoms in the actively dying patient as well as with advanced pain and symptom management, with knowledge of how and when to enlist the assistance of hospice or home care, and with how to customize treatment plans will allow the hospice provider the skill set necessary to provide effective patient-centered end-of-life care.

References

1. Dame Cicely Biography – Cicely Saunders International. Home – Cicely Saunders International. http://www.cicelysaundersfoundation.org/about-us/dame-cicely-biography. Web 10 July 2011.
2. National Hospice Foundation. The history of hospice. http://www.nationalhospicefoundation. org/i4a/pages/index.cfm?pageid=218. Web 10 July 2011.
3. Sullivan P. Florence S. Wald, 91; U.S. Hospice Pioneer. Washington Post. http://www.washingtonpost.com/wp-dyn/content/article/2008/11/12/AR2008111202953.html. 13 Nov 2008.
4. The Hospice and Palliative Care Association (HPCAI). NHPCO Facts & Figures. http://www.nhpco.org/files/public/Statistics_Research/NHPCO_facts_and_figures.pdf. Web 10 July 2011.
5. The National Hospice and Palliative Care Organization. What is hospice and palliative care? http://www.nhpco.org/i4a/pages/index.cfm?pageid=4648. Web 16 July 2011.
6. The National Hospice and Palliative Care Organization. Levels of care. http://www.nhpco.org/i4a/pages/index.cfm?pageid=5504. Web 16 July 2011.
7. Medicare Payment Advisory Commission. A Data Book: Healthcare spending and the Medicare Program, June 2010. 2010.
8. Office of the Assistant Secretary for Planning and Evaluation, HHS. Important questions for hospice in the next century: appendices. http://aspe.hhs.gov/daltcp/reports/impquesa.htm. Web 21 May 2011.
9. Mitchell SL, Kiely DK, Hamel MB, et al. Estimating prognosis for nursing home residents with advanced dementia. JAMA. 2004;291:2734–40.
10. Crooks V, Waller S, et al. The use of the Karnofsky Performance Scale in determining outcomes and risk in geriatric outpatients. J Gerontol. 1991;46:M139–44.
11. Schag CC, Heinrich RL, Ganz PA. Karnofsky performance status revisited: reliability, validity, and guidelines. J Clin Oncol. 1984;2:187–93.
12. Levy WC, Mozaffarian D, Linker DT, et al. The Seattle Heart Failure Model. Prediction of survival in heart failure. Circulation. 2006;113:1424–33.

13. Celli BR, Cote CG, Marin JM, et al. The body-mass index, airflow obstruction, dyspnea, and exercise capacity index in chronic obstructive pulmonary disease. N Eng J Med. 2004;350(10):1005–12.
14. Said A, et al. Model for end stage liver disease score predicts mortality across a broad spectrum of liver disease. J Hepatol. 2004;40:897–903.
15. Celli Beddhu S, Bruns FJ, Saul M, Seddon P, Zeidel ML. A simple comorbidity scale predicts clinical outcomes and costs in dialysis patients. Am J Med. 2000;108:609–13.
16. Miskulin DC, Martin AA, Brown R, et al. Predicting 1-year mortality in an outpatient hemodialysis population: a comparison of comorbidity instruments. Nephrol Dial Transplant. 2004;19:413–20.
17. Wright AA, Katz IT. Letting go of the rope – aggressive treatment, hospice care, and open access. N Engl J Med. 2007;357:324–7.
18. Candy B, Jones I, Drake R, Leurent B, King M. Interventions for supporting informal caregivers of patients in the terminal phase of a disease (Review). Cochrane Libr. 2011;9:1–75.
19. Downing M, Lesperance M, Lau F, Yang J. Survival implications of sudden functional decline as a sentinel event using the palliative performance scale. J Palliat Med. 2010;13:549–57.
20. Lunney J, Lynn J, Hogan C. Profiles of older Medicare decedents. J Am Geriatr Soc. 2002;50:1108–12.
21. Guralnik J, LaCroix A, Branch L, Kasl S, Wallace R. Morbidity and disability in older person in the years prior to death. Am J Public Health. 1991;81:443–7.
22. Teno J, Weitzen S, Fennell ML, Mor V. Dying trajectory in the last year of life: does cancer trajectory fit other diseases? J Palliat Med. 2001;4:457–64.
23. Minino A, Smith B. Deaths preliminary data for 2000. Natl Vital Stat Rep. 2001;49:1–40.
24. Lynn J. Serving patients who may die soon and their families: the role of hospice and other services. JAMA. 2001;285:925–32.
25. Kasven-Gonzalez N, Souverain R, Miale S. Improving quality of life through rehabilitation in palliative care: case report. Palliat Support Care. 2010;8(3):359–69.
26. Marin M, Laviano A, Pichard C. Nutritional intervention and quality of life in adult oncology patients. Clin Nutr. 2007;26(3):289–301.
27. Cline D. Nutrition issues and tools for palliative care. Home Healthc Nurse. 2006;24(1):54–7.
28. Clary P, Lawson P. Pharmacologic pearls for end-of-life care. Am Fam Physician. 2009;79(12):1059–65.
29. Adam J. ABC of palliative care: the last 48 hours. Br Med J. 1997;315(7122):1600–3.
30. Grond S, Zech D, Diefenbach C, Bischoff A. Prevalence and pattern of symptoms in patients with cancer pain: a prospective evaluation of 1635 cancer patients referred to a pain clinic. J Pain Symptom Manage. 1994;9:372–82.
31. Skaer T. Transdermal opioids for cancer pain. Health Qual Life Outcomes. 2006;4(24):1–9.
32. Kornick C, Santiago-Palma J, Moryl N, Payne R, Obbens E. Benefit-risk assessment of transdermal fentanyl for the treatment of chronic pain. Drug Saf. 2003;26:951–73.
33. Evans H, Easthope S. Transdermal buprenorphine. Drugs. 2003;63:1999–2010.
34. LeGrand S, Walsh D. Scopolamine for cancer-related nausea and vomiting. J Pain Symptom Manage. 2010;40(1):136–41.
35. Altman R, Barthel H. Topical therapies for osteoarthritis. Drugs. 2011;71(10):1259–79.
36. Payne R, Chandler S, Einhaus M. Guidelines for the clinical use of transdermal fentanyl. Anticancer Drugs. 1995;6:50–3.
37. Fonzo-Christe C, Vulkasovic C, Wasilewski-Rasca A, Bonnabry P. Subcutaneous administration of drugs in the elderly: survey of practice and systematic literature review. Palliat Med. 2005;19:208–19.
38. Leppert W. Role of intranasal fentanyl in breakthrough pain management in cancer patients. Cancer Manag Res. 2010;2:225–32.
39. Nagda C, Chotai N, Nagda D, Patel S, Patel U. Development and characterization of mucoadhesive microspheres for nasal delivery of ketorolac. Pharmazie. 2011;66(4):249–57.
40. Stote R, Miller M, Marbury T, Shi L, Strange P. Enhanced absorption of Nasulin, an ultrarapid-acting intranasal insulin formulation, using single nostril administration in normal subjects. J Diabetes Sci Technol. 2011;5(1):113–9.

41. Reid C, Hatton R, Middleton P. Case report: prehospital use of intranasal ketamine for pediatric burn injury. Emerg Med. 2011;28(4):328–9.
42. Mystakidou K, Tsilika E, Tsiatas M, Vlahos L. Oral transmucosal fentanyl citrate in cancer pain management: a practical application of nanotechnology. Int J Nanomedicine. 2007;2(1): 49–54.
43. Anderson M, Tambe P, Sammons H, Mulla H, Cole R, Choonara I. Pharmakinetics of buccal and intranasal lorazepam in healthy adult volunteers. Eur J Clin Pharamacol. 2012;68(2): 155–9.
44. Van Hoogdalem E, De Boer A, Breimer D. Pharmacokinetics of rectal drug administration. Part I. General considerations and clinical applications of centrally acting drugs. Clin Pharmacokinet. 1991;21(1):11–26.
45. Plonk W, Arnold R. Terminal Care: the last weeks of life. J Palliat Med. 2005;8(5):1042–54.
46. Ferris F, von Gunten C, Emanuel L. Competency in end-of-life care: last hours of life. J Palliat Med. 2003;6:605–13.
47. Morita T, Tsunoda J, Inoue S, Chihara S. Risk factors for death rattle in terminally ill cancer patients. Palliat Med. 2000;14:19–23.
48. Back I, Jenkins K, Blower A, Beckhelling J. A study comparing hyoscine hydrobromide and glycopyrrolate in the treatment of death rattle. Palliat Med. 2001;15:329–36.
49. Casarett D, Inouye S. Diagnosis and management of delirium near the end of life. Ann Intern Med. 2001;135:32–40.
50. Ingham J, Breitbart W. Epidemiology and clinical features of delirium. In: Portenoy RK, Bruera E, editors. Topics in palliative care, vol. 1. New York: Oxford University Press; 1997. p. 7–20.
51. Morita T, Hirai K, Sakaguchi Y, Tsuneto S, Shima Y. Family perceived distress from delirium-related symptoms of terminally ill cancer patients. Psychosomatics. 2004;45:107–13.
52. Morrison R, Magaziner J, Gilbert M, Koval K, McLaughlin M, Orosz G, Strauss E, Siu A. Relationship between pain and opioid analgesics on the development of delirium following hip fracture. J Gerontol. 2003;58:76–81.
53. Lawlor P, Gagnon B, Mancini I, Pereira J, Hanson J, Suarez-Almazor M, Bruera E. Occurrence, causes, and outcomes of delirium in patients with advanced cancer: a prospective study. Arch Intern Med. 2000;160:786–94.
54. Breitbart W, Marotta R, Platt M, Weisman H, Derevenco M, Grau C, Corbera K, Raymond S, Lund S, Jacobson P. A double blind trial of haloperidol, chlorpromazine, and lorazepam in the treatment of delirium in hospitalized AIDS patients. Am J Psychiatry. 1996;153:231–7.
55. Finucane T. Delirium at the end of life. Ann Intern Med. 2002;137:295.
56. Glare P, Virik K, Jones M, Hudson M, Eychmuller S, Simes J, Christakis N. A systematic review of physicians' survival predictions in terminally ill cancer patients. BMJ. 2003;327:195.
57. Morita T, Ichiki T, Tsunoda J, Inoue S, Chihara S. A prospective study on the dying process in terminally ill cancer patients. Am J Hosp Palliat Care. 1998;15:217–22.
58. Wildiers H, Menten J. Death rattle: prevalence, prevention, and treatment. J Pain Symptom Manage. 2002;23:310–7.
59. Mercandante S, Casuccio A, Fulfaro F. The course of symptom frequency and intensity in advanced cancer patients followed at home. J Pain Symptom Manage. 2000;20:104–12.
60. Ellershaw J, Ward C. Care of the dying patient: the last hours or days of life. BMJ. 2003;326:30–4.
61. Lynn J, Teno J, Phillips R, Wu A, Desbiens N, Harrold J, Claessens M, Wenger N, Kreling B, Connors Jr A. Perceptions by family members of the dying experience of older and seriously ill patients. Ann Intern Med. 1997;126:97–106.
62. Hickman S, Tilde V, Tolle S. Family reports of dying patients distress: the adaptation of a research tool to assess global symptom distress in the last week of life. J Pain Symptom Manage. 2001;22:565–71.
63. Addington-Hall J, McCarthy M. Dying from cancer: results of a national population-based investigation. Palliat Med. 1995;9:295–305.

Review Questions

1. An 83 year-old man with end stage COPD comes to your office to discuss goals of care. His breathing has deteriorated over the last few months, and he has been hospitalized four times this year. He states that he would like to avoid returning to the hospital if he were to get sick again and would like to focus on comfort. He heard that hospice can offer him the opportunity to have symptom management to focus on comfort for his remaining days. Which of the following describes the covered services and items he could receive?

   (a) Daily in-home caregiver
   (b) Room and board at a nursing facility
   (c) Hospital bed, oxygen, and commode for home use
   (d) Homemaking assistance with cooking and light housework

2. Which of the following statements regarding Hospice care is *false*?

   (a) Hospice care includes coverage for durable medical equipment, medications, and home visits for pain and symptom management
   (b) Once signed on to the Medicare Hospice benefit, patient visits to their Primary Care Physician (PCP) for a hospice related diagnosis are not covered
   (c) Hospice care is revoked if a patient elects to go to the Emergency department for an acute health issue related to their hospice diagnosis
   (d) In order to receive Hospice benefits, the patient must agree to "Do Not Resuscitate" Status

3. A 73 year-old patient with end stage dementia and failure to thrive on Hospice begins to stabilize. Her oral intake is fair with hand feeding, she has not had pneumonia or a urinary infection in over 1 year, and she continues to have periods of lucidity where she can hold a limited conversation. Which of the following actions is most appropriate?

   (a) Discharge the patient from Hospice; she may re-enroll in the future as her condition progresses
   (b) Keep her on hospice but provide her with a reduced number of nurse visits, as she is doing well enough with only a bath aid visiting weekly
   (c) Keep her on hospice for a limited period of 1 month and monitor her for disease progression
   (d) Discuss her case with her former primary care physician before making a decision

4. A patient with stage IV liver cancer is in under home hospice care, with her husband as her primary caregiver. She has intense pain and nausea, and is significantly encephalopathic and agitated. Her husband and nurse are having difficulty controlling her symptoms. Which of the following is *false* regarding treatment options?

   (a) This patient could benefit from a home visit from the hospice physician for evaluation

   (b) The patient could be transferred via EMS to the emergency department for a few hours of intensive symptom management while remaining on hospice care

   (c) The patient would qualify for general inpatient care due to her refractory symptoms

   (d) The patient's uncontrolled symptoms qualify her for continuous nursing care in the home for continuous pain control and monitoring

5. What is the current average length of stay on hospice?

   (a) 10–20 days
   (b) 3–4 months
   (c) Over 8 months
   (d) 80–100 days

6. A 72-year-old terminally ill female is showing decreased awareness of his surroundings, decreased oral intake of solids or liquids, and is no longer able to get out of bed. The most likely explanation for this constellation of findings is:

   (a) Loss of hope
   (b) Impending death
   (c) Depression
   (d) Uremia

7. A 24-year-old palliative care patient with terminal breast cancer with metastasis to bone takes oral narcotics regularly for bone pain. The patient is no longer able to swallow. What is an alternative route of medication administration while under hospice care at home?

   (a) Topical salicylates
   (b) Transdermal scopolamine
   (c) Transdermal buprenorphine
   (d) Topical capsaicin

8. A 61-year-old male is in his final stages of death and now under palliative "terminal" sedation. The primary goal with this type of sedation is:

   (a) Relief of intractable pain or suffering
   (b) Hasten the onset of death
   (c) Improved tissue oxygenation
   (d) Reduction in opioid medication usage

9. An 87-year-old home hospice patient becomes increasingly less mobile and is physically limited to lying in her bed. A common complication of immobility while caring for a patient like this is:

   (a) Joint laxity
   (b) Hamstring hypertrophy
   (c) Pressure ulcers
   (d) Cerebral vascular accidents

10. A terminally ill patient has advanced disease due to pancreatic cancer. The patient is cachectic and now lost the ability to swallow. The patient's family is concerned for the patient's nutritional status. The following are reasons to withhold nutrition *except*:

   (a) There are metabolic derangements associated with total parenteral nutrition
   (b) Aspiration and infections are possible with tube feeds
   (c) Starvation produces a euphoric state that increases comfort
   (d) Forcing food and fluids will help to prolong or enhance life

Answers

1. (c)
2. (d)
3. (a)
4. (b)
5. (d)
6. (b). While caring for someone with a terminal illness, the terminal phase of the illness can be one of the most challenging times. The terminal phase of an illness is defined as the time when a person's disease process is incurable and their health deteriorates to the point where he or she is not expected to live more than a few days, weeks, or months. The signs and symptoms of impending death are often very similar, even in patients with very different terminal illnesses. Those caring for patients during this stage should be familiar with the common signs and symptoms of impending death so that he or she can educate the patient and caregivers about the dying process and support patients and caregivers through the patient's death. With impending death, the patient has decreasing interest and awareness of his/her surroundings and a reduced desire or ability to move around. The patient will have a marked decrease in food or fluid intake and often develops difficulty with swallowing.
7. (c). Pharmacologic symptom management can improve the quality of life of patients with a severe life-limiting illness. Although pharmacotherapy is only one component of end-of-life care, ensuring timely access to needed medication is a fundamental component of effective palliative care with increasing importance as death approaches. The loss of an oral intake route is a possibility that can occur at any time; therefore, the need for an effective alternate route for administering medication may become more urgent due to the inability to swallow. Additionally, since parenteral medications may not be available emergently, medications delivered via alternate routes should be made accessible for immediate administration. Transdermal buprenorphine is now being prescribed in the USA, but was initially used in Europe and Australia for chronic and cancer pain management. Buprenorphine's mixed agonist/antagonist activity, dosage ceiling, and high affinity to the opiate receptor limit its use to those patients who do not already require large daily doses of opioids. Thus, buprenorphine may not be an appropriate medication for some patients with advanced unremitting cancer pain. Transdermal scopolamine is effective for severe drug-resistant nausea and vomiting in advanced cancer. It is most appropriate for vestibular causes of nausea and vomiting precipitated or exacerbated by head or body movement, with or without dizziness. Topical salicylates and capsaicin are available in the US without a prescription, but neither has shown substantial efficacy in clinical trials, and both have the potential to cause serious adverse reactions. Accidental poisonings have been reported with salicylates, and concerns exist that capsaicin-induced nerve desensitization may not be fully reversible and that its autonomic nerve effects may increase the risk of skin ulcers in diabetic patients.

8. (a). The main goals of palliative care involve the relief of pain and suffering in the dying patient. Terminal/palliative sedation describes the use of sedative agents to treat pain or suffering in the dying patient when other treatment measures are ineffective. This type of sedation is used to relieve intractable symptoms in the dying patient, not to expedite the dying process.

9. (c). As a patient becomes progressively less mobile with advanced stages of his/her disease, there are numerous complications associated with immobility. Complications include muscle atrophy, constipation, joint stiffness and pain, urinary tract infection, increased clotting risk, and pressure ulcers. Pathologic fractures are not increased with immobility. Prevention of pressure ulcers can be maximized with the use of turning and positioning techniques.

10. (d). Starvation and dehydration are not caused by lack of intake but by the disease process itself. Providing or even forcing food and fluids will not prolong or enhance life and may be a burden or detrimental. A healthy individual has an anabolic metabolism, which can use nutrients to build and repair tissue. However, during the dying process, the body shifts from an anabolic to a catabolic state. It is this catabolic condition that leads to starvation and dehydration. This shift is a natural part of the dying process and occurs whether or not food and fluids are provided. Furthermore, there is a possibility of additional problems due to complications of central line infections and metabolic derangement associated with total parenteral nutrition (TPN). Even tube feeding is not without risks, which include dislodgement, infection, discomfort, and aspiration. It is often not realized that starvation produces a euphoric state that increases comfort. As the body uses fat as the main energy source and ketones build up, the resulting ketonemia causes euphoria.

Chapter 5
Communication in Palliative Care

Dominique Anwar, Sean Ransom, and Roy S. Weiner

Introduction

Good communication skills are obviously important for any health professional, but they are especially essential when taking care of patients facing a life-threatening disease. It is never easy to give news about a diagnosis and/or prognosis that will give patients a perspective of death far closer than imagined. Not only are these communication skills important when breaking news initially and through patient follow-up, but such skills also allow effective collaboration with other involved health professionals. In the palliative context, these skills do not only facilitate the proper management of physical symptoms, but also assist in other dimensions, such as social, spiritual, and psychological, which all must be addressed. The patient remains, of course, at the center of care with involvement of family/loved ones, but each member of the healthcare team has specific competencies that must be acknowledged and shared.

D. Anwar, M.D. (✉)
Section of General Internal Medicine and Geriatrics,
Tulane University School of Medicine, New Orleans, LA, USA
e-mail: danwar@tulane.edu

S. Ransom, Ph.D.
Department of Psychiatry and Behavioral Sciences,
Tulane University School of Medicine, New Orleans, LA, USA

R.S. Weiner, M.D.
Tulane Cancer Center, Tulane University School of Medicine, New Orleans, LA, USA

N. Vadivelu et al. (eds.), *Essentials of Palliative Care*,
DOI 10.1007/978-1-4614-5164-8_5,
© Springer Science+Business Media New York 2013

In addition, distressed, exhausted family members may sometimes be difficult to manage. Family caregivers may show dysfunction, aggressiveness, or denial, but their needs also must be addressed as these behaviors may be signs of intense suffering. Finally, it is important to ensure that the needs of a "difficult" family do not bring team members to exhaustion. This, also, is the role of a coordinated, communicative team approach.

In complex medical situations, the patient usually receives care not only by the primary care provider, but also by several specialists, sometimes in various locations. If healthcare providers involved in the patient's care fail to coordinate their efforts, patients and their family members may hear several "stories" regarding the patient's present and future condition, which may be distressing or confusing. Implementing a smooth transition and a relation of trust between the patient, family, and healthcare providers can be achieved only if there is real collaboration/communication between these healthcare providers, with understanding of the roles of each professional involved.

Breaking bad news is not an easy task and will never be, whatever our professional training, experience, or level of empathy. Some individuals may have natural communication skills, but one can always improve. Students and professionals from various disciplines (physicians, nurses, medical school and nursing school students, psychologists, social workers, chaplains) may learn how to better communicate at any stage of their career. Observing skilled communicators is a good way to learn, but observation will never take the place of "hands-on" training. Working with standardized patients or role playing may promote improvement without the fear of "hurting" a patient; thus, training in a formal, resourced environment is optimal. Several communication skills training programs have been described in the medical literature and have proven to be highly effective, including training models for medical students [1, 2]and for oncologists [3, 4]. One Cochrane review confirmed that several training models, both those for physicians and for nurses, appear to be effective [5].

We will mainly focus on a very important aspect of communication in palliative care: Breaking bad news. We will also explore briefly issues that are of special interest too in this area: dealing with "difficult" families and communicating with other health professionals.

Breaking Bad News

Throughout time, there has been an evolution from Hippocrates' recommendation (late fifth century BC) [6]: *"Conceal most things from the patient while you are attending to him. Give necessary orders with cheerfulness and serenity…revealing nothing of the patient's future or present condition. For many patients … have taken a turn for the worse … by forecast of what is to come"* and those from the American Medical Association in the nineteenth century [7]: *"The life of a sick person can be shortened not only by the acts, but also by the words or the manner of a physician. It is, therefore, a sacred duty to guard him carefully in this respect and to avoid all things which have a tendency to discourage the patient and to depress his spirits.*" Closer to us, in the 1960s, when oncological options were still scarce, physicians tended to consider it inhumane to break bad news to a patient while knowing that there would be no treatment option to offer [8]. Today, however, finds a tremendous emphasis on the patient's autonomy and right to know everything about his or her condition and to make his or her own decisions. Physicians also face the challenge of tailoring the delivery of bad news, depending on the assessment of the specific patient's wishes, needs, culture, and resources.

"*I left my house on October 2, 1996, as one person, and came home another*" [9]: this quote from Lance Armstrong after being informed of his advanced oncological condition illustrates how stressful and life-changing receiving bad news is.

Four key points need to be considered while delivering bad news:

1. Address the patient first, even if the patient appears confused or unwilling to participate. If comatose, never talk to the family as if the patient were not present. The patient must remain the center of care in all circumstances [10]
2. Ask the patient, if able to communicate, if and how the family/loved ones should be involved in the discussion, to emphasize the right to privacy if desired [10]
3. Demonstrate that you and all the healthcare providers involved are going to team with the patient and the patient's caregivers/loved ones in this difficult period. Fine et al. demonstrated that even though the first thing that the patient requests is good symptom management, "companionship," which means an active "partnership" not only with his family members but with the healthcare providers too, is very high in the list of needs [11]
4. Do you need to get more involved in the patient's decision-making process? This is a rather provocative concept as today's Western societies emphasize patient-centered decision making and the concept of autonomy. Nevertheless, patients may prefer their doctors to be partners and may sometimes ask physicians to take difficult decisions for them. A recent study conducted by Chungon more than 8,000 hospitalized patients showed that even though 97% of respondents wanted doctors to offer them choices and to consider their opinion, two out of three preferred however to leave medical decisions to their physician [12]

Several guidelines on the sequence to follow when delivering bad news have been published, some of which being available in a convenient format, which are worth having in the lab coat pocket for a quick double-check before a meeting, especially at the beginning of training. Some are based on simple mnemonic (*ABCDE*) [6],on steps [13, 14]or acronyms (SPIKES) [15, 16].All account for the important elements of a good discussion not only while breaking bad news, but also while discussing other important issues, such as advanced care planning or treatment goals. One of these guidelines, SPIKES, was also assessed as an education tool for the ED residents to ease the discussions with the family members after a patient's death [17].

Table 5.1 Checklist of key elements for a successful meeting while breaking bad news

Getting ready for the meeting
- Determine who will be present (a)
- Obtain/review all necessary information regarding the patient's condition and plan of care *before* the meeting
- Discuss briefly with the professionals who will be present, what the main point(s) to discuss are, who will lead, and who will answer questions of various topics
- Determine the amount of time necessary to dedicate to the meeting
- Prepare an appropriate environment
- Minimize distractions from cell phones, pagers, disruptions. Ensure that every medical team member is physically and mentally prepared

Initiating the meeting
- Be on time
- Introduce everybody; be sure that everybody is sitting comfortably
- The meeting leader will set up the timing and explain the goal of the meeting, and suggest some "rules" (e.g., only one person speaks at a time, with no interruptions)

During the meeting
- Start by addressing the patient: "Mr. X, how are **you** feeling **now**?"
- Briefly assess patient understanding: "What do **you** know about your situation?" (b)
- Assess patient readiness for receiving the bad news, and the level of detail necessary to provide: "What do **you** want to know" (c)
- Break the news (d)
- Respond to emotion (e)
- Be attentive (especially to the patient and the family reactions, nonverbal language, and interactions)
- Plan the follow up (f)

After the meeting
- Create a written summary of the meeting, including date, participants' names, decisions, problems, plan of care, and specific elements of meeting
- Determine if the team achieved its initial goals
- Assess what went well and what did not
- Determine who is going to perform necessary follow-up tasks
- Reflect on your own and the team members' limits (e.g., bad personal period, fatigue, feelings of medical team members toward patients and patient family members) (g)
- Assess availability and access to our resources (h)

Table 5.1 presents a series of the main elements to consider in order to facilitate communication when bad news is to be presented. Additional information regarding some of these key points are detailed afterwards.

(a) Determine who will be present

It is important to determine how many family members are expected or are key persons, and which team members' presence would be helpful. It is better to be accompanied by another member of the healthcare team, especially if not experienced, not knowing the situation well, or feeling uncomfortable or unready. The patient needs to know that his or her physician will not neglect treatable aspects of health, diabetes, hypertension, nutritional deficiencies, etc. There is no shame in asking for help! Do not hesitate to send reminders of the meeting and to request a confirmation from the participants, especially if you will meet several key family members.

(b) Briefly assess patient understanding

Some possible questions

- "Could you describe your medical situation for me in your own words?"
- "When you first had this symptom, what did you think it might be?"
- "Are you worried about your illness or symptoms?"
- "What did my colleague (oncologist, PCP, radiologist…) tell you about your condition or the procedure you underwent?"

In a study conducted by Rowland Morin, it has been shown that some of the factors of satisfaction of the patients during initial interviews with physicians was their use of silence or the reaction time latency between speakers [18]. As it has been demonstrated that most patients take two minutes to answer your questions, but that an average medical doctor interrupts the patient within 18–23 s, so hold on!

This important step may allow you to understand:

- What the patient knows (*"I have lung cancer, and I need surgery"*)
- What he understands about his disease (*"the doctor said something about a spot on my chest x-ray"*)
- His level of technical sophistication (*"I've got a T2N0 adenocarcinoma"*)
- His emotional state (*"I've been so worried I might have cancer that I haven't slept for a week"*)
- His relations with his family members (*"Let me talk for a change, I'm the sick one"*)

(c) Assess patient readiness for receiving the bad news, and the level of detail necessary to give

Some possible questions:

- "If this condition turns out to be something serious, would you want to know?"
- "Do you want me to go over the test results now and to explain exactly what they mean?"
- "Some patients want me to cover every medical detail, but other patients want only the big picture. What would you prefer now?"
- "Some persons prefer not to be told what is wrong with them, but would rather have their family told instead. Both solutions are perfectly OK. What do you prefer?"

(d) Break the news

The topics you would like/need to cover during the meeting may be extensive and address the diagnosis, potential additional investigations, treatment options, prognosis, and/or advanced directives.

It is very important to:

- Use softening language as you begin to prepare for the delivery of bad news. You may say: "I feel badly to have to tell you this," "I'm afraid the news is not good," "The report is back, and it is not what we hoped for."
- Talk in a sensitive but straightforward manner.
- Avoid the single, steady monologue. Give pieces of information in small chunks and pause frequently ("I'm going to stop for one minute to see if you have some question at this point.").
- Avoid technical jargon (no pathophysiology course) or euphemisms (the "mass," the "problem").
- Check for understanding. ("You just received news that is not what you expected. There is a lot going on right now for you and your family. Please tell me if you understood everything I told you or if you want me to go back to some specific issues.").

(e) Respond to emotion:

- Be ready to face a broad range of reactions (e.g., denial, blame, intellectualization, disbelief, acceptance, anger).
- Wait and be there. Silence and the use of nonverbal language are great tools that we underuse.
- Have tissue papers available.
- Acknowledge the emotions.
- "I'm sorry" and "I don't know" are OK!
- Avoid defensiveness regarding the medical care. Do not criticize other healthcare professionals.
- If things turn bad and you face an aggressive reaction, do not take it personally and do not respond in the same way.

(f) Plan the follow-up:

- Give additional information on potential treatments options, further necessary investigations, and appropriate referrals. ("We'll go step-by-step.").
- Maintain realistic hope. "There is nothing we can do for you" is the worst thing we can tell our patients from an emotional standpoint, in addition to being completely wrong. Palliative/EOL care has much to offer regarding symptom management and can address the various dimensions specific to the patient.
- Allow extra time for final questions (while respecting the time allocated). Help break the news to the family if no member is present during the meeting.
- Never leave the patient without having organized a follow-up appointment or a phone call contact. Reiterate that you will be there to help in difficult moments.
- Always double check: Is the patient alone? Driving? Depressive? Suicidal? Living alone? Does he have former or current addictions?
- Organize, if needed, prompt social, psychological, and/or spiritual support.
- If the patient has been admitted, try to avoid holding the discussion at the time of discharge. The patient may need the supportive environment of the hospital to make his or her initial accommodations.

(g) Reflect on your own and the team members' limits:

Breaking bad news may be challenging and may bring us above our limits. We can experience a sense of failure and frustration with the inability to help more or by judging our performance while breaking the news. Some professionals may even desire to avoid a specific patient and family to escape these feelings. These feelings can be exacerbated if we have simultaneously developed a close relation and start to identify with the patient (e.g., patient who looks like our own father, young patient with children the same age than ours, etc.), undergo a difficult personal period, or are overwhelmed by a huge work load. These emotions may affect both the patient's care and our well-being. Such unexamined emotions may lead to disengagement, poor judgment, distress, and burnout [19]. It is said that approximately one of every three physicians will experience burnout at any given time, which could lead in the worst cases to substance abuse, intent to leave medical practice, and suicide [20]. Even though a recent review failed to demonstrate that burnout levels were higher in palliative care health workers than in other contexts [21], we may imagine that in this specific context with a constant immersion in a field where patients of all ages present very advanced conditions, the risk of being overwhelmed may be higher than in other medical areas. For this reason teamwork is so important. A health professional should not be the only one to carry the weight of this difficult moment. Discussing with colleagues after the meeting about what was said, what happened in the meeting, the plans for patient care, and making plans to share responsibilities can be tremendously helpful.

(h) Access to our availabilities and resources

Also, it is important to make sure that you have personal resources and to know that you can access them. For some of us, it is just our family circle, for others, such resources can include extreme sports, nature, arts, meditation, or any of a number of other sources of coping. Whatever it is, we need to know what can help us. Seeking professional help can also be an asset in difficult moments. There is no shame to request help from our peers, from our mentors, or from professionals. Remember that if you arrive in the stage of burn-out, you will not only hurt yourself, but you will not be of any help to your patients and your team!

Other Important Issues

"Doc, how much time do I still have?" Physicians are not good prognosticators. A 2000 study conducted by Christakis et al. asked 343 doctors to provide survival estimates for 468 terminally ill patients (<6 months to live if disease ran expected course). For this population, which finally had a median survival of 24 days, 63% of the physicians were overoptimistic, and 17% overly pessimistic, a long relationship with the patient being associated with overestimation [22]. Over-optimism as well as unnecessary pessimism may harm, it may be wise to remain vague at the beginning and to reassess on a regular basis rather than to cite a bunch of statistics. If a specific

patient requests statistics, it is important while giving them to emphasize that each patient is unique, and that it is almost impossible to predict where in these statistics the particular patient will fall.

"To touch or not to touch?" We are often concerned about being disrespectful of the patient's private sphere if we touch his hand or his shoulder. Usually, patients with oncological situations, especially ones presenting with mutilating lesions, may feel rejected and find comfort in being touched. Holding a patient's hand may also give you important clues: Is the patient cold? Shaking? Myoclonic? If the patient does not find comfort in being touched, the patient will tell you, either directly, or through nonverbal signs.

What Does the Patient Remember?

Several studies have shown that the patient may not remember points physicians addressed. In a recent study, Olson et al. interviewed patients on their discharge day. Among the patients, only 57% knew their present diagnosis while 77% of the physicians were sure that they were aware of it [23]. Even more relevant, when a new medication had been prescribed, 20% of the patients said their physician never told them about it, while all the physicians said they had told them about it. Regarding the side effects, only 10% of the patients said they were told about them while 81% of the physicians said they had described them. This discrepancy is probably even more present when the patient has to assimilate bad news.

The Importance of the Body Language

Four components are important:

– The first impression: Shake hand, make eye contact, be seated
– The physician's nonverbal language
– The patient's nonverbal language
– The family members' nonverbal language

The first two components will help you create a good relation with your patient and family members. These elements should be addressed in any communication training. The last ones will bring you invaluable elements which may help you to obtain a global vision necessary to build up a strategy of care.

Cultural and Spiritual Issues

As society becomes more pluralistic, physicians will face increasing numbers of patients from various cultures or religious backgrounds. The more we know about the different needs of diverse patient groups, the more tools we will have to deal appropriately with situations involving them. Studies have shown that people from many different cultures are more likely to believe discussing death can bring death closer, including Native Americans and immigrants from Africa, China, Korea, and Mexico [24]. Even though patient autonomy is a strong cultural value in the USA and other Western cultures, it is not the same in some non-Western cultures, such as those found in Asia and Latin America, where primary decision makers are often supposed to be the family members. The more we know about these different visions, and the more we respect them as well as their spiritual beliefs, the more it will help build a relation of trust between the patients and us. It is often rewarding for the patients and their families when physicians ask questions about their culture and their beliefs. It is also always possible to contact a spiritual leader or an influential member of a specific community to obtain as much relevant information as possible—all within the requisite of patient confidentiality and trust.

Communicating with "Difficult" Families

Integrating families and loved ones in patient care is a mandatory part of good palliative medicine as defined by the most recent WHO definition [25]. The patient needs to know that we take care of the needs of loved ones, too, and that these loved ones can be part of the decision-making and care process if the patient so wishes. Also, it is often extremely difficult for patients to know they are leaving behind beloved ones after death, and the patient sometimes worries more about them than about him or herself. For this reason special emphasis is placed on end-of-life family conferences. Several guidelines have been developed to help organize these conferences [26, 27].

It can likewise be extremely difficult for family members to see their beloved one decline and sometimes suffer or be confused. Family members may feel guilty because they cannot help the patient more. Often, these family members are themselves on the verge of exhaustion. Sometimes family members and loved ones are left in terrible distress, and for this reason bereavement services are offered as part of regular hospice care for up to 13 months following the patient's death.

Relationships physicians develop with the patient's family members and loved ones are often excellent, rewarding, and helpful. The longer physicians interact with these caregivers and the more the family trusts the physician, the better this relation may become. Especially effective physicians consistently emphasize the important role family members play in their beloved one's care, gather family members' opinions on this care, and allow them to ask any question they may have [10].It is also important to ask family members on a regular basis how they are feeling and coping with this terrible situation. It may be useful for the physician to acknowledge that this caring may be a physical and emotional drain on family caregivers. Proactively suggesting "respite" may relieve guilt and promote better relationships between the patient and the family caregivers as well as between the family and the physician.

In some occasions however, the communication with the family may be more challenging than the patient's care himself, whether the patient is still able or not to communicate accurately. Some family members may express their suffering in various ways that can be difficult for the healthcare providers to handle. This may be the family members' way trying to deal with a reality they find intolerable. Physicians must understand that unpleasant reactions may only be the expression of an intense suffering. Family members may be extremely demanding, come back again and again with unrealistic expectations and hopes, interfere with best care practices ("no morphine, I don't want him to receive dangerous medications," even while the patient is in excruciating pain or severe dyspnea), or sometimes be very aggressive and question the physician's every suggestion. Healthcare professionals may also face the occasional pathologic personality among family members, such as narcissistic, antisocial, or other personality disorders. Some family members may also present with active addictions that will also interfere with the patient's care.

If the patient's family members had very disappointing interactions previously with other healthcare providers, sometimes believing that the patient has been not diagnosed on time, or did not receive the care they would have desired, they may not be quickly willing to trust any doctor again, and the medical team may need more time and a united effort to gain their trust again.

Past or ongoing conflicts among family members are sometimes exacerbated in the end-of-life period. Some family members, who may not have been present and involved in the patient's care previously, may feel a form of guilt and aggressively manifest these feelings by trying to exert control in the situation, which may upset other family members. There may also be financial concerns or interests. And family members may inappropriately expect members of the healthcare team to determine who is right or wrong, which may put physicians and others into difficult situations [27].

Some important points:

1. If a scheduled family meeting is expected to be difficult, it is important to prepare the meeting carefully. Make sure that all the main family members will be present and ask them confirm their presence. Prepare a team approach and have all the relevant team members available before starting the meeting. If you expect six family members, try not to be alone; show a coherent interdisciplinary approach. On the other hand, with one or two family members only, having them to face a whole healthcare team may be overwhelming.

2. Try to figure out as soon as possible who holds the patient's power of attorney, whether there is a living will if the patient is not able to communicate, and determine clearly who will be the main contact among the family members.

3. Be especially clear in your expectations during this meeting. Difficult family members often lead to difficult meetings. Expectations regarding meeting time, how the meeting is led, as well as ground rules on participation—that all members participate in turn and that shouting, cursing, and violent behavior are not accepted. When situations are expected to be particularly tense, be sure to have prompt access to security. If you see that you do not have any more control of the situation, and the discussion arrives at a dead end, it is better to call for a "time-out" and to reschedule another meeting.

4. No member of the healthcare team should be recruited to judge family conflicts. Likewise, family conflicts should not be mirrored by healthcare team members. Dysfunctional family members may be highly skilled at recruiting others into their orbit and thus splitting the healthcare team. In some occasions, it is worth asking an angry person to address you rather than another member of the family to avoid a spiral of discord or violence.

5. Before the meeting, try to gather as much information regarding the specific cultural and spiritual context of the present family as possible. Showing your knowledge, your interest and, most importantly, your respect for other cultures and religions may help improve communication and create trust relations with the family members [28].

6. As usually, remember that it is always better to ask for help if needed: a more experienced colleague, a palliative care physician, or an ethics committee consultation may be of help.

7. After the meeting, take time to debrief the situation within the team. Document all possible elements, the family and team members present, what was discussed and the decisions taken. Do not forget that there is always a risk of lawsuit, particularly when family members are angry, excessively distressed, or otherwise highly emotional.

Communication Among Health Professionals

Patients and their loved ones with advanced disease face numerous, well-documented problems—the poor prognosis, symptom burden, and suffering, as well as the logistical difficulties of a heavy schedule of appointments, sometimes in various locations, with conflicted schedules, heavy costs, and long waiting times—but such difficulties are only exacerbated when the patient and his loved ones receive conflicted opinions from various healthcare professionals. It is especially difficult if one professional questions openly the attitude of another one.

Another difficult situation when the patient switches abruptly from a primary care provider to a specialist like an oncologist, and the switch can be even more distressing when going from the specialist from whom he expected potential cure to palliative or hospice care.

In these terrible moments when the patient faces death, the patient needs even greater trust in the healthcare providers, and to know that they will work all together to offer the best option appropriate to the specific situation, adjusting to changes in the disease state and goals of care. If we go back to Fine's survey conducted among hospice patients and asking the simple question: "What would be the most useful way I can be of help to you today?", symptoms relief came first of course, but close to this came the request of companionship [11].

It is also well represented in this African proverb quoted by Spruyt: "If you want to travel quickly, go alone. But if you want to travel far, you must go together" [29].

In fact, there is a lot to do in the travel toward death in a palliative condition, and the way is sometimes long. We need to join our efforts to help our patient and the patient's loved ones to go through this travel as smoothly as possible. We need to collaborate and communicate better, whether among team members, or the various physicians involved.

Interdisciplinary Team Communication

A well-conducted hospice team meeting is a wonderful example of the effectiveness of interdisciplinarity. Medical students or young residents who attend these meetings for the first time are very often surprised to see that the physician is not the "leader" of the team. Each team member, physician, nurse, psychologist, social worker, chaplain, pharmacist, volunteer, is important, as each of them has a specific expertise and unique skills and values that work in synergy with those of the other team members. We know the importance of close communication, respect, shared team philosophy, as well as good interpersonal relationships among the team members if we want to offer the best care to our patient [30].

Communication Among Physicians

This is as important as the interdisciplinary communication. It is not rare at the hospital to have a patient assessed by several specialists, sometimes giving contradictory opinions regarding treatment options or global attitudes, without discussing with their colleagues, leaving the patient feeling powerless and confused. The first question at any moment should always be: "Who will take the decisions and organize the care offered to the patient." This "captain" should obtain information from all the specialists and organize the plan of care accordingly. Regular meetings among all involved specialists are ideal of course, but due to the busy schedule of all the physicians such meetings are difficult to coordinate sometimes. The communication between the primary care physician, the specialists, and then the palliative care or hospice physician must be maintained to avoid the patient distressing transitions. It is also a good way to gather new information, to have a better idea of the "reality of the other," and to demonstrate our respect for our colleagues. Finally, the technology that surrounds us is wonderful, but sometimes a simple phone call or a visit to a colleague will be more helpful and personalized that the most sophisticated electronic letter.

References

1. Rosenbaum ME, Ferguson KJ, Lobas JG. Teaching medical students and residents skills for delivering bad news: a review of strategies. Acad Med. 2004;79(2):107–17.
2. Rider S, Hinrichs MM, Lown BA. A model for communication skills assessment across the undergraduate curriculum. Med Teach. 2006;28(5):e127–34.

 3. Stiefel F, Barth J, Bensing J, et al. Communication skills training in oncology: a position paper based on a consensus meeting among European experts in 2009. Ann Oncol. 2010;21:204–7.
 4. Kissane DW. Communication skills training for oncology professionals. J Clin Oncol. 2012;30(11):1242–7.
 5. Moore PM, Wilkinson SSM, Rivera Mercado S. Communication skills training for health care professionals working with cancer patients, their families and/or carers. Cochrane Database Syst Rev. (2):CD003751. doi:10.1002/14651858. Published online: 21 Jan 2009.
 6. Vandekieft G. Breaking bad news. Am Fam Physician. 2001;64(12):1975–8.
 7. King LS. Medicine in the USA: historical vignettes. IX. The AMA sets a new code of ethics. JAMA. 1983;249(10):1338–42.
 8. Oken D. What to tell cancer patients. A study of medical attitudes. JAMA. 1961;175:1120–8.
 9. Armstrong L. It's not about the bike: my journey back to life. New York: Putnam; 2000.
10. Mitnick S, Leffler C, Hood VL. Family caregivers, patients and physicians: ethical guidance to optimize relationships. J Gen Intern Med. 2010;25(3):255–60.
11. Fine P, Peterson D. Caring about what dying patients care about caring. J Pain Symptom Manage. 2002;23(4):267–78.
12. Chung GS, et al. Predictors of hospitalized patients' preferences for physician-directed medical decision-making. J Med Ethics. 2012;38(2):77–82.
13. Buckman R, Baile W. Truth telling: yes, but how? J Clin Oncol. 2007;25(21):3181.
14. Von Gunten CF, Ferris FD, Emanuel LL. The patient-physician relationship. Ensuring competency in end-of-life care: communication and relational skills. JAMA. 2000;284:3051–7.
15. Bailey W, et al. SPIKES-A six-step protocol for delivering bad news: application to the patient with cancer. Oncologist. 2000;5:302–11.
16. Back AL, Arnold RM, Baile WF, et al. Efficacy of communication skills training for giving bad news and discussing transitions to palliative care. Arch Intern Med. 2007;167:453–60.
17. Park I, et al. Breaking bad news education for emergency medicine residents: a novel training module using simulation with the SPIKES protocol. J Emerg Trauma Shock. 2010;3(4):385–8.
18. Rowland-Morin PA, Carroll JG. Verbal communication skills and patient satisfaction. A study of doctor-patient interviews. Eval Health Prof. 1990;13(2):168–85.
19. Meier DE, Back AL, Morrison RS. The inner life of physicians and care of the seriously ill. JAMA. 2001;286(23):3007–14.
20. Shanafelt TD, Sloan JA, Habermann TM. The wellbeing of physicians. Am J Med. 2003;114(6):513–9.
21. Pereira SM, Fonseca AM, Carvalho AS. Burnout in palliative care: a systematic review. Nurs Ethics. 2011;18(3):317–26.
22. Christakis NA, Lamont EB. Extent and determinants of error in doctors' prognoses in terminally ill patients: prospective cohort study. BMJ. 2000;320:469–72.
23. Olson DP, Windish DM. Communication discrepancies between physicians and hospitalized patients. Arch Intern Med. 2010;170(15):1302–70.
24. Curtis JR, Patrick DL, Caldwell ES, Collier AC. Why don't patients and physicians talk about end-of-life care? Barriers to communication for patients with acquired immunodeficiency syndrome and their primary care clinicians. Arch Intern Med. 2000;60:1690–6.
25. Ventafridda V. According to the 2002 WHO definition of palliative care…. Palliat Med. 2006;20(3):159.
26. Lautrette A, Ciroldi M, Ksibi H, Azoulay E. End-of-life family conferences: rooted in the evidence. Crit Care Med. 2006;34(11):S364–72.
27. King DA, Quill T. Working with families in palliative care: one size does not fit all. J Palliat Med. 2006;9:704–15.
28. Crawley LM, Marshal PA, Koenig BA. Respecting cultural differences at the end of life. In: Snyder L, Quill T, editors. Physician's guide to end of life care. Philadelphia: American College of Physicians; 2001. p. 35–8.
29. Spruyt O. Team networking in palliative care. Indian J Palliat Care. 2011;17:S17–9.
30. Junger S, Pestinger M, Elsner F, et al. Criteria for successful multiprofessional cooperation in palliative care teams. Palliat Med. 2007;21(4):347–54.

Review Questions

1. In a global population discharged from the hospital, how many patients can tell you their current diagnosis?

    (a) 90%
    (b) 75%
    (c) 57%
    (d) 35%

2. For how long does a "standard" physician let a patient talk before interrupting him?

    (a) 18–23 s
    (b) 30–60 s
    (c) 2–3 min
    (d) Usually does not interrupt him

3. When you have to break bad news to a patient, what is one of the most important initial step?

    (a) To be sure that you will have time to address all the important issues, such as diagnosis, prognosis, treatment, advanced directives
    (b) To find somebody willing to do this for you
    (c) To discuss in the corridor, standing, to avoid to spend too much time with the patient
    (d) To try to have all the relevant information available

4. Is Palliative Care a medical specialty with higher risk of burn-out than others?

    (a) Yes
    (b) No, it is ICU
    (c) No, it is surgery
    (d) No, the risk is the same in all medical specialties

5. The best way to improve your communication skills is:

    (a) There is no way to improve, either you are an innate good communicator, or you are not
    (b) To observe skilled colleagues or mentors
    (c) To learn from our mistakes
    (d) To follow a formal communication training

Answers

1. (c) 57%
2. (a) 18–23 s
3. (d) To try to have all the relevant information available
4. (d) No, the risk is the same in all medical specialties
5. (d) To follow a formal communication training

Chapter 6
Guidance with Complex Treatment Choices

Sukanya Mitra and Nalini Vadivelu

Introduction

Rightly or wrongly, good or bad, we take decisions and make choices every day, in almost all aspects of life. These choices are made in response to questions that range from the apparently simple ("which dress to wear tonight for the evening party") to perhaps the more complex ("which one to marry from the three prospective suitors"). In terms of treatment choices too, decisions need to be made, again ranging from the relatively mundane ("does the patient need an antibiotic? If so, which one, which route, what dose, for how long?") to relatively complex ("does the patient, with extensive metastasis and limited survival probability, one who himself does not wish to undergo any further surgery and simply wants to die 'in peace and dignity,' but whose family and friends want him to 'live as long as possible and at any cost' and consider that the patient may not have decision-making capacity now because of brain metastasis related cognitive impairment, and finally where there are several intervention options but none with a clear advantage over another, need a specific intervention? If so, which one, what type, with what intensity, for how long?"). Decision making and treatment choices can be extremely complex and uncertain, especially in the context of a serious and life-threatening illness or in the terminal stages. This is where, in the setting of palliative care, decision making may need guidance or sharing.

S. Mitra, M.D. (✉)
Department of Anaesthesia and Intensive Care,
Government Medical College and Hospital,
Chandigarh, India
e-mail: Drsmitra12@yahoo.com

N. Vadivelu, M.D.
Department of Anesthesiology,
Yale University School of Medicine,
New Haven, CT, USA

N. Vadivelu et al. (eds.), *Essentials of Palliative Care*,
DOI 10.1007/978-1-4614-5164-8_6,
© Springer Science+Business Media New York 2013

There are three general stages in any decision making. The first and foremost essential stage is that of information. This information is necessarily about the patient's diagnosis, current condition, complications, other relevant background information (e.g., allergy to certain drugs, other medications, coexisting conditions, etc.), and scientific information regarding the effectiveness and safety of particular interventions available in the current situation as well as the doctor's clinical experience-based information under the particular circumstances. However, this "medical" or "objective" information, though clearly necessary for the decision making to proceed further, may not be sufficient for this purpose, and there can be a vital role played by information of another nature, that based on the values, principles, priorities, and feelings of the patient, at times his family, and even rarely the doctor (e.g., whether conducting a medical abortion is "right").

This latter, "value" or "preference" based information becomes very important during the second stage of decision making, the stage of deliberation. It is at this stage that the information from the different sources mentioned above are analyzed, their pros and cons weighed, and attempts are made to negotiate conflicting issues if any (e.g., between medical information and patient preference). Finally the actual stage of decision making is arrived at, when the final decision to be implemented is made based on the previous two stages [1].

Models of Decision Making

In the general healthcare setting, the differences between these three stages described above become apparent when we consider the models of decision making. Three broad models of decision making have been described, with shades of gray in between [1–3] (Table 6.1).

The first, "paternalistic model," is the traditional model that has held its sway over centuries of medical care and is still the dominant model in many parts of the world. This is the "Doctor knows the best and hence decides" model. The patient may receive some information and seek clarification but remains the passive person in "receiving" the decision regarding treatment or any other intervention. Thus, there is no actual partnership between the doctor and the patient. The information is medical is nature, the deliberation is between different options but without the patient taking any active role in it, and decision making is done solely by the doctor or the treating team. The guiding basic bioethical principles behind this model are beneficence ("do what is good for the patient") and nonmaleficence ("do not do any harm to the patient").

The other extreme of decision-making models is called the "informed choice model." This model arose in response to the growing waves of consumerism, patient-centered medicine, and patient rights movement, especially fuelled by the bioethical principle of patient autonomy. Here the doctor informs, the patient deliberates and decides. During the deliberation stage, it is the patient who weighs the medical information provided by the doctor against his own values and preferences, which

Table 6.1 Models of decision making

Characteristics	Paternalistic model	Informed choice model	Shared decision-making model
Underlying bioethical principle	Beneficence; nonmaleficence	Patient autonomy	Combination of autonomy and beneficence
"Center" of orientation	Person centered (doctor)	Person centered (patient)	Relationship centered
Partnership or collaboration	No	No	Yes
Decision-making stage			
Information base	Medical	Medical (personal information not shared with doctor)	Medical and personal (shared)
Deliberation between doctor and patient	No	No	Yes
Decision making	Unilateral (doctor)	Unilateral (patient)	Bilateral (mutually agreed)

he is not obligated to share with the doctor. Based on this, the patient makes the final decision. The doctor may or may not agree with this final decision, but nonetheless is obligated to implement it provided the patient is understood to retain decision-making "capacity," i.e., he can receive the relevant medical information provided by the doctor, can retain the information long enough to weigh the pros and cons of different intervention (including the choice of no intervention at all), can arrive at the final treatment choice, and can communicate this choice to the treating team. Note that in this model the principle of patient autonomy (what the patient thinks is best for him) may conflict with the principle of beneficence (what the doctor thinks is best for the patient). In case of such a conflict, under this informed choice model for a patient with decisional capacity, patient autonomy wins. In a sense then, again there is no true partnership or collaboration between the doctor and the patient.

The third, intermediate form is best known as the "shared decision model" (SDM). This model is placed in between the other two. As the term suggests, here information is shared, deliberation is interactive, and the final decision is mutually agreed upon. The information domains cover both medical (objective) and personal (subjective), where the patient shares his part of the "information" with the doctor. The deliberation is a two-way process unlike both the earlier models. The negotiations can be iterative and dynamic, and can involve—other than the doctor and the patient—other members of the patient's family, other members of the treating team, and other staff of a multidisciplinary team (MDT) such as nursing staff and social worker. The final decision is mutually agreed upon. Here the principles of autonomy, beneficence, and nonmaleficence are all attempted to be accommodated, and conflicts are resolved by discussion. In this sense, the SDM is a truly partnership-based collaborative model [3].

It is to be noted that there is no inherent "superiority" of any of these models, and that intermediate forms ("shades of gray") exist in real-life applications. For example, in a case where there is a clear-cut treatment option with proven efficacy (e.g., antibiotic choice of known efficacy as determined by culture and sensitivity) the paternalistic model would work fine. In another case where there are multiple treatment options of proven efficacy but differing tolerability issues, the informed choice model may be suitable. On the other hand, when there are multiple options in a complex situation, with no clear-cut efficacy of one over another but with varying pros and cons, the patient's preference may be negotiated with the medical information and a mutually agreeable final choice is finalized. This is the SDM, and it is especially suitable for palliative care and end-of-life scenarios.

Preference-Sensitive Treatment Decisions in Palliative Care

"The need for some form of doctor patient partnership is most compelling when the patient presents with a serious or life threatening illness; different treatment options exist, with different benefits and risks; and outcomes are uncertain. In this situation, the stakes are high and there is no one 'right' treatment. Since the patient will bear the consequences of whatever treatment is implemented, it is important that his or her values and preferences are known and respected.

Patients in this situation are likely to feel vulnerable and may not initiate such a discussion; it is the doctor's responsibility to ensure that this occurs" [3].

Palliative care involves a mix of complex medical information, a personal emotional dimension, and options of care whose outcomes can be uncertain. Under these circumstances, the dilemma of choosing between life-prolonging treatments with potential side effects or maximizing quality of life can become accentuated. Patients are faced with difficult decisions about a wide range of issues, such as place of care, various options to treat symptoms, the use of opioids, palliative treatments such as chemotherapy, advance directives, etc. [4]. Many of these decisions are known as "preference-sensitive" decisions, where, because there is no one "right answer," patient (or family's) preference to follow one course of action over another gains priority and becomes the final deciding factor.

Not only this, but more importantly and to complicate matters further, the decisions to be taken during palliative care keep on changing along the trajectory of the life-threatening disease: from its diagnosis, through multiple points of curative or disease-modifying treatments, remissions and relapses, through life-prolonging or life-sustaining treatments, through comfort care, till the issue of where, when, and how to die in order to have a "good death." Each of these "decision transition points" brings with it new questions, new dilemmas, and new priorities. Particularly towards the end of this trajectory, patient's and his family's values, preferences, and priorities tend to become progressively more meaningful and important that shape the treatment choice. Eventually, end-of-life decisions arise, such as "Do not resuscitate" orders, withdrawal or withholding of life-prolonging measures and where to receive end-of-life care.

The types of decisions that are needed to be made depending upon the decision transition points could be [5]:

- Selecting a surrogate and other advance care planning decisions
- Making various decisions regarding aspects of disease-modifying therapies
- Treatment choices when cure is not possible
- Whether or not to be admitted to intensive care unit (ICU) and receive life-prolonging treatments or to focus on comfort care
- Where to receive end-of-life (EOL) care and other EOL decisions

A partial list of the goals of palliative care where decisions need to be made include:

- Cure
- Slowed progression
- Remission
- Prolonging life span
- Achievement of life goals
- Maximizing normal life experience
- Maximizing periods of lucidity
- Maximizing comfort
- Minimizing pain and other symptoms
- Maximizing family access
- Having care and/or death occur in their preferred location

As mentioned above, these goals shift depending upon the decision transition points. The important point to note is that in many of these decisions to be made one needs to move beyond the narrow medical model of a disease and its treatment. The choices to be made depend not only upon the medical circumstances of the "case" but also center around increasing or at least optimizing the quality of life of the "person," which is the ultimate overarching goal of palliative care as defined by the World Health Organization [6].

Guidance with Complex Treatment Choices

It follows that the SDM as described earlier intuitively appeals as the suitable model to be followed in making complex decisions, given the uncertainty and multidimensional nature of the situations, nonsuperiority of any particular interventions at times, adverse effects of many of the interventions, and the need to take into account the values, personal goals, feelings, and priorities of the patient and the family.

However, these same factors outlined above, and especially the complex treatment choices with their own pros and cons, can be quite overwhelming for the patient. Information overload can occur; the patient may feel perplexed and daunted; and each "arm" of the decision-making process may come into conflict with one another. This is true even in case of the so-called preference-sensitive decisions, because at times the patient may not be clear as to what is "preference" is, because of conflicting values, wishes, and needs. This can give rise to a state of "decision conflict," which is defined as "a psychological state of uncertainty around which course of action to pursue. Decisional conflict occurs when choices are uncertain, involving value trade-offs between patient judged benefits and harms and individually valued health states, when there is no clear 'right choice.' Unresolved decision conflict may result in regret over the decision" [5]. In the worst-case scenario, this may even lead to "decisional paralysis," rendering the patient passive and choiceless, leading the patient to defer to the clinician because he or she considers the decision "too complicated" for the lay person.

Starting with the patient's goals and values early in the consultation and tailoring the presented options to those goals and values, one can individualize and narrow the wide array of options to those most consistent with the patient's values. It is important to avoid burdening patients and families under stress with options that are not desired, are unrealistic, or are presented in an array may simply be overwhelming or cause decisional "paralysis" as mentioned above. Hence it is important first to sit together, discuss the various options, narrow down the possibilities, and then present the information to the patient and family in a distilled and tailored fashion.

For all these reasons, the MDT remains an invaluable asset in guidance of patients with complex choices. The MDT, in its multidisciplinary meeting, can discuss various findings, options, their pros and cons, and can reach a consensus or at least narrow down the options, which can then be discussed with the patient to arrive at a final decision [7].

Decision Support, Decision Aids, Decision Coaching

As mentioned above, decision making can be quite daunting for patients at times and can lead to decision conflict. Health care providers can develop patients' and families' skills in SDM resulting in a preference for more active involvement. In this connection, decision science and its application in healthcare can be of great help. Decision scientists have designed techniques to promote SDM and relieve decisional conflict that are collectively called "decision support." Decision support is really an umbrella term that encompasses a broad range of skills, interventions, strategies, and processes that help the patient in making a choice based on the options available and his personal values and preferences.

It is to be noted that decision support strategies do not make the decisions for the patient; they only help or guide the patient through a structured process to clarify different aspects of the difficult question that the patient has to answer ultimately. Thus, they are adjuncts to the decision-making process. These support strategies include, on one hand, focused counseling by a health practitioner, and on the other hand, computerized interactive program modules. This term recognizes that, irrespective of the nature of the delivery system, any method that attempts to support individuals facing decisions, either in dialogue with an agent, such as a health care professional, or independently of such dialogues, is a patient-orientated decision support intervention [8].

Table 6.2 Definitions

Decision science	Study of understanding and improving the process and quality of decision making
Decisional conflict	Psychological state of uncertainty around which course of action to pursue. Decisional conflict occurs when choices are uncertain, involving value trade-offs between patient judged benefits and harms and individually valued health states, when there is no clear "right choice"
Decision support	An umbrella term referring to clinical skills, strategies, interventions, and other processes whereby patients are provided with structured support during an explicit process of decision making that includes focused counseling, and in some cases employs a patient "decision aid" to enable them to make informed health care choices
Decision aids	Tools that help people become involved in decision making by providing information about the options and outcomes and by clarifying personal values. They are designed to complement, rather than replace, counseling from a health practitioner
Decision coaching	Individualized support provided through the decision process by a clinician who guides a patient to consider the information relevant to a particular decision and the patient's values to reach an informed preference
Shared decision making (SDM)	A process by which a healthcare choice is made jointly by the practitioner and the patient and is said to be the crux of patient-centered care. Briefly, SDM rests upon knowing and understanding the best available evidence of the risks and benefits across all available options while ensuring that the patient's values are taken into account

Sources: [5, 9, 10]

[See Table 6.2 for various definitions used in this and other sections of this chapter.]

Various decision support interventions can include: direct focused counseling; use of several adjuncts such as leaflets, pamphlets, flip charts, question prompt sheets, "issues cards," "decision boards," hand-held information tools, information displayed on computer screens, video, DVD, etc.; and interactive instrumental media via computer software or Internet where the patient may be guided through successive interactive steps so as to clarify the final decision or narrow down the choices.

Elwyn et al. [8] have classified the multitude of decision support interventions into three broad categories:

Category 1: Those That Are Used by Clinicians in Face-to-Face Encounters

These interventions are specifically designed for use by healthcare professionals when they wish to involve patients in decisions. They typically display information using short statements or graphics so that they act as materials that can be easily shared across a desktop in a clinical encounter. They act as catalysts to SDM by acting as prompts and props, typically by making options visible and by organizing information according to attributes that patients find relevant. They help the clinician engage the patient in a discussion about preferences. Examples include risk communication tools, display boards, issues cards, etc. It is to be noted that these are not stand-alone tools, but rather help to focus the clinician–patient dialogue.

Category 2: Those That Can Be Used Independently from Clinical Encounters

These are also more commonly known as "patient decision aids" or simply "decision aids." (The term "decision aid" is also broadly used as a generic term for all the decision support interventions, but here it is used in reference to Elwyn's Category 2) [8]. Decision aids are by far the most common type of decision support interventions used. They are used by the patients independent of the actual clinical encounter, either before (when the patient wants to come "prepared" for the discussion in SDM) or after (if, following an initial consultative meeting, the patient wishes to make the final choice).

Decision aids are defined in a broad way as "interventions designed to help people make specific and deliberative choices among options by providing information about the options and outcomes that are relevant to a person's health status" [8]. Because this definition is very broad and practically synonymous with "decision support" as defined above, a narrow definition has been offered: "Tools that help people become involved in decision making by providing information about the options and outcomes and by clarifying personal values" [9]. Most trials to date have been undertaken with this type of intervention. Standards have been developed to assess the quality of these decision aids: The International Patient Decision Aids Standards (IPDAS) [11]. There are a number of websites that feature various decision aids, and the decision aids website of Ottawa Hospital Research Initiative hosts an "A–Z" inventory of such tools [9].

Table 6.3 A partial list of online resources for patient decision aids and other decision support interventions

http://decisionaid.ohri.ca/AZinvent.php
http://decisionaid.ohri.ca/decaids.html#poc
http://decisionaid.ohri.ca/index.html
http://pennstatehershey.org/web/humanities/home/resources/advancedirectives
http://www.americanbar.org/groups/law_aging/resources/health_care_decision_making.html
http://www.fraserhealth.ca/
http://www.healthdialog.com/Main/Personalhealthcoaching/Shared-Decision-Making/
http://www.healthwise.net/cochranedecisionaid/Content/StdDocument.aspx?DOCHWID=tu1430
http://www.acpdecisions.org
http://www.calgaryhealthregion.ca/programs/advancecareplanning/
http://www.fimdm.org
http://www.healthdialog.com
http://www.healthlinkbc.ca/kb/
http://www.healthwise.org
http://www.mayoclinic.org

Table 6.3 gives a partial list of this and other resources.

In general, decision aids guide the patient through the following steps [12]:

Step 1: Clarify the specific decision involved
Step 2: Explore the options, with their pros and cons (benefits and harms)
Step 3: Clarify the values, beliefs, and wishes of the patient
Step 4: Screen for decisional difficulties (decisional uncertainty, need for more information, clarity for conflicting values, etc.)
Step 5: Arrive at patient's choice (which may include no intervention)

Decision aids have already been developed for some of the common decisions faced in hospice and palliative care such as completing advance directives, appointing a surrogate decision maker, receiving a feeding tube, cardiopulmonary resuscitation (CPR), artificial nutrition and hydration, and place of care.

Category 3: Those That Are Mediated by More Interactive and Social Technologies

Decision coaching is a term often used in this context. This refers to individualized support provided through the decision process by a clinician (usually a nurse or other professionals trained in decision support techniques) who guides a patient to consider the information relevant to a particular decision and the patient's values to reach an informed preference [5, 13]. Decision coaches are health professionals who (a) assess patients' decisional conflict and related needs; (b) tailor decision support to address patients' needs by offering patient decision aids and/or providing evidence-based information, verifying understanding, clarifying values, and building skills in accessing support; (c) guide patients through the decision-making process; and (d) monitor for factors that can influence implementing the decision (e.g., motivation, self-efficacy, barriers). Often conducted over the telephone, the coach provides and discusses information with the patient, guides him to find other resources, helps explain the issues, and supports the deliberation process. Decision coaching goes beyond decision aids in that the individualized one-to-one discussion is often iterative and is followed up once a specific choice has been made.

Newer modes of decision coaching can utilize computer technologies in what is called "interactive health communication systems" (IHCS). An IHCS offers one platform for providing the information, communication, and coaching resources that cancer patients and their families need to understand the disease, find support, and develop decision-making and coping skills. A particular IHCS called Comprehensive Health Enhancement Support System, Lung Cancer module (CHESS-LC) has been developed for patients with advanced lung cancer and their family caregivers. CHESS-LC provides information, communication, and coaching resources. In particular, it provides web-based interactive decision aids and follows the decisions through coaching. Unlike decision aids that stop at the decision itself, CHESS-LC also extends decision support to implementing and evaluating the decision [14].

A large amount of literature is available on the effectiveness of using decision support interventions, or decision aids in a broad way, in several outcome parameters of decision making. A number of reviews, both narrative and systematic, have attested to the general effectiveness of decision aids. A series of Cochrane reviews has been published on this subject, starting from 2001. The latest updated review, published in October 2011, included 86 randomized controlled trials involving more than 20,000 participants from eight countries (Australia, Canada, China, Finland, Germany, Netherlands, the UK, and the USA) [10]. The primary outcomes were defined according to IPDAS. Decision aids performed better than usual care interventions by increasing knowledge, reducing decisional conflict, and increasing participation in the decision-making process. Further, people exposed to decision aids chose major elective invasive surgery less often than conservative options. There was no evidence of increased anxiety or other adverse effects of exposing people to decision aids. This is important because one often anticipates that increasing patient involvement in difficult decision making and imparting "bad news" regarding disease and its complications and outcome may adversely affect the patients. The authors concluded that: "Consistent with findings from the previous review, which had included studies up to 2006: decision aids increase people's involvement, and improve knowledge and realistic perception of outcomes; however, the size of the effect varies across studies. Decision aids have a variable effect on choices. They reduce the choice of discretionary surgery and have no apparent adverse effects on health outcomes or satisfaction" [10]. Similar results are available specifically in the cancer setting where a meta-analysis of 23 randomized controlled trials found that patients exposed to decision aids are more likely to participate in decision making and achieve higher quality decisions [15].

Guidance with End-of-Life Decisions

Many of the issues regarding the decision-making process come into sharper focus, at times with a sense of urgency, as the disease trajectory moves toward end of life. Such end-of-life (EOL) issues are of two overlapping categories: clinical and non-clinical. Clinical decisions that occur near the end of life further fall into two broad categories: decisions to use potentially life-prolonging treatments for emergency conditions such as respiratory failure or cardiac asystole (e.g., mechanical ventilation, CPR, ICU admission), and decisions for situations that are nonemergent and typically involve the use of treatment modalities that emphasize quality of life (e.g., opioid use for pain, palliative sedation, other "comfort care") [16]. The general goals of treatment focus on relative emphasis on life prolongation vis-à-vis preservation of quality of life. The specific areas of decision making may include:

1. Advance directives (what the patient does or does not want in terms of nature or location of treatment ["Living will"]; proxy or surrogate decision maker when the patient loses decisional capacity ["Durable power of attorney"])
2. Do not (attempt) resuscitation (DN(A)R) orders
3. Other life-sustaining therapies, such as mechanical ventilation; feeding tube or, in general, artificial nutrition and hydration; antibiotics; hemodialysis
4. Palliative care issues, such as management of pain and other symptoms; relief of psychological, social, spiritual, and existential suffering
5. Creating opportunity to address unfinished business [17]

Although a detailed discussion of all these issues is beyond the scope of this chapter, some general directions can be given regarding the guidance for complex choices in the EOL care setting. The basic principles discussed in the earlier sections all apply. Based on these, the following sections are focused particularly on guidance with EOL related decision making. The steps underlined below are not exactly discrete "steps" but rather represent a "flow" of sequences in waves that merge with one another.

The first step in providing such guidance is initiating the process. Clinical indications for discussing EOL care include (a) Urgent Indications, such as imminent death; talk about wanting to die; inquiries about hospice or palliative care; recently hospitalized for severe progressive illness; severe suffering and poor prognosis; and (b) Routine Indications, such as discussing prognosis; discussing treatment with low probability of success; discussing hopes and fears; physician would not be surprised if the patient died in 6–12 months [17]. The person ideally suited to initiate such discussions is the physician with a long-standing professional relationship with the patient. In the absence of such a relationship, a single physician should be designated to coordinate and communicate the medical aspects of each patient's overall care throughout his stay in a given facility, including disease-related and palliative care issues. This physician should encourage full participation by the entire team, including nurses, social workers, pharmacists, clergy, and family members, as desired by the patient, to maximize the development of a trusting context for subsequent decision making. The role of the MDT assumes paramount importance in this context.

The second step is assessment of the patient's needs and the values and goals. Physicians can help patients to make critical end-of-life decisions by first assessing the patient's current physical symptoms and psychological and spiritual needs, assessing family and social support system, estimating and communicating prognosis, and asking the patient to define his or her end-of-life goals. In one study, the five most important components of quality EOL care identified by patients were:

1. Adequate pain and symptom management
2. Avoiding inappropriate prolongation of dying
3. Achieving a sense of control
4. Relieving burden
5. Strengthening relationships with loved ones [18]

The third step is providing critical information to the patient and family. The physician needs to be truthful and clear, at the same time not appearing blunt, intimidating, or noncaring. Physicians need to avoid giving false hope of cure or of greater benefit than likely or expected. On the other hand, physicians should avoid painting the situation worse than it is in order to get the patient to decide what the physician feels to be in his/her best interests. Goal is to hope for the best course of illness or for best quality of life for the longest possible time but we need to plan for the worst or the unexpected.

The fourth step is advanced care planning. Advance care planning is a process whereby the patient, with the help of his/her health care providers, family members, and loved ones, makes decisions about his/her future medical care. Advance Care Planning involves discussion of the diagnosis, prognosis, the expected course of the illness and the possible treatment alternatives, their risks and benefits and should be placed in the context of the patient's goals, expectations, fears, values, and beliefs [19].

It must be remembered that care planning is a process and not a single event. The issues of advance directive, assessment of decisional capacity, appointment of surrogate decision maker in the later event of patient losing capacity, and such issues take time, and the patient (and family) may need time and support from the MDT or its members to resolve these issues.

The fifth step is decision making for specific situations likely to arise during EOL care, such as the need for mechanical ventilation, CPR, artificial nutrition and hydration, other life support measures, admission in ICU, and location of care in the final days of life. Several decision aids or decision support interventions discussed above specifically address these issues. The A–Z decision aids inventory of the

Ottawa Hospital Research Initiative (http://decisionaid.ohri.ca/AZlist.html), for example, mentions the following under the section "Guidance with End-of-Life Decisions" [9]:

- End-of-life care: Should I have artificial hydration and nutrition?
- End-of-life care: Should I receive CPR and life support?
- End-of-life care: Should I stop kidney dialysis?
- End-of-life care: Should I stop treatment that prolongs my life?
- Making choices: Long-term feeding tube placement in elderly patients
- Understanding the options: Planning care for critically ill patients in the intensive care unit
- When you need extra care, should you receive it at home or in a facility?

Another palliative care approach to aid decision making is a "time-limited trial (TLT)." "A TLT is an agreement between clinicians and a patient/family to use certain medical therapies over a defined period to see if the patient improves or deteriorates according to agreed-on clinical outcomes" [20]. Examples include: offering a time-limited trial of dialysis for patients with renal failure considering dialysis; mechanical ventilation for patients suffering from hypoxic ischemic encephalopathy, initial treatment of severe stroke and end-stage congestive heart failure; and dialysis/renal failure in presence of limited functional or cognitive status. If the patient improves, the therapy continues. If the patient deteriorates, the therapies involved in the trial are withdrawn, and goals frequently shift more purely to palliation. If significant clinical uncertainty remains, another TLT might be renegotiated. During such a trial, there are many opportunities for health care professionals to provide effective decision support. TLTs help establish mutual expectations, guidance, and a regular dialogue about how the patient is progressing, lessening the chance of conflict among treatment teams and the patient or family. Also, patients and families may see this as a "middle ground" to satisfy them that "everything possible" has been tried before "giving up."

Conclusion

Palliative care often involves making difficult choices for the patient, the family, and the treating team. As the disease progresses and the evidence of scientifically robust effective therapeutic options becomes less certain, decisions tend to become more preference sensitive, where the values, goals, and priorities of the patient (and the family) gain increasing importance. In such a situation, the shared decision-making model is more appropriate. The physician or the multidisciplinary team can provide guidance with complex decisions with the help of various decision support interventions, or decision aids, which help to clarify the patient's knowledge regarding the decisions to be taken vis-à-vis personal preferences and values.

References

1. Charles C, Gafni A, Whelan T. Shared decision making in the medical encounter: what does it mean? (Or, it takes at least two to tango). Soc Sci Med. 1997;44:681–92.
2. Charles C, Gafni A, Whelan T. Decision making in the physicianpatient encounter: revisiting the shared treatment decision making model. Soc Sci Med. 1999;49:651–61.
3. Charles C, Whelan T, Gafni A. What do we mean by partnership in making decisions about treatment? BMJ. 1999;319:780–2.
4. Bélanger E, Rodríguez C, Groleau D. Shared decision-making in palliative care: a systematic mixed studies review using narrative synthesis. Palliat Med. 2011;25:242–61.
5. Bakitas M, Kryworuchko J, Matlock DD, Volandes AE. Palliative medicine and decision science: the critical need for a shared agenda to foster informed patient choice in serious illness. J Palliat Med. 2011;14(10):1–8.
6. World Health Organization. WHO definition of palliative care. Geneva: WHO. http://www.who.int/cancer/palliative/definition/en/. Updated 24 Oct 2011; cited 25 Oct 2011
7. Devitt B, Philip J, McLachlan S-A. Team dynamics, decision making, and attitudes toward multidisciplinary cancer meetings: health professionals' perspectives. J Oncol Pract. 2010;6:e17–20.
8. Elwyn G, Frosch D, Volandes AE, Edwards A, Montori VM. Investing in deliberation: a definition and classification of decision support interventions for people facing difficult health decisions. Med Decis Making. 2010;30:701–11.
9. Ottawa Hospital Research Initiative. Patient decision aids. http://decisionaid.ohri.ca/. Updated 2011; cited 31 Oct 2011.
10. Stacey D, Bennett CL, Barry MJ, Col NF, Eden KB, Holmes-Rovner M, et al. Decision aids for people facing health treatment or screening decisions. Cochrane Database Syst Rev. 2011;(10):CD001431. doi:10.1002/14651858. CD001431.pub3.
11. Elwyn G, O'Connor A, Stacey D, Volk R, Edwards A, Coulter A, et al. Developing a quality criteria framework for patient decision aids: online international Delphi consensus process. BMJ. 2006;333:417–23.
12. O'Connor AM, Légaré F, Stacey D. Risk communication practice: the contribution of decision aids. BMJ. 2003;327:736–40.
13. O'Connor AM, Stacey D, Légaré F. Coaching to support patients in making decisions. BMJ. 2008;336:228–9.
14. DuBenske LL, Gustafson DH, Shaw BR, Cleary JF. Web-based cancer communication and decision making systems: connecting patients, caregivers, and clinicians for improved health outcomes. Med Decis Making. 2010;30:732–44.
15. Stacey D, Samant R, Bennett C. Decision making in oncology: a review of patient decision aids to support patient participation. CA Cancer J Clin. 2008;58:293–304.
16. Weissman DE. Decision making at a time of crisis near the end of life. JAMA. 2004;292:1738–43.
17. Quill TE. Initiating end-of-life discussions with seriously ill patients: addressing the "elephant in the room". JAMA. 2000;284:2502–7.
18. Singer PA, Martin DK, Kelner M. Quality end-of-life care: patient's perspectives. JAMA. 1999;281:163–8.
19. Hawryluck L, Wahl J. Ian Anderson Program in end-of-life care. Module 4: end-of-life decision-making. Toronto: University of Toronto; 2000.
20. Quill TE, Holloway R. Time-limited trials near the end of life. JAMA. 2011;306:1483–4.

Review Questions

1. The following statement is *not* true of the paternalistic model of decision making:

   (a) Patient autonomy is the dominating bioethical principle
   (b) The shared information is primarily medical in nature
   (c) The deliberation and decision making is one way (doctor)
   (d) There is no true partnership between doctor and patient

2. The following statement is *not* true of the informed choice model of decision making:

   (a) Patient autonomy is the dominating bioethical principle
   (b) The shared information is primarily medical in nature
   (c) The deliberation and decision making is one way (doctor)
   (d) There is no true partnership between doctor and patient

3. The following statement is *true* of the shared decision making (SDM) model:

   (a) Patient autonomy is the dominating bioethical principle
   (b) The shared information is primarily medical in nature
   (c) The deliberation and decision making is one way (doctor)
   (d) There is a true partnership between doctor and patient

4. In the "preference-sensitive" decisions, as opposed to "effectiveness-based" decisions:

   (a) There is no single "right" decision
   (b) The paternalistic model works best
   (c) The "preference" refers to the doctor, not the patient
   (d) Is more important in the early stage of disease rather than at end-of-life care

5. A preference-sensitive decision becomes more important in the context of:

   (a) Disease modifying treatment
   (b) End-of-life care
   (c) Evidence-based care
   (d) Diagnosis of cancer

6. For guidance with complex treatment choices in palliative care, the best model is:

   (a) Paternalistic model
   (b) Informed choice model
   (c) Shared decision-making model
   (d) None of the above

7. The various decision support interventions have been categorized into

    (a) 3 categories
    (b) 4 categories
    (c) 5 categories
    (d) 6 categories

8. The International Patient Decision Aids Standards (IPDAS) is concerned with:

    (a) Classifying the numerous decision aids into coherent categories
    (b) Formulating guidelines for decision aids
    (c) Establishing an internationally approved set of criteria to determine the quality of patient decision aids
    (d) All of the above

9. Decision coaches are:

    (a) Computer programs
    (b) Web-based applications
    (c) Resource materials
    (d) Human beings

10. Specific areas of decision making at the end of life may include any of these *except*:

    (a) Disease-modifying therapy
    (b) Advance directives
    (c) Do not (attempt) resuscitation (DN(A)R) orders
    (d) Management of pain and other symptoms

Answers

1. (a)
2. (c)
3. (d)
4. (a)
5. (b)
6. (c)
7. (a)
8. (c)
9. (d)
10. (a)

Chapter 7
Symptom Management

Angèle Ryan

Introduction

The definition of palliative care is subject to different interpretations by various groups and organizations. Services such as assistance with decision making, defining goals of care, and facilitating communication and continuity of care across diverse care settings are frequently promoted, but symptom management remains a prominent element of this type of care [1]. Indeed, untreated symptoms are what generate numerous hospital admissions, utilization of healthcare resources, and crisis referrals to palliative care teams. With control of physical symptoms, patients are better equipped to address other components of suffering.

Pain

The most dramatic and feared symptom in advanced disease is pain [2] and is a common stimulus for palliative care consultation [3]. It is estimated that up to 90% of patients with advanced cancer report pain [4–6], 40–50% with moderate to severe pain, and 25–30% with very severe pain [7]. This symptom has attracted much attention in the medical literature and public media. Much of this attention is a result of historical under treatment of this distressing accompaniment to illness.

A. Ryan, M.D. (✉)
Department of Anesthesiology, Keck School of Medicine,
University of Southern California,
Los Angeles, CA, USA
e-mail: angel@ix.netcom.com

N. Vadivelu et al. (eds.), *Essentials of Palliative Care*,
DOI 10.1007/978-1-4614-5164-8_7,
© Springer Science+Business Media New York 2013

Table 7.1 Drugs commonly used in pain management

Analgesics	Adjuvants
Nonopioids	Augment analgesia
• Acetaminophen	• Antidepressants
• Aspirin and other NSAID's	• Anticonvulsants
Opioids	• Muscle relaxants
Weak opioids	• Corticosteroids
• Codeine	Control side effects
• Hydrocodone	• Laxatives
Strong opioids	• Antiemetics
• Morphine	• Psychostimulants
• Hydromorphone	
• Fentanyl	
• Methadone	

Despite the consensus that most end of life pain can be managed by noninvasive tools available to most physicians [8–11] pain remains undertreated [12]. This is likely due to physicians' inexperience in the use of appropriate analgesics, accompanied by a unique fear of opioids from practitioners, patients, and families. This knowledge deficit causes a dilemma for physicians who wish to continue providing care for terminally ill patients while lacking the necessary confidence to provide the aggressive treatments required. A systematic approach to the use of pharmacological tools for the treatment of pain will allow successful control even in severe cases. Expertise from pain and palliative care physicians will supplement the management of routine problems by primary care providers.

The pharmacologic tools used for pain management consist of two general categories, analgesics and adjuvants (see Table 7.1). Analgesics are a familiar category for most practitioners, consisting of nonopioids and opioids. Adjuvants are medications often with labeled indications other than treatment of pain, but nonetheless useful as part of a comprehensive pain regimen. This adjuvant category is further classified into those agents that enhance analgesia by alternate mechanisms, and those medications that proactively treat anticipated side effects of the analgesic drugs, thus allowing for optimal dosing.

The World Health Organization (WHO) has provided guidelines for pain management specifically for cancer pain (see Fig. 7.1), based on the simple premise of choosing an analgesic based on patient self-report pain score, essentially matching the level of pain with the potency of the analgesic. The guidelines continue to provide directions for the use of these medications: by the mouth, around the clock, with attention to detail. The oral route is preferred for convenience, efficacy, and ease of administration across multiple care settings. Around the clock dosing provides uninterrupted analgesia for a chronic pain disease, and attention to detail requires a custom regimen for each patient.

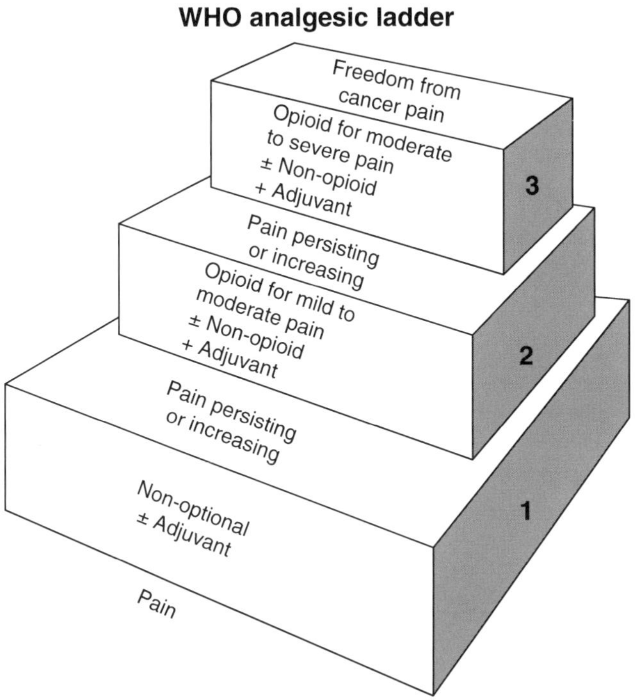

WHO analgesic ladder

Fig. 7.1 WHO analgesic ladder

Nonopioids

The nonsteroidal anti-inflammatory drugs (NSAIDs) provide a useful tool as part of comprehensive pain regimen in end-of-life care. Noncancer diagnoses may present with mild or moderate pain which responds to these medications. In more severe pain associated with cancer diagnosis, these medications provide coanalgesia with opioids via anti-inflammatory action [13], and are particularly potent for treating the pain of bone metastasis in cancer [14, 15], thus providing synergistic opioid sparing benefits.

Therapeutic effects arise from blockade of Type II cyclo-oxygenase (COX-II) enzymes that facilitate the formation of deleterious inflammatory products. The adverse effects of NSAIDs arise from the blockade of type I cyclo-oxygenase enzymes (COX-1) that are responsible for the formation of beneficial prostaglandins that are gastrointestinal, platelet, and renal protective. This results in gastropathy, disruption of platelet function, and renal impairment [16]. Congestive heart failure [17] and bronchospasm can occur in susceptible individuals. These undesirable effects may be minimized by use of prophylactic measures such as careful patient selection, co-treatment with gastrointestinal protecting agents such as proton pump inhibitors, and assuring adequate renal perfusion. Consideration may also be given to using a nonacetylated salicylate such as choline magnesium trisalicylate for GI and platelet sparing benefit [18]. Newly available selective COX-II inhibitors claim reduced toxicities and may be beneficial in high-risk patients. Individual tolerance to NSAIDs is variable, likely as a result of the unique relative degree of COX-1 vs. COX-II inhibition of each drug. Therefore, sequential trial of different agents is warranted if a patient does not tolerate an initial choice of NSAID. Although the majority of NSAIDs require oral route, new formulations are available via topical gel or transdermal route for patients who are not able to swallow. Ketorolac, generally recommended for short-term use only, has been successfully used via parenteral route for longer periods if other options are not feasible [19].

Acetaminophen, despite minimal anti-inflammatory effects, is beneficial in treating mild to moderate pain and should be considered for additional opioid sparing mechanism of action. It is felt to have centrally active effect [20]. Lacking the antiplatelet effect and GI toxicity associated with NSAIDs, it is a reasonable alternative to other nonopioids. Risk of hepatotoxicity in high doses limits use to 4 g daily. Dosing of all nonopioids is limited by end organ toxicities, producing a ceiling effect. This is not of concern when prescribing opioids.

Opioids

Cancer is the prototype end-of-life diagnosis that presents with the most significant pain treatment challenges. Opioids are the mainstay of treatment for this type of severe pain.

Much of the mystery for the average practitioner in providing pain therapies involves the escalation of medication to the category of pure opioids, step three in the WHO stepladder.

The class of medications categorized as weak opioids is often combined with a nonopioid. The toxicities of the nonopioid component of the formulation limit titration of the opioid component. For example, hydrocodone, an opioid frequently classified in conversion charts as equipotent to morphine, is only available in the US in combination with nonopioids, limiting dose escalation to optimal levels. Despite this limitation, practitioners' familiarity and comfort with these medications frequently result in continued use of step 2 medications when step 3 agents are indicated based on WHO stepladder guidelines. The narrow dose ranges of these combination drugs, with clearly defined upper limits, promote physician comfort and continued use of these medications despite lack of efficacy in more severe pain. Mixed agonist/antagonists such as nalbuphine or butorphanol, are also not recommended due to their ceiling effect, risk of psychotomimetic side effects, and potential to provoke a withdrawal reaction when given to opioid tolerant individuals [21].

If good pain control is to be achieved, the practitioner must quickly move past the familiar comfort zone and use pure opioids. It is often at this stage of a patient's disease, when pain levels exceed the level that can be controlled with nonopioids and weak opioids, that expert consultation is requested. In many communities,

Table 7.2 Conversion table for common opioid medications based on Morphine 10 mg intravenous as standard for comparison[b]

Original drug	Oral route dose (mg)	Intravenous route dose (mg)
Morphine	30	10
Hydromorphone	7.5	1.5
Methadone[a]	20	10
Oxycodone	20	n/a
Hydrocodone	30	n/a
Oxymorphone	10	1

[a]Based on single dose
[b]Aloysi AS, Bryson EO (2012) Prescription drugs: implications for the chronic pain patient. New York: Springer

however, if this resource is not available, the practitioner can use a methodical approach to the use of opioids. The unique trait of opioids in lacking toxic effects on end organs allows the prescriber to customize the analgesic regimen to the patient's precise needs. Thus, the feature of opioids that cause initial discomfort for the prescriber also allows unlimited range in dosing (see Table 7.2). The dose is only limited by physiologic side effects, which are frequently transient and manageable. The following is a systematic plan for initiating and managing the use of opioids.

Let us take the example of the patient who has experienced only mild to moderate pain, managed by combination drugs according to step one and step two of the ladder, but are no longer effective despite maximum recommended dosing. The first step to continue pain control for this patient is to uncouple the opioid and nonopioid of this compound drug and initiate dose titration with a pure opioid. Conversion to an opioid alone allows self-titration by the patient to a satisfactory level of relief unencumbered by a dose limited nonopioid. The initial dose may remain conservative. A conversion to 5 mg. oral morphine is not a significant deviation from the previously administered medication either in dose or duration of action, providing reasonable assurance that the medication will be tolerated without side effects. The use of an immediate short acting agent allows for rapid and frequent dose change based on efficacy. Dose finding may be achieved by increases of 5 mg increments until effective. This technique duplicates the more familiar intravenous patient controlled analgesia (PCA) method, applying the same titration principles using oral route instead [22]. Self-titration by the patient provides his own pain relief, and defines for the prescriber the dose required to achieve 24-h analgesia. After several days of patient self-titration, the provider now has accurate information for conversion to sustained action formulations (see Table 7.3). During this time it is essential to stress upon the patient that this cycle of frequent medicating is merely a trial period of dose finding and titration that will ultimately be replaced by a more palatable

Table 7.3 Systematic titration of opioid doses

1. Uncouple nonopioid and opioid compound drug
2. Start short acting pure opioid in frequent intervals to allow self-titration. Adjust dose as needed and tolerated
3. Allow patient to self-titrate to comfort
• Provide assurance that frequent medicating schedule is temporary intended for dose finding only
• Aggressive treatment and education about side effects
• Education regarding misconceptions and fear of opioids
4. Conversion of cumulative 24-h dose to sustained acting formulation
5. Provide short acting rescue medication equal to 5–15% of baseline opioid
6. Consider appropriate adjuvants for opioid sparing benefits
7. Monitor and maintenance for ongoing titration

dosing schedule. Education and aggressive treatment of anticipated transient side effects are an essential element in assuring patient compliance and acceptance of opioid therapy. Misconceptions regarding this class of medications are common and may compromise therapy if not addressed.

Once a stable 24-h dose is established by the patient, the provider can convert the total dose to the convenient long-acting formulations generally administered every 12 h. For example, if the patient self-administered a total of 210 mg oral morphine in a 24-h period, this may translate to 100 mg every 12 h of long acting morphine to provide continuous baseline analgesia. Titration continues in this manner until pain control is achieved. Astute monitoring of patient self-dosing will allow timely adjustments in the regimen. Judicious incremental increases in opioid dosing will prevent uncontrolled pain exacerbations while allowing gradual tolerance to side effects to develop [20].

Breakthrough Pain

Initiating a long acting opioid to provide 24-h analgesic coverage does not preclude the continued use of a short-acting agent. This provides rescue treatment for incidents of pain that breaks through the analgesia provided by the long acting agent and allows for continued titration. In general, this is approximately 5–15% of the 24-h dose [23].

Once the pain is stable on a regimen of this sort, it is essential to continue to monitor the use of rescue medications. An acceptable level is no more than 3–4 doses of short acting agents in a 24-h period [6]. The increased use of rescue medications signals increasing pain levels and warns of an imminent loss of pain control. A pain crisis, and unnecessary hospital admission, can be avoided by a timely increase in the baseline long acting opioid. The increase is estimated as originally calculated in the original titration. That is, to add all the doses of opioid in a 24-h period, convert to a new baseline dose, and provide the proportionally appropriate dose of the short acting opioid for rescue. This process can be applied at any time that pain is not controlled and analgesic use escalates. If pain is well controlled, or adverse effects are present, and no rescue doses are used, a trial of reduced baseline dosing is justified.

Pain Emergencies and the Emergency Department

In end-of-life care, visits to emergency departments for treatment of uncontrolled pain frequently generate a hospital admission. With judicious application of titration principles, this can be avoided, and what is considered a dire situation may be resolved in as quickly as 90 min using intravenous route [24]. The successful achievement of pain control using rapid titration under the guidance of the practitioner allows the patient to experience first hand the efficacy of opioids while avoiding the dreaded side effects. This promotes patient confidence for continued self-titration and long-term control of pain.

Side Effects

The adverse effect endpoint of opioids is defined by physiologic limits rather than by end organ toxicity. Generally all opioids in equianalgesic doses produce the same side effects, exerting greatest pharmacologic action on the central nervous system and gastrointestinal system. Addressing these side effects proactively and aggressively will assist greatly in promoting patient adherence to the prescribed opioid regimen. It is important to stress upon the patient that the typical opioid side effects that frighten patients, the mental clouding and nausea and vomiting, are short lived and treatable [25]. Tolerance develops within several days to these side effects [26]. The side effect that frightens providers is respiratory depression. Although serious, it is generally rare, occurring in less than 2% of appropriate opioid applications. Additionally, tolerance to this side effect occurs rapidly [27]. Of significant note, the one side effect to which tolerance develops extremely slowly if at all is constipation. This distressing symptom is predictable and treatment must be initiated concurrent with opioid therapy. Less common side effects include urinary retention, generally more a problem with spinal route than with oral or parenteral routes, and myoclonus which occurs as a result of accumulation of metabolic by-products when high doses of morphine are used.

In the event that the therapeutic window between adequate analgesia and unacceptable side effects is excessively narrow, rotation to an alternate agent is indicated. The basis for this technique is the variable affinities of the individual opioids for the different opioid receptors in the central nervous system. A new opioid provides analgesia by binding to different receptors while toxic metabolites of the previous opioid dissipate. This provides increased effect without the burdens of dose escalation [28]. In fact, in stable pain conditions, reduction of opioid equivalent dose is typically indicated. A general rule is 25–50% reduction of the calculated equianalgesic dose of the new opioid [20, 29]. Another option is rotation of the short acting rescue drug. Titration principles continue to apply to the new medications. Typical alternatives to sustained release morphine include sustained release oxycodone or hydromorphone, or fentanyl patch. There are numerous equianalgesic tables available, and they provide a guideline for opioid dosing. The choice of conversion mathematics is secondary to the judicious monitoring of patient response. A word of caution, patients and families may confuse initial side effects with allergic reaction. Timely education will prevent unnecessary labels of "allergies" that may compromise later treatments.

Meperidine is not indicated for long-term treatment of pain due to its short half life, low bioavailability, and accumulation of neurotoxic metabolites [20].

Caution is advised if methadone is considered for opioid rotation. Despite benefits of high potency, long duration of action, cost effectiveness, and absence of metabolites, this drug possesses characteristics that make it problematic for routine use [30], such as drug interactions, variability of half life, and prolongation of QT interval on electrocardiogram. The most significant concern with methadone, however, is the nonlinear conversion ratio with other opioids which produces greater potency at higher levels of opioid tolerance. Although this feature allows an effective rotation in highly tolerant individuals (e.g., greater than 1,000 mg oral morphine daily), it may also result in overdose due to effect on NMDA receptors and significant reduction of tolerance. If rotation to methadone is considered, expert consultation is recommended.

Adjuvants

The complexity of severe pain provides a challenge to the practitioner seeking a practical treatment plan. The various components of pain do not all respond to the familiar analgesics in medical practice, including the strong opioids. Drugs generally labeled for other indications have been found to provide benefit in these conditions.

The most common indication for the use of adjuvants is the presence of a neuropathic component of pain. This pain is caused by damage and pathologic hyperexcitability of nerve issue, either by physical injury or by disease process, and results in anatomical, physiological, and functional distortion of normal pain pathways. Pain is generally described as burning, shooting, and pins and needles. Classic examples are diabetic neuropathy and postherpetic neuralgia. This pain is less responsive to opioids than nociceptive pain which results from injury to peripheral tissue. The two major classes of medication that treat this pain are antidepressants and anticonvulsants.

Antidepressants

Some psychotropic medications have been shown to be effective in the treatment of some pain chronic pain syndromes, not only for treatment of concurrent emotional components of pain such as anxiety or depression, but also for their analgesic enhancing properties when a neuropathic component of pain is suspected. One of the first adjuvants considered in such circumstances is an antidepressant medication. The most studied agent for this indication is amitriptyline, a tricyclic antidepressant (TCA). The role of TCAs in the management of neuropathic pain is well established [31, 32]. The mechanism of analgesia is a nonspecific inhibition on the reuptake of norepinephrine and serotonin, providing analgesia in doses lower than the antidepressant doses. This drug, however, is associated with adverse effects which include cardiotoxity, such as conduction disorders and arrhythmias, orthostatic hypotension, somnolence, and altered mentation, particularly in patients with previous dementia, brain metastasis, or concurrent use of other centrally acting drugs. The anticholinergic side effects such as urinary retention, constipation, dry mouth, and blurred vision also can add to the symptom burden. Other agents of this category, such as nortriptyline or desipramine, although less studied, may be better tolerated.

The selective serotonin reuptake inhibitors (SSRIs) have not been shown to be sufficiently effective in the treatment of neuropathic pain to justify their use over tricyclics.

Serotonin norepinephrine reuptake inhibitors (SNRIs) are a newer class of medications that offer promise. The commonly used agents in this category are venlafaxine and duloxetine.

Anticonvulsants

Traditionally, the use of anticonvulsant agents such as carbemazepine and phentoin for treatment of lancinating pain of neuropathic origin has been based on these agents' presumed effect on neural hyperexcitability [33]. Despite the benefits, high incidence of side effects with these drugs led to a preference for newer agents. Gabapentin is a current popular choice with a pharmacological profile that offers a relatively high degree of safety, including no hepatic metabolism, and no drug–drug interaction. Mechanism of action is believed to be action on GABA receptors. If an anticonvulsant is considered, gabapentin is a logical first-line choice due to its efficacy in treating pain of neuropathic origin in cancer patients [34, 35]. The most common adverse effect from gabapentin is sedation, which may be a benefit if the patient also experiences insomnia. Daytime sedation may be minimized by slow upward titration to effect. Doses up to 3,600 mg daily have been reported [36]. Although gabapentin is generally well tolerated, it may be necessary to consider an alternate agent in some patients. Clonazepam [37] or pregabalin [38] offer additional options.

NMDA Antagonists

N-methyl-D-aspartate (NMDA) receptors are located on the second order neurons in the dorsal horn of the spinal cord. They are generally dormant and only activated after repeated stimulation by nociceptive input from peripheral tissues. This excitation is believed to be involved in the development of neuropathic pain and tolerance to opioids. NMDA antagonists offer promise in treating neuropathic pain as these medications directly target this specific trigger. A trial of currently available agents in this category, despite limited practical application, may offer benefit.

The anti-NMDA effect of dextromethorphan, the popular ingredient in numerous cough medicines, has attracted attention for the additional indication of analgesia. The higher doses required for pain indication, however, are associated with unacceptable side effects consisting of nausea, vomiting, mental clouding, and dizziness and therefore limit its usefulness [39].

Ketamine is a dissociative anesthetic with analgesic properties in subanesthetic doses. Although psychotomimetic effects are seen when used in anesthetic doses, this is less common in the low doses used for pain control. The low risk of respiratory depression from ketamine coupled with the significant opioid sparing effect results in an improved balance between analgesia and side effects. Creative use of oral route using parenteral solution has been used and generally well tolerated in doses of 10–25 mg up to qid with upward titration up to 500 mg daily [40]. Sublingual route is also an option if compromised swallowing is present. Continuous subcutaneous or intravenous infusions in combination with other agents have been used in cases of refractory pain with good results [41–43]. Doses may start at 1–2.5 mg/kg/24 h with upward titration as needed. Infusions as high as 600 mg/day have been reported without untoward effects [44] and effective for long-term use [45]. The addition of benzodiazepines or haloperidol may attenuate psychotomimetic effects that may occur at high doses [39].

Nonspecific Adjuvants

Corticosteroids

There is evidence that corticosteroids are beneficial in reducing pain [46–48]. Mechanism of action of corticosteroids is unknown, but may include reduction of peritumor edema and decompression on pain sensitive structures, in steroid responsive neoplasms, reduction of tumor mass themselves, reduction of inflammatory mediators, specifically prostaglandins and leukotrienes, tempering of aberrant electrical activity in damaged nerves. Like NSAIDs they are beneficial for bone metastasis. The side effects of corticosteroids, such as gastrointestinal disturbances, fluid retention, osteoporosis, hypertension, neuropsychological effects, and myopathy, are well known and physicians are wary of using these medications, but in the palliative care setting, long-term treatment with relatively low doses is generally well tolerated and often provides symptom relief that outweighs the burdens. For short-term use, doses as high as 100 mg daily may be necessary for control of acute episodes of pain such as that arising from superior vena cava syndrome or spinal cord compression [49].

Intravenous infusion of lidocaine, a sodium channel blocker, has been shown to be effective for several pain situations, but most notably for neuropathic pain [50, 51]. Oral agents originally intended for cardiac arrhythmias have played a role in pain management but their use has been curbed by high incidence of side effects, most notably nausea. A more practical application of this mode is likely the local anesthetic patch of lidocaine.

Biphosphonates are commonly used for disease-modifying treatments of bone metastases. In addition, they have efficacy in modulation of pain [52] and prevention of fractures.

Radiotherapy has particular benefit in providing relief of pain caused by bone metastases [53, 54], compression of neural structures [55], obstruction, and cerebral metastases [56]. Surgical interventions are justified for debulking, venting. The role of chemotherapy is less defined but there are promising agents that offer symptom relief as well as life-prolonging benefit. Examples include gefitinib [57] and gemcitabine [58].

GI Symptoms

Xerostoma

Dry mouth is a common complaint in advanced disease and predisposes a patient to more distressing symptoms such as ulceration, infections, and compromised ingestion of food and drink, leading to worsening of anorexia, nutritional deficiencies, and weight loss. The ability to take nourishment is a strong emotional need for many patients and families and is associated with fundamental well-being. As with most symptoms afflicting patients in end of life, the causes are multiple and all potentially treatable causes should be addressed. Commonly, this distressing condition may be the result of treatments such as radiotherapy, medications, or dehydration. Direct insult to oral mucosa may arise from disease-modifying chemotherapy as well.

Management consists of stimulation of natural saliva by mechanical chewing or sucking on gum or sugarless candy, by a cholinergic stimulant such as pilocarpine, or several saliva substitutes available [59].

Nausea and Vomiting

Despite the prevalence of this symptom and the current knowledge regarding receptor-specific therapies, it remains undertreated [60], and the prescribing of

Table 7.4 Antiemetic choices

Clinical clue	Site of action	Drug class	Example
Serum toxins (chemo-therapy, opioids) Tumor toxins Hypercalcemia, uremia	Dopaminic Seratonergic Chemoreceptor trigger zone	Antidopamine Antiseratonin	Prochlorperazine 10 mg po or 25 mg rectal suppository q. 6 h as needed Haloperidol 0.5–2 mg po q 6 h prn Ondansetron 8mg po bid-tid
Bowel distention	Cholinergic Vomiting center	Anticholinergic	Scopolamine up to 3 patches q. 3 days
Dizziness	Histaminic Inner ear	Antihistamine	Promethazine 12.5–25 mg q. 4–6 h Cyclizine
Increased intracranial pressure	Cerebral cortex	Corticosteroid	Dexamethasone 2–4 mg po daily
Emotional factors pain, fear Anticipatory nausea	Higher brain center	Benzodiazepine	Lorazepam 0.5–1 mg po or iv q. 6 h as needed

antiemetics is often sporadic, possibly limited by formulary and third party payer restrictions. With known knowledge about the mechanisms for nausea and vomiting, successful control of this unpleasant symptom is readily attainable when the inciting factor is known (e.g., chemotherapy, radiation therapy) [61, 62]. In advanced disease, however, when treating a patient in the absence of clearly identifiable etiologies, a logical approach based on clinical response is indicated, a technique not unlike the titration of pain medications (see Table 7.4).

A clinical systematic approach is suggested [63]:

1. Make a best educated guess regarding etiology.
2. Choose most likely neurotransmitter and receptors responsible.
3. Provide antiemetic most likely to counteract the responsible cause by route that will be absorbed.
4. Encourage pt. to self-titrate to relief.
5. Reassess for efficacy. If partially effective, provide ATC.
6. Add second agent with new mechanism for as needed use for "breakthrough" nausea.
7. Continue in this manner with subsequent agents for optimal coverage of all mechanisms.

Inoperable bowel obstruction.

This unique etiology of nausea and vomiting is often encountered in end-of-life care. In general practice, the occurrence of this complication typically initiates plans for gastric decompression, hydration, and immediate surgical correction. This may not be a realistic solution if the patient has advanced disease [64]. A patient is deemed to have a poor prognosis if intraabdominal carcinomatosis, ascites is present, and the patient has poor performance status. In such a case, the recommendation is for pharmacologic treatment of symptoms instead. Insertion of a nasogastric tube is indicated only for temporary use for emergency gastric decompression, with percutaneous gastrostomy tube as the preferred method for venting. There is ample support in the literature for the benefit of pharmacologic treatments for inoperable bowel obstruction [65–67]. The goal of treatment is to alleviate the symptoms caused by the sequence of increased gastric secretions, distention of bowel, and motor activity against obstruction, specifically pain and nausea and vomiting. A classic triad of treatments is described:

1. Morphine for pain, doses titrated to patient needs
2. Haloperidol for nausea, 2–4 mg daily orally, sublingually, or parenterally
3. Somatostatin for reduction of secretions and motility, starting at 200–600 mcg subcutaneously in divided doses

The addition of corticosteroid may alleviate periluminal edema. This pharmacologic regimen can be effective in controlling symptoms but may also correct the obstruction and permitting oral intake [68].

Constipation

Patients approaching end of life often require medications with constipating side effects, most notably opioids, although other medications and other illness factors may contribute to this common symptom. Stool softeners are often prescribed as monotherapy for constipation when opioid therapy is initiated, but this is inadequate as a softener alone does not adequately treat the compromised peristalsis, that occurs in the severely ill patient [69] (see Table 7.5). An effective first-line therapy is the combination of softener and stimulant. If necessary, an osmotic agent provides more stimulation by increasing the fluid content of stool. The addition of lubricant laxatives will provide easier evacuation. Bulking agents containing indigestible fiber require substantial fluid intake which may be difficult in the seriously ill patient and should be avoided in this patient population. In addition, immobility and gastrointestinal effects of medications compound this problem and this class of laxative should be avoided in this patient population. The traditional opioid receptor antagonists such as naloxone have been used in oral form for treatment of refractory constipation with some success, but the potential for analgesia reversal limits the usefulness of these agents. The recent introduction of peripherally active opioid receptor antagonists that do not cross the blood–brain barrier represents a promising new mechanism for treatment of opioid-induced constipation without compromise of analgesic effect [70]. The currently available parenteral formulation of methylnaltrexone offers a unique solution for patients unable to tolerate oral intake, filling a void in current palliative medicine formulary where most bowel preparations require oral or rectal route.

Table 7.5 Bowel regimen

General measures
Hydration
Diet
Exercise
Stool softener
Docusate sodium 100–300 mg po daily
Stimulants
Senna 2 tabs (17 mg) qd up to 4 tabs bid
Bisacotyl 5 mg po or 10 mg pr
Cascara 325 mg po
Magnesium citrate 240 ml po
Milk of magnesium 15–30 ml po
Serotonin agonists prokinetic agents
Metaclopramide 10 mg AC and HS
Osmotic agent
Lactulose 15–30 ml po qd-tid
Sorbitol 15–30 ml po qd-tid
Lubricants
Mineral oil
Opioid receptor blockers
Methylnaltrexone 8–12 mg qod based on weight administered subcutaneously
Enemas, suppositories

Cachexia Syndrome and Fatigue

Cachexia is a significantly distressing and most commonly encountered symptom in advanced disease. Weakness and fatigue are predominant features of this syndrome and is reported as the most troublesome and most common symptom in palliative care patients [71]. The insidious nature of this disturbance in a patient's function often makes it secondary to more dramatic symptoms such as pain. It is not the sort of symptom that generates emergency visits or hospitalizations, and yet it compromises a patient's sense of self in a profound manner.

Cachexia is defined by the group of symptoms consisting of fatigue, asthenia, anorexia, muscle wasting, and weight loss [72]. It is essential to remember and provide education for patients and family that anorexia is a component of the syndrome, and not the cause. It is important to stress that availability of nutrients is not the culprit, but rather the reduced assimilation of those nutrients caused by the underlying disease. Cachexia is a systemic inflammatory response that is caused by host generated cytokines and tumor factors that detrimentally alter carbohydrate, lipid, and protein metabolism. Tumor toxins and cytokines from immune system cause deleterious effects, increase skeletal muscle catabolism, decrease skeletal muscle synthesis, and decrease glycogen and lipid stores. A common misconception is that lack of nutrients is the culprit in this condition which leads to the initiation

Table 7.6 Reversible causes for cachexia

Mouth pain, compromised swallowing
Oral hygiene
Address mouth lesions and xerostoma
Dyspepsia, gastroparesis
Coating agents—carafate 1 g suspension
Proton pump inhibitors, antacids
Prokinetic agents
Relief of nausea and vomiting, constipation
Pain and other physical symptoms affecting appetite and interest in food
Emotional distressing
Anger, stress, depression, anxiety
Treatment of comorbidities
Anemia
dehydration
Infections
Insomnia
Beneficial medications for cachexia and fatigue
Prokinetic agents
Metaclopramide 10 mg AC and HS
Appetite stimulants
Megasterol up to 800 mg daily
Corticosteroids
Dexamethasone 4 mg qd-qid
Psychostimulants [77]
Methylphenidate 2.5–5 mg qd-bid prior to noon
Dextroamphetamine 2.5–5 mg in AM
Modafinil 100–400 mg in AM
Armodafinil 150–250 mg in AM
Antidepressants
Mirtazepine 15–45 mg daily
Thalidamide
Tetrohydrocannabinol (THC) 2.5 mg tid
Melatonin dose variable
Eicosapentaenoic acid, NSAIDs

of artificial nutrition. Although optimal nutritional status leads to improved benefit from disease-modifying therapies, it is not always indicated and may often lead to side effects more burdensome than beneficial. In 1989, the American College of Physicians issued a position paper refuting the wisdom of artificial feeding in severe disease [73]. Therefore when contemplating artificial nutrition, it is of paramount importance to weigh benefits and burdens of what is a medically invasive treatment. As with all symptoms, management begins with aggressive treatment of underlying factors that contribute to the compromised nutritional state (see Table 7.6). Starting with the oral cavity, efforts to treat bacterial, viral, and fungal infections as well as ulcerations will ease any discomfort of oral ingestion. Antacids, prokinetic drugs, and coating preparations will provide relief of dyspepsia and early satiety. An aggressive antiemetic regimen may be necessary to control nausea and vomiting, as well as a solid bowel regimen to address constipation. Control of any other physical or emotional symptoms will improve sense of well-being and promote increased appetite.

Depending on the prognosis, more aggressive measures may prove beneficial. Appetite stimulants are indicated if life expectancy is estimated to be 3 months or more and should be initiated early in the course of the disease to allow for desired effect. Weight gain may not be achieved, but improvement of appetite will contribute to sense of well-being and quality of life. Megastrol acetate in doses 160–800 mg daily may be helpful. In cases with shorter prognosis, a course of corticosteroid is useful for a state of well-being as well as addressing other symptoms that may be present, such as nausea, vomiting, pain, respiratory distress. Dexamethasone 10–20 mg daily is preferred for reduced mineralocorticoid activity. Mirtazepine is a promising agent for treatment of cachexia and improved quality of life [74]. Additional benefits of this medication are improved sleep and appetite, reduced nausea, and antidepressant effect. There are reports of the therapeutic benefits attained with medical marijuana for improvement in appetite and relief of nausea and vomiting [75, 76]. Psychostimulants such as methylphenidate [77] may be helpful in treating fatigue, as well as associated depression, sedation, and concentration [78]. Modafinil, a nonamphetamine psychostimulant, combats fatigue and depression by an alternate mechanism of action on the hypothalamus [79]. Armodafinil, a newer addition to the market, is composed of the active isomer of the racemic mixture of modafinil.

There are additional medications that offer promise. Thalidomide, despite the historical baggage as a teratogenic agent associated with its use as an antiemetic, is an agent currently receiving attention for its anti-inflammatory antitumor effects for treatment of some cancers, most notably multiple myeloma [80] but has also made an impression in the palliative medicine literature for treatment of multiple symptoms [81]. Administered at bedtime, the sedating side effects contribute to improved sleep and relief of nausea in cancer patients [82], there is evidence that this agent offers promise for weight gain and sense of well-being in AIDS patients [83]. The most significant side effects include deep vein thrombosis and neuropathy, but the short-term low dose regimen applied in end-of-life care may provide a favorable benefit/burden result. Melatonin, a naturally occurring hormone, is gaining attention, not only for its sleep-inducing properties, but also for benefit in cachexia [84]. Promising agents that target the inflammatory nature of cachexins include omega 3 fatty acids, particularly eicosapentaenoic acid and nonsteroidal anti-inflammatory drugs [85–87]. The continued quest for agents to promote appetite stimulation and well-being underscores the principles of aggressive treatment of symptoms even in the face of limited disease-modifying options.

Dyspnea

One of the prevailing mantras of palliative medicine is the assertive use of disease-modifying treatments as a means of treating symptoms, and there are few symptoms that exemplify this concept as dramatically as dyspnea. Dyspnea is defined as the subjective sensation of difficulty breathing, not necessarily with

Table 7.7 Treatment of reversible causes of dyspnea

Examples of reversible causes of dyspnea	Treatment options
Cancer tumor invasion of lungs, bronchi, lymphangitis carcinomatosis, pleural effusions	Radiation, surgical debulking corticosteroids, stenting, chemotherapy
Cardiopulmonary disease	Bronchodilators, corticosteroids, cardiac strengthening drugs, diuretics
Anemia, fatigue, electrolyte abnormalities	Transfusions, optimal nutritional support
Infections	Antimicrobial therapies
Pleural effusions, ascites	Aspiration, pleurodesis
Pulmonary embolism	Anticoagulants
Pain	Analgesic regimen

correlation to observed signs such as respiratory rate or arterial oxygenation. Diagnosis is made by patient self-report. It occurs in up to 90% of terminally ill patients with cancer, pulmonary disease, or cardiac disease [88, 89]. Although the mechanisms regulating respiration are known, this distressing symptom brings therapeutic challenges, as the causes are multifactoral and the physical sensation is frequently accompanied by patient perceptions and emotions, much like the experience of pain, and is often interpreted as the harbinger of decline by patients and families [90].

The numerous causes for dyspnea provide an extensive source of treatment options based on the underlying pathology (see Table 7.7). Even slight improvements of physiological components may bring significant relief and all therapies should be considered regardless of disease stage or prognosis at the time of presentation.

Despite the medical efforts to reverse underlying pathology, there will be a point where disease has progressed to advanced stage with increasing resistance to curative measures. As dyspnea is a symptom with physical, emotional, and spiritual components, an interdisciplinary treatment plan that addresses all these components will likely produce the most successful result. Education and advice regarding activity adjustments, positioning, cool air, psychological support are simple initial methods. Counselors on palliative care teams can play a significant role in addressing nonphysical components of the dyspneic experience, providing coping tools and anxiety reduction training that will empower patients with control over the dyspnea. Caregivers who observe what appears to be signs of distress require attention and explanations to ease anxiety. It is important to provide reassurance that the patient's sensation of dyspnea does not necessarily correspond to distress as is perceived by observers [91].

Although the pathophysiology of dyspnea is not fully understood, there are empirical therapies that have been effective. The mainstay of pharmacologic treatment is systemic opioid. Mechanism is not entirely known but theories suggest both central and peripheral activity. There is a good body of evidence to support this therapy which is beneficial and well tolerated in patients with cancer and pulmonary disease [92–94] and is considered a first-line therapy. Optimal dosing is achieved by titration to patient response. In opioid naive patients with mild symptoms, weak opioids such as hydrocodone or codeine may provide relief. In more severe cases, a strong opioid such as morphine is the rational choice. A low dose of 5 mg orally every 4 h is a reasonable initial dose with titration as needed to provide relief. In patients who are opioid tolerant as a result of an analgesic regimen, an increase in baseline dose of 25–50% may be indicated for antidyspneic effect.

As emotional factors may play a role in patient's perception of respiratory discomfort, anxiolytics have been shown to provide additional benefit in patients with COPD [95]. Oral Lorazepam or diazepam may be provided as needed, in combination with haloperidol if fear is present. Midazolam is a parenteral option if respite sedation is needed for severe breathlessness [96]. Corticosteroids are often used for treatment of specific pathology such as COPD, but for empirical treatment of dyspnea, may provide a broad spectrum of effects through reduced edema and for sense of well-being. Dexamethasone is a popular choice in palliative medicine due to the lower mineralocorticoid activity. Concerns regarding the well-known side effects are weighed against the comfort benefit in a terminally ill individual. While oxygen is a valid treatment of reversible hypoxemia, the value in treating dyspnea empirically is less clear. Patients and families view the administration of oxygen as a potent symbol of medical intervention and, as such, this treatment may exert a strong influence on the psychological components of dyspnea. The flow or air may be the factor that is providing the relief and should be considered. Simple apparatus should be used to avoid the cumbersome and intrusive mask devices. Careful patient selection will identify individual who will derive benefits from oxygen therapy, and the advantages must be weighed against the unfavorable burdens of cost, fire hazard, psychological dependence, and equipment constraints [97]. Nebulized medications such as morphine [98, 99] hydromorphone [100] have been reported to be effective in certain cases, but there is insufficient evidence to justify this route.

In extreme cases of dyspnea, it may be necessary to provide sedation for relief of the distress. At this point the principles of Double Effect would dictate continued titration of medications to desired effect.

Cough

Cough is often a debilitating symptom that contributes to worsening of other symptoms such as increased pain episodes, provoking vomiting, anxiety, and insomnia. As in all symptoms in end-of-life care identification of the underlying cause will dictate initial therapy. The causes of cough parallel the pathology in dyspnea and include primary pulmonary or cardiac disease, irritation from infections, obstructions, or tumor invasion. It may be productive or nonproductive. In addition to definitive disease-modifying treatments of underlying causes, there are general measures that may be helpful.

Cough suppressants are an initial treatment that may abate an irritating dry cough. Opioids are the most potent cough suppressants and offer first-line therapy. A weak agent such as codeine is a logical first choice in opioid naive patients. Hydrocodone has been shown to have a positive effect in treating cough when used as a single agent, or when added to an ineffective opioid regimen, suggesting a specific antitussive action when compared to other opioids and offers additional benefit for dyspnea, which may often be a coexisting symptom [101]. In general, however, if a patient is currently treated with opioids for pain, it is prudent to simplify the regimen and remain with the same agent using upward titration of 20–25% [102], similar to the process described for dyspnea. Expectorants are frequently used with benefit if liquification of sputum is desired and the patient has strength to expectorate. In debilitated patients, however, preferential use of cough suppressants is indicated.

Dextromethorphan, a centrally acting opioid derivative, has long been used as an antitussive agent and provides an alternative to opioids as it is not associated with the adverse mental clouding and gastrointestinal effects of opioids. Benzonatate, also a nonopioid has been shown to be of benefit [103]. Humidified air, nebulized saline, and chest physiotherapy can be used to supplement pharmacologic treatments.

Delirium

Delirium is a common occurrence in end of life and represents a poor prognostic sign. It is caused by a medical condition and characterized by a fluctuating course of:

1. Disturbance of consciousness manifested by detached awareness of environment and difficulty maintaining or shifting attention.
2. Cognitive impairment, manifested by disorientation, memory deficit, perceptual disturbances.

Subtypes of delirium are categorized as hyperactive, hypoactive, or mixed, a combination of both hyperactive and hypoactive types. Despite the prevalence of this symptom toward the end of life, this is a symptom that is often undertreated [104, 105]. The reasons for underrecognition are several. Although an agitated hyperactive patient presents the most familiar picture and draws rapid attention from care providers, the hypoactive or mixed type may elude diagnosis, as these less disruptive symptoms receive less notice and may be confused with depression, withdrawal, anxiety, or pain behaviors and may be missed by casual observation up to 50% of cases [106]. The fluctuating nature of delirium and periods of lucidity further compound the diagnostic insight. All subtypes of delirium have the potential of being distressing for the patient. Decision to delay treatment of delirium empirically may be made based on perceived degree or lack of distress, such as a pleasant vision of a previously deceased relative or friend. Although this experience is not uncommon during terminal stages of life, the variable course of this symptom dictates judicious monitoring for rapid development of a more disturbing experience. Therefore, any patient who presents with new onset of changes in behavior, perception, or function should be screened for delirium to assure prompt treatment.

In management of delirium, as with all symptoms, efforts should be made to assess for reversible causes, with appropriate diagnostic tests as tolerated by patient's condition (see Table 7.8). With advanced disease, however, multiple factors may play a role and treatable etiology may not be found. In less than 50% of cases it is

Table 7.8 Common causes of delirium

Drug or poison intoxication
  Opioids
  Sedatives and hypnotics
  Substance withdrawal
  Chemotherapy agents
  Corticosteroids
Metabolic disturbances
  Encephalopathies
    Hepatic
    Renal
  Hypoxemia
  Electrolyte imbalance
  Hypercalcemia
  Dehydration/poor nutrition
  Infective process/fever
Direct tumor invasion in central nervous system
Presence of unrelieved symptoms
  Pain
  Fecal impaction/urinary retention
  Spiritual distress/fear

Table 7.9 Pharmacologic treatment of delirium

Haloperidol 1–2 mg q 2 h titrate until settled
  Risperdone 0.5–1 mg po as alternative
Benzodiazepine if agitation is present
  Diazepam 2–5 mg po or iv q 1–4 h
  Midazolam 1–2 mg hourly iv or sq
Chlorpromazine 25–50 mg tid to qid
Olanzepine 2.5–5 mg q 12 h po
Phenobarbital 90–180 mg tid po or iv
Propofol 10–50 mg hourly iv

possible to identify a treatable source [107]. Several nonpharmacologic supportive interventions may be initiated, including relaxation, reductions in environmental distractions at night, familiar surroundings. If pharmacologic treatment is required (see Table 7.9), a neuroleptic antipsychotic is the drug of choice in treating delirium. Haloperidol is generally well tolerated, is available in oral or parenteral formulation, and the wide therapeutic window allows for titration to effect. In the presence of agitation, benzodiazepines are commonly used, but they are not beneficial when used alone, and may paradoxically aggravate symptoms. If the sedating properties of benzodiazepine are indicated, the combination of a benzodiazepine with a neuroleptic agent may provide a synergistic benefit as the benzodiazepine protects against the potential extrapyramidal effects of the neuroleptic and the neuroleptic protects against the possible paradoxical effect of the benzodiazepine [104]. Other agents that may be used include resperidone, a nursing facility-friendly alternative to haloperidol. Olanzepine offers the advantage of fewer extrapyramidal effects than haloperidol. In cases where the delirium is not responsive to standard therapies, a trial of respite sedation may be necessary. Short acting agents such as propofol or midazolam offer opportunity for rapid titration as well as reversibility.

Insomnia

Insomnia is defined as a disorder of poor or inadequate sleep generally accompanied by daytime fatigue and adverse effect on daytime function. It is a symptom that exerts a major impression on any patient who suffers from it, as lack of sleep impairs physical and mental well-being, with significant impact on function and quality of life. Although insomnia is prevalent in the general population [108], sleep disturbance is even more problematic in patients with advanced disease who already have compromised function from other multiple symptoms [109], but frequently remains undertreated [110]. Patients with advanced disease have multiple contributory pathologies that may contribute to insomnia. Features may include difficulty initiating sleep, failure to stay asleep, or premature waking. Tools are available for detailed assessment of insomnia [111].

A typical assessment of causes for insomnia consists of determination of underlying factors, physical, emotional, environmental, with goal of treating underlying problem. In patients with advanced disease these morbidities are multiple and heightened [112, 113]. In keeping with the general principles of palliative medicine, aggressive approach toward reversal of causative triggers is warranted. Medical conditions that are responsible for primary insomnia such as sleep apnea or restless leg syndrome should be excluded.

Therapy will vary depending on contributory causes. Initially it is essential to assure that optimal physical comfort is provided, emotional and spiritual suffering is addressed, and assistance offered with difficult care settings and caregiver concerns, all the services typically associated with an interdisciplinary palliative care team. Interventions include sleep hygiene training and behavioral-cognitive therapies. A thorough questioning regarding patients' bedtime habits, environment, and patterns will provide an opportunity to focused education aimed toward the elimination of habits that perpetuate insomnia. Although such behavioral treatments have been shown to be effective [114] and offer an integral component of treatment, the patient with advanced disease with limited prognosis should also be considered for the more rapid pharmacologic solution (see Table 7.10). The first line of therapy is a hypnotic agent, either a benzodiazepine or benzodiazepine-like agents. The typical concerns of benzodiazepine use in other populations, such as dependence, cognitive impairment, and increased risk of falls, are weighed against the immediate anxiolytic and sedative benefits in the palliative care setting. The favorable side effect profile of the benzodiazepine-like "Z" agents, zolpidem and zaleplon, and eszopiclone may be preferred for shorter metabolic half life, reducing the risk of

Table 7.10 Approach to insomnia

Treat contributory symptoms
Physical nausea, pain, dyspnea, psychological e.g., anxiety, depression
Sleep hygiene education
Cognitive behavioral therapy (e.g., guided imagery, meditation) if warranted by prognosis
Pharmacologic
Hypnotics
Benzodiazepine
Lorazepam 0.5–2 mg po
Clonazepam 0.25–1 mg po
Nonbenzodiazepine-"Z" drugs are preferred for their short metabolic half life
Zolpidem 5–10 mg po
Zaleplon 5–10 mg po
Eszopiclone 2 mg po
Sedating antidepressants
Mirtazepine (low dose) 15 mg po
Tricyclics, e.g., amitriptyline 10–25 mg po
Melatonin receptor agonist
Ramelteon 8 mg po

residual daytime sedation. They are generally well tolerated [115]. Both classes exert effect via the gabaminergic system.

Sedating antidepressants such as tricyclics or mirtazepine or an antineuropathic medications such as gabapentin will provide dual benefit for a patient with neuropathic pain or depression. Neuroleptics such as olanzepine may be added if there is a component of delirium present. Older agents such as chloral hydrate or barbiturates are problematic due to side effects and have limited use. Over-the-counter aids exert action via antihistamine mechanism. The benefit for insomnia in these patients is short lived and use should be limited to situations where an antihistamine may benefit other symptoms such as nausea.

Melatonin, a hormone secreted at night by the pineal gland, is a popular medication in the public media, and a preparation of ramelteon, a derivative of melatonin, is now available for sleep onset disturbance. It is a selective melatonin receptor agonist with rapid onset and short duration. It is felt that the specificity of action at the melatonin receptors rather than the gabaminergic system is the feature that limits side effects typical of the benzodiazepines [116].

Conclusion

When a clinician is faced with the suffering patient, exhibiting a multitude of symptoms, it presents a difficult challenge to determine the most effective evidence-based therapies. This field of medical study is in its infancy and the research that has been conducted in this discipline frequently offers the conclusion that "more studies are needed". With growing interest and continued emphasis on end-of-life care, the knowledge base will continue to expand as our profession embraces this area of medical practice.

References

1. Aspinal F, Hughes R, Dunckley M, Addington-Hall J. What is important to measure in the last months and weeks of life?: A modified nominal group study. Int J Nurs Stud. 2006;43(4):393–403.
2. Bonica JJ. The management of pain. 2nd ed. Philadelphia: Lea & Febiger; 1990. p. 400–60.
3. Ryan A, Carter J, Lucas J, Berger J. You need not make the journey alone: overcoming impediments to providing palliative care in a public urban teaching hospital. Am J Hosp Palliat Care. 2002;19(3):171–80.
4. Lairda B, Colvin L. Fallon management of cancer pain: basic principles and neuropathic cancer pain. Eur J Cancer. 2008;44:1078–83.
5. Foley KM. The treatment of cancer pain. New Engl J Med. 1985;313:84–95.
6. Mays TA. Antidepressants in the management of cancer pain. Curr Pain Headache Rep. 2001;5:227–36.
7. Jost L, Roila F. Management of cancer pain: ESMO Clinical Practice Guidelines. Ann Oncol. 2010;21 Suppl 5:v257–60.
8. Zech DF, Grond S, Lynch J, et al. Validation of the World Health Organization guidelines for cancer pain relief: a 10-year prospective study. Pain. 1995;63:65–76.
9. Schug SA, Zech D, Dorr U. Cancer pain management according to WHO analgesic guidelines. J Pain Symptom Manage. 1990;5:27–32.
10. Ventafridda V, Caraceni A, Gamba A. Field testing of the WHO guidelines for cancer pain relief: summary report of demonstration projects. In: Proceedings of the second international congress of cancer pain. Vol 16 of Advances in pain research and therapy. New York: Raven; 1990. p. 451–64.
11. Walker VA, Hoskin PJ, Hauks GW, et al. Evaluation of WHO analgesic guidelines for cancer pain in a hospital-based palliative care unit. J Pain Symptom Manage. 1988;3:145–9.
12. Cleeland CS, Gonin R, Hatfield AK, Edmonson JH, Blum RH, Stewart JA, Pandya KJ. Pain and its treatment in outpatients with metastatic cancer. N Engl J Med. 1994;330(9):592–6.
13. Vane JR, Botting RM. Anti-inflammatory drugs and their mechanism of action. Inflamm Res. 1998;47 Suppl 2:S78–87.
14. Eisenberg E, Berkey CS, Carr d, et al. Efficacy and safety of non steroidal anti-inflammatory drugs for cancer pain: a meta-analysis. J Clin Oncol. 2004;22:1975–92.
15. Sabino MA, Mantyh PW. Pathophysiology of bone cancer pain. J Support Oncol. 2005;3:15–24.
16. Davies NM, Reynolds JK, Undeberg MR, Gates BJ, Ohgami Y, Vega-Villa KR. Minimizing risks of NSAIDs: cardiovascular, gastrointestinal and renal. Expert Rev Neurother. 2006;6(11):1643–55.
17. Abrahm JL. Advances in pain management for older adult patients. Clin Geriatr Med. 2000;16:269–311.
18. Rothwell KG. Efficacy and safety of a non-acetylated salicylate, choline magnesium trisalicylate, in the treatment of rheumatoid arthritis. J Int Med Res. 1983;11(6):343–8.
19. Gordon RL. Prolonged central intravenous ketorolac continuous infusion in a cancer patient with intractable bone pain. Ann Pharmacother. 1998;32(2):193–6.
20. Piletta P, Porchet HC, Dayer P. Central analgesic effect of acetaminophen but not of aspirin. Clin Pharmacol Ther. 1991;49:350–4.
21. Levy MH. Pharmacologic treatment of cancer pain. N Engl J Med. 1996;335(15):1124–32.
22. Mercadante S, Sapio M, Serretta R, Caligara M. Patient-controlled analgesia with oral methadone in cancer pain: Preliminary report. Ann Oncol. 1996;7:613–7.
23. Portenoy RK, Hagen N. Breakthrough pain: definition, prevalence and characteristics. Pain. 1990;41:273–81.
24. Hagen NA, Elwood T, Ernst S. Cancer pain emergencies: a protocol for management. J Pain Symptom Manage. 1997;14(1):45–50.
25. Bruera E, Fainsinger R, MacEachern T, Hanson J. The use of methylphenidate in patients with incident cancer pain receiving regular opiates. A preliminary report. Pain. 1992;50:75–7.

26. Mercadante S. Management of cancer pain. Intern Emerg Med. 2010;5 Suppl 1:S31–5.
27. Foley KM. Clinical tolerance to opioids. In: Basbaum AI, Besson JM, editors. Towards a new pharmacotherapy of pain: report of the Dahlem Workshop. New York: Wiley; 1991. p. 181–204.
28. de Stoutz ND, Bruera E, Suarez-Almazor M. Opioid rotation for toxicity reduction in terminal cancer patients. J Pain Symptom Manage. 1995;10:378–84.
29. Indelicato RA, Portenoy RK. Opioid rotation in the management of refractory cancer pain. J Clin Oncol. 2002;20(1):348–52.
30. Plummer JL, Gourlay GK, Cherry DA, Cousins MJ. Estimated of methadone clearance: application in the management of cancer pain. Pain. 1988;33:313–22.
31. Dworkin RH, Backonja M, Rowbotham MC, et al. Advances in neuropathic pain: diagnosis, mechanisms, and treatment recommendations. Arch Neurol. 2003;60:1524–34.
32. Saarto T, Wiffen PJ. Antidepressants for neuropathic pain. Cochrane Database Syst Rev. 2007;(4):CD005454.
33. Killian JM, Fromm GH. Carbamazepine in the treatment of neuralgia: use and side effects. Arch Neurol. 1968;19:129–36.
34. Plaghki L, Adriaensen H, Morlion B, et al. Systemic overview of the pharmacological management of postherpetic neuralgia. An evaluation of the clinical value of critically selected drug treatments based on efficacy and safety outcomes from randomized controlled studies. Dermatology. 2004;208:206–16.
35. Rowbotham M, Harden N, Stacey B, et al. Gabapentin for the treatment of postherpetic neuralgia: a randomized controlled study. JAMA. 1998;280:1837–42.
36. Rowbotham M, Harden N, Stacey B, Bernstein P, Magnus-Miller L. Gabapentin for the treatment of postherpetic neuralgia. JAMA. 1998;280(21):1837–42.
37. Swerdlow M, Cundill JG. Anticonvulsant drugs used in the treatment of lancinating pain. A comparison. Anaesthesia. 1981;36(12):1129–32.
38. O'Connor AB, Dworkin RH. Treatment of neuropathic pain: an overview of recent guidelines. Am J Med. 2009;122(10 Suppl):S22–32.
39. Siu A, Drachtman R. Dextromethorphan: a review of N-methyl-D-aspartate receptor antagonist in the management of pain. CNS Drug Rev. 2007;13(1):96–106.
40. Enarson MC, Hays H, Woodroffe MA. Clinical experience with oral ketamine. J Pain Symptom Manage. 1999;17(5):384–6.
41. Mercandante S, Lodi F, Sapio M, Calligara M, Serretta R. Long-term ketamine subcutaneous continuous infusion in neuropathic cancer pain. J Pain Symptom Manage. 1995;10(7):564–8.
42. Berger JM, Ryan A, Vadivelu N, Merriam P, Rever L, Harrison P. Ketamine-fentanyl-midazolam infusion for the control of symptoms in terminal life care. Am J Hosp Palliat Care. 2000;17:127–34.
43. Mitchell AC, Fallon MT. A single infusion of intravenous ketamine improves pain relief in patients with critical limb ischaemia: results of a double blind randomised controlled trial. Pain. 2002;97(3):275–81.
44. Yentür EA, Yegül I. High dose ketamine in management of cancer-related neuropathic pain. J Pain Symptom Manage. 2000;19(6):405–8.
45. Mercadante S, Lodi F, Sapio M, Calligara M, Serretta R. Long-term ketamine subcutaneous infusion in neuropathic cancer pain. J Pain Symptom Manage. 1995;10(7):564–8.
46. Wooldridge JE, Anderson CM, Perry MC. Corticosteroids in advanced cancer. Oncology. 2001;15(2):234–6.
47. Watanabe S, Bruera E. Corticosteroids as adjuvant analgesics. J Pain Symptom Manage. 1991;9(7):442–5.
48. Rousseau P. The palliative use of high-dose corticosteroids in three terminally ill patients with pain. Am J Hosp Palliat Care. 2001;18(5):343–6.
49. Rousseau P. The palliative use of high-dose corticosteroids in three terminally ill patients with pain. Am J Hosp Palliat Care. 2001;18(5):343–6.
50. Viola V, Newnham HH, Simpson RW. Treatment of intractable painful diabetic neuropathy with intravenous lignocaine. J Diabetes Complications. 2006;29:34–9.
51. Carroll I. Intravenous lidocaine for neuropathic pain: diagnostic utility and therapeutic efficacy. Curr Pain Headache Rep. 2007;11:20–4.

52. Wong R, Wiffen PJ. Bisphosphonates for the relief of pain secondary to bone metastases. Cochrane Database Syst Rev. 2002;(2):CD002068.
53. Sze W, Shelley M, Held I, Wilt T, Mason M. Palliation of metastatic bone pain: single fraction versus multifraction radiotherapy – a systematic review of randomised trials. Clin Oncol. 2003;15:345–52.
54. Janjan NA. Radiation for bone metastases: conventional techniques and the role of systemic radiopharmaceuticals. Cancer. 1997;80:1628–45.
55. Bates T. A review of local radiotherapy in the treatment of bone metastases and cord compression. Int J Radiat Oncol Biol Phys. 1992;23:217–21.
56. Vermeulen SS. Whole brain radiotherapy in the treatment of metastatic brain tumors. Semin Surg Oncol. 1998;14:64–9.
57. Promme E. Gefinitib: a new agent in palliative care. Am J Hosp Palliat Care. 2004;21(3):222–7.
58. Haller DG. New perspectives in the management of pancreas cancer. Semin Oncol. 2003;30(4 Suppl 11):3–10.
59. Sweeney MP, Bagg J. The mouth and palliative care. Am J Hosp Palliat Care. 2000;17(2):118–24.
60. Greaves J, Glare P, Kristjanson LJ, Stockler M, Tattersall MHN. Undertreatment of nausea and other symptoms in hospitalized cancer patients. Support Care Cancer. 2009;17:461–4.
61. Lichter I. Nausea and vomiting in patients with cancer. Hematol Oncol Clin North Am. 1996;10(1):207–20.
62. Baines MJ. Nausea, vomiting, and intestinal obstruction. BMJ. 1997;315(7116):1148–50.
63. Lichter I. Which antiemetic? J Palliat Care. 1993;9(1):42–50.
64. Ripamonti C, Twycross R, Baines M, Bozzetti F, Capri S, De Conno F, Gemlo B, Hunt TM, Krebs HB, Mercadante S, Schaerer R, Wilkinson P. Clinical-practice recommendations for the management of bowel obstruction in patients with end-stage cancer. Support Care Cancer. 2001;9:223–33.
65. Jatoi A, Podratz K, Gill P, Hartmann L. Pathophysiology and palliation of inoperable bowel obstruction in patients with ovarian cancer. J Support Oncol. 2004;2:323–37.
66. Baines M. ABC of palliative care: nausea, vomiting, and intestinal obstruction. BMJ. 1997;315:1148.
67. Prommer E. Established and potential therapeutic applications of octreotide in palliative care. Support Care Cancer. 2008;16:1117–23.
68. Mercadante S, Ferrera P, Villari P, Marrazzo A. Aggressive pharmacological treatment for reversing malignant bowel obstruction. J Pain Symptom Manage. 2004;28(4):412–6.
69. Herndon CM, Jackson KC, Halli PA. Management of opioid-induced gastrointestinal effects in patients receiving palliative care. Pharmacotherapy. 2002;22:240–50.
70. Kurz A, Sessler DI. Opioid-induced bowel dysfunction pathophysiology and potential new therapies. Drugs. 2003;63(7):649–71.
71. Hoekstra J, Vernooij-Dassen M, de Vos R, Bindels PJE. The added value of assessing the 'most troublesome' symptom among patients with cancer in the palliative phase. Patient Educ Couns. 2007;65:223–9.
72. Bruera E. ABC of palliative care: Anorexia, cachexia, and nutrition. BMJ. 1997;315:1219.
73. McGeer AJ, Detsky AS, O'Rourke K. Parenteral nutrition in patients receiving cancer chemotherapy. Ann Int Med. 1989;110(9):734–5.
74. Riechelmann RP, Burman D, Tannock IF, Rodin G, Zimmermann C. Phase II trial of mirtazapine for cancer-related cachexia and anorexia. Am J Hosp Palliat Med. 2010;27(2):106–10.
75. Walsh D, Nelson KA, Mahmoud FA. Established and potential therapeutic applications of cannabinoids in oncology. Support Care Cancer. 2003;11(3):137–43.
76. Beal JE, Olson R, Laubenstein L, Morales JO, Bellman P, Yangco B, et al. Dronabinol as a treatment for anorexia associated with weight loss in patients with AIDS. J Pain Symptom Manage. 1995;10:89–97.

77. Sarhill N, Walsh D, Nelson KA, Hornsi J, LeGrand S, Davis MP. Methylphenidate for fatigue in advanced cancer: a prospective open-label pilot study. Am J Hosp Palliat Care. 2001;18(3):187–90.
78. Homsi J, Walsh D, Nelson KA, LeGrand S, Davis M. Methylphenidate for depression in hospice practice: a case series. Am J Hosp Palliat Care. 2000;17(6):393–413.
79. Scammell TE, Estabrooke IV, McCarthy MT, et al. Hypothalamic arousal regions are activated during modafinil-induced wakefulness. J Neurosci. 2000;20:8620–8.
80. Eleutherakis-Papaiakovou V, Bamias A, Dimoulos MA. Thalidomide in cancer medicine. Ann Oncol. 2004;15:1151–60.
81. Davis MP, Dickerson ED. Thalidomide: dual benefits in palliative medicine and oncology. Am J Hosp Palliat Care. 2001;18(5):347–51.
82. Peuckmann V, Fisch M, Bruera E. Potential novel uses of thalidomide focus on palliative care. Drugs. 2000;60(2):273–92.
83. Kaplan G, Thomas S, Fierer DS, et al. Therapy with thalidomide for the treatment of AIDS-associated wasting. AIDS Res Hum Retroviruses. 2000;16(14):1345–66.
84. Mahmoud F, Sarhill N, Mazurczak MA. The therapeutic application of melatonin in supportive care and palliative medicine. Am J Hosp Palliat Med. 2005;22(4):295–309.
85. MacDonald N. Cancer cachexia and targeting chronic inflammation: a unified approach to cancer treatment and palliative/supportive care. J Support Oncol. 2007;5:157–62.
86. Dewey A, Baughan C, Dean T, Higgins B, Johnson I. Eicosapentaenoic acid (EPA, an omega-3 fatty acid from fish oils) for the treatment of cancer cachexia. Cochrane Database Syst. 2007;(1):CD004597.
87. Lai V, George J, Richey L, Kim HJ, Cannon T, Shores C, Couch M. Results of a pilot study of the effects of celecoxib on cancer cachexia in patients with cancer of the head, neck, and gastrointestinal tract. Head Neck. 2008;30(1):67–74.
88. Davis CL. ABC of palliative care: breathlessness, cough, and other respiratory problems. BMJ. 1997;315:931.
89. Chandler S. Nebulized opioids to treat dyspnea. Am J Hosp Palliat Care. 1999;16(1):418–22.
90. Zeppetella G. The palliation of dyspnea in terminal disease. Am J Hosp Palliat Care. 1998;15(6):322–30.
91. Burns BH, Howell JB. Disproportionately severe breathlessness in chronic bronchitis. Q J Med. 1969;151:277–94.
92. Bruera E, MacEachern T, Ripamonti C, Hanson J. Subcutaneous morphine for dyspnea in cancer patients. Ann Intern Med. 1993;119:906–7.
93. Thomas JR, von Gunten CF. Clinical management of dyspnoea. Lancet Oncol. 2002;3:223–8.
94. Light RW, Muro JR, Sato RI, Stansbury DW, Fischer CE, Brown SE. Effects of oral morphine on breathlessness and exercise tolerance in patients with chronic obstructive pulmonary disease. Am Rev Respir Dis. 1989;139:126–33.
95. Man GCW, Sproule BJ. Effect of alprazolam on exercise and dyspnea in patients with chronic obstructive pulmonary disease. Chest. 1986;90:832–6.
96. Booth S, Moosavi SH, Higginson IJ. The etiology and management of intractable breathlessness in patients with advanced cancer: a systematic review of pharmacological therapy. Nat Clin Pract Oncol. 2008;5(2):90–100.
97. Booth S, Anderson H, Swannick M, Wade R, Kite S, Johnson M. The use of oxygen in the palliation of breathlessness. A report of expert working group of the scientific committee of the association of palliative medicine. Respir Med. 2004;98:66–77.
98. Hayes Jr D, Anstead MI, Warner RT, Kuhn RJ, Ballard HO. Inhaled morphine for palliation of dyspnea in end-stage cystic fibrosis. Am J Health Syst Pharm. 2010;67:737–40.
99. Ripamonti C. Management of dyspnea in advanced cancer patients. Support Care Cancer. 1999;7:233–43.
100. Sarhill N, Walsh D, Khawam E, Propiano P, Stahley MK. Nebulized hydromorphone for dyspnea in hospice care of advanced cancer. Am J Hosp Palliat Care. 2000;17(6):389–91.

101. Homsi J, Walsh D, Nelson KA, Sarhill N, Rybicki L, LeGrand SB, Davis MP. A phase II study of hydrocodone for cough in advanced cancer. Am J Hosp Palliat Med. 2002;19(1):49–56.
102. Bonneau A. Cough in the palliative care setting. Can Fam Physician. 2009;55:600–2.
103. Doona M, Walsh D. Benzonatate for opioid-resistant cough in advanced cancer. Palliat Med. 1997;12:55–8.
104. Breitbart W, Strout D. Delirium in the terminally ill. Clin Geriatr Med. 2000;16(2):357–72.
105. Inouye SK. The dilemma of delirium: clinical and research controversies regarding diagnosis and evaluation of delirium in hospitalized elderly medical patients. Am J Med. 1994;97:278–88.
106. Gustafson Y, Brannstrom B, Norberg A, Bucht G, Winblad B. Underdiagnosis and poor documentation of acute confusional states in elderly hip fracture patients. J Am Geriatr Soc. 1991;39:760–5.
107. Bruera E, Miller L, McCallion J, Macmillan K, Krefting L, Hanson J. Cognitive failure in patients with terminal cancer: a prospective study. J Pain Symptom Manage. 1992;7(4):192–5.
108. Anderson WM. Top ten list in sleep. Chest. 2002;122:1457–60.
109. Passik SD, Whitcomb LA, Kirsh KL, Theobald DE. An unsuccessful attempt to develop a single-item screen for insomnia in cancer patients. J Pain Symptom Manage. 2003;25:284–7.
110. Savard J, Morin CM. Insomnia in the context of cancer: a review of a neglected problem. J Clin Oncol. 2001;19:895–908.
111. Holcomb SS. Recommendations for assessing insomnia. Nurse Pract. 2006;31(2):55–60.
112. Shuster Jr JL, Breitbart W, Chochinov HM. Psychiatric aspects of excellent end-of-life care. Ad Hoc Committeeon End-of-Life Care. The Academy of Psychosomatic Medicine. Psychosomatics. 1999;40:1–4.
113. Stark D, Kiely A, Smith A, Velikova G, House A, Selby P. Anxiety disorders in cancer patients: their nature, associations, and relation to quality of life. J Clin Oncol. 2002;20:3137–48.
114. Friedman L, Benson K, Noda A, et al. An actigraphic comparison of sleep restriction and sleep hygiene treatments for insomnia in older adults. J Geriatr Psychiatry Neurol. 2000;13:17–27.
115. Schenck CH, Mahowald MW, Sack RL. Assessment and management of insomnia. JAMA. 2003;289(19):2475–9.
116. Simpson D, Curran MP. Ramelteon: a review of its use in insomnia. Drugs. 2008;68(13):1901–19.

Review Questions

1. Tolerance develops rapidly to all the following opioid side effects except:

    (a) Respiratory depression
    (b) Sedation
    (c) Dysphoria
    (d) Constipation
    (e) Nausea

2. All the following drugs provide antineuropathic benefit in the treatment of pain, with the exception of:

    (a) Tricyclic antidepressants
    (b) Nonsteroidal anti-inflammatory drugs (NSAIDs)
    (c) Serotonin norepinephrine reuptake inhibitors (SNRIs)
    (d) Anticonvulsants
    (e) Ketamine

3. Which of the following statements about dyspnea is true:

    (a) Nebulized opioids are an established treatment for this symptom
    (b) Emotional factors contribute to the severity of dyspnea
    (c) The extent of dyspnea is reliably measured by respiratory rate and arterial oxygenation
    (d) Anxiolytics may result in respiratory depression and should be avoided
    (e) Disease-modifying therapies are rarely beneficial in treating dyspnea

4. For the management of delirium in advanced disease, which of the following statements is false:

    (a) Aggressive use of benzodiazepines is required to treat the agitation typically associated with delirium
    (b) Review of medications is essential to assess for reversible causes
    (c) Periods of lucidity do not rule out the presence of delirium
    (d) Depression and pain behaviors may mimic the signs of delirium
    (e) The provision of supportive familiar surroundings is an effective treatment

5. Beneficial interventions for the treatment of symptoms associated with inoperable bowel obstruction include all the following except:

    (a) Somatostatin analog
    (b) Percutaneous gastric venting
    (c) Haloperidol
    (d) Corticosteroids
    (e) Parenteral nutrition

Answers

1. (d). This symptom remains throughout the treatment course, tolerance developing very slowly, if at all, thus requiring vigilance and treatment. The other side effects dissipate within several days.
2. (b). Although anti-inflammatory drugs provide significant co-analgesia in many pain states, the most commonly used agents for neuropathic pain include the antidepressants, N-methyl-D-aspartate (NMDA) antagonists such as ketamine, and anticonvulsants.
3. (b). Similar to the pain symptom, dyspnea is accompanied by fear and apprehension regarding physical discomfort as well as the prognostic implications. Anxiolytics are an important tool for alleviating the distress. Although nebulized drugs are used in limited circumstances, the mainstay of pharmacological treatment is systemic opioids. Since this is a subjective symptom, external measures are of little value in assessing dyspnea. Correction of any underlying pathology is beneficial in alleviating the symptom burden.
4. (a). Although agitation is a component of the hyperactive category of delirium, benzodiazepines, when used alone, may aggravate delirium. Review of medications is important as drugs are a reversible etiology of this symptom. The variable course of delirium which includes periods of lucidity and signs that mimic other disease states (e.g., depression, pain) should be considered when making the diagnosis of delirium. Nonpharmacologic modalities are an important component of therapy.
5. (e). The goal of treatment in this condition is to reduce the symptoms caused by increased secretions and motility in the gut. Artificial nutrition adds to the metabolic and fluid load and worsens symptoms. The other choices are all valid for treatment of the associated nausea.

Chapter 8
Nutrition in Palliative Care

M. Khurram Ghori and Susan Dabu-Bondoc

Introduction and Epidemiology

Malnutrition is an immense problem in palliative care. It occurs in about a third of all patients newly diagnosed with cancer. It is an independent risk factor for increased morbidity and mortality, and is a primary cause of death in about 20 % of patients with cancer [1]. Worldwide statistics have revealed that malnutrition can develop in as much as 30–90 % of the time over the course of a malignancy [2]. It has been a second leading cause of death in developed countries [3]. Cachexia is a debilitating and distressing condition. It can prolong hospital stay and can cause delayed, missed, or decreased tumor treatments and decrease cost–benefit and risk–benefit ratios of anticancer therapies [4].

Cachexia is most commonly associated with tumors of the head and neck, lung and central nervous system, pancreas and gastrointestinal (GI) tract. Patients with tumors of the head and neck and of the upper digestive tract such as the esophagus, stomach, pancreas, etc., often present with moderate to severe malnutrition at time of diagnosis. On the other hand, patients with hematological tumors, such as leukemia, develop the lowest rates and severity of weight loss. This may be due in part to the rapid development of such tumors in relatively young patients.

Nutritional interventions have been developed in an attempt to prevent or counteract the deleterious effects of cancer cachexia during different stages of the disease and its therapy that often compromise nutritional status. With expanding knowledge and understanding of the pathophysiology of cancer cachexia, research and investigations have focused on the efficacy and efficient use of pharmaco-immunological nutrients, and on the development of new strategies for nutritional planning and counseling.

M.K. Ghori, M.D. • S. Dabu-Bondoc, M.D. (✉)
Department of Anesthesiology, Yale University School of Medicine,
New Haven, CT, USA
e-mail: susan.dabu-bondoc@yale.edu

N. Vadivelu et al. (eds.), *Essentials of Palliative Care*,
DOI 10.1007/978-1-4614-5164-8_8,
© Springer Science+Business Media New York 2013

Nutritional Care in Cachexia

Definitions

Anorexia is loss of appetite. Cachexia is defined as a significant weight loss due to disease. Although cachexia often occurs with anorexia, cachexia is not caused merely by decreased nutritional intake. It is a catabolic state that results from an imbalance between nutritional demand and nutrient availability. Such imbalance can be a result of multiple factors, such as metabolic and pathophysiological changes, induced inability to ingest or utilize nutrients, social or psychological factors, or to toxicity resulting from treatment. Cachexia is characterized by increased resting energy expenditure, preferential loss of skeletal muscle and fat, and increased proteolysis and lipolysis. Chronic systemic inflammation and circulating tumor-derived factors have also been implicated as possible causes [5, 6].

Palliative care is medical treatment that aims to relieve suffering and improve the quality of life of patients with advanced disease. It encompasses the relief of physical, emotional, and existential suffering, as well as the support for best quality of life for both patient and family caregivers. Palliative care has grown since the start of the hospice movement in the USA in 1970s and in the UK in the 1960s. The Medicare Hospice Benefit was created, in 1983, by US federal legislation. This has since provided palliative care services to more than seven million terminally ill patients. Under current regulatory and compensatory Medicare rules, patients are eligible for hospice if their physician states that death is likely within 6 months, and the patient is willing to forego attempts at curative or life-prolonging therapies.

Pathophysiology and Mechanisms of Cachexia

Cancer cachexia is multifactorial. It can be due to (a) inadequate food intake, (b) metabolic disturbances leading to a wasting medical condition, and/or (c) humoral/anti-inflammatory factors or responses. Anorexia and metabolic alterations are considered most important in the development of nutritional declension. In addition, the adverse effects of interventions often compound the underlying organic causes of the condition. Malnutrition develops as a result of the "parasitic" activity of the tumor at the expense of the host, the impact of the tumor on the metabolism of the host, and the adverse effects of cancer interventions.

Anorexia and Decreased Food Intake

Loss of appetite is a general effect of cancer. It is considered the most common and most crucial contributing factor in the development of nutritional decline and weight loss in cancer patients. It occurs in approximately 70 % of patients with advanced cancer and is often worsened by the cytotoxic effects of cancer therapy causing nausea, mucositis, and/or dysphagia [7].

Several complex interrelated pathophysiological mechanisms are implicated in the development of anorexia [2]. Depression and other psychological factors are often present. Alterations in taste and smell exist in approximately 50 % of patients. About a third of patients experience alterations in recognizing sweet taste; while sourness, saltiness, and bitterness (responsible for dislike of meat) are less commonly altered. Several investigations have indicated that such changes in taste and smell correlated with poor response to treatment, reduced intake of nutrients, and tumor extension and spread.

A variety of factors affect the GI tract. These include delayed digestion which can cause early satiety, and gastric or intestinal atrophy, which leads to appetite loss. GI obstruction due to tumors of the digestive and hepato-biliary tracts, as well as external compression from metastatic masses, can all lead to early satiety, nausea, vomiting, or GI obstruction. "Blind loop syndromes," typically presenting with relapsing episodes of bowel obstruction, can critically impair nutrient absorption. In several wasting diseases, small bowel mucosa often atrophies and results in malabsorption. Several other factors have been implicated in the etiology of anorexia, including altered plasma levels of amino acids, cytokines or free fatty acids, resistance to insulin, elevated plasma lactate due to anaerobic metabolism of cancer cells, etc.

Anticancer interventions such as chemotherapy can cause abdominal cramping, bloating, nausea, vomiting, mucositis, malabsorption, and/or paralytic ileus. Despite the availability of a variety of pharmacologic antiemetic therapies, vomiting remains a common cause of malnutrition in cancer patients. Chemotherapeutic agents, particularly adriamycin, cysplatin, fluorouracil, and methotrexate are known inducers of serious GI toxicity. Lined by rapidly dividing cells, known as enterocytes, the GI tract is particularly susceptible to the cytotoxic effects of chemo- or radiotherapeutic agents. Erosive lesions including mucositis, tongue ulceration, and esophagitis can all severely impair food intake. Enteropathies, combined with ulcerations, necrosis, and mucosal atrophy could be harbingers of marked radiation enterocolitis that can be complicated by peritonitis, obstruction, or fistulas. Advances in radiation technology, such as bowel shielding, fractioning, dosing and timing, and use of high energy, have been applied in an attempt to prevent radiation-induced small bowel complications.

It should be noted that anorexia is often a major primary contributing factor of cachexia. Its severity can vary as the cancer progresses and the toxic effects of disease intervention complicate the former. Given that nutrient intake is not always impaired during the course of cancer, the degree of food intake may not necessarily correlate with the nutritional status. This highlights the fact that cancer-associated malnutrition involves not only systemic but also metabolic changes.

Metabolic Perturbations and Cachexia

Perturbations that alter energy expenditure (EE), as well as, metabolism of carbohydrate, protein, fat, and vitamins have all been associated with cancer [2].

Regardless of the nutritional status of the host, the tumor grows and maintains a high degree of metabolic activity at the expense of the host. Cancer cells sustain a high level of glycolysis producing significant levels of lactate. The presence of a net uptake of amino acids by the tumor tissue, as demonstrated by scientific investigations, has proved that cachexia is caused by increased tumor metabolic requirements. However, despite the increased tumor metabolic demands, the host responds by decreasing nutrient intake, which is not a normal mechanism of metabolic regulation. Furthermore, cachexia may not necessarily be readily reversible by provision of adequate nutrient. Evidently, abnormal tumor metabolism and associated anorexia as well as alterations in host metabolism are all major contributory factors in the development of cachectic syndrome.

Despite the initial controversy over whether cancer patients had elevated EE relative to cachectic noncancer patients, normalization of EE following tumor removal has favored the hypothesis that EE elevation is cancer driven. Depending upon the type of neoplasm, EE appears to be related to an increased adrenergic state and/or the presence of an inflammatory process. For example, patients with lymphomas are not metabolically different from healthy patients, while patients with myeloproliferative tumors, and some, but not all hematologic cancers, demonstrate major metabolic abnormalities. EE elevations in cancer, although usually modest (10–15 %), can give rise to critical weight loss over time.

Apart from neoglucogenesis, the trapping of glucose and its conversion to lactate and subsequent recycling of lactate to glucose by tumor cells, the carbohydrate metabolism of the cancer patient is also characterized by glucose intolerance, due to resistance of peripheral tissues to the effects of insulin. In addition, the pancreas secretes reduced amounts of insulin in response to food intake.

Loss of fat mass in tumor patients may not only result from anorexia, but also from a primary imbalance between lipolysis and lipogenesis. In cachectic but not normal weight cancer patients, stored lipids are rapidly depleted due to increased peripheral fat mobilization, and excessive fatty acids oxidation. This is reflected by increased plasma levels of glycerol and FFA by-products of triglyceride hydrolysis. Studies demonstrating the possible role of decreased lipogenesis in malnutrition remain inconclusive.

Adaptive mechanisms that decrease protein catabolism to preserve functional lean body mass in conditions of starvation are absent in cancer patients. This explains the rapid protein depletion and/or marked muscle atrophy that develop in cancer states. The most common protein metabolism abnormalities found in cancer include (1) increase in protein turnover, e.g., increased protein synthesis plus increased muscle protein breakdown, (2) decrease in muscle protein synthesis, (3) elevation of inflammatory hepatic protein synthesis, (4) a constantly negative nitrogen balance due to a relative greater reduction of protein synthesis, and (5) various alterations in plasma amino acid profile. Some of these amino acid level changes have been studied as potential markers of extent of cancer and as a basis for nutritional intervention. Alterations in protein metabolism are regionally distributed. This is evident by the presence of marked hypoalbuminemia in cachectic cancer patients. A shift from peripheral to visceral redistribution of protein synthesis occurs in either or both the host and the neoplasm.

Inflammatory and Humoral Activities in the Host–Neoplasm Interaction

Various humoral and inflammatory factors have been implicated in anorexia, metabolic perturbations, or weight loss associated with cancer. The role of cytokines and other mediators in appetite regulation and in metabolic abnormalities are poorly understood. Elevated cytokine (e.g., IL-1, IL-6, gamma interferon, tumor necrosis factor-alpha) activity, abnormal eicosanoid production, excessive monocyte and macrophage activation and TNF production, altered lymphocyte functions, abnormal IL-2, or peptidoglycan production have all been described. Various interrelationships exist among these factors and perturbations in inducing and maintaining a state of catabolism. Development of new therapeutic interventions against cancer cachexia has targeted such inflammatory and humoral responses.

Effects of Nutritional Support on Tumor

An ideal nutritional support would be one that nourishes the patient but not the tumor. There have been attempts to modulate tumor growth by nutritional manipulation, both in animal and human models, but conclusive results are yet to be achieved. Results of several trials performed in GI and head and neck malignancies placing subjects on enteral or parenteral nutrition consisting of varying amounts of protein and calories favored a lack of increase in cancer size with nutritional support. Different approaches of nutritional component manipulation to limit metabolism by cancer cells have been investigated. These include restriction of protein, use of halogenated carbohydrates, 2-deoxyglucose or pentoses, and use of medium-chain triglycerides and omega-3 fatty acids. Regimens consisting of high nonprotein calories (e.g., 90 % medium chain [MCT] and long chain [LCT] triglyceride lipid mixtures) were found to maintain stable patient weight and tumor volume for several months. Studies involving the use of inhibitors of neoglucogenesis, such as hydralazine sulfate have yet to demonstrate improved clinical outcome. Newer pharmaconutrients such as arginine, glutamine, and omega-3 fatty acids have been target of research for their impact on immune status.

Evaluation of Nutritional Status and Diagnosis

Nutritional assessment is an essential tool in palliative care. There are several reasons why nutrition is a very important component in the management of patients with advanced, incurable cancer. First, anticancer treatments often lead to deterioration of energy intake [8, 9]; second, chemotherapeutic agents can directly affect skeletal muscle [10], and third, tumor responses to cancer therapy are often associated with cachexia-related symptoms [11, 12]. Therefore, continuous monitoring of patients' nutritional intake, weight, and other symptoms such as fatigue or early satiety are valuable.

Nutritional assessment is important in order to:

1. Identify patients who may benefit from dietary counseling
2. Determine the severity and cause(s) of malnutrition
3. Identify patients at risk of complications from surgery, chemo- or radiation therapy
4. Assess the efficacy of nutritional support

Nutritional assessment warrants periodic evaluation and reassessment as malnutrition evolves over the course of a malignant or advanced chronic disease and its intervention. Nutritional parameters to assess nutritional status during the course of the disease, from baseline at diagnosis to remission or cure, are available. Such parameters have sufficient sensitivity and specificity to reliably assess nutritional status. Nutritional management should be tailored to the patient's needs by combining nutritional assessment and monitoring of performance status and quality of life.

A standardized, easy to use, validated, and accepted tool to evaluate nutritional status must be applied [13]. Nutritional indexes or scores have been developed to evaluate and to triage patients according to need for counseling or immediate nutritional support. Subjective global assessment (SGA) [14, 15] estimates the degree of nutritional depletion and identifies patients at risk of malnutrition. It correlates closely with objective parameters (e.g., serum protein levels, anthropometric measurements) and predicts postsurgical clinical outcome accurately (82 % sensitivity, 72 % specificity) [16]. A training period of a few days is typically needed to minimize an inter-observer variability and satisfy reproducibility.

Validated for adults and children, nutritional risk score (NRS) is a 5-item questionnaire that classifies severity of malnutrition. Assessing weight loss, body mass index, appetite, ability to eat spontaneously, and intercurrent diseases, it compares favorably with clinical judgment and other nutritional risk indices. It is fairly reproducible among different nutrition professionals, including nurses, nutritionists, and dieticians. Other indexes and screening tools for the community, hospital, and geriatric care homes (9-item questionnaire, Zeno Stanga's MUST/NRS/MNA), all with moderate to substantial inter-rater reliability, were created to identify patients who are malnourished or at risk of malnutrition. These tools should be utilized as part of the global initial assessment to guide nutritional management.

Weight change is a good indicator of nutritional deficit. A weight loss of 10 % or more within the prior 6 months, or 5 % or more within the prior month, indicates malnutrition and correlates well with clinical outcome. Use of other variables such as subscapular/triceps skinfold, mid-arm muscle area/circumference to estimate body fat, and fat-free mass have poor inter-rater reproducibility, and have not been validated in cancer patients. Biological measurements such as use of anabolic protein, e.g., transferrin, transthyretin, and albumin plasma levels are more utilized than nutritional/immunological (lymphocyte, IGF-1) proteins, which are generally expensive and have impractical clinical utility. Changes in muscle function such as hand grip strength and impedancemetry measurements require well-trained and highly motivated operators.

In many institutions, appetite and rehabilitation clinic teams have been created and are responsible for completing medical, nutritional, speech, swallowing and physical therapy evaluations for cachectic or terminally ill patients. The goal is to create an individualized program that will meet patients' needs and improve overall quality of life.

Management of Anorexia and Cachexia

The main goals of intervention in palliative patients include nutritional management, pain control, home recuperation support, and relief of spiritual pain.

Development of a variety of nutritional interventions has evolved, along with the expanding knowledge on the pathophysiology of anorexia and cachexia and the results of clinical application investigations.

Nutritional Counseling

Nutritional management in cachexia or palliative care commences with dietetic counseling. Depending upon the severity of malnutrition or its risk, different levels of nutritional support can be designed. Individual patient's needs, preferences, and eating habits are important considerations for the nutritionist, both for the purposes of assuring satisfaction and/or for controlling symptoms [17].

Nutritional counseling is an important aspect of care in cancer or advanced chronic disease. Simple dietary recommendations can significantly increase oral protein-energy intake by cancer patients even when the beneficial effect on weight is not so apparent [18]. There is good evidence that individualized nutritional counseling improves outcome. In patients with GI and head and neck malignancies, for example, results of investigations favor the use of intensive dietary counseling to prevent weight loss and treatment interruptions [19]. In addition, Ravasco and his group, have demonstrated improvement of diarrhea, flatulence, and abdominal distention during the late effects of radiotherapy in the nutrition intervention group (group 1), compared with the less-intensive counseling groups (group 2-nutritional supplements, group 3-control). Furthermore, 4-year survival rate was reported to be astoundingly 100 % in group 1, when compared with groups 2 and 3 (88 % and 75 % 4-year survival rate, respectively). Malnutrition has been shown to be a risk factor for decreased survival and postoperative complications in cancer patients [20–23]. Despite this risk, however, few interventions, as that one in Ravasco's trial, exist to improve poor outcomes.

The impact of systematic nutritional assessment and counseling on cancer relevant outcomes has also been documented by other investigations. One [24] randomized controlled trial of oncology outpatients, compared nutritional counseling plus oral nutrition supplementation versus a less aggressive approach, and demonstrated improved energy intake and quality of life with the former. Another study [25] showed that the inclusion of enteral nutrition support in a comprehensive symptom control and pain management can lead to improved nutritional status and increased rates of completion of palliative anticancer therapy. Overall et al. [26], in a study involving 21 palliative home care services as well as telephone interviews with 621 patients, a high frequency of utilization of both combined oral nutrition and oral supplements (41 %), and artificial nutrition (14 %) was reported. Conducted qualitative interviews indicated that patients and family member gain physical, social, and psychological benefits from home nutritional support. Some of the concerns raised by majority of patients with advanced cancer include eating less and weight loss [27]. Based on this, interventions have been developed utilizing , and authorizations of patient to "support eating well," and "self-action."

The dietician is responsible for calculating food consumption, evaluating nutritional status, and anticipating the nutritional risk of both cancer and its therapy. The main goals are to maintain adequate nutrition in the normo-nourished and to minimize or prevent cachexia in the malnourished. Type of tumor, its extension and planned treatments, as well as, patient's socioeconomic background are typically all accounted. Working in collaboration with the oncologist, surgeon, anesthesiologist, nutritional team members, dieticians monitor the patient's nutritional status and intake, the efficacy of dietary advice or treatments, recommend possible needs for enteral or parenteral support, and participate in training staff on nutritional management.

The importance of early detection of nutritional risk and malnutrition must also be recognized. Screening tools are available in daily clinical practice and have been discussed in the previous section. Nutrition guidelines have been formulated by the American Society of Parenteral and Enteral Nutrition, the American Cancer Society, and the European Society of Parenteral and Enteral Nutrition (the ACS webpage can be found at http://www.cancer.org/acs/groups/cid/documents/webcontent/002577-pdf.pdf).

Oral Nutritive Supplements

Several oral nutritive supplements (ONS) are used when oral calorie-protein intake is insufficient. Preparations vary according to osmolarity, energy density, type of protein content, lactose/gluten/fiber content, flavor, and formulation. Addition of immunonutrients, such as arginine, nucleotides, and n-3 fatty acids to ONS to increase their cost–benefit ratio have been studied but results are inconclusive.

Normo-nourished cancer patients undergoing treatment stress have a resting energy expenditure (REE) of 20–25 kcal/kg of usual weight per day. Calorie (non-protein) amounts of 100–200 % of their REE should typically maintain the nutritional status of these patients. Normally, no restrictions are required while oral feeding is intact other than in the presence of coexisting medical condition(s). The optimum ratio of carbohydrates and lipids in oral nutritional support is still up to debate.

Progestogens and Corticosteroids

Over the years, there has been a shift of cancer treatment response assessment from traditional to symptomatic oncological outcomes, including functional status and quality of life. Consequently, symptomatic treatments have been on the rise in recent years.

Orexigens, such as progestogens (megestrol acetate [MA], medroxy-progesterone acetate [MPA]) and corticosteroids, are the most studied treatments used to improve appetite in the terminally ill with anorexia. Orexigens reduce the action of cytokines at the level of both monocytes and the central nervous system. Systematic reviews (11 RCTs, 1,767 subjects: RR 1.74) [7, 28] have found high-quality evidence that progestins increase appetite and weight gain in cancer patients when compared to placebo. However, they also increase the risk of adverse effects such as lower limb edema, deep vein thrombosis, and vaginal bleeding in up to 30 % of patients. On the contrary, a retrospective case–control study of 2,127 elderly nursing home residents with cachexia did not find a significant difference in median weight at 6 months between subjects with and without MA [29]. Furthermore, same study showed that the median survival of residents receiving MA was significantly decreased (23.9 months vs. 31.2 months) compared with untreated subjects.

Corticosteroids have been shown to offer benefits in the terminally ill. Although side effects have been found with their prolonged administration, six RCTs of 647 patients have demonstrated that prednisolone, methylprednisolone, or dexamethasone were shown to improve appetite in the short term (but benefit may decrease after several weeks of use) compared with placebo [7]. In this study no results on survival were reported. Adverse effects from prolonged intake of corticosteroids included delirium, proximal muscle weakness, skeletal muscle atrophy, osteoporosis, and immunosuppression.

To improve appetite in cancer patients, treatment of other symptoms such as pain, depression, and side effects of cancer interventions may provide benefit. Opiates can complicate food intolerance by causing or worsening constipation. Antidepressants such as imipramines or fluoxetine can further reduce appetite and nutrient intake.

Other Pharmacologic Approaches

Most of these agents still warrant further clinical research, and no firm recommendations for use in clinical practice are made at this time.

1. Hydralazine sulfate—inhibition of gluconeogenesis: a systematic review found no significant benefit with use of hydralzine sulfate.
2. Metoclopramide—attenuation of nausea and vomiting
3. 5HT3 receptor antagonists
4. Cyproheptadine—reduction of serotoninergic transmission
5. Other—melatonin, fatty acids, erythropoietin, androgenic steroids, NSAIDS, interferon, cannabinoids, eicosapentaenoic acid, thalidomide, ghrelin, pentoxifylline

Artificial Nutrition

Enteral Nutrition

Artificial nutrition is recommended when oral intake is less than 60 % of nutritional needs. The main goal of the use of artificial nutrition is to correct metabolic perturbations of malnourished cancer patients over the course of the disease and disease treatment. Functional lean body mass must be preserved through replenishment and maintenance of active muscle and visceral cell mass. Artificial nutrition makes it possible to limit the nutritional decline of cancer patients, the biological aggressiveness of the tumor, and or improve efficacy of cancer therapy [2]. Improved general well-being and comfort and resumption of activity are the best evidences of efficacy of artificial nutrition.

Enteral artificial nutrition (EN) is used if the digestive tract is intact and functional, otherwise, parenteral nutrition (PN, also known as TPN) is utilized. EN and PN are both safe and effective methods of administering nutrients. Neither route of nutrition is indicated in well-nourished or mildly malnourished cancer patients.

Volitional nutritional support (VNS), i.e., orally consumed supplements, may improve survival in the malnourished geriatric population, however, neither VNS nor EN via a tube feeding can be *routinely* recommended in individuals with cancer or other advanced chronic diseases, as some studies report no results in improved appetite or weight gain [30]. Cancer patients undergoing major visceral surgery who are severely malnourished may benefit from enteral nutritional support.

Parenteral Nutrition

Unless there are prolonged durations of GI toxicity (e.g., bone marrow transplant patients), EN or PN is often not clinically efficacious for patients treated with chemotherapy or radiotherapy. Current research has focused on the impact of nutrition interventions and nutritional pharmacology on the clinical outcome of cancer patients. Shang et al. [31], in a randomized controlled trial of 152 subjects with advanced cancer, found that combining parenteral nutrition (PN) to enteral nutritional (EN) support significantly increased mean BMI at 4 months (21.9 vs. 20.5) and cumulative survival, when compared with EN alone. Similarly, Lundholm et al. [32], also in a randomized controlled trial of 309 cancer patients with cachexia who were followed for up to 24 months, demonstrated that combining oral and home PN to the cyclooxygenase-1 (COX-1) selective inhibitor indomethacin plus erythropoietin increased energy balance, however, no statistically significant differences between groups in intention-to-treat analysis were found. Glutamine-supplemented PN appears to be beneficial in bone marrow patients.

For both EN and PN, the recommended regimen includes a daily intake of 20–35 kcal/kg, consisting of a balanced proportion of glucose and lipids (50:50 or 60:50 glucose to fat ratio), and of a 0.2–0.35 g nitrogen/kg (~1.2–2 g protein/kg/day), as well as, adequate provision of electrolytes, vitamins, and trace elements [2]. In clinical practice, carbohydrate or glucose is commonly administered using 5 mg/kg/min, and lipids at no more than 2.5 g/kg/day and no more 60 % of total calories from fat is used. For patients who have no difficulty tolerating proteins, the common dose given to "nonstressed" patients is 0.8 g/kg/day and 1.2–2.5 g/kg/day in critically ill patients. The main goal of nitrogen supply is to limit muscle catabolism, while also maintaining adequate supply, particularly the essential amino acids, to the liver to maintain synthesis of proteins needed for immune defenses.

For obese patients, an adjusted body weight, about 120 % of ideal body weight (IBW), is used to estimate calorie requirements. Lean body mass accounts for about 25 % of excess weight in obese people, using the formula:

$$\left[\left(\text{Actual weight} - \text{IBW}\right) \times 0.25\right] + \text{IBW} = \text{adjusted weight}$$

For patient whose weight is less than 90 % IBW, an average weight can be used to estimate calorie needs as follows:

$$\left(\text{Actual weight} + \text{IBW}\right)/2 = \text{average weight}$$

Parenteral nutrition is known to carry a higher risk of line infection and associated sepsis. Therefore, nutritional support in palliative care should be based on the potential risks and benefits of EN and PN, as well as the patient's and the family's wishes.

In far advanced cancer, there is controversy on whether the use of enteral or parenteral nutritional support improves outcome. In terminally ill cancer patients, enteral and parenteral nutrition appear to be overused, as reported by one recent review [33]. This review also indicated that education, implementation of guidelines, and shared decision making could decrease the use of nutritional support. Another study reported that gastrostomy tube feeding use is as high as 90 % in patients with advanced dementia despite paucity of evidence that it improves clinical outcome [34]. There was also a report of a preference against tube feeding by many patients and that about 15 % of them had feeding tubes inserted regardless of documented refusal by the patient(s).

Physician education, in combination with palliative care consultation, has been reported to decrease feeding tube insertion rates by half.

Other strategies of nutritional interventions:

1. Modification of taste and smell
2. Calorie and protein modifications
3. Use of lipid emulsions
4. Immunonutrition

Supplementation with zinc sulfate can improve metallic taste and other taste alterations during head and neck irradiation. Antiemetics, setrons, and corticosteroids are regimens that can have beneficial effects on taste disorders. Dietary adaptation to changes in taste is considered the most effective measure, e.g., avoidance of unpleasant foods and rein-forcement of salt and sweet depending upon level of sensitivity. It has been shown that the outcome of taste disorders tends to follow that of the disease, i.e., reversal of abnor-malities occur within a few days to weeks after the last cycle of chemotherapy. The data on the benefit and/or risk of using lipid emulsions in cancer patients is conflicting.

Immunonutrition

It has been demonstrated that immunonutrition could improve the beneficial effects of nutritional support during cancer, chemotherapy, or radiotherapy [1]. Immune diets also appear to decrease the rate of infectious complications and the length of hospital stay after GI surgery [2]. The immunonutrition substances, omega-3 fatty acids, and amino acids such as glutamine, arginine, polyamines, antioxidant micro-nutrients, are tested mainly for their effects. Megestrol acetate and corticosteroids demonstrated their efficacy in short-term cures.

Clinical Indications of Nutritional Support

Nutritional support can be utilized during one or more of the following:
1. Perioperative period
2. Chemotherapy
3. Bone marrow transplantation
4. Radiotherapy
5. Palliative care

Complications of Nutritional Support

Nutritional interventions are often assumed to be safe; however, nutritional thera-pies are not without potentially detrimental effects.

Refeeding syndrome is characterized by a series of clinical manifestations related to electrolyte changes typically associated with the restarting of the nutritive contribution of either enteral or parenteral regimens. It is not an uncommon entity in malnourished patients placed on parenteral or enteral nutrition. In one study, it occurred in about half of subjects, and it was associated with increased mortality rate and hospital stay [35].

Management of Dehydration

Decreased fluid intake is common in palliative care patients. Dehydration can be due to a variety of factors such as anorexia/cachexia syndrome, loss of desire to drink, nausea, generalized weakness, decreased level of consciousness, mechanical bowel obstruction, or occasionally, no specific etiology could be identified. Routine practice on management of dehydration varies widely geographically and between care settings and, high quality evidence from the literature is scant [36]. Observational evidence exists that terminally ill individuals may not experience suffering from terminal dehydration, provided that good mouth hygiene is maintained [37, 38]. A small prospective study of 32 comfort care patients [37] showed that thirst or dry mouth could be alleviated usually by application of ice chips and lubrication to the lips or with small amount of fluids. And in this trial, 62 % of patients experienced either no thirst or thirst only initially during their terminal condition. Perception of thirst has been associated with, as demonstrated in a small prospective trial of 88 terminally ill cancer patients [39], hyperosmolality (300 mosmol/kg or more), oral breathing, stomatitis, use of opioids, and poor general condition.

Hydration can be performed either via gastrostomy, intravenously, or subcutaneously (hypodermoclysis). But among palliative care physicians, medically assisted hydration remains an issue of much debate. A systematic review in 2008 identified only five studies including two RCTs (93 patients) on the effects of short-term hydration in terminal cancer. Such studies seemed insufficient to make recommendations as trials were either underpowered or of insufficient quality [40]. Although evidence was weak, there was indication that artificial hydration may improve sedation and myoclonus. However, artificial hydration showed no beneficial effect on other outcomes and there was increased fluid retention (e.g., pleural effusion, peripheral edema, and ascites) compared with no artificial hydration.

Management of Nausea and Vomiting

Nausea occurs in up to 68 % of patients with incurable cancer and vomiting in about 13 % [41, 42]. Nausea and vomiting (NV) can adversely affect the patients' quality of life as it causes tremendous discomfort and lead to dehydration and electrolyte disturbances. Chemotherapy induced nausea and vomiting and other chemotherapy-associated toxic effects have been shown to delay chemotherapy in up to 50 % of patients, and lead to longer hospitalizations and increased financial cost [43].

Effective treatments of nausea and vomiting have utilized treating the cause of nausea and or vomiting. There are four main mechanism-based causes of nausea and/or vomiting which have been coined by the so-called VOMIT acronym [44]: V for vestibular etiology, O for obstructive (e.g., bowel obstruction), M for motile or dysmotility of the gut, and I for infectious or inflammatory causes. Vestibular and obstructive NV, as they involve histaminic, cholinergic receptors, they could be best treated by anticholinergic/antihistaminic regimens such as promethazine, diphenhydramine, scopolamine patch. Obstructive NV also involves 5HT3 receptors, so are also best treated by senna products. Prokinetics such as metoclopramide are best administered to motility-related NV. Treatment for infectious or inflammatory NV should include anticholinergic scopolamine, antihistaminic (promethazine, diphenhydramine), 5HT3 inhibitor (ondansetron, granisetron), neurokinin 1 inhibitors (aprepitant), and anti-inflammatory agents (corticosteroids).

There is weak evidence that supports the consensus-based guidelines for treatment of nausea and vomiting in advanced cancer [45]. This emetic pathway neuropharmacology-based approach to treatment of NV, however, may not necessarily be always appropriate in the setting of far advanced cancer. On the contrary, the empirical approach (trying various antiemetics regardless of the cause of NV), though can be highly effective, has not been compared to its mechanistic counterpart in a scientific manner. Nevertheless, it is recommended that the mechanistic approach should be utilized as a basis in choosing first-line antiemetic agents. While uncontrolled studies demonstrated a high (75–95 %) response rate to such standard regimens, randomized controlled studies reported much lower (18–52 %) response to these therapies. Although these approaches are practical and simplistic, well-designed studies to find its impact on outcome of such standard management on NV in the palliative setting need to be done. There is strong evidence for the use of steroids in malignant bowel obstruction, and for metoclopramide in cancer-related dyspepsia. Evidence is conflicting with regard to the efficacy of serotonin antagonists compared with standard agents such as metoclopramide, dexamethasone, and dopamine antagonists. Novel neurokinin antagonists are a new class of antiemetic agents that hold potential promise for the future.

Management of Constipation

While the prevalence of constipation in patients using opioid for noncancer pain is about 15–90 %, that of patients following WHO guidelines for cancer pain treatment is about 23 % [46, 47]. Constipation prophylaxis is generally recommended in all individuals placed on opioid agents. Commonly prescribed treatments for constipation include oral laxatives, opioid antagonists, or rectally administered agents.

Laxatives

Lactulose is an osmotic laxative that is used to decrease hard stools in patients on opioid treatment. Lactulose has been shown as equally effective as polyethylene glycol 3350/electrolyte solution (PEG) in decreasing constipation [48].

Macrogels (e.g., PEG) are osmotic agents used to improve stool consistency and their efficacy have been demonstrated in a placebo controlled trial.

Senna (a stimulant laxative) is another commonly prescribed oral anticonstipation agent. Unlike Docusate, Senna has been shown in controlled trials [49] to be as efficacious as lactulose or herbal preparations for decreasing frequency of hard stools in patients who are on opioids, or who have advanced cancer.

Docusate is a stool softener that is also prescribed in patients on opioid therapy. However, literature does not show good evidence to back up its use [50].

Other oral laxatives that have been used for constipation include: Bisacodyl, methylcellulose, magnesium salts, sodium picosulfate, ispaghula husk.

Opioid Antagonists

Opioid acts on peripheral opioid receptors in the GI tract. Opioid antagonists can be used to block GI receptors to prevent constipation; however, they could also potentially reverse the analgesic effects of opioids [51]. Commercially available opioid antagonists include methylnaltrexone (MNTX) and alvimopan. The efficacy in increasing the rate of bowel movements of subcutaneous MNTX in palliative care or hospice patients with terminal cancer has been demonstrated in placebo-controlled trials [52]. In these trials, constipation improved without interference of analgesia. Alvimopan, in 0.5 mg and 1.0 mg doses, has significantly improved bowel movements in patients treated with opioid for chronic back pain.

Rectally Administered Medications

Various rectally applied agents such as phosphate enemas, liquid paraffin, glycerol suppositories, sodium citrate micro-enemas, and arachis oil enemas have been used in patients on opioid treatment. However, no clinically important results about the effects of these medications are found in the literature [53].

Care Facilities for the Palliative Patient

The palliative patient can be cared for in a hospice, hospital, nursing home, or in a home health care setting. Financial, personal, personnel availability, or medical factors impact which facility the palliative patient is cared in. Hospice utilization has been on the rise in the USA, and at least 20 % of patients have received hospice care [54]. More than 80 % of hospice care in the USA is provided through Medicare. Typically, patients are referred to hospice care at later phases of their disease. As availability of palliative care services is limited, patients who wish to pursue life-long treatments or those who have undetermined prognosis are ineligible for hospice services.

Nonhospice palliative care has been increasingly available in US hospitals, but access to nursing homes or community settings remains uneasy. Hospitals have progressively invested in palliative care services not only to reduce ICU and total bed days but also to facilitate transitions from high-costs hospitals to more appropriate settings such as the home [55, 56]. By the early part of this decade, at least a quarter of US hospitals had a palliative care program.

Palliative patients on a stable general condition can be cared in a nursing home or at their home provided that mobile palliative team or home health care support is available. Such teams or family must be able to provide adequate or reasonable amount of nutrition, hydration, and adequate control of symptoms and pain. Tube feedings are utilized if it is the sole criterion that denies patient admission to nursing home [57]. To avoid ethical or lawful dispute situations, comprehensive information and advance directives on management and full power to the nursing personnel who will provide care to the palliative patient must be in place. Goal directed therapy that calls for improved quality of life of palliative patients may allow patient's desire to recuperate at home if possible.

Nutritional Care in Patients with Noncancer Chronic Illnesses

Nutritional support is important in critically ill patients. In acute lung injury (ALI) and acute respiratory distress syndrome (ARDS), for example, characteristic pro-inflammatory processes and excess catabolism can result in substantial nutritional deficits. Nutritional support is essential to prevent significant caloric deficits, lean body mass loss, muscle strength decline, and malnutrition [58]. In these patients early administration of enteral nutrition was demonstrated to be associated with modulation of stress and immune response, and attenuation of disease severity.

In patients with chronic diseases other than cancer, the role of palliative care is often unrecognized [59]. In patients with heart failure, as prognostication is often not easy, integrating patients' preferences into goals of care becomes very important. Despite disability and poor prognosis, patients with advanced heart failure and chronic obstructive pulmonary disease (COPD) often do not receive palliative care services. Similarly, because dementia is rarely viewed as a terminal illness, many dementia patients suffer and die in pain due to little or no palliative care received.

Occurring in about five million Americans, dementia in advanced stages is a leading cause of death in individuals older than 65 in the USA [60]. After the age of 85 years, about 50 % of individuals suffer from memory loss secondary to dementia. During the most advanced stage of dementia, severe functional impairment, eating problems, and malnutrition typically occur. Decisions to direct care towards either to palliation or to invasive measures like placement of feeding tubes should be made in these patients. Barriers to the provision of palliative care to these patients, pharmacological or other treatment options for feeding problems are critical issues that need discussion. Strategies to help clinicians provide effective support to patients with advanced dementia and their family are crucial [61].

Enteral Tube Feeding in Advanced Dementia Patients

At least one-third of nursing home residents with advanced dementia have a feeding tube inserted [61]. However, there is insufficient evidence to suggest that enteral tube feeding is always beneficial in patients with advanced dementia. The use of feeding tubes (FT) in patients with advanced dementia has been found, in two systematic reviews, not to improve survival, prevent aspiration pneumonia, heal or prevent decubitus ulcers, or improve other clinical outcomes [62, 63].

Characteristics associated with higher rates of feeding tube (FT) insertion in nursing home residents with advanced cognitive impairment who were admitted to US acute care hospitals have been evaluated (2,797 acute hospitals), 163,000 nursing home residents with advanced cognitive impairment [64]. Approximately two-thirds of nursing home residents in the USA who are tube fed had their feeding tube placed during an acute care hospitalization, usually for an infection. In this study, the rate of FT insertion was as high as 40 % per 100 hospitalizations; the mean rate of FT insertions has been decreasing from year 2000 to 2007; higher insertion rates being associated with hospital features such as: (1) for profit ownership versus government owned, (2) larger hospital size, and (3) greater ICU use in the last 6 months of life. Also in this study, advance care planning such as having written advance directives, do not resuscitate (DNR) orders, and orders to forego artificial nutrition and hydration were reported to be associated with lower rates of FT placements.

Advance care planning is often lacking in nursing homes [65, 66]. Only about 6 % of hospitalized nursing home residents with advanced cognitive impairment had an order to forgo artificial hydration and nutrition. Advance care planning is apparently essential to ensure that feeding tube placements are based on informed patient preferences [67, 68].

Ethical Aspects of Nutrition in Palliative Care

Nutritional support at the end of life is a critical decision. It is important that decision making be transparent. If the decision is documented as part of an initial long-term care planning, with involvement of patients and family members, then decision making becomes transparent. The decision to stop or continue nutritional support becomes an issue when there is no written or implied directive from the patient. At this point consultation with palliative care physicians, hospital ethics committee, or legal system of the state or country comes into play. Palliative care physicians are trained to improve quality of end of life days. They use nutritional support as one of the most important tools to improve quality of life. Nutritional support should be used to improve symptoms and to enhance patient satisfaction. In special circumstances like advanced stages of dementia or cachexia, family members are faced with critical decision making on whether aggressive tube feeding should be maintained or nutritional support be withdrawn. Under such circumstances, previous examples of complex cases are used to guide decision making. The most popular court cases of Terri Schiavo, Quinlan, Nancy Cruzan, and others may be utilized as examples during the critical decision-making process made by care providers and family members.

There is a lack of national or international guidelines for nutritional decision making at the end of life. Differences of opinion exist among physicians and nursing staff regarding withdrawal of nutritional support. Each group has different views regarding the use of nutritional support to improve quality of care versus prolongation of life. Medical literature has not kept pace with the need of merging palliative care with curative care. Cancer-related cachexia is a primary cause of death in 20 % of all patients. Though its cause is multifactorial, nutritional causes are most important, where supply has to overcome increased demands of cancer-related malnutrition. It is a consensus that provided that the risks, benefits, and alternatives are discussed with both patient and relatives, the care provider's personal judgment of conscience can be used. The nephrology team can lead the patient and family through this process by providing timely, realistic information to help them make the best decisions.

End-of-life decision making should be a part of an initial long-term care planning that is shared with every patient and family. When conflicts persist and the need for initiation of dialysis is urgent, it is necessary to initiate and continue treatment until the resolution of these conflicts, making sure that a record of this decision is in place. In certain circumstances, the use of advanced decision making by patients and family members resolves many conflicts. If discrepancies arise in hospitals, care should be continued until hospital ethics committee makes an informed ethical decision. Ethics committee help decide whether to use or not to use ventilators, nutritional or hydrational support. The availability of end-of-life care services was reviewed with respect to strategies adopted by few administrators in Japan. It was concluded from the survey that when patients become unstable in a long-term care (LTC) facility, referral to hospitals becomes necessary. Palliative care consultants were necessary to manage these patients in LTC facilities. In cancer patients, appropriate models are necessary for good death. Once appropriate interventions are established from such models, future LTC decision making may become easier to establish.

The psychiatrists of Oregon are divided into two groups for physician-assisted suicide on compassionate grounds. Euthanasia and physician-assisted suicide are punishable acts under Canadian criminal law. It is a critical decision when the burden of nutrition support outweighs the benefit to the patient. Open and effective communication, and respect of patient's wishes, should be communicated effectively. According to US DHHS survey, nursing home patients were more likely to be old, have dementia and have other noncancer primary diagnosis, receive dietary/nutrition service, medication management and physician services, than home hospice patients. These challenges may be overcome by the creation of clear language that stresses the patient's goals of care. "Comfort feeding only," an order that states what steps are to be taken to ensure the patient's comfort through an individualized feeding care plan, has been proposed. Through careful hand feeding, "comfort feeding only," when possible, offers a clear goal-oriented alternative to tube feeding and, eliminates the "care-no care" dichotomy imposed by orders to forgo artificial hydration and nutrition.

The increasing number of patients suffering from Alzheimer's disease has led to growing issues relating to the withholding and withdrawing of life-prolonging treatments. In these patients, the most important factors influencing the withholding or withdrawing of life-prolonging treatments include (1) advanced directives, (2) the family intention, and (3) futility of treatment [69]. Furthermore, the availability of advanced directives and family's consent for hospice care were found to facilitate critical decision making in the care of end-stage Alzheimer's disease.

References

1. Demoor-Goldschmidt C, Raynard B. How can we integrate nutritional support in medical oncology? Bull Cancer. 2009;96(6):665–75.
2. Nitenberg G, Raynard B. Nutritional support of the cancer patient: issues and dilemmas. Critic Rev Oncol Hematol. 2000;34:137–68.
3. World Health Organization. National cancer control programmes: policies and managerial guidelines. Geneva: World Health Organization; 2002.
4. Granda-Cameron C, DeMille D, Lynch MP, Huntzinger C, Alcorn T, Levicoff J, Roop C, Mintzer D. An interdisciplinary approach to manage cancer cachexia. Clin J Oncol Nurs. 2010;14(1):72–80.
5. Couch M, Lai V, Cannon T, Guttridge D, Zanation A, George J, Hayes DN, Zeisel S, Shores C. Cancer cachexia syndrome in head and neck cancer patients: part I. Diagnosis, impact on quality of life and survival, and treatment. Head Neck. 2007;29:401–11.
6. Moses AW, Slater C, Preston T, Barber MD, Fearon KC. Reduced total energy expenditure and physical activity in cachectic patients with pancreatic cancer can be modulated by an energy and protein dense oral supplement enriched with n-3 fatty acids. Br J Cancer. 2004;90:996–1002.
7. Yavuzsen T, Davis MP, Walsh D, LeGrand S, Lagman R. Systematic review of the treatment of cancer-associated anorexia and weight loss. J Clin Oncol. 2005;23:8500–11.
8. van den Berg MG, Rasmussen-Conrad EL, Gwasara GM, Krabbe PF, Naber AH, Merkx MA. A prospective study on weight loss and energy intake in patients with head and neck cancer, during diagnosis, treatment and revalidation. Clin Nutr. 2006;25(5):765–72.

9. Ohno T, Kato S, Wakatsuki M, Noda SE, Murakami C, Nakamura M, Tsujii H. Incidence and temporal pattern of anorexia, diarrhea, weight loss and leukopenia in patients with cervical cancer treated with concurrent radiation therapy and weekly cisplatin: comparison with radiation therapy alone. Gyncol Oncol. 2006;103(1):94–9.

10. van Norren K, van Helvoort A, Argiles JM, van Tuijl S, Arts K, Gorselink M, Laviano A, Kegler D, Haagsman HP, van der Beek EM. Direct effects of doxorubicin on skeletal muscle contribute to fatigue. Br J Cancer. 2009;100(2):311–4.

11. Geels P, Eisenhauer E, Bezjak A, Zee B, Day A. Palliative effect of chemotherapy: objective response is associated with symptom improvement in patients with metastatic breast cancer. J Clin Oncol. 2000;18(12):2395–405.

12. Koeberle D, Saletti P, Borner M, Gerber D, Dietrich D, Caspar CB, Mingrone W, Beretta K, Strasser F, Ruhstaller T, Mora O, Hermann R, Swiss Group for Clinical Cancer Research. Patient-reported outcomes of patients with advanced biliary tract cancers receiving gemcitabine plus capecitabine: a multicenter phase II trial of the Swiss Group for Clinical Research. J Clin Oncol. 2008;26(22):3702–8.

13. Delmore G. Assessment of nutritional status in cancer patients: widely neglected? Support Care Cancer. 1997;5(5):376–80.

14. Baker JP, Detsky AS, Wesson DE, et al. Nutritional assessment: a comparison of clinical judgement and objective measurements. N Engl J Med. 1982;306(16):969–72.

15. Ottery FD. Definition of standardized nutritional assessment and interventional pathways in oncology. Nutrition. 1996;12(1):S15–9.

16. Detsky AS, McLaughlin JR, Baker JP, et al. What is subjective global assessment of nutritional status? JPEN J Parenter Enteral Nutr. 1987;11(1):8–13.

17. Benarroz MO. Bioethics and nutrition in adult patients with cancer in palliative care. Cad Saude Publica. 2009;25(9):1875–82.

18. Ovesen L, Allingstrup L, Hannibal J, et al. Effect of dietary counseling on food intake, body weight, response rate, survival, and quality of life in cancer patients undergoing chemotherapy: a prospective, randomized study. J Clin Oncol. 1995;11:2043–9.

19. Ravasco P, Monteiro Grillo I, Camilo M. Cancer wasting and quality of life react to early individualized nutritional counseling! Clin Nutr. 2007;26(1):7–15.

20. Meyerhardt JA, Tepper JE, Niedzwiecki D, Hollis DR, McCollum AD, Brady D, O'Connell MJ, Mayer RJ, Cummings B, Willett C, MacDonald JS, Benson 3rd AB, Fuchs CS. Impact of body mass index on outcomes and treatment-related toxicity in patients with stage II and III rectal cancer: findings from Intergroup Trial 0114. J Clin Oncol. 2004;22(4):648–57.

21. Tewari N, Martin-Ucar AE, Black E, Beggs L, Beggs FD, Duffy JP, Morgan WE. Nutritional status affects long term survival after lobectomy for lung cancer. Lung Cancer. 2007;57(3):389–94.

22. Pacelli F, Bossola M, Rosa F, Tortorelli AP, Papa V, Doglietto GB. Is malnutrition still a risk factor of postoperative complications in gastic cancer surgery? Clin Nutr. 2008;27(3):398–407.

23. Bachman J, Heiligensetzer M, Krakowski-Roosen H, Buchler MW, Friess H, Martignoni ME. Cachexia worsens prognosis in patients with resectable pancreatic cancer. J Gastrointest Surg. 2008;12(7):1193–201.

24. Rufenacht U, Ruhlin M, Wegmann M, Imoberdorf R, Ballmer PE. Nutritional counseling improves quality of life and nutrient intake in hospitalized undernourished patients. Nutrition. 2010;26(1):53–60.

25. Sharma R, Singh DP, Sharma OP, Sharma S. Improvement of nutritional status in advanced head and neck cancer patients. In: ESMO symposium nutrition and cancer; 2009. Abstract 17PD.

26. Overall Y, Tishelman C, Permert J, Cederholm T. Nutritional support and risk status among cancer patients in palliative home care services. Support Care Cancer. 2009;17(2):153–61.

27. Hopkinson JB, Wright DN, McDonald JW, Corner JL. The prevalence of concern about weight loss and change in eating habits in people with advanced cancer. J Pain Symptom Manage. 2006;32(4):322–31.

28. Barenstein EG, Ortiz Z. Megestrol acetate for treatment of anorexia-cachexia syndrome. Cochrane Database Syst Rev 2005;(2):CD004310.
29. Bodenner D, Spencer T, Riggs AT, Redman C, Strunk B, Hughes T. A retrospective study of the association between megestrol acetate administration and mortality among nursing home residents with clinically significant weight loss. Am J Geriatr Pharmacother. 2007;5:137–46.
30. Koretz RL, Avenell A, Lipman TO, Braunschweig CL, Milne AC. Does enteral nutrition affect clinical outcome? A systematic review of the randomized trials. Am J Gastroenterol. 2007;102:412–29.
31. Shang E, Weiss C, Post S, Kaehler G. The influence of early supplementation of parenteral nutrition on quality of life and body composition in patients with advanced cancer. JPEN J Parenter Enteral Nutr. 2006;30:222–30.
32. Lundholm K, Daneryd P, Bosaeus I, Korner U, Lindholm E. Palliative nutritional intervention in addition to cyclooxygenase and erythropoietin treatment for patients with malignant disease: effects on survival, metabolism, and function. Cancer. 2004;100:1967–77.
33. Morss S. Enteral and parenteral nutrition in terminally ill cancer patients: a review of the literature. Am J Hosp Palliat Med. 2006;23:369–77.
34. Lorenz K, Rosenfeld K, Wenger N. Quality indicators for palliative and end-of-life care in vulnerable elders. J Am Geriatr Soc. 2007;55:S318–26.
35. Hernandez-Aranda JC, Gallo-Chico B, Luna-Cruz ML, Rayon-Gonzales MI, Flores-Ramirez LA, Ramos Munoz R, Ramirez-Barba EJ. Malnutrition and total parenteral nutrition: a cohort study to determine the incidence of refeeding syndrome. Rev Gastroenterol Mex. 1997;62((4):260–5.
36. Lanuke K, Fainsinger RL. Hydration management in palliative care settings: a survey of experts. J Palliat Care. 2003;19:278–9.
37. McCann RM, Hall WJ, Groth-Juncker A. Comfort care for terminally ill patients. The appropriate use of nutrition and hydration. JAMA. 1994;272:1263–6.
38. van der Riet P, Good P, Higgins I, Sneesby L. Palliative care professionals' perceptions of nutrition and hydration at the end of life. Int J Palliat Nurs. 2008;14:145–51.
39. Morita T, Tei Y, Tsunoda J, Inoue S, Chihara S. Determinants of the sensation of thirst in terminally ill cancer patients. Support Care Cancer. 2001;9:177–86.
40. Good P, Cavenagh J, Mather M, Ravenscroft P. Medically assisted hydration for palliative care patients. Cochrane Database Syst Rev. 2008;(2):CD006273.
41. Teunissen SC, Wesker W, Kruitwagen C, de Haes HC, Voest EE, de Graeff A. Symptom prevalence in patients with incurable cancer: a systematic review. J Pain Symptom Manage. 2007;34:94–104.
42. Solano JP, Gomes B, Higginson IJ. A comparison of symptom prevalence in far advanced cancer, AIDs, heart failure, chronic obstructive pulmonary disease, and renal disease. J Pain Symptom Manage. 2006;31:58–69.
43. Grunberg SM. Antiemetic activity of corticosteroids in patients receiving cancer chemotherapy: dosing, efficacy, and tolerability analysis. Ann Oncol. 2007;18:233–40.
44. Hallenbeck J. Palliative care perspectives. New York: Oxford University Press; 2003. p. 75–86.
45. Glare P, Pareira G, Kristjanson LJ, Stockler M, Tattersall M. Systematic review of the efficacy of antiemetics in the treatment of nausea in patients far-advanced cancer. Support Care Cancer. 2004;12(6):432–40.
46. Clemens KE, Klaschik E. Managing nausea, emesis, and constipation in palliative care. Dtsch Arztebl. 2007;104:A269–78.
47. Pancha SJ, Muller-Schwefe J, Wurzelmann JI. Opioid-induced bowel dysfunction: prevalence, pathophysiology and burden. J Clin Pract. 2007;61:1181–7.
48. Van Der Spoel JIO, Zandstra DFV. Laxation of critically ill patients with lactulose or polyethylene glycol: a two-center randomized, double-blind, placebo-controlled trial. Crit Care Med. 2007;35:2726–31.
49. Miles CL, Fellowes D, Goodman ML, Wilkinson S. Laxatives for the management of constipation in palliative care patients. Cochrane Database Syst Rev. 2006;(4):CD003448.

50. Hurdon V, Viola R, Schroder C. How useful is ducosate in patients at risk for constipation? A systematic review of the evidence in the chronically ill. J Pain Symptom Manage. 2000;19:130–6.
51. Becker G, Galandi F, Blum HE. Peripherally acting opioid antagonists in the treatment of opiate-related constipation: a systematic review. J Pain Symptom Manage. 2007;34:547–65.
52. Yuan CS. Methylnaltrexone mechanisms of action and effects on opioid bowel dysfunction and other opioid adverse effects. Ann Pharmacother. 2007;41:984–93.
53. Mendoza J, Legido J, Rubio S, Gisbert JP. Systematic review: the adverse effects of sodium phosphate enema. Aliment Pharmacol Ther. 2007;26:9–20.
54. Plonk WM, Arnold RM. Terminal care in the last weeks of life. J Palliat Med. 2005;8: 1042–54.
55. Meier DE. Palliative care in hospitals. J Hosp Med. 2006;1:21–8.
56. Lorenz KA, Lynn J, Dy SM, Shugarman LR, Wilkinson A, Mularski RA, Morton SC, Hughes RG, Hilton LK, Maglione M, Rhodes SL, Rolon C, Sun VC, Shekelle PG. Evidence for improving palliative care at the end of life: a systematic review. Ann Intern Med. 2008;148(2):147–59.
57. Schmidt E. Percutaneous endoscopic gastrostomy tube for a patient with glioblastoma to enable his admission into a nursing home. Wien Med Wochenschr. 2010;160(13):328–30.
58. Krzak A, Pleva M, Napolitano LM. Nutrition therapy for ALI and ARDS. Crit Care Clin. 2011;27(3):647–59.
59. Rodriguez KL, Barnato AE, Arnold RM. Perceptions and utilization of palliative care services in acute care hospitals. J Palliat Med. 2007;10:99–110.
60. Alzheimer's Association. Alzheimer's disease facts and figures. 2009. http://www.alz.org/national/documents/report_alzfactsfigures2009.pdf. Accessed 28 Oct 2011.
61. Mitchell SL, Teno JM, Roy J, Kabumoto G, Mor V. Clinical and organizational factors associated with feeding tube use among nursing home residents with advanced cognitive impairment. JAMA. 2003;290(1):73–80.
62. Gillick MR. Rethinking the role of tube feeding in patients with advanced dementia. N Eng J Med. 2000;342(3):206–10.
63. Finucane TE, Christmas C, Travis K. Tube feeding in patients with advanced dementia: a review of the evidence. JAMA. 1999;282(14):1365–70.
64. Teno JM, Mitchell SL, Gozalo PL, Dosa D, Hsu A, Intrator O, Mor V. Hospital characteristics associated with feeding tube placement in nursing home residents with advanced cognitive impairment. JAMA. 2010;303(6):544–50.
65. Rich SE, Gruber-Baldini AL, Quinn CC, Zimmerman SI. Discussion as a factor in racial disparity in advance directive completion at nursing home admission. J Am Geriatr Soc. 2009;57(1):146–52.
66. Mitchell SL, Teno JM, Intrator O, Feng Z, Mor V. Decisions to forgo hospitalization in advanced dementia: a nationwide study. J Am Geriatr Soc. 2007;55(3):432–8.
67. Molloy DW, Guyatt GH, Russo R, Goeree R, O'Brien BJ, Bedard M, Willan A, Watson J, Patterson C, Harrison C, Standish T, Strang D, Darzins PJ, Smith S, Dubois S. Systematic implementation of an advance directive program in nursing home: a randomized controlled trial. JAMA. 2000;283(11):1437–44.
68. Volandes AE, Paasche-Orlow MK, Barry MJ, et al. Video decision support tool for advance care planning in dementia: randomized controlled trial. BMJ. 2009;338:b1259. doi:10.1136/bmj.b2159.
69. Minooka M. The withholding and withdrawing of life-prolonging treatment for end-stage Alzheimers disease patients. Gan To Kagaku Ryoho. 2007;34 Suppl 2:203–4.

Review Questions

1. Cachexia is most commonly noted in patients suffering from all of the following cancers except

   (a) Head and neck
   (b) Pancreas
   (c) Leukemia
   (d) Lungs

2. Cachexia in cancer patients is found to be related to imbalance of one of the following factors

   (a) Carbohydrates
   (b) Proteins
   (c) Energy expenditure
   (d) Fats

3. The following interventions have shown promising results to maintain weight in cancer patients except

   (a) High medium chain triglyceride and long chain triglyceride mixture nutrition
   (b) Arginine and glutamine-rich diets
   (c) Halogenated carbohydrate diets
   (d) Omega 6 fatty acid rich diets

4. Nutritional assessment tools most commonly used are the followings except

   (a) Subjective global assessment (SGA)
   (b) Nutritional risk score (NRS)
   (c) MUST/MNA/NRS
   (d) Subscapular/triceps skin fold measurement

5. Nutritional interventions in cancer-related cachectic patients includes all except

   (a) Modification of taste and smell
   (b) Calorie and protein modification
   (c) Use of lipid emulsion
   (d) Use of high dose narcotic agonists

6. Enteral tube feeding in hospitalized patients with advanced cognitive impairment is increased in all of the followings except

   (a) For profit ownership vs. government owned hospitals
   (b) Large hospital size vs. small hospital
   (c) Greater ICU use in last 6 months of life
   (d) Presence of advance directives for DNR orders

7. Complications of enteral and parenteral therapy include

    (a) Dehydration
    (b) Constipation
    (c) Refeeding syndrome
    (d) All of the above

8. The decision to withhold nutritional support in advanced Alzheimer patients includes all of the following factors except

    (a) Advanced directives
    (b) Family intentions
    (c) Futility of treatment
    (d) Age of the patient

9. In the USA, the approximate prevalence of malnutrition as a primary cause of death in cancer patients is about

    (a) 2 %
    (b) 20 %
    (c) 60 %
    (d) 90 %

10. Ethical decision making for nutritional support of cancer patients is highly influenced by

    (a) Local State laws in the USA
    (b) Physician training and belief
    (c) Advance directive
    (d) WHO ethical committee

Answers

1. (c) Leukemia
2. (c) Energy expenditure
3. (d) Omega 6 fatty acid rich diets (correct answer Omega 3)
4. (d) Subscapular/triceps skin fold measurement
5. (d) Use of high dose narcotic agonists
6. (d) Presence of advance directives for DNR orders
7. (d) All of the above
8. (d) Age of the patient
9. (b) 20 %
10. (c) Advance directive

Chapter 9
Nursing Perspective and Considerations

Ena M. Williams and Tong Ying Ge

Introduction

Palliative Care is defined by the World Health Organization (WHO) as an approach that improves the quality of patients and their families facing the problem associated with life threatening illnesses, through the prevention and relief of suffering by means of early identification and impeccable assessment and treatment of pain and other problems, physical, psychosocial and spiritual. [1]

Palliative Care aims to:

- Affirm life and regard dying as a normal process
- Provide relief from pain and other distressing symptoms
- Integrate the psychological and spiritual aspects of patient care
- Offer a support system to help patients live as actively as possible until death
- Offer a support system to help the family cope during the patient's illness and in their own bereavement

Palliative Care is provided by those providing the day-to-day care to patients and carers in their homes and hospitals as well as those who specialize in palliative care (consultants, medicine, and clinical nurse specialists, for example).

E.M. Williams, R.N., M.S.M., M.B.A. (⊠)
Department of Perioperative Services, Yale-New Haven Hospital,
New Haven, CT, USA
e-mail: ena.williams@ynhh.org

T.Y. Ge, R.N., M.S.N. (Master Degree of Nursing)
Pain Advanced practice nurse, Sir Run Run Shaw Hospital,
Hangzhou, China

N. Vadivelu et al. (eds.), *Essentials of Palliative Care*,
DOI 10.1007/978-1-4614-5164-8_9,
© Springer Science+Business Media New York 2013

This chapter will focus on the role of the nurse in palliative care and working with the multidisciplinary team. The main practice areas for the nurse involved in palliative care can be summarized into the following main focus areas:

1. Coordinating the program and treatment plan for patients and their families
2. Working with the multidisciplinary team
3. Symptom management
4. Education and research

The nurse spends the most time with the patient and therefore his or her role is to ensure the following:

1. Relief of physical symptoms
2. Helping the patient to achieve the highest quality of life
3. Assist the patient in maintaining his or her independence
4. Provide relief for mental anguish and social isolation
5. Support patient and family members
6. Assist the patient to reduce isolation, fear, and anxiety
7. Support the process of dying well

The nurse should be available to enable convenience, respond to anger, respond to colleagues, respond to family, and be present or available when death occurs. The importance of palliative care has led to a new field of Palliative Care Nursing. This type of nursing differs in essence from other areas of nursing care and reflects a "whole *person*" philosophy of care across the lifespan and across diverse health settings. It focuses on the patient and family as the unit of care.

In palliative nursing, the "*individual*" is recognized as a very important part of the healing relationship. This relationship of the nurse with the patient and family is crucial. Together with knowledge and skills, is the essence of palliative care nursing and sets it apart from other areas of nursing practice. However, palliative care as a therapeutic approach is appropriate for all nurses to practice. It is an integral part of many nurses' daily practice, as is clearly demonstrated in work with the elderly, the neurologically impaired, and infants in neonatal units. The palliative care nurse frequently cares for patients with major stressors, such as physical, psychological, spiritual, or existential [2]

In caring for the suffering, the role of the nurse is one of coaching. "Coaching is an interpersonal intervention that requires therapeutic use of self, involving one's own mind, past experiences, words, heart, and hand-to comfort those who suffer". In coaching, the nurse:

- Establishes a trusting partnership
- Assesses those who are at risk for suffering or who are vulnerable; reassures patients that although their suffering may not disappear, they will not be abandoned
- Identifies factors that may be eliminated or modified to alleviate suffering
- Intervenes to facilitate expression of feelings, find meaning in suffering, help patients and families redefine the quality of life

Table 9.1 Six ways the nurse/health professional can relieve suffering

1. Being a companion to sufferers by identifying the pain of their losses and exploring the circumstances and extent of their loss
2. By listening for statements of meaning from sufferers and allowing the person's natural instincts and energy to surface the issue of higher meaning
3. By valuing any self-disclosure on meaning that a sufferer offers, by analyzing the meaning of the statements and learning what the statements reveal about the sufferer's point of view of him or herself
4. By encouraging the sufferer's interpretation of their own experience
5. By validating the sufferer's interpretation of their own experience while clarifying the meaning and
6. The nurse can identify supportive resources and hope for the sufferer to extend his or her identity and meaning in the future

The nurse must be self-accepting, secure in his or her own self-concept, and feel confident in strengthening others.

Nurses and other health professionals can relieve suffering in six ways (see Table 9.1).

Palliative Nurse and Interdisciplinary Care Team

The team design and composition varies depending on the needs of the patient and available resources. What is most common is the presence of a nurse and a physician on the team. The nurse normally serves as the primary liaison between team members, patient, and family and also brings the team's plan to the bedside, whether at home, in the clinic of inpatient setting. The nurse can also work with the physician to adjust and determine changes in treatment. This is due to the fact that the nurse spends much time with the family and patient, and becomes intimate with the patients condition. Other members of the team often include the chaplain and social worker. No single discipline can meet the needs of most patients and their families; an interdisciplinary team (IDT) is highly preferred.

Apart from assessment and management of pain, in which the nurse's key role has been clearly recognized, the other most important process in palliative care is the family meeting to establish goals and objectives. This is a standard of practice in institutions and especially in the Intensive Care Unit where sometimes the outcome may be unknown for some time. It is in this meeting that families received clarification, have their questions answered and are helped to understand the patient's condition and prognosis, can share their knowledge of the patients values and preferences along with their concerns as well as receive emotional and practical support. This meeting is the backbone of the informed, patient-focused, decision-making about care goals and treatment. Nurses can contribute to these meetings in many important ways:

- The nurse usually has the most current and up-to-date information about the patient's condition.
- This nurse is usually the clinician with the best knowledge of the strongest relationship with the family.
- He/she has the most continuous presence, seeing and hearing interactions with patients and families by clinicians from all disciplines, including the many specialties that are involved in the patient's care.
- Following the family meeting, the nurse is the connectivity to all individuals who may not have been present at the family meeting to ensure continuity of care and treatment.
- Nurses are great at providing information that patients and families can understand.
- Palliative Care Nurse Specialists are specially trained to address communication and other needs of the patient and family in the context of complex and life-threatening situations.
- The nurse is usually the one who needs to carry out the orders decided on at the family meeting.

The essential role of the nurse cannot be understated in palliative care [3].

The Nurse and Hospice Care

Another area where nurses are essential and important is in hospice care of patient. Chapter 3 provides more details on the hospice care. The role of the nurse in hospice care which may occur at home or as inpatient involves three broad areas: (1) approaching care from a patient and family-based, interdimensional care focus; (2) expertise in end-stage disease symptom management; and (3) applying nursing process as a member of the hospice IDT through a critical thinking approach that supports the Hospice Experience Model. The hospice's nurse initial role in end-of-life care is to work with the patient and family to prevent or minimize the suffering that results from physical and functional decline of advancing age or from end-stage disease progression [2].

Nursing Pain Management of the Palliative Care Patients

Nursing Assessment of Pain

Pain is one of the most common but also one of the most feared symptoms that palliative care patients experience during the terminal phase of their lives. The cornerstone of adequate pain management of the palliative care patient is a thorough patient assessment and frequent reassessment. Nurses usually spend more time with a patient than any other health care professional and therefore have the ability and responsibility to perform a holistic pain evaluation. Pain is "whatever the experiencing person says it is, existing whenever and wherever the person say it does". According to the Agency of Healthcare Research and Quality (AHRQ), the most reliable indicator of the existence and intensity of pain is the patient's self-report. Pain is affected most importantly by physiological, psychological, and spiritual factors. The evaluation of pain must consider the evaluation of these factors. When the clinician needs to assess pain, there are some key areas or questions that are recommended (Table 9.2) [4].

The information obtained will help determine the cause of pain and the design of an appropriate pain management plan. It may help the clinician to determine if the pain is caused by disease (e.g., direct invasion by cancer), treatment (e.g., constipation with opioids), debility (e.g., pressure sores), or other unrelated pathology (e.g., arthritis). Pain management should always encompass a holistic approach to treat the cause of pain, including spiritual perspectives.

Care from Family Members and Education of Family and Patient

In some cultures, for instance in Chinese, Asian, as well as several other cultures, interactions with family are extremely important and family members value being able to help with each other. Family members play important roles in meeting both the patient's physical and psychosocial needs as well as accomplishing treatment goals. They perform a wide range of tasks and invest huge amounts of time in taking care of the patient. When the patient can no longer sit, walk, eat, or perform activities of daily living such as bathing, feeding, toileting, dressing, and turning they require total support and physical strength from the family members. In addition, family caregivers may be needed to assist with other necessary activities such as preparing meals, managing medications, observing disease progression, and building links with health professionals. Family caregivers could be parents, spouse, children, children-in-law, and relatives. Some of them may provide 24 h help when the patient has terminal cancer.

People who are dying need care in four areas:

1. Physical comfort
2. Mental and emotional needs
3. Spiritual issues and
4. Practical tasks

Pain is one of main causes of physical discomfort. Pain can affect mood. Being in pain can make someone seem angry or short-tempered. Irritability resulting from pain might make the patient hard to talk, hard to share thoughts and feelings. Experts believe that care for someone who is dying should focus on relieving pain without worrying about possible long-term problems, such as opioids dependence or abuse [5]. Family members should not be afraid of giving pain medicine as is prescribed by the doctor. Pain is easier to prevent than to relieve, and overwhelming pain is hard to manage. If the pain is not controlled well, the patient and his family members should communicate with the doctor. It can be relieved safely and rapidly.

Table 9.2 Pain assessment terminology

Term	Definition	How to use clinically
Duration	How long the pain has been experienced and continues to be present (lasting minutes or hours)	• This information is critical for evaluating the effectiveness of the treatment plan • Duration of pain can be gathered as part of a comprehensive history of the pain as well as each time pain is assessed
Frequency	The number of occurrences in a specified period of time; how often the pain is experienced in a given time period	• Knowing the frequency of pain is useful in developing treatment strategies and for individualized scheduling of care activities
Intensity (or severity)	The descriptive rating of the pain experience	• Usually helpful to identify intensity for the older adult's "worst pain" over a specified period of time as well as "the best the pain gets" in a particular time period • Assessing the present pain rating and an identified pain rating acceptable to the patient is also important • Use the most appropriate scale individualized to the patient's cognitive and sensory abilities (see Figs. Fig. 9.1 Example of a Numeric Pain Intensity Instrument/Scale Fig. 9.2 Example of a Pain Assessment Tool/Scale. Reprinted from Stuppy DJ. The faces pain scale: reliability and validity with mature adults. Appl Nurs Res. 1998;11(2):84–9. Copyright 1998, with permission from Elsevier 9.1 and 9.2)
Location	Anatomic site(s) of pain	• Older adults often have pain in more than one location • Identify and document all sites with corresponding intensity and character • Pain maps are very useful in documenting all pain locations, guiding therapy, and as a tool in providing daily care (e.g., CNAs can use the pain map to establish the least painful ways to turn and/or ambulate the person they are working with)
Onset	Description of the experience of the beginning of the pain	• The patient may describe a sudden or gradual development of the pain, associated with a known injury or illness • Asking about onset can also help identify pain triggered by specific movement or activity

| Pattern (or rhythm) | The course of the pain over time including variations, often influenced by times of day (e.g., certain hours of the day, night or day, monthly patterns), periods of rest, or specific or general activity/movement | • Older adults can experience constant and/or episodic pain
• Analgesic therapy should be tailored to these patterns
• For example, short-acting analgesics are most appropriate for episodic pain, whereas long-acting agents are best for constant pain. Routinely dosed, short-acting agents may work well as an alternative to long-acting opioids in older adults
• Older adults with both constant pain and episodic increases in pain (breakthrough pain) need both short-acting and long-acting medications |
| Quality (or character) | Description of the characteristics of the pain, preferably in the words used patient to describe the pain | • Helpful in determining the type of pain to guide the most appropriate analgesic
• If the older adult has difficulty describing the pain, it may be helpful to offer examples of descriptions
• These may include the following: aching, sore, cramping, pounding, sharp, throbbing, dull, nagging, penetrating, shooting, numb, tingling, spasm, burning, gnawing, pressure-like, radiating, stabbing, tingling, tender, knife-like, etc. |

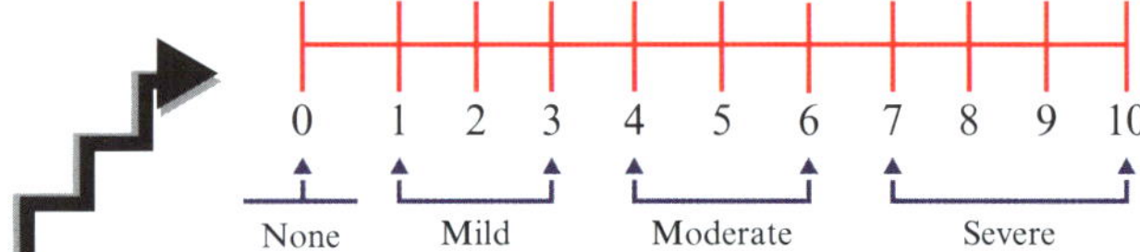

Fig. 9.1 Example of a Numeric Pain Intensity Instrument/Scale

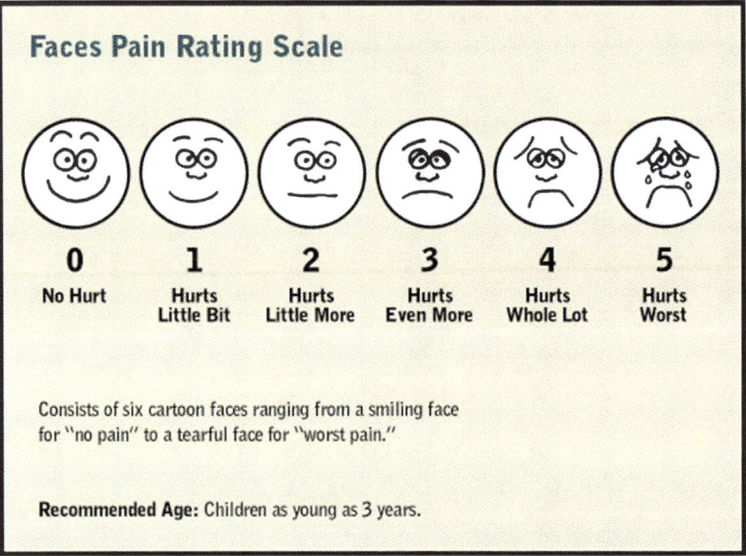

Fig. 9.2 Example of a Pain Assessment Tool/Scale. Reprinted from Stuppy DJ. The faces pain scale: reliability and validity with mature adults. Appl Nurs Res. 1998;11(2):84–9. Copyright 1998, with permission from Elsevier

There are some myths about pain, which can hinder effective pain management. Nurses should attach great importance to these myths when they educate patients and their families (see Table 9.3).

Treatment Modalities for Pain

PCA and Other Treatment for Palliative Cancer Pain Patient

There are several treatment modalities that can be used to deliver effective pain management. One of these methods is the use of a patient controlled analgesia (PCA).

This is the technique whereby patients can self-administer small doses of parenteral analgesics by means of a simple push button mechanism. PCA is an effective and

Table 9.3 Common myths about dying and pain management

1. Myth: Dying is always painful	Not everyone who is dying experiences pain. Many people die without experiencing pain
2. Myth: There are some types of pain that cannot be relieved	Recent advances in medical area assure that all pain can be relieved by using combined approaches, such as medications and nerve block
3. Myth: If I get morphine, I will stop breathing	Morphine does slow down respirations in many people, however, proper doses of morphine usually do not cause someone to stop breathing
4. Myth: To get good pain relief, you have to take injections	We used to think that opioids were not effective unless administered by injection. We now know that morphine is effective when given orally or even by suppository. There are some long-acting preparations of morphine which can be given every 12 h, or some skin patches which can be applied every 72 h, to simply the route of pain control
5. Myth: People should wait until their pain is bad to take morphine so it will be effective when it is really needed	Using it when it is needed in the early phases of the disease does not mean that opioids and morphine will be ineffective in the advanced phases of the disease
6. Myth: Once you start taking morphine, the end of your life is always near	Morphine does not always cloud consciousness. It does not initiate the final phase of life or lead directly to death
7. Myth: Patients have to stay in a hospital to get effective pain relief	Patients can get safe and effective relief of severe pain at home. If treating the pain at home does not work, the patient may need further treatment in a hospital or outpatient setting or by a visiting nurse

safe treatment for cancer pain. PCA allows for more immediate relief of breakthrough pain and can provide patients with a greater sense of person control over their pain.

A number of parameters on the PCA pump can be set, including:

- **Drug concentration** in the drug reservoir.
- **Bolus dose** can be delivered by a permitted request.
- **Lockout time** is the interval between two bolus doses is set to allow time for the effect of the previous dose before the subsequent dose.
- **Rate of background infusion** is the amount of the continuous infusion. This feature is optional.
- **Hour limit** is set as the maximum amount the patient can receive in 1 or 4 h.

Patient and family education is critical for safe, effective use of PCA. Education must be provided to patients prior to initiation of PCA and must address their role in pain management. The family also needs to be educated on the use, dosage, and should be provided with answers and clarifications to questions they may ask. Education needs to both written and verbal and must include the following information:

- Definition of PCA and patient's responsibility in PCA therapy
- Pump operation

- PCA by proxy
- Description of when to alert the nurse include the following symptoms:
    - Inadequate pain relief
    - Side effects of nausea
    - Vomiting, constipation
    - Urinary retention
    - Itching

There are intravenous and subcutaneous routes of PCA. IV infusions require the need for an intravenous access. As death nears, the burden of maintaining IV access, especially in the home setting, can be enormous. The subcutaneous PCA route is an acceptable alternative to intravenous PCA.

Pain Team

In many countries, if a terminal ill inpatient needs a complex pain management, it is customary for the physician to refer the patient to a pain team. A pain team consists of pain doctors and pain management advanced practice nurses (APN). The pain doctor prescribes PCA orders based on the patient's current total daily opioid dose, and the pain management APN assesses the patient's cognitive function to determine if the patient is able to understand and participate in PCA therapy. In palliative care, pain management therapies including PCA therapy are often conducted in patient's homes. Nurses are a vital part of pain therapy at home since they are the liaison between patients and physicians in this setting.

After the initiation of PCA therapy, registered nurses assess the vital signs, pain, sedation, and respiratory rate and quality frequently. Assessment results are documented in the patient's chart. If the patient has any side effects related to pain treatment, registered nurses will contact the pain team [6].

The pain team will perform follow-up assessments every day and prescribe adjustments of PCA orders based on the patient's response to treatment. Meanwhile, a multimodal approach is combined with PCA therapy. The pain team will communicate strategies of pain treatment with the patient, family members, oncologists, and nurses.

Cultural and Spiritual Considerations

Losses and difficulties in life can challenge faith and philosophical systems. Those experiencing loss and grief may differ regarding religious and spiritual perspectives from which they seek answers, search for meaning, and to which they turn for ritual, comfort, and support [7]. It is important that the nurse understand the ways that spirituality or religion plays a role or not, facilitates or complicates the experience. The nurse also needs to be aware of his or her own beliefs and experiences and be careful not to allow those beliefs to negatively impact the patient and families in their care [8].

References

1. Jocham HR, Dassen T, Widddershoven G, Halfens R. Evaluating palliative care – a review of literature. Palliat Care Res Treat. 2009;3:5–12.
2. Ferrell B, Coyle N. Textbook of palliative nursing, vol. 355. New York: Oxford University Press; 2006.
3. Nelson J, Cortez TB, Curtis JR, Lustbader DR, Mosenthal AC, Mulkerin C, et al. Integrating Palliative care in the ICU: the nurse in a leading role. J Hosp Palliat Nurs. 2011;13(2):89–94.
4. Cancer pain management in children. http://www.childcancerpain.org/frameset.cfm?content=assess01. Accessed 22 Jan 2012.
5. Oliver DP, Wittenberg-Lyles E, Demiris G, Washington K, Porock D, Day M. Barriers to pain management: caregiver perceptions and pain talk by hospice interdisciplinary teams. J Pain Symptom Manage. 2008;36(4):374–82.
6. Nalini V, Urman R. Essentials of pain management. New York: Springer; 2011.
7. Matzo M, Sherman L, Witt D. Palliative care nursing: quality care to the end of life. New York: Springer; 2005.
8. White KR, Coyne PJ. Nurses's perceptions of educational gaps in delivering end-of-life care. Oncol Nurs Soc. 2011;38(6):711–7.

Review Questions

1. Palliative Care is focused on only the care of the dying patient

   (a) False
   (b) True

2. Palliative care is defined by:

   (a) JCAHO
   (b) WHO
   (c) The state
   (d) Nurses
   (e) Physicians

3. Palliative nursing is a new field of nursing that

   (a) Differs in essence from other areas
   (b) Reflects a whole person philosophy
   (c) Focuses on the patient and family as a unit
   (d) a, b, & c
   (e) b only

4. The nurse can relieve suffering in the following ways

   (a) By listening for statements of meaning from sufferers and allowing the person's exploring circumstances to surface the issue of higher meaning
   (b) By encouraging the sufferer's interpretation of their own experience
   (c) By validating the sufferer's interpretation of their own experience while clarifying meaning
   (d) a & c only
   (e) All the above

5. What is the most common palliative team design

   (a) A nurse and a physician
   (b) A nurse only
   (c) A nurse and social worker
   (d) A physician and chaplain
   (e) A physical therapist and a nurse

6. Pain is defined as whatever the patient says it is

   (a) True
   (b) False

7. The healthcare provider should be worried about patients becoming addict because they need to take pain medicine over a period of time

   (a) True
   (b) False

Answers

1. (a)
2. (a)
3. (d)
4. (e)
5. (a)
6. (a)
7. (b)

Chapter 10
Physical and Occupational Therapy in Palliative Care

Kais Alsharif and Justin Hata

Introduction

Rehabilitation in palliative care addresses physical limitations caused either by a severely debilitating or life-threatening illness. Physical limitations may be caused by tumor mass effects or by the treatments used for palliation of that illness. Palliative rehabilitation can be divided into three categories: preventative, restorative, and supportive. Preventative rehabilitation attempts to address and prevent functional decline by addressing and correcting morbidity caused by cancer or its treatment. When long-term impairment can be avoided, restorative rehabilitation attempts to return patients to their premorbid functional status. Supportive rehabilitation attempts to maximize function after permanent impairments caused by cancer and/or its treatment [1].

Rehabilitation in palliative care can be challenging due to the various types of pathologies encountered in this field of medicine. The varied presentations, the generally poor prognosis, and the patient-specific response to disease and disease treatments all represent challenges for the treating medical team. There is evidence to suggest that therapy referrals are uncommon and underutilized in the palliative care setting [2]. At the same time, palliative care patients express interest and are willing to undergo therapy, especially walking and home-based programs [3]. Furthermore, there is strong evidence that physical activity has a significant and positive impact on the quality of life in palliative patients with advanced cancer [4], multiple sclerosis [5, 6], Alzheimer's disease, spinal cord injury (SCI), brain injury (BI) [7–10], cardiopulmonary disease [11, 12], and human immunodeficiency virus (HIV) [13–18]. There is strong evidence that hospice patients participating in palliative rehabilitation show decreased pain, decreased dyspnea, improved leg edema, better

K. Alsharif, M.D. (✉) • J. Hata, M.D.
Department of Anesthesiology and Perioperative Care, University of California,
Irvine School of Medicine, Irvine, CA, USA
e-mail: fastkais@hotmail.com

N. Vadivelu et al. (eds.), *Essentials of Palliative Care*,
DOI 10.1007/978-1-4614-5164-8_10,
© Springer Science+Business Media New York 2013

mood, enhanced motor function, improved cognitive function from admission to discharge, as well as increased mobility and better quality of life [19, 20]. In this chapter, we will discuss the use of physical and occupational therapy in palliative medicine, including the reported benefits and evidence behind their use.

Physiologic and Functional Changes in the Palliative Patient

Fatigue, cachexia, anorexia, and muscle wasting are very common in the palliative patient. Fatigue is the most common symptom, and has many causes in the palliative patient, including primary and secondary etiologies [21]. Primary fatigue is often due to the tumor itself and can occur through alterations in ATP and muscle metabolism [21]. Tumor load and subsequent proinflammatory cytokine production, including interleukin-1, interleukin-6, and tumor necrosis factor-α, interact to contribute to cancer-related fatigue (CRF) in the end stages of cancer [22]. Primary fatigue can also be due to central mechanisms including dysregulated hypothalamic–pituitary–adrenal axis, serotonin metabolism, circadian rhythm disruption, vagal afferent activation, or reduced recruitment of motor units [21]. Comorbidities contribute to secondary fatigue and include anemia, infections, depression, pain, dyspnea, sleep disorders, as well as prolonged physical inactivity. Medications—such as opiates and anxiolytics, often used to palliate symptoms—can also contribute to fatigue [21, 22].

Cachexia is often accompanied by decreased muscle strength, often due to both decreased muscle protein synthesis and increased proteolysis [23]. Skeletal muscle protein turnover in cachectic patients is significantly reduced [23]. In addition, a large percentage of palliative patients are elderly with lower lean muscle mass and less maximal power output compared with younger populations. Other causes of decreased muscle strength in the palliative setting include myopathies and neuropathies. These can be induced by the cancer itself or more often due to toxic and metabolic sequelae of antineoplastic treatments [24–26].

Progressive fatigue and anorexia–cachexia syndrome can contribute to loss of physical function in the palliative cancer patient and to the detriment of overall quality of life [22]. Up to one-third of all cancer deaths are related to poor exercise and nutrition [27, 28]. The primary goal of palliative care is to maximize overall quality of life for patients and their families [29], and physiotherapy does so by maintaining optimum respiratory and circulatory function; preventing muscle atrophy; preventing joint contractures; improving pain control; and optimizing independence and function [30]. In addition, physiotherapy plays a role in the education and participation of caregivers, as well as reducing the burden of care for families and caregivers [2, 30]. It should be emphasized that in the palliative patient, group exercise therapy, regular therapy, and energy conservation therapies become more important in managing fatigue. Similarly, relaxation training and guided imagery play important roles in decreasing nausea associated with palliative treatments [31].

Rehab Team and Setting

The palliative rehabilitation team should consist of a physiatrist, physical therapist, occupational therapist, a speech/respiratory therapist, recreational therapist, nutritionist, a nurse, and a social worker. All team members should be trained and be familiar with hospice and palliative care. The setting can be inpatient or outpatient or home based, and will depend on the need for hospitalization for other palliative treatment. Inpatient rehabilitation is suited for patients able to tolerate at least 3 h of rigorous therapy, and who also have potential for significant functional improvement [1]. Subacute inpatient rehabilitation, or "slow paced rehabilitation," often at a skilled nursing facility provides less intense rehabilitation for patients who can tolerate at least 1 h each day. Subacute inpatient rehabilitation can serve as a transitional program for palliative care patients before discharge from a medical or surgical unit [1]. Most importantly, palliative patients tend to adhere to and respond better to programs designed to address their own specific physical activity interests and preferences [32].

The physiatrist should perform a complete initial historical and physical assessment, paying special attention to the musculoskeletal and neurologic systems. Further evaluation should include information on pathology location, staging, estimated life expectancy, comorbidities, as well as pain symptoms. Several functional scales can be used for prognosis of the palliative patient and are summarized in Table 10.1 [1]: The team should be aware of previous and anticipated treatments and therapies. Adequate pain control should be attempted to achieve appropriate levels of analgesia without causing undue side effects such as nausea and sedation, which can limit participation in therapy. Achieving this delicate balance requires close cooperation between all team members, under the guidance and supervision of the physiatrist or team leader.

Rehabilitation Strategies and Types of Therapy

Exercise is used to improve or maintain strength, to maintain flexibility, to improve range of motion (ROM) of the joints and prevent contractures, and improve proprioception and balance. Exercises used include passive, active, active-assisted, resistive exercises, flexibility (stretching) exercises, and aerobic conditioning [1]. Walking, cycling, and aerobic devices utilized include treadmills, rowing machines, and ergometers. Resistive exercises can include performing a set of 8–12 repetitions at 60–70 % of one maximal over a 12-week program in upper and lower extremities. In prostate cancer patients receiving chemotherapy, such a resistive program was shown to result in decreased fatigue and improvement in strength and quality of life, without changes in body composition and with good patient tolerance [33]. Proprioceptive and balance training can include use of the biomechanical ankle platform system (BAPS) board.

Table 10.1 Rehabilitation of the hospice and palliative care patient

Category	Assessment tools	Scoring system
Physical function	Karnofsky Performance Scale (KPS) [39, 40]	– 100-point scale (100=normal function; 0=death) – KPS score of 50 or lower is associated with a limited survival
	Palliative Performance Scale (PPS) [41]	– 100-point scale (100=normal function and activity; 0=death) – Lower scores are associated with limited survival
	Eastern Cooperative Oncology Group (ECOG) Functional Index [42]	– 5-point scale (0=perfect health; 5=death – ECOG scores of 3 and 4 are associated with limited survival
	Edmonton Functional Assessment Tool (EFAT) [43, 45]	– 4-point rating scale (0=functionally independent; 0=total loss of function)
	Katz Activities of Daily Living (ADLs) [46, 47]	– Measures six domains of function – Each domain is rated as 0 (dependent) or 1 (independent) – Total scores; 6=full function; 4=moderate impairment; and 2=severe impairment – Dependency in two or more ADLs contributes to clinical decline and limited prognosis
	Lawton Instrumental Activities of Daily Living (IADLs) [48, 49]	– Measures eight domains of function – Each domain is scored either 0 (impairment) or 1 (normal function) – Higher scores indicate higher functional status
	Barthel Index (BI) [51]	– Measures patients' performance in 10 ADL tasks – Each task is scored in increments of 5 points (5–10–15) – Scores range from 100 (full independence) to 0 (bedridden state)
	Functional Independence Measure (FIM) [52, 53]	– Yields a total score, motor score, and a cognitive score – The scores vary from 18 to 126; higher scores indicate higher independence levels

Balance/fall risk	Berg Balance Scale [54]	– 14-item performance based measure of balance – Each task in measured on a 5-point scale ranging from 0 (lowest level of function) to 4 (higher levels of function) (total maximum score = 56) – Scores correlate with fall risk; 41–56 = low fall risk; 21–40 = medium fall risk; and 0–20 = high fall risk
	Tinetti Assessment of Balance and Gait [55]	– Nine items for balance and seven items for gait – Each task is scored on a 3-point scale from 0 (complete impairment) to 2 (independence) – Maximum score for gait is 12 and balance is 16 (total of 28) – Risk for falls if total score 19–24; high risk for falls if total score < 19
	Timed Up and Go (TUG) [56-57]	– High risk for falls if time to complete the task is ≥20 s
Endurance	6 Minute Walk Test (6MWT) [58]	– Primary measurement is total distance waked in 6 min

From: Javier NS, Montagnini ML. Rehabilitation of the hospice and palliative care patient. J Palliat Med. 2011;14(5):638–48. doi: 10.1089/jpm.2010.0125

Table 10.2 Activities of daily living (ADLs)

Bathing and showering
Bowel and bladder management
Personal hygiene and grooming
Toilet hygiene
Dressing
Eating
Feeding
Functional mobility
Personal device care
Sexual activity

Pulmonary rehabilitation includes programs to improve cardiopulmonary capacity utilizing inspiratory muscle re-training, noninvasive mechanical ventilation, breathing techniques, management of secretion, and postural drainage [1]. Aerobic conditioning has been shown to reduce symptom burden [34]. In bone marrow transplant patients, performance of cycling at 50 % heart rate reserve reduces: declines in speed and walking distance, neutropenia, thrombocytopenia, and psychologic distress [34].

Physical modalities for pain control can supplement medical treatments (discussed in full elsewhere) and contribute to improved physical function. These modalities include massage, heat, cold, ultrasound, transcutaneous electrical nerve stimulation (TENS), manual lymphatic drainage, soft tissue mobilization, and diathermy [1].

Occupational therapy addresses and treats deficits in activities of daily living (ADLs) (Table 10.2), work activities and employment, with the use of adaptive equipment, as well as recreational activities. Therapists provide home assessment evaluations and prescriptions for equipment, as well as provide education and strategies for caregivers. Environmental modification may include the removal of throw rugs from areas that cause falls, adding railings in staircases and bathrooms, having a high stool in the kitchen to reach a cupboard, and adjusting the height and arms of the chair to assist in transfers [1]. Adaptive equipment used to assist with activities of daily living (ADLs) include reachers, rocker knives, cutting boards, and holders for assistance with cooking and eating [1], as well as raised toilet seats and shower chairs for assistance with toileting and bathing. Assistive devices such as canes, crutches, walkers, wheelchairs, and scooters can be used to assist with ambulation. Lifts, ramps, and transfer boards help with transfers. In addition to helping balance and ambulation, these assistive devices also decrease load on weight-bearing joints helping with joint instability, balance, and relieving weight bearing on affected extremities. Orthotics can also be used to improve and optimize best joint mechanics and compensate for motor deficits. Examples include ankle foot orthosis (AFO) used for treatment of foot drop, or thoracolumbosacral orthosis (TLSO) in spinal compression fractures to limit spinal flexion.

Specific Strategies

Rehabilitation of Specific Cancers or Related Complications

Head and Neck Cancer

Treatments for head and neck cancers include conservative and radical surgical resection, as well as postsurgical irradiation. Complications from surgical procedures include damage to muscles and nerves within the zone of resection. Furthermore, external beam radiation is associated with tissue necrosis and fibrosis. The combination of surgical and radiation treatment can thus alter normal anatomy, often leading to nerve palsies, weak cervical musculature with contracture and subsequent exaggerated thoracic kyphosis. Aggressive ROM should be initiated following surgical healing (usually within 3–7 days depending on the type of surgery), and should be continued during the radiation treatment and for at least 2 years following treatment. Spinal accessory nerve palsy is another complication, and can lead to trapezius muscle weakness, with winging of the scapula and frozen shoulder. Active and passive ROM exercises, strengthening of the remaining scapular stabilizers, and postural modification are some of the rehabilitation techniques available.

Breast Cancer

Treatment of breast cancer often involves surgical treatments including modified radical mastectomy (MRM), lumpectomy, axillary lymph node resection (ALND), and transverse rectus abdominus flap breast reconstruction (TRAM-flap). These procedures result in anatomic changes that require rehabilitation. Deficits in shoulder ROM following ALND are well documented, and the time course for rehabilitation has been studied. Early exercises following ALND were initially discouraged due to the possibility of lymphedema and seroma formation. However, a systemic review [35] showed that early rather than delayed onset training did not affect the incidence of postoperative lymphedema. Post-TRAM-flap rehabilitation to correct abdominal muscle weakness and stabilize the trunk is essential, has been shown to have long-lasting benefits and is well tolerated. Finally, axillary web syndrome is the presence of a taut palpable cord originating in the axilla and the upper arm following ALND. Therapy to increase ROM, along with manual therapy to soften the cords can be helpful.

Lymphedema

Lymphedema can develop following irradiation or resection of lymph nodes and vessels as lymphatic congestion develops in the affected areas. Complete decongestive therapy (CDT) is an intensive treatment tool available for managing lymphedema. It combines manual lymphatic drainage followed by compressive bandaging, therapeutic exercise, and elastic compressive garments. Manual lymphatic drainage is performed for 45–60 min, which is followed by the application of a compressive bandage which can be left for up to 24 h. Following improvement (usually after 3–7 days), the patient is then transitioned to a maintenance phase in which compressive garments are used during the day, followed by compressive bandaging at night, and manual lymphatic drainage as needed. CDT has been shown to be effective in decreasing swelling, improving lymphatic flow and venous return, maintaining skin integrity, and protecting the limb from trauma [36, 37].

References

1. Javier NS, Montagnini ML. Rehabilitation of the hospice and palliative care patient. J Palliat Med. 2011;14(5):638–48. doi:10.1089/jpm.2010.0125.
2. Montagnini M, Lodhi M, Born W. The utilization of physical therapy in a palliative care unit. J Palliat Med. 2003;6:11–7.
3. Lowe SS, Watanabe SM, Baracos VE, Courneya KS. Physical activity interests and preferences in palliative cancer patients. Support Care Cancer. 2010;18(11):1469–75.
4. Lowe SS, Watanabe SM, Courneya KS. Associations between physical activity and quality of life in palliative cancer patients: a pilot survey. J Pain Symptom Manage. 2009;38(5):785–96.
5. Motl RW, McAuley E. Pathways between physical activity and quality of life in adults with multiple sclerosis. Health Psychol. 2009;28:682–9.
6. Motl RW, McAuley E, Snook EM. Physical activity and quality of life in multiple sclerosis: possible roles of social support, self-efficacy and functional limitations. Rehabil Psychol. 2007;52:143–51.
7. Ginis KA, Latimer AE, McKechnie K, Ditor DS, McCartney N, Hicks AL, et al. Using exercise to enhance subjective well-being among people with spinal cord injury: the mediating influences of stress and pain. Rehabil Psychol. 2003;48:157–64.
8. Katz JF, Adler JC, Mazzarella NJ, Ince LP. Psychological consequences of an exercise training program for a paraplegic man. Rehabil Psychol. 1985;30:53–8.
9. Nayak S, Wheeler BL, Shiflett SC, Agostinelli S. Effect of music therapy on mood and social interaction among individuals with acute traumatic brain injury and stroke. Rehabil Psychol. 2000;45:274–83.
10. Holmes PS. Theoretical and practical problems for imagery in stroke rehabilitation: an observation solution. Rehabil Psychol. 2007;52:1–10.
11. Lanken PN, Terry PB, DeLisser HM, Fahy BF, Hansen-Flaschen J, Heffner JE, et al. An official American Thoracic Society policy statement: palliative care for patients with respiratory diseases and critical illnesses. Am J Respir Crit Care Med. 2008;177:912–27.
12. LeGrand SB. Dyspnea: the continuing challenge of palliative management. Curr Opin Oncol. 2002;14:394–8.
13. Harding R, Karus D, Easterbrook P, Raveis VH, Higginson IJ, Marconi K. Does palliative care improve outcomes for patients with HIV/AIDS: a systematic review of the evidence. Sex Transm Infect. 2005;81:5–14.
14. Cade WT, Peralta L, Keyser RE. Aerobic exercise dysfunction in human immunodeficiency virus: a potential link to physical disability. Phys Ther. 2004;84:655–64.
15. Nixon S, O'Brien K, Glazier R, Tynan AM. Aerobic exercise interventions for adults living with HIV/AIDS. Cochrane Database Syst Rev. 2005;(2):CD001796.

16. O'Brien K, Nixon S, Tynan AM, Glazier RH. Effectiveness of aerobic exercise in adults living with HIV/AIDS: systematic review. Med Sci Sports Exerc. 2004;36:1659–66.

17. O'Brien K, Nixon S, Glazier R, Tynan AM. Progressive resistive exercise interventions for adults living with HIV/AIDS. Cochrane Database Syst Rev. 2004;(4):CD004248.

18. O'Brien K, Tynan AM, Nixon S, Glazier RH. Effects of progressive resistive exercise in adults living with HIV/AIDS: systematic review and meta-analysis of randomized trials. AIDS Care. 2008;20:631–53.

19. Yoshioka H. Rehabilitation for the terminal cancer patient. Am J Phys Med Rehabil. 1994;73:199–206.

20. Sabers SR, Kokal JE, Girardi JC, Philpott CL, Basford JR, Therneau TM, Schmidt KD, Gamble GL. Evaluation of consultation-based rehabilitation for hospitalized cancer patients with functional impairment. Mayo Clin Proc. 1999;74:855–61.

21. Strasser F. Diagnostic criteria of cachexia and their assessment: decreased muscle strength and fatigue. Curr Opin Clin Nutr Metab Care. 2008;11(4):417–21.

22. Kumar SP, Anand J. Physical therapy in palliative care: from symptom control to quality of life: a critical review. Indian J Palliat Care. 2010;16:138–46.

23. Dworzak F, Ferrari P, Gavazzi C, et al. Effects of cachexia due to cancer on whole body and skeletal muscle protein turnover. Cancer. 1998;82:42–8.

24. Oettle H, Richards D, Ramanathan RK, et al. A phase III trial of pemetrexed plus gemcitabine versus gemcitabine in patients with unresectable or metastatic pancreatic cancer. Ann Oncol. 2005;16:1639–45.

25. Colson K, Doss DS, Swift R, et al. Bortezomib, a newly approved proteasome inhibitor for the treatment of multiple myeloma: nursing implications. Clin J Oncol Nurs. 2004;8:473–80.

26. Schrag D, Chung KY, Flombaum C, Saltz L. Cetuximab therapy and symptomatic hypomagnesemia. J Natl Cancer Inst. 2005;97:1221–4.

27. Pate RR, Pratt M, Blair SN, Haskell WL, Macera CA, Bouchard C, et al. Physical activity and public health: a recommendation from the centers for disease control and prevention and the American college of sports medicine. J Am Med Assoc. 1995;273:402–7.

28. Bryan A, Hutchinson KE, Seals DR, Allen DL. A transdisciplinary model integrating genetic, physiological and psychological correlates of voluntary exercise. Health Psychol. 2007;26:30–9.

29. Borgsteede SD, Deliens L, Francke AL, et al. Defining the patient population: one of the problems for palliative care research. Palliat Med. 2006;20:63–8.

30. Kumar SP, Jim A. Physical therapy in palliative care: from symptom control to quality of life: a critical review. Indian J Palliat Care. 2010;16(3):138–46.

31. Lyles JN, Burish TG, Krozely MG, Oldham RK. Efficacy of relaxation training and guided imagery in reducing the aversiveness of cancer chemotherapy. J Consult Clin Psychol. 1982;50:509–24.

32. Jones LW, Courneya KS. Exercise counseling and programming preferences of cancer patients. Cancer Pract. 2002;10(4):208–15.

33. Segal RJ, Reid RD, Courneya KS, et al. Resistance exercise in med receiving androgen deprivation therapy for prostate cancer. J Clin Oncol. 2003;21:1653–9.

34. Dimeo F, Fetscher S, Lange W, et al. Effects of aerobic exercise on the physical performance and incidence of treatment-related complications after high-dose chemotherapy. Blood. 1997;90:3390–4.

35. Chan DN, Lui LY, So WK. Effectiveness of exercise programmes on shoulder mobility and lymphedema after axillary lymph node dissection for breast cancer: systemic review. J Adv Nurs. 2010;66(9):1902–14.

36. Ko DS, Lerner R, Klose G, et al. Effective treatment of lymphedema of the extremities. Arch Surg. 1998;133:452–8.

37. Moseley AL, Carati CJ, Pillar NB. A systemic review of common conservative therapies for arm lymphoedema secondary to breast cancer treatment. Ann Oncol. 2007;18(4):639–46.

Review Questions

1. The most common complaint experienced by cancer patients resulting in decreased physical function is?

   (a) Pain
   (b) Depression
   (c) Fatigue
   (d) Weakness

2. Which of the following are physiologic changes contributing to fatigue in the palliative patient?

   (a) Alteration in, or decrease in ATP
   (b) Tumor load resulting in tumor proinflammatory cytokine production, including interleukin-1, interleukin-6, and tumor necrosis factor-a
   (c) Alterations in muscle metabolism
   (d) All of the above are true

3. Physical modalities for pain control include all except?

   (a) Massage
   (b) Heat/cold
   (c) Ultrasound
   (d) Transcutaneous electrical nerve stimulation (TENS)
   (e) Epidural injection

4. Regarding breast cancer rehabilitation following lumpectomy, axillary lymph node dissection or modified radical mastectomy, which of the following is true?

   (a) Early rehabilitation is associated with seroma formation and is discouraged
   (b) Rehab usually begins 2–3 months following surgery
   (c) Early rehabilitation results in better outcomes and is not associated with postoperative seroma formation
   (d) None of the above are true

5. Which of the following is true regarding axillary web syndrome?

   (a) It is a congenital disorder
   (b) It is a taut palpable cord in the axilla occurring following lymph node dissection
   (c) It does not respond to manual therapy
   (d) It is a vascular malformation of the axillary artery

6. A 78-year-old female with history of metastatic breast cancer on hospice care is having difficulty reaching for objects in her kitchen, as well as more frequent falls at home. Which of the following can an occupational therapist help with?

   (a) Environmental modification such as removal of throw rugs to prevent falls, addition of railing to staircase, etc.

    (b) Evaluating for adaptive equipment such as a reacher
    (c) Providing a high stool in the kitchen
    (d) Providing a cane or walker to assist with ambulation
    (e) All of the above

7. Which of the following are essential to a successful evaluation of a palliative patients' rehabilitation needs?

    (a) Close attention to the neurologic and musculoskeletal systems
    (b) Awareness of previous therapies and treatments received
    (c) Information on pathology location, staging, estimated life expectancy, and other comorbidities
    (d) Adequate pain evaluation and treatment
    (e) All of the above

8. What is subacute rehabilitation?

    (a) An outpatient rehab program for palliative patients
    (b) An inpatient program for patients who can tolerate at least 3 h of vigorous physical and occupational therapy
    (c) Slow paced rehab, often at a skilled nursing facility which provides less intense rehabilitation for patients who can tolerate at least 1 h each day, but less than 3 h
    (d) Another name for a nursing home

9. All of the following are true, except:

    (a) There is evidence to suggest that therapy referrals are uncommon and underutilized in the palliative care setting
    (b) Palliative care patients are not interested and feel unable or unwilling to undergo therapy
    (c) There is strong evidence that physical activity has a significant positive impact on the quality of life in palliative patients with advanced cancer, multiple sclerosis, Alzheimer's disease, spinal cord injury, brain injury, cardiopulmanry disease, and HIV
    (d) There is strong evidence that hospice patients show decreased pain, dyspnea, leg edema and better mood, motor function, cognitive function from admission to discharge as well as increased mobility and better quality of life

10. Rehabilitation in the palliative setting is associated with all of the following except:

    (a) Maintaining optimum respiratory and circulatory function
    (b) Preventing muscle atrophy
    (c) Preventing joint contractures
    (d) Prolonging life expectancy
    (e) Improving pain control
    (f) Optimizing independence and function

Answers

1. (c) Fatigue
2. (d) All of the above are true
3. (e) Epidural injection
4. (c) Early rehabilitation results in better outcomes and is not associated with postoperative seroma formation
5. (b) It is a taut palpable cord in the axilla occurring following lymph node dissection
6. (e) All of the above
7. (e) All of the above
8. (c) Slow paced rehab, often at a skilled nursing facility which provides less intense rehabilitation for patients who can tolerate at least 1 h each day, but less than 3 h
9. (b) Palliative care patients are not interested and feel unable or unwilling to undergo therapy
10. (d) Prolonging life expectancy

Chapter 11
Social Work in Palliative Care

Janet Lucas, Bill Mejia, and Anne Riffenburgh

*You matter to the last moment of your life, and we will do all we can
to help you not only die peacefully, but also to live until you die.*

– Dame Cicely Saunders

Introduction

Palliative care has a unique place in medicine. It calls us to acts of compassion,
touches our deepest fears, raises profound questions of life and death, and offers the
possibility of transcendence. Social work, with its rich tradition of understanding
and assisting individuals in extreme circumstances, is well positioned to address the
special challenges faced by patients, families, and medical team members.

As palliative care social workers, we combine "what we know" with "what we
do" to contribute our specialized skills and services in three major ways:

- Collaboration with fellow members of the medical team
- Interaction with patients and families
- Promotion of social work ideals through research and training.

J. Lucas, L.C.S.W., B.S., M.S.W. (✉)
Family Practice Residency Program,
Glendale Adventist Medical Center, Glendale, CA, USA
e-mail: jclucas11@aol.com

B. Mejia, L.C.S.W., B.S., M.S.W.
Palliate Care Consult Service, Huntington Hospital, Pasadena, CA, USA

A. Riffenburgh, L.C.S.W., B.S., M.S.W.
Huntington Cancer Center, Huntington Hospital, Pasadena, CA, USA

N. Vadivelu et al. (eds.), *Essentials of Palliative Care*,
DOI 10.1007/978-1-4614-5164-8_11,
© Springer Science+Business Media New York 2013

What We Know

The palliative care social worker uses a variety of skills and tools to enhance collaboration and therapeutic interventions. The National Association of Social Workers (NASW) has established essential areas of knowledge for social workers in palliative care. These include:

- Recognition of the complex roles and functions of the clinical social worker
- Familiarity with the biopsychosocial stages of the dying process
- Understanding of the physical, psychological, and spiritual aspects of pain
- Expertise in a wide range of psychosocial interventions to alleviate suffering
- Recognition of the biopsychosocial needs of patients and family members
- Awareness of the effect of ethnic, religious, and cultural differences
- Capacity to navigate the health care system, interact effectively with health care providers, and facilitate health care decision making
- Coordination of care and facilitation of communication among patient, family, and health care providers
- Ability to operate in a wide range of settings that provide palliative and end-of-life care, including hospitals, home care, nursing homes, and hospice settings
- Knowledge of available community resources and discharge planning options
- Sensitivity to the financial impact of illness and end-of-life
- Recognition of cross-cultural and socioeconomic disparities in accessing palliative care services
- Adherence to guidelines established by accreditation and regulatory standards in all palliative care settings
- Competence in working with diverse populations, including those with special physical, mental, emotional, and developmental needs (NASW 2011).

What We Do

Palliative care social workers intervene in a wide range of settings, such as hospitals, clinics, freestanding hospices, nursing homes, and private homes. We work with a variety of individuals and populations, including children, adults, the frail elderly, caregivers, and families. We are adept at creating a therapeutic environment to enhance trust, promote communication, and alleviate suffering. The palliative care social worker will:

- Assume leadership in promoting compassionate end-of-life care
- Assist with end-of-life decision making and care planning
- Assist with the resolution of ethical dilemmas
- Act as a liaison between the patient/family and medical staff
- Promote cultural competency
- Participate in/facilitate family conferences

- Educate healthcare professionals, patients, and family members in the psychosocial aspects of end-of-life care
- Conduct and document psychosocial assessments
- Provide psychosocial interventions (crisis intervention, supportive counseling, and grief counseling)
- Advocate for patients' and families' wants and needs
- Provide community resource information
- Supervise social work interns
- Provide lectures, presentations, and training
- Conduct and publish research that promotes evidence-based practice in palliative and end-of-life care (NASW 2011).

The Palliative Care Social Worker and the Team

Although palliative care social workers demonstrate a high degree of autonomy, our care and practice skills are enhanced by our participation as members of an interdisciplinary team. In the palliative care arena, multiple team configurations exist, ranging from the simple, such as:

- Physician/nurse
- Physician/palliative care social worker
- Physician/nurse/palliative care social worker

  …to the more comprehensive, such as:

- Physician/nurse/palliative care social worker/ward or unit social worker/chaplain/ music therapist/art therapist/volunteer

Evolution of the Team

Much has been written about the process by which a team evolves from disorganization to cohesiveness. Tuckman's model [2] describes a fledgling team as uncertain about roles, responsibilities, and team mission, further complicated by a lack of trust and a heightened level of anxiety. During this stage, the physician is often the de facto team leader. As the team begins to mature, cliques may form and power struggles may occur. In this formative stage, the palliative care social worker plays an active role in facilitating communication, clarifying goals, and building consensus.

In the example below, a palliative care social worker describes the growing pains of forming a cohesive team.

Our program began with a physician, nurse practitioner, and social worker. The first few weeks were productive and exciting. Staff members were supportive of this new venture and eager to help us succeed. As we began to establish our roles, challenges emerged. During consultations, the physician dominated the discussion, and the nurse and I believed that our expertise wasn't being utilized. We felt irritated and frustrated. We also felt anxious about addressing the issue. I felt especially unnerved because I'm supposed to be the "communication expert" on the team. At our next team meeting, the nurse and I expressed our concerns to the physician about his sense of control. He was surprised but receptive. He shared his own nervousness about the success of the program and acknowledged his habit of "taking over" in order to cope. He shared his intention to pay attention to his controlling tendencies. There was such relief after this discussion that we decided to meet regularly to air our concerns. We found that creating an atmosphere of honesty and trust was paramount in developing a cohesive and effective team.

As the team matures, consensus is achieved more easily, roles and responsibilities are clear and defined, and important decisions are reached as a group. Smaller decisions may be delegated to individuals or subgroups. The team feels an increased sense of commitment and unity. Leadership is shared and the group hierarchy becomes more fluid. The fully mature team is characterized by a shared vision and commitment to strategic goals. Each member enjoys a high degree of autonomy. Disagreements occur but are resolved through open communication and consensus. Trust, mutual support, and team pride are well developed [2].

The Palliative Care Social Worker and the Consult

The team is often called upon to assist with complex aspects of palliative and end-of-life care. Common consult requests include managing pain and symptoms, establishing goals of care and care planning, discussing code status, and addressing ethical issues.

During the initial consult, the social worker focuses upon the psychosocial issues affecting the patient and family. However, the social worker may meet with referring medical staff first to clarify patient and family issues or to address the emotional needs of the staff members themselves. A comprehensive social work assessment may include:

- Mental status, mood, affect, willingness to engage
- Presence of suicidal/homicidal ideation
- Problems, questions, and concerns of the patient and/or family/caregiver
- Patient and/or family/caregivers' understanding of diagnosis and prognosis
- Current medical concerns
- Patient and family goals
- Patient and family dynamics
- Developmental/life stage issues
- Patient's living situation
- Psychosocial strengths and coping strategies
- Psychosocial stressors and vulnerabilities

- Past experience with illness, death, and loss
- End-of-life wishes (advance directive)
- Support network
- Spiritual needs
- Cultural values and beliefs
- Ethical concerns

Care Planning and the Patient–Family Meeting

The social worker's assessment provides valuable input which deepens the team's clinical understanding of the patient. The palliative care team communicates with the referring medical team and other involved staff to review the patient's current status and goals of care. Considering each treatment, relative to care plan goals allows practitioners to evaluate the burdens and benefits of a particular regimen [3]. In palliative care, with its focus on relieving symptoms and maximizing quality of life, evaluating the burdens and benefits of treatment is paramount.

The palliative care team meets with the patient and family to present recommendations. One end-of-life care planning model, the Seven "Cs", was developed by social workers at the Keck School of Medicine in Los Angeles. The checklist below provides a framework for developing a care plan in which interventions are consistent with goals of care.

The Seven "Cs"

1. Condition

   - Current status
   - Diagnosis
   - Treatments

   The first step is to establish the patient's immediate medical status: "What's happening right now?" This is an opportunity to determine whether the patient is stable, deteriorating, in crisis, improving, or imminently dying. The team notes the various medical conditions that are affecting the patient and the treatments that he or she is receiving.

2. Capacity

   - With capacity: The patient will participate in care planning
   - Without capacity: The team identifies a surrogate decision maker

If the physician determines that the patient lacks capacity, the social worker assists with establishing the patient's surrogate decision maker. The social worker determines if an advance directive exists; if not, the social worker begins to explore the question of decision making with family members.

3. Clinical course expectations—what is the patient's prognosis for:

  - Surviving the hospitalization?
  - Weaning from the mechanical ventilator?
  - Achieving an acceptable quality of life (as defined by the patient or decision maker)?

  Relying on general descriptions for prognosis such as, "fair," "poor," and "grave" can be vague and unhelpful. Linking a patient's prognosis to relevant areas of care can help patients and family members develop realistic expectations.

4. Care goals

  - CURE the disease
  - SLOW the progression of the disease
  - ALLOW DEATH to proceed, and palliate symptoms exclusively

  Once the team has established clinical course expectations, goals of care can be considered. Goal setting becomes particularly important when cure is no longer possible. One of the tasks for the palliative care team is to assess whether a proposed treatment is consistent with the care goal. For example, if the goal is to allow death to proceed naturally, then attempting CPR would not be consistent with a peaceful death. Likewise, maintaining blood draws or initiating TPN feeding might be inappropriate.

5. Care plan

  - Assess each treatment in terms of the care goal
  - Assess each treatment in terms of its burden and benefits to the patient

  Recommend to:

  - INITIATE a treatment
  - FORGO a treatment
  - MAINTAIN a treatment
  - WITHDRAW a treatment

6. Conference

  - Discuss care plan recommendations with interdisciplinary staff involved with the patient's care.
  - Discuss care plan recommendations with the patient and/or decision maker and other involved family members

7. Chart

  - Document the agreed upon care plan [4]

The Care Planning Model and the Role of the Palliative Care Social Worker

During the team meeting, the palliative care social worker facilitates the team's progression through each of the seven steps in the care planning model. The social worker helps provide the patient and family with a cohesive, structured discussion. The overarching focus is to develop a care plan that is clinically consistent with the agreed upon goals of care. Scheduled times may be established to review the care plan. The social worker helps to clarify and justify the care plan recommendations to initiate, forgo, maintain, or withdraw treatments, highlighting the burdens and benefits to patients.

Cultural Awareness

A natural tension exists between recognition of our common human bonds and our individual differences. In palliative care, understanding and honoring individual differences help create an atmosphere of trust and rapport that contribute to optimal communication and care planning. Researchers have found significant differences in how cultural groups view illness, grief, death, and dying, and end-of-life decision making. In addition, even within specific cultural groups, individual differences exist [5, 6].

The first step in developing cultural awareness lies in the Oracle's admonition, "Know thyself." Palliative care social workers must make conscious their own beliefs, attitudes, and assumptions. When working with patients and families whose values and traditions differ from our own, unconscious biases can creep into interactions via body language, facial expressions, and speech, unintentionally alienating those we seek to help. Those who feel judged often retreat physically and emotionally, inhibiting open communication and a willingness to solicit or accept support. Self-knowledge is a vital tool for palliative care social workers as we strive to remain professionally objective, compassionate, and helpful.

A second step in promoting cultural awareness is recognizing that great diversity exists, even within the same cultural group. Asking, not merely assuming, is paramount to gaining an understanding of patients' and families' values and beliefs [6, 7].

Sample questions may include:

- What do you know about your condition?
- How did this happen?
- What do you know about your treatment options?
- Tell me about your life before you got sick.
- Would you like us to give medical information to you or a family member?

- Do you want to make medical decisions about your care or would you prefer to have a family members do so?
- Do you have any spiritual beliefs or traditions that are important to you?
- Tell me what else I should know about you (and your family) in order to understand and help you.

While such questions may yield useful information, the possibility exists that not every question may be culturally appropriate for a particular patient or family member. It may be considered rude or disrespectful for a younger social worker to query an older person, for a woman to question a man, or a stranger to seek personal information. Developing cultural awareness takes courage, curiosity, and a willingness to make mistakes. If a patient of family member finds a question rude or inappropriate, rapport can often be reestablished if the social worker demonstrates willingness to apologize or atone for the breach. In addition, patients and families can be remarkably forgiving when they recognize that the social worker has a genuine desire to help [7].

Communication and the Care Plan

Thoughtful and accurate use of language is vital when communicating with patients and families to develop a care plan. The palliative care social worker strengthens clarity by promoting terminology used by the team that is specific, descriptive, and consistent. Examples include:

Avoid saying: "We recommend that the patient be DNR".

Do say: "We do not recommend attempting cardiopulmonary resuscitation (CPR) or putting the patient on a breathing machine/mechanical ventilator".

Rationale: The word "attempting" introduces the idea that resuscitation is not always successful. The recommended language deliberately links CPR to the use of a ventilator and opens the door to clarifying what a DNR order entails.

Avoid saying: "Life support" or "life sustaining treatment".

Do say: "Mechanical ventilation" or "breathing machine"

Rationale: Euphemistic or vague terms can provide a false impression that artificial treatment is promoting or sustaining life as opposed to prolonging death and suffering.

Avoid saying: "Futile".

Do say: "Not helpful" or "harmful" when describing a proposed treatment or intervention.

Rationale: The word "futile" implies that a treatment or intervention has neither harm nor benefit, when in fact many potential end-of-life options can lead to trauma and suffering, reducing quality of life and impeding a peaceful death.

Avoid saying: "There's nothing more we can do".

Do say: "We will provide ongoing supportive care/symptom management/comfort care…."

Rationale: Patients and families commonly fear abandonment by medical personnel and may choose invasive treatment to ensure ongoing contact and care. The palliative care team seeks to emphasize that care never stops, although the focus will shift from curative treatment to comfort and quality of life. The recommended terminology provides a starting point for discussion of what this ongoing care will look like.

Avoid saying: "What do you want us to do?"

Do say: "We recommend…" or "The treatment is/is not medically indicated"

Rationale: The question "What do you want us to do?" is likely to elicit the following response, "We want everything done!" It is incumbent upon the palliative care team to provide appropriate recommendations based upon the team's expertise and recognized standards of care. Patients and families can be overwhelmed if they are asked to make end-of-life decisions without appropriate education and guidance.

Do say: "We are *hopeful* that we'll be able to help you leave the hospital to spend time tending your garden." "We are *hopeful* that you will be able to spend Christmas with your grandchildren." "We are *hopeful* that you'll be able to sit on your horse, Zephyr, and maybe even take him for a couple of turns around the corral".

Rationale: Redefinition of hope can help ease the transition from curative to palliative care [8]. When cure is no longer possible, linking the word "hopeful" to a patient's realistic and achievable goals helps shift the focus from emphasizing medical intervention to fulfilling meaningful last wishes.

Tools for the Family Meeting: Integrating a New Reality

Ideally, a family meeting results in consensus. Often, however, conflicts arise. One primary reason for conflict is the inability of one or more family members to accept the reality of the patient's functional decline or grave prognosis. The social worker can use several strategies to help families gain understanding and acceptance of the patient's diagnosis and prognosis. Family members can be encouraged to:

- Share stories and memories about the patient before he or she became ill
- Participate in bedside care
- Meet regularly with the palliative care team for updates and discussion.

The use of narrative is recognized as an important tool in creating meaning and guiding the care plan [9, 10]. Sharing stories about the patient allows family members to compare and contrast the patient's former status with his or her current condition, shedding light on the new reality. In addition, family members, as well as the team, may gain insights into patient's wishes and preferences regarding care plan goals. Participating in bedside care allows family members to witness the patient's physical and mental changes firsthand, enabling a better understanding of the care plan recommendations. Meeting regularly with the palliative care team enhances trust and communication, which can prevent or mitigate conflict.

The following vignette illustrates the effective use of care planning strategies.

Mary G

Mary G. was a 74-year-old female with end stage lung cancer. She was in the ICU on a ventilator. The team determined that Mary would not likely survive the hospitalization. The team's recommended care plan goal was to allow death to proceed as peacefully and comfortably as possible. The care plan included forgoing CPR and withdrawing the vent, tube feedings, blood transfusions, and regular blood draws. The team also recommended that IV pain medications and anti-anxiety drugs be maintained and titrated as needed. The social worker arranged a meeting with Mary's daughter, the designated decision maker, and other family members to discuss the team's recommendations. Although the family intellectually understood Mary's grave prognosis, recommendations to withdraw the ventilator and tube feedings met with resistance. The social worker arranged the meeting in Mary's room on the ICU. While the physician provided education about the ventilator and tube feedings, Mary's bedside nurse performed suctioning. The family found this difficult to watch. The social worker asked the daughter to share a favorite memory of her mother. She tearfully described how the two of them enjoyed hiking on the trails behind Mary's home. There was silence for a moment, and then the daughter added, "She wouldn't want this, but I'm afraid." The social worker asked, "What are you afraid of?" The daughter responded, "I don't want my mother to suffocate and starve to death." Once this fear was expressed, the physician was able to successfully educate the family regarding the use of opiates and anti-anxiety medications to treat any sensation of shortness of breath. She was also able to explain the body's limited need for nutrition at the end-of-life. The following day the family reached consensus, agreeing that the doctor should implement a "comfort care measures only" care plan.

Ramona F

Ramona F. was a 38-year-old woman with vaginal cancer admitted to the hospital for symptom control. She had several treatment options, including radiation and chemotherapy with the possibility of an aggressive, potentially curative surgery. During the initial meeting, Ramona presented as frail, fatigued, severely underweight and emotionally overwhelmed. Through tears, she told the palliative care physician and social worker, "I want to live." In the next breath, however, she confided, "I don't know how I'm going to get through the chemo and radiation. My partner and my parents are pushing me to not only have the chemo and radiation but the surgery too." Despite her expressed ambivalence, Ramona stated her wish to pursue the first two treatment options. Surgery, however, was another matter. "Look at me! If I had surgery now I KNOW I would die on the table. Even if I survived, the complications might kill me." She felt anxious and fearful about the reaction of her loved ones. Together, the physician and the social worker affirmed that their role was to help her understand the treatment options, including the potential risks and benefits, and provide a safe environment where she could express her wishes. The social worker offered to arrange a family meeting in which these issues could be openly shared and discussed. Ramona reiterated her fear about communicating her wishes in the presence of her partner and family. The social worker then presented examples of some of the language that might be used in the family meeting. Ramona shared her relief and hopefulness that her wishes would be honored and heard.

Core Therapeutic Interventions

Palliative care social workers have the unique privilege of spending time with patients and families at the bedside. Through our use of key therapeutic interventions, we facilitate adjustment to illness and disability along the continuum from new diagnosis to impending death. As rapport and trust develop, opportunities emerge to enhance coping and heal psychosocial wounds. Interventions include:

- Providing supportive listening
- Normalizing/validating feelings
- Asking open-ended questions
- Enabling patients and family members to "tell their story"
- Assisting patients in "finding their voice"
- Presenting options and facilitating decision making
- Identifying areas of resilience and coping
- Providing cognitive behavioral reframing
- Integrating the reality of diagnosis and prognosis
- Providing individualized therapeutic techniques, such as:

  - Working with dreams and visions
  - Breathing and meditation
  - Relaxation and guided imagery
  - Journaling

- Providing bereavement follow-up

The use of core therapeutic interventions helps elicit valuable information and facilitates psychosocial healing. A comprehensive understanding of the patient and family is a vital component in the development of an individualized and targeted care plan. One challenge for palliative care social workers is that we must intervene in a fast-paced environment, sometimes with just one or two interactions. In the example below, the palliative care social worker used therapeutic interventions to help the patient explore concerns about her family and her own spiritual care needs. This therapeutic process allowed the patient to more fully accept her prognosis and her need for hospice care.

Marcia R

The palliative care team received a referral to see Marcia R., a 42-year-old wife and mother, with advanced ovarian cancer. Hospital staff had expressed concern that the patient was "in denial" because she refused to consider hospice, despite her deteriorating status. The social worker met with Marcia at the bedside. His assessment showed that she was well aware of the serious nature of her prognosis. Marcia shared her fear that accepting hospice would signal to her family that she was giving up. Her plan was to try to maintain as much normalcy as possible for her husband and two school-age daughters, by avoiding, for as long as possible, the trappings of illness. She identified durable medical equipment and having strangers in the house as her two most pressing concerns. She also revealed her need to "make peace with Jesus" before she could fully acknowledge that death was near. The social worker thought that the most immediate need was spiritual. He asked her, "What does making peace with Jesus look like for you?" She immediately responded, "He would let me know that I was forgiven." She spent some time discussing the importance of faith in her life. As trust grew between Marcia and the social worker, he was able to introduce the concept of hospice and show the ways in which the hospice team could support her medical and faith needs as well as the needs of her family. After leaving the bedside, the social worker made a referral to chaplain services. During their next encounter, Marcia told the social worker of Jesus coming to her in a dream. She described a loving presence, full of forgiveness. Later that day, Marcia said, "I'm ready," and accepted hospice care.

The palliative care social worker's involvement is not limited to the patient and family. In many settings, social workers are a key source for emotional support for staff members. Palliative care social workers are routinely called upon to help staff members process difficult emotions and circumstances. In the example below, a medical resident sought out the palliative care team to process an emotional reaction to a difficult case.

Dr. L

Dr. L was a young resident caring for a 22-year-old patient with end-stage anorexia, who had dwindled to 75 pounds. Her organ systems were failing.

She remained a full code. Although the patient's mother had a realistic under-standing of her daughter's condition, Dr. L struggled to reconcile the patient's failing status with her youth. He asked the palliative care social worker and physician for help. The first step was to help Dr. L understand that the patient's death was inevitable and that resuscitative measures would be traumatic and without benefit. While Dr. L knew this intellectually, the emotional impact of the patient's youth impeded his ability to establish a "comfort measures only" care plan. The palliative care social worker helped the resident to label his feelings, which he described as "despair" and "helplessness." By reframing that a peaceful death was both "medically sound and compassionate," the social worker and physician helped the resident gain a new perspective. This interaction not only addressed Dr. L's emotional reservations but also provided the language with which he could effectively engage the mother.

Keeping the Fire Burning: How Not to Burnout

Palliative care social workers are routinely asked, "How do you do your job? Isn't it depressing?" and "How do you keep from burning out?" Sometimes it is difficult for people on the outside to comprehend the many gifts and rewards that come from working with the ill and the dying. Nonetheless, there is a toll. Those who work in palliative care are susceptible to a form of pervasive exhaustion called compassion fatigue. Figley [11] has described compassion fatigue as "a deep physical, emotional, and spiritual exhaustion," which affects "those who do their work well." Researchers have distinguished between burnout and compassion fatigue. Burnout is characterized by a withdrawal from patients and a depletion of empathy. Those suffering from compassion fatigue, however, continue to dedicate themselves to their work, often finding it difficult to balance their empathy and compassion with healthy boundaries and adequate self-care [12].

Warning signs of compassion fatigue may include:

- Abusing drugs, alcohol, or food
- Increased anger/irritability
- High self-expectations/low self-esteem
- Depression/hopelessness/exhaustion
- Chronic lateness
- Physical symptoms, i.e., headaches, gastrointestinal complaints, hypertension
- Inability to maintain a balance of empathy and objectivity [12]

Palliative care social workers can engage in self-care activities to prevent or mitigate compassion fatigue:

- Acknowledge that palliative care is stressful work that carries an emotional toll
- Recognize that self-care is a professional responsibility
- Find an understanding peer or colleague who can listen

- Practice healthy behaviors: rouvtine exercise, good nutrition, adequate sleep, rewarding leisure activities, etc.

The cornerstone of professional enthusiasm rests upon the balance between caring appropriately for others as well as oneself. Appropriate boundaries come with recognizing the limitations of the social work role. One palliative care social worker notes, "My patients are in an incredibly difficult situation, my job is to offer them support, guidance, and resources to make their situation a bit better." Another says, "I understand that I'm stepping into someone else's journey. It's not my journey."

Noted psychologist Jonathan Young, who counsels those in the helping professions, uses DaVinci's powerful image of God and Adam in the Sistine Chapel as a metaphor for the mutuality of the helping relationship. In Dr. Young's view, God reaches for Adam with the same committed intensity with which Adam reaches for God. The lesson for palliative care social workers is that patients have the choice as to whether they want to accept support and intervention. In the words of one palliative care social worker, "I know I'm overstepping my boundaries if I'm working harder than the patient or family."

In the same vein, Father Gregory Boyle, founder of Homeboy Industries and the author of *Tattoos on the Heart: The Power of Boundless Compassion*, shares the dream of a boy he worked with, which led him to a deeper understanding of boundaries and burnout [13]. In the boy's dream, Father Boyle is holding a flashlight in a darkened room. There is a light switch on the wall. The boy feels grateful for the flashlight. He knows Father Boyle will shine the flashlight on the light switch, but he also knows that he alone must walk over and turn on the light. Father Boyle's definition of burnout: "…to always be trying to turn on the light switch for others." His antidote: "OK, I own a flashlight, I can aim it. That has to be enough. The rest is up to you. I can't turn the light on for you."

These two anecdotes remind us that maintaining clear professional boundaries is a crucial aspect of self-care and an important prerequisite for remaining inspired and passionate, allowing us to bring our best to the patients and families we serve.

Promotion of Palliative Care and Social Work Ideals

Palliative care social workers are well positioned to promote the core principles of both social work and palliative care. Modeling social work ideals begins with how we conduct ourselves professionally. As experts in the areas of communication, conflict resolution, and consensus building, social workers can lead by example as well as explore the nuances of interpersonal dynamics in a variety of settings: as part of a team, at the bedside, on the ward, and in the community.

As palliative care social workers, we have a responsibility to be the voice on the team that provides insights into the psychosocial and spiritual aspects of end-of-life care. Our presence ensures that the patient and family's psychosocial needs and concerns are integrated into the team's consciousness. Misconceptions still exist about the social work role. Bedside introductions can be met with, "No thank you,

I already have insurance" or "I don't need welfare." These interactions provide a direct opportunity to educate patients and families about social work's role in providing emotional support, finding useful community resources, and navigating the challenges of illness and end-of-life. Our presence on the ward enables us to interact with members of other disciplines—doctors, nurses, physical therapists, dietitians, discharge planners, and chaplains—sharing what we do, and learning from their experience and expertise as well.

Seasoned social workers can share their knowledge and wisdom through supervising, educating, and training social work students. Supervision enables students to learn through a combination of observation, practice, and in-service training. In addition, providing an opportunity for students to process their experiences helps them to cope with the emotional intensity of participating in end-of-life care.

Finally, the need to advance social work and palliative care ideals goes beyond the clinical setting into the greater community. As leaders in this new and innovative field, we are called upon to promote our professional ideals through public speaking, conference presentations, and published research.

Participating in the Mystery

Palliative care creates a portal that invites patients, family members, and social workers to share an intimate journey along the continuum from illness to end-of-life. The work is demanding, rewarding, heartfelt, and occasionally heartbreaking. As palliative care social workers, we ask the hard questions and listen to the hard answers. We help find solutions in the most difficult of circumstances. We strive to alleviate suffering and promote healing, be it physical, emotional, or spiritual. Sharing the end-of-life journey provides encounters that few experience in a professional setting. We offer a safe place where patients and family members can express deeply held hopes, fears, regrets, and achievements. We listen as patients recount dreams of the hereafter, interactions with deceased loved ones, and visions of the sacred. Through these intimate connections, we bear witness to the power of faith, hope, courage, and transcendence. We are the recipients of gifts beyond measure.

References

1. National Association of Social Workers. Standards for social work practice in palliative and end-of-life care. Washington, DC: National Association of Social Workers; 2011.
2. Tuckman BW. Developmental sequence in small groups. Psychol Bull. 1965;63(6):384–9.
3. Harrington SE, Smith TJ. The role of chemotherapy at the end-of-life: "When is enough, enough?". J Am Med Assoc. 2008;299(22):2667–78.
4. Crary J, Lucas J, Carter J. A journey through the seven "C's", a care plan model. Keck School of Medicine; 2000. Unpublished.

5. Blackhall LJ, Murphy ST, Frank G, Michel V, Azen S. Ethnicity and attitudes toward patient autonomy. J Am Med Assoc. 1995;274(10):820–5.
6. Fadiman A. The spirit catches you and you fall down: a Hmong child, her American doctors, and the collision of two cultures. 1st ed. New York: Noonday; 1997.
7. Rosenblatt PC. The culturally competent practitioner. In: Doka KJ, Tucci AS, editors. Diversity and end-of-life care. Washington, DC: Hospice Foundation of America; 2009. p. 21–32.
8. Evans WG, Tulsky JA, Back AL, Arnold RM. Communication at times of transitions: how to help patients cope with loss and re-define hope. Cancer J. 2006;12(5):417–24.
9. Charon R. Narrative medicine: a model for empathy, reflection, profession, and trust. J Am Med Assoc. 2001;286(15):1897–902.
10. Farber S. Difficult choices: making decisions when cure is not possible. In: Doka KJ, Tucci AS, editors. Cancer and end-of-life care. Washington, DC: Hospice Foundation of America; 2010. p. 25–38.
11. Figley CR, editor. Compassion fatigue: coping with secondary traumatic stress disorder in those who treat the traumatized. New York: Brunner/Mazel; 1995.
12. Pfifferling JH, Gilley K. Overcoming compassion fatigue. Fam Pract Manag. 2000;7(4):39–44.
13. Boyle G. Tattoos on the heart: the power of boundless compassion. New York: Free Press; 2010.

Review Questions

1. Palliative care social workers contribute their specialized skills and services in the following way(s):

   (a) Collaboration with fellow members of the medical team
   (b) Interaction with patients and families
   (c) Promotion of social work ideals through research and training
   (d) All of the above

2. Which of the following is *not* an example of the skills and tools used by palliative care social workers:

   (a) Familiarity with the biopsychosocial stages of the dying process
   (b) The pros and cons of various pain medications
   (c) Awareness of the effect of ethnic, religious, and cultural differences
   (d) Knowledge of available community resources and discharge planning options

3. Duties of the palliative care social worker include:

   (a) Witnessing durable power of attorney documents
   (b) Facilitating family conferences
   (c) Acting as a liaison between the patient/family and medical staff
   (d) Both b and c

4. In the formative stage of team building, which of the following is *not* a responsibility of the palliative care social worker?

   (a) Clarifying goals
   (b) Facilitating communication
   (c) Supporting a power hierarchy
   (d) Building consensus

5. A comprehensive social work assessment may include:

   (a) Developmental/life stage issues
   (b) Psychosocial strengths and coping strategies
   (c) Patient and/or family/caregivers' understanding of diagnosis and prognosis
   (d) All of the above

6. In the seven "Cs" care planning model, which of the following is *not* considered a care goal?

   (a) CURE the disease
   (b) SLOW the progression of the disease
   (c) WITHDRAW all care
   (d) ALLOW DEATH to proceed, and palliate symptoms exclusively

7. Researchers have found significant differences in how cultural groups view:

    (a) Illness
    (b) Grief, death, and dying
    (c) End-of-life decision making
    (d) All of the above

8. The palliative care social worker strengthens clarity by promoting terminology used by the team that is specific, descriptive, and consistent. Examples of recommended language include:

    (a) "Mechanical ventilation" or "breathing machine"
    (b) "Not helpful" or "harmful" (when describing a proposed treatment or intervention)
    (c) "Futile"
    (d) "We are hopeful"

9. Which of the following is *not* a therapeutic intervention employed by palliative care social workers?

    (a) Enabling patients and family members to "tell their story"
    (b) Providing a timeline for grief
    (c) Presenting options and facilitating decision making
    (d) Integrating the reality of diagnosis and prognosis

10. Which of the following would *not* be considered a self-care activity?

    (a) Develop strategies to distract yourself from disturbing emotions
    (b) Find an understanding peer or colleague who can listen
    (c) Acknowledge that palliative care is stressful work that carries an emotional toll
    (d) Practice healthy behaviors: routine exercise, good nutrition, adequate sleep

Answers

1. (d)
2. (b)
3. (d)
4. (c)
5. (d)
6. (c)
7. (d)
8. (c)
9. (b)
10. (a)

Chapter 12
The Healthcare System: More Questions than Answers

Jackie D.D. Carter

As the USA continues to struggle with how healthcare will look in the next 10–15 years, it is the patients and their families who will look toward their practitioner to guide them through the maze known as healthcare. The healthcare system can be frustrating to a relatively healthy person, but for a patient and their family dealing with end-of-life issues the healthcare system can be overwhelming. It is important to listen to their questions, assess their needs, and ascertain what services are available to them.

The patients and their family will have questions and will want you, as their provider, to answer them. Questions may arise in the areas of the disease process, insurance, and available resources. It is important to understand that you will not have all the answers. Be honest and keep the lines of communication open. Key issues in the care plan will revolve around communication with the patient and their ability to access care.

Communication

Questions Asked of the Provider

As the provider, the patient and family will look to you to answer all kinds of questions, from "are you sure to how come you can't fix it?" This is not intended to be

J.D.D. Carter, R.N., M.S.N., C.N.S. (✉)
2537 Millbrae Ave, Duarte, CA 91010, USA

Department of Nursing, LAC+USC Medical Center, 1200 N. State Street,
Los Angeles, CA 90033, USA
e-mail: jsacar11@yahoo.com; jdcater@dhs.lacounty.gov

N. Vadivelu et al. (eds.), *Essentials of Palliative Care*,
DOI 10.1007/978-1-4614-5164-8_12,
© Springer Science+Business Media New York 2013

personal attack. "How can it be when they know nothing about you?" You are the provider and as the provider you are expected to know all the answers. This, of course is a myth. What you can do, however, is be accessible, answer questions to the best of your ability, explain, prepare, do not waive (be consistent), and provide resources. At times it will be uncomfortable, frustrating, and depressing. It can also be peaceful, rewarding, and affirming.

Questions that you may initially receive are "how and why? How did this happen?" Give them the history as you know it. It may be a history of genetics versus environment. It may involve a history of high blood pressure, aging, smoking, drug abuse, etc. It may be none of the above. It may be that you do not know. As much as possible try to alleviate the patients' and families' fears. Know that these fears may be real or imaginary. Some family members will want to believe that they can prevent this from happening to them. If possible, answer the questions. Be as honest and compassionate as possible. It is normal for the patient and family members to be scared, frustrated, and angry.

Be clear and concise. Do not use euphemisms. Families can hear the phrase "everyday he lives is a miracle" and the family will believe their family member will survive. Why not? They believe in miracles. It is not for you to give them hope or take it away, but provide them with the needed information to make educated decisions.

Questions You Should Ask Yourself

Prior to meeting with the patient and their family you need to ask yourself what is your goal? What is the purpose of the goal? How do you plan to accomplish the goal? It has been found that providers in the USA are aggressive in their care [1]. Any procedure that you may want to do needs to reflect the patients' comfort and goal of quality of life. Will the therapy be painful? What are the expectations of the therapy? What are the risks and benefits? Are there any cultural barriers that may prevent your plan from going forward? Alert the patient of the option of stopping therapy at anytime.

There are aspects of the patient life you need to know prior to making these decisions. Is the patient in the hospital? Will the patient realistically leave the hospital? If so, where will the patient go? What are the resources? This is when you will need the aid of social workers and financial workers. They will be able to give you a picture of the options prior to initiating therapy. What are the post-therapy resources that are needed? Again, will they be available? Can the family provide them? Do they have the space for the needed equipment? Other resources that may be available to you in assisting in the care plan of the patient include the visiting nurse and chaplain. They will help to provide a clearer picture of the patient and family.

The ultimate goal for any patient receiving hospice is the control of symptoms and a peaceful death. Any therapy initiated should reflect that therapy. Culture should always be examined. A large portion of the African-American community has preconceived concepts of palliative care and hospice. There is the thought that hospice hastens death. Therefore, not many in that community utilize the services [2]. The cultural that needs to be examined the closest is "the family." The family will have their own problems which might influence the plan of care. Some of the problems may need addressing, others will not. Acknowledgment of the issues and recognizing when you are out of your depth is essential in building a trusting and rewarding relationship.

Questions the Provider Should Ask

Questions that should concern you as the provider include what the future plans are for the patient? What treatment plan is the patient following? Palliative care can incorporate many aspects of care including palliative chemotherapy and radiation therapy. What is the family expectation of therapy? Never assume that the family is on the same page as you. Their plan may include for the patient to continue the same course of therapy whereas your plan was to transition the patient to supportive therapy and send the patient home. Be clear in your expectations. Listen to theirs. When possible, mesh the two conversations into plan all can agree with. Does the patient have a support system? Is it available 24 hours a day? Are they dependable? Never assume that the family understands the goal of therapy. When all aggressive therapies toward cure are complete and the patient is receiving supportive therapy, reassure the family that the goal is to be just as aggressive in the management of the patients' symptoms.

What resources do the patient and family have? What will be needed? Will they need a hospital bed? Is there room for one? What about a bedside commode? Does the family have access to a restroom when needed? Never assume. Does the patient require oxygen? Does anyone in the house (euphemism for all dwellings) smoke? Is the patient's plan of discharge realistic? Does the family want to take the patient home? Some families will feel guilty if they do not take the patient home. Let the family know if it does not work out what procedure is needed to have the patient re-hospitalized. Utilize the social worker or case manager to assist with care plan. Some families will not want to have someone to die in their home. Discuss this with the family. Let them know there is no wrong choice.

Another issue that may arise when transitioning a patient from curative therapy to comfort care is a feeling of desertion. A smooth transition from their primary care to hospice care reassures the family that all is not lost. The care will continue but the focus of the care has shifted.

Access

Information

The information age and the internet have allowed for anyone with a computer access to a variety of information. The patient and family will have access to physician's history, hospital ratings, and complaints that may have been made against the physician or hospital. Computers are providing the layperson with a wealth of access to information on diagnoses, medications, end-of-life decisions, and patients' rights [3]. The information may or may not be accurate. It will be your job to weed through the information presented by the patient and family and inform them of what is and what is not true. It is not your job to convince them but provide them with the information.

Patients and their family may present with a plan of care that may or may not be realistic with their available resources. It is important to know what information they have and do they really understand the patients' situation. This may or may not give the patient and family confidence in the care plan. The key to gaining and maintaining trust is to provide accurate and consistent information at all times. It is all right to say you want to consult with a colleague and get back to them. It is better for the family to feel that you can be trusted than for you to give information and the family find information to the contrary.

Resources

What level of healthcare does the patient have access to? What are the goals of the therapies being provided? This cannot be stressed enough. There is a belief that as long as the patient is still going to the doctor, a cure exists.

Access to healthcare is something we assume everyone has, yet it is the level of access that will determine what is available to the patient. It is very important to be aware of the patients' type of insurance. What will it pay for? Patients with unlimited resources are easier to ensure care for than those with no or minimal insurance. This does not mean that patients with unlimited resources should not be given the same courtesy and honesty when it is time to transition their care from cure to comfort.

There are several different levels to insurance. The list includes those who have money as well as access to anything that healthcare can provide, those with private insurance who need referrals from their provider to access other specialists (this includes PPO's and HMO's), those with state aid insurance (i.e., Medicare/Medical), and those with no insurance to name a few. There are extreme's at each end of the financial spectrum and all will have questions and require guidance.

Resources could be as limited. Limitations could include patient and family living outside an area serviced by hospice. If so, what are the viable options? Will home health services support the patient? Will the patient need a skilled nursing facility instead? What care is realistic considering the insurance or lack thereof?

Insurance will also affect the medications and what is payable versus what is not. Certain medications may not be available and if available at what price? What is the reasonable alternative? Has the patient trialed the medication for efficacy prior to discharge? Some insurance programs have restrictions on the amount of medication for which they will pay [4]. Contact the pharmacist to assist in the amount of medication available per billing cycle of the insurance. Is there an institutional policy that limits the number of medications prescribed to the patient? Discharging a patient with pain medications still has many taboos. Some physicians will not give a complete month supply, leaving the patient vulnerable to running out of medication, prior to the next billing cycle. Provide the appropriate amount of medication to the patient so that the patient will have one less concern during this time.

A trip to the doctor's office is not necessarily easy for all patients. Some do not drive and will rely on friends or family to get them to appointments. What appointments, if any, are really needed? Again, know the available resources. Does a family member have to miss a day of work to bring the patient to an appointment? Does the family have a car? Are they using taxi? Are they taking the bus? How are they getting to the appointment and are there resources available to assist with transportation. When more than one appointment, what works best for the patient and family? Get the case manager and the social worker involved. You are not expected to know all of the ins and outs of the system. You need to learn and develop a working relationship with your resources for the best interest of the patient.

As the number of people growing older continues to increase so does the number of people requiring hospice [5]. Caring for a patient at the end of life can be just as complex as that of a patient in an intensive care unit. The outcome will still be loss of a loved one, but the care received during this difficult period can make all the difference to the patient and their family. Knowing that you are a part of a momentous event should make the experience more important. It is not necessarily about providing all the answers as much as it is about knowing the questions. All that is possible is to make the hospice experience the best possible and provide resources when needed. Utilize your resources; you are not in this alone.

References

1. McBride D. End of life care for advanced lung cancer differs between U.S. and Canadian patients. ONS Connect. 2011;26(8):21.
2. Pullis B. Perceptions of hospice care among African Americans. J Hosp Palliat Nurs. 2011;13(5):283–7.
3. Healthnet. Navigating the health care system: a resource guide for consumers. 2008; Apr 1–14.
4. Brant JM. Practical approaches to pharmacologic management of pain in older adults with cancer. Oncol Nurs Forum. 2010;37(5):S17–26.
5. Martz K, Gerding A. Perceptions of coordination of care between hospice and skilled nursing facility care providers. J Hosp Palliat Nurs. 2011;13(4):210–9.

Review Questions

1. In order to assist the patient and family is important to

    (a) Listen to their questions
    (b) Assess their needs
    (c) Determine services available
    (d) All of the Above

2. Patients and their families will ask questions that include all the following *except*:

    (a) Are you sure of the diagnosis?
    (b) Why is the treatment not working?
    (c) You know all the answers, don't you?
    (d) How did this happen?

3. Emotions that the provider might experience include:

    (a) Comfortable
    (b) Peaceful
    (c) Happy
    (d) Content

4. The provider should use euphemisms in order to make the patient and family feel more comfortable?

    (a) True
    (b) False

5. Questions the providers should ask themselves prior to meeting with the patient and family include all of the following

    (a) What will the procedure accomplish?
    (b) What is the patient and families goal?
    (c) Will the therapy or procedure be painful?
    (d) All of the above

6. What resource can best assist the provider with the care plan?

    (a) Patient
    (b) Chaplain
    (c) Social workers
    (d) Case managers

7. What questions should the providers ask the patient and their family

    (a) What is your understanding of the patients' condition?
    (b) What is the expectation of therapy
    (c) What treatment plan is the patient following
    (d) All of the above

8. All families are more comfortable if their family member can die at home amongst family?

   (a) True
   (b) False

9. The availability of information via the computer can provide patients and their families with a wealth of accurate information?

   (a) True
   (b) False

10. The type of insurance the patient has does not limit the care that is available to the patient?

   (a) True
   (b) False

Answers

1. (d)
2. (c)
3. (b)
4. (b)
5. (d)
6. (a)
7. (d)
8. (b)
9. (b)
10. (b)

Chapter 13
Vascular Access: Ostomies and Drains Care in Palliative Medicine

Patricia L. Devaney

Palliative care began with the hospice movement, where hospices were originally places of rest for travelers in the fourth century. Hospices were established in the nineteenth century in Ireland and London for the dying by a religious order [1]. They have grown from a volunteer-led movement to an important component of the health care system, providing improved care for people dying alone, isolated, or in hospitals. Hospital-based palliative care programs in the USA began in the late 1980s at a handful of institutions, Cleveland Clinic and Medical College of Wisconsin. There are now more than 1,400 hospital-based palliative care programs [1]. Hospital palliative care programs care for nonterminal patients as well as hospice patients. Both represent two different aspects of care with similar philosophy, but different payment systems and location of services.

Palliative care is most often provided in acute care hospitals structured around an interdisciplinary framework and focused on optimizing the patient's comfort. Patient's comfort includes life-limiting, advanced disease, and catastrophic injury; relief of distressing symptoms; coordination of patient- and family-centered care in diverse settings; use of specialized care systems including hospice; management of the imminently dying patient; and legal and ethical decision making in end-of-life care [2].

Nurses who practice in the palliative care areas are responsible for managing and alleviating pain and other physical symptoms—along with satisfying the emotional, social, cultural, and spiritual needs of patients who are facing life-threatening illness [3]. Of all the symptoms experienced, pain is the most common and also the most feared. A thorough evaluation of the patient's complaint of pain is necessary

P.L. Devaney, R.N., B.S., M.S. (✉)
Department of Diagnostic Radiology, Yale-New Haven Hospital,
New Haven, CT, USA
e-mail: Patricia.Devaney@ynhh.org; nursepatdi@yahoo.com

N. Vadivelu et al. (eds.), *Essentials of Palliative Care*,
DOI 10.1007/978-1-4614-5164-8_13,
© Springer Science+Business Media New York 2013

to manage and maintain adequate pain control. Gastrointestinal symptoms, nausea, and vomiting, are frequently experienced with advanced disease which lead to nutritional depletion and dehydration. Anorexia and cachexia syndrome generate a negative energy balance in which the food intake is inappropriately less than the energy output, resulting in the net effect of loss of body weight. Delirium is not uncommon in dying patients and can have many causes both metabolic and structural; examples are dehydration, infections, opioid analgesia, hypoxia, and electrolyte imbalances. Psychological problems, especially depression, are not uncommon when patients are initially diagnosed. For some, this acute stress response may persist and interfere with medical management.

Certain general principles in the evaluation of a patient's pain are important. Believe the patient's complaint and intensity of pain. Occasionally, family members may be summoned to corroborate the patient's description of pain. Obtain a careful history of the pain, when it occurs, its intensity, duration, character, as well as precipitating and alleviating factors. Assign a pain intensity scale to determine objective changes as various therapies are initiated. Social and psychological factors need to be addressed when evaluating if the therapy is achieving adequate pain control. It is critical to determine the cause of the pain. Always remember pain is a symptom.

Pain Service and Palliative Care specialties should be consulted when available for a therapy plan that is individualized for each patient [4]. Usually non-opioid analgesics are the first-line agents for mild to moderate pain and include acetaminophen and non-steroidal anti-inflammatory drugs. They are used orally with no tolerance or physical dependence with repeated dosing. After the maximum effect is attained, drug-related toxicity or advancement of the disease is evident by the variation of pain control; opioid analgesics are the next line of therapy (Table 13.1). They are used for moderate to severe pain and are distinguished by their complex interaction with multiple opioid receptors in the nervous system. The opioid-agonist drugs, morphine, bind to specific opioid receptors, producing analgesia. The opioid-antagonist drugs block the effects of morphine at its receptor. There are the mixed agonist–antagonist drugs, which demonstrate either agonist or antagonist properties [5].

There are guidelines when using opioid analgesics to individualize therapy. Avoid dosing "as needed" which produces sporadic blood levels and ineffective pain control [5]. Scheduled around-the-clock dosing will provide a constant blood level of the analgesic. Start with a low dose and titrate until desired control is reached, avoiding drugs that increase sedation without enhancing analgesia. Drug combinations that enhance analgesia may reduce drug side effects and limit the need to titrate the opioid component in combination. Adjuvant or supplementary analgesic agents represent a third group of drugs used to treat chronic pain. Their analgesic mechanism of action is not known and not directly related to the opioid receptor system. These include anticonvulsants, phenothiazines, antidepressants, antihistamines, steroids, and antibiotics. Concerns about opioid addiction have not been scientifically proven.

Other specialties may be consulted to assist with palliative therapies. For a patient with interstitial lung disease or end-stage COPD, a tracheotomy may be considered.

Table 13.1 Opioids commonly prescribed [5]

Generic name	Trade name	Applicant/sponsors
Fentanyl	Duragesic Extended Release Transdermal System	Ortho McNeil Janssen
Hydromorphone	Palladone Extended Release Capsules[a]	Purdue Pharma
Methadone	Dolophine Tablets	Roxanne
Morphine	Avinza Extended Release Capsules	King Pharms
Morphine	Kadian Extended Release Capsules	Actavis
Morphine	MS Contin Extended Release Tablets	Purdue Pharma
Morphine	Oramorph Extended Release Tablets	Xanodyne Pharms
Oxycodone	OxyContin Extended Release Tablets	Purdue Pharma
Oxymorphone	Opana Extended Release Tablets	Endo Pharma

http://www.fda.gov/SiteIndex/ucm148521.htm. Page last updated: 05/04/2010
[a]No longer being marketed, but is still approved

This is a minor surgical procedure that creates an opening in the trachea allowing the patient to be weaned from the ventilator, decrease the work of breathing, and clear secretions. Failure to be weaned from the ventilator requires lengthy intubation and care in an intensive care unit [6]. Extended length of intubation can cause erosion of the trachea and damage to the vocal cords, which can be avoided if a tracheotomy is performed. Tracheotomy patients could then transfer out of the intensive care unit and eventually be discharged with home care or to an extended care facility. Patients and caregivers are trained to care for the tracheotomy tube prior to leaving the hospital [7]. Some tubes have inner cannulas that are disposable and replaced every twenty-four hours. For those that are not disposable, the inner cannula is removed and soaked in an aseptic manner, dried and re-inserted. This needs to be done every eight hours and as needed. The area around the insertion site needs to be cleaned using warm water daily and as needed. The tracheostomy tube is secured with ties around the neck for safety, ensuring skin integrity and changed weekly. The use of supplemental humidified air or oxygen facilitates secretions to be thin enough to be cleared by coughing and suctioning. An appropriate sized suction catheter is used with the suction regulator set between 80 and 120 mmHg [8].

The catheter is placed into the tracheotomy tube gently advancing until meeting the end of the airway. As you pull back, slowly apply suction by intermittently holding the thumb over the open side of the catheter. Make note of the secretion's characteristics.

Esophageal, head, and neck cancer patients lack sufficient nutrition measured by serum albumin levels. Surgical intervention does not allow the patient to take anything by mouth postoperatively; radiation treatment may cause esophageal strictures and head and neck tissue changes. All of these issues, inclusive of depression, can cause anorexia or failure to thrive syndrome. Other sources contributing to malnutrition may be the development of an oral candida infection commonly called thrush or mucositis; both may be due to antibiotic therapy, poor oral hygiene, dehydration, and chemotherapy.

Each patient will require a nutritional evaluation to maximize his or her dietary requirements. Many patients who are still able to eat are ordered an unrestricted diet with high caloric and protein supplements despite other medical conditions such as diabetic or cardiac restrictions. Patients not able to eat due to oral lesions or esophageal strictures may require enteral feedings via a temporary gastric tube placed nasopharyngeal or, in more severe cases, a gastrostomy tube.

There are several kinds of nasogastric tubes and are selected according to the type of feeding to be delivered, gastric or jejuna [9]. The tube is lubricated and gently passed into the nares asking the patient to swallow to assist tube insertion. Positioning the head forward with chin on chest opens the esophageal tract and closing off the airway so that the tube is not inserted into the bronchial tubes. Many opinions as to the technique used to safely confirm tube placement have been examined with chest X-ray seemingly always the most reliable. Securing the tube also has been debatable, to preserve skin integrity, prevent dislodgement, and safely instilling feedings and medications. Most frequently adhesive tape is used to secure the tube on the nose and occasionally a tegaderm may further secure it on same-sided check.

A gastrostomy tube is placed when the patient can no longer swallow food due to aspiration, esophageal strictures, surgery, or the effects of radiation.

PEG is an acronym for percutaneous endoscopic gastrostomy [9]. The tube is placed endoscopically assisted through the abdominal wall into the stomach. There are high and low profile type tubes. High-profile tubes are not flush to the skin but extend out while low-profile tubes are flush to the skin and are called buttons. High-profile tubes are secured to the skin to prevent trauma at the insertion site or inadvertent dislodgement. The insertion sites of all gastrostomy tubes are inspected daily for skin integrity and any sign of complications. When the base of the tube is too snug against the skin, an irritation or breakdown of the skin may occur allowing gastric contents to leak. There may be a small amount of greenish mucous type drainage around the insertion site that is normal. Cleanse the site and thoroughly dry to avoid irritation. Feedings and medications can be administered after checking for residual stomach contents and follow the doctor's orders for withholding feedings. Insufficiently crushed and dissolved medications may obstruct the tube. A small amount of warm water in a plunger type syringe may clear the clogged area. If still obstructed, try a carbonated liquid such as club soda or coca cola.

Other patients with gastrointestinal or urinary tract obstructions or diseases: Crohn's, ulcerative colitis, small bowel obstructions, perforations, trauma, or cancer may be faced with the decision to have a fecal or urinary diversion [10, 11]. Fecal diversion may be required on either a temporary or permanent basis and is classified according to the segment of bowel utilized. A colostomy or ileostomy [11] is where a portion of the bowel is brought up through the abdominal wall to drain stool.

Urinary diversion, an ileal conduit or ileal loop [10], is performed for bladder cancer where a piece of ileum is resected, one end sewn shut, ureters are attached, and the open end brought up through the abdominal wall as a stoma. The ostomy serves to allow urine and mucous to drain out. Most medical centers have ostomy nurses that are consulted to support and teach the patient and family members the maintenance and care of their ostomy. The bedside nurse's role is to reinforce teachings and clarify any uncertainties through collaboration with the ostomy nurses and the patient's physician.

Patients are instructed to monitor stoma color, care of the skin around the stoma, fecal, or urinary output, proper application of the stoma pouch, to empty the pouch when one-third to half full, and how to change the pouch every 3 days and as needed [12–14]. Normal stoma color is pink to red. The mucocutaneous junction is observed for signs of separation or infection and surrounding skin to be intact. There may be several days before fecal material begins to pass from the stoma. Dietary considerations need to be discussed especially if a patient has an ileostomy. The recommendation for these patients is to take at least 1.5 l of fluid daily to prevent stoma blockages. Many foods such as nuts, raw fruits, and grains may not be compatible with an ostomy. Patients need to trial their food choices to determine which are the least disturbing to their gastrointestinal tract.

Pleural effusion is excess fluid that accumulates in the pleura, the fluid-filled space that surrounds the lungs. Excessive amounts of such fluid can impair breathing by limiting the expansion of the lungs during respiration.

Pleural effusion is usually diagnosed on the basis of medical history, physical exam, and confirmed by chest X-ray. Once accumulated fluid is more than 500 ml, there are usually detectable clinical signs in the patient, such as decreased movement of the chest on the affected side, stony dullness to percussion over the fluid, diminished breath sounds on the affected side, decreased vocal resonance, and pleural friction rub. Above the effusion, where the lung is compressed, there may be bronchial breathing and egophony. In a large effusion, there may be tracheal deviation away from the effusion. Recurrent pleural effusions can be malignant or nonmalignant in nature and caused by left ventricular failure, cirrhosis, nephrotic syndrome, pneumonia, pulmonary embolism, and cancer. Pleural fluid accumulation can be managed long term with a drainage system called the Pleurex catheter [15]. It requires a procedure that can be performed by a physician or licensed independent practitioner and is used for intermittent drainage of symptomatic, recurrent pleural effusions that do not respond to medical management of the underlying disease. The catheter is placed under the skin into the pleural space and referenced as a tunneled catheter. Once the catheter is placed, the fluid is drained as prescribed and then closed with a new sterile cap at the conclusion of each drainage. Frequency of drainage must be ordered by a physician or licensed independent practitioner and performed using sterile technique. Removal of pleural fluid should be no more than one liter per lung per day, using only the drainage lines and bottles included in the Pleurx kit. Pleurx catheters should only be flushed by a physician or licensed independent practitioner trained in the use of these catheters [16].

Symptoms that need to be reported to the physician include infection at the catheter insertion site, changes in the appearance or integrity of the catheter, severe pain, shortness of breath, coughing, fever, decreased oxygen saturation, leaking of fluid around the catheter, or less than 50 ml obtained for three consecutive drainage attempts. Dressing changes are performed with each drainage procedure. Patient and family education is completed before discharge and provided with a Carefusion folder and DVD, with additional resources found at http://www.carefusion.com. Homecare is prescribed using a registered nurse to reinforce care of the catheter and supervise the drainage as well as aseptic technique.

There is a growing population of heart failure patients that become increasingly symptomatic not due to an acute event or another chronic disease. Biventricular pacemakers [17] are a consideration and have been shown to improve quality of life. Three leads are placed: right atrial, right ventricular, and an additional lead into the coronary sinus. The lead in the coronary sinus will pace the left ventricle in synchrony with the right ventricle. It has been shown that single chamber, right ventricular pacing, weakens the cardiac muscle where synchronized pacing actually remodels the cardiac muscle improving cardiac output. Patient's symptoms improve enhancing their quality of life and return to activities previously unable to achieve.

Patients with chronic heart failure who have a very poor long-term prognosis and are not transplant candidates due to factors such as advanced age, end-stage renal disease, malignancy, non-compliance, or chronic obstructive pulmonary disease may be considered for a left ventricular assist device [18, 19] and these are referred to as destination devices. The left ventricular assist device offers a better treatment for advanced-stage heart failure patients who require hemodynamic support and become refractory to medical management. It has demonstrated the ability to restore hemodynamics, increase survival, and dramatically improve functional status and quality of life. Such patients will most likely die from their heart failure unless a mechanical assist device is offered.

The patient who suddenly presents with acute heart failure, unable to be weaned from cardiopulmonary bypass, massive acute myocardial infarction, acute myocarditis, or severe cardiac decompensation, may be implanted for a short term until improvement in cardiac function or implanted as bridge to transplant. Left ventricular assist devices are surgically implanted by a credentialed cardiothoracic surgeon. After implantation, they are cared for by the heart failure and cardiac surgery teams in most centers. Patients with devices remain in the hospital until either a compatible heart can be transplanted or cardiac function improves. When a compatible heart cannot be found and cardiac function stabilizes, patients can be discharged home but only after thorough education. Education consists of detailed information about the technical principles, system set-up, function, maintenance, infection control, and risks. Post implant, the most important education is directed towards infection control strategies including strict hand washing, sick visitor restrictions, and using aseptic technique when performing daily driveline dressing change. Discuss signs and symptoms of infection and immediate reporting. Anticoagulation therapy is also an important consideration and requires a strict regimen following the vendor's recommendations.

The domain of autonomy reflects the patient's degree of informed participation in decision making and planning concerning their illness. Rigorous research has demonstrated that open communication about advanced illness does not compromise the patient's psychological distress [2, 20, 21].

Direct assessment of autonomy can be measured by the following questions:

- Are we doing all but only the things you desire?
- Do you feel in control of your care?
- Do you feel heard and listened to?
- Have you been told of the nature of your illness and what to expect of it?
- Are we following your wishes to your satisfaction?
- What worries you the most?

It is important to select an environment for these discussions and to facilitate communication eliciting the patient's knowledge of their condition and desire to know about their condition. Open-ended questions and actively listening to the answers tend to minimize the patient's worries and concerns. This approach can aide in the resolution of conflicts, minimize anxiety, enhance the sense of dignity, and depression in the patient and their family.

Patients are encouraged to communicate with their loved ones about completion of life affairs, contribution to others, life review, and legacy [3, 20, 21].

While only about one-fourth of the patients with advanced cancer consider themselves to be suffering, a significant fraction attribute their suffering to closure-related problems, such as a pervasive sense of struggle, dependency, loss of identity, control, or their role in the family, or society in general. In contrast, advanced cancer patients who have a higher degree of peaceful acceptance of their terminal illness suffer from less depression, anxiety, and post-traumatic stress disorder. Where appropriate, opening a dialogue about closure may involve tactfully asking any of the following questions:

- How would you want to be remembered?
- Is there anyone whom you have not seen in a long time and need to talk to?
- Is there anyone to whom you wish to offer (and/or ask for) forgiveness?
- What do you feel most proud of (in your life)?
- Are there things or times you regret?
- Is there anyone who you can talk to about your fears and plans?
- Do you feel prepared for what is still ahead of you?
- Have you been able to share important things or thoughts with others?
- What do you still want to accomplish in your life?
- What would be left unfinished if you were to die today?

One successful palliative intervention, Dignity Therapy [2], invites patients to address issues that matter most to them or speak about things that they would most want remembered. An edited "Legacy" transcript of the dialogue is then returned to the patients for their review and sharing with others. Patients with advanced illness and their caregivers frequently experience profound financial and social strain. Family and friends provide most of the end-of-life assistance, for a mean of 43 hours per week. Almost one-third of the families report loss of all or most savings due to the illness and care giving. Furthermore, economic burden may profoundly impact health care decisions. In one study, economic hardship on the family was associated with a preference for comfort care over life-extending care in another; substantial care giving needs were associated with endorsement of euthanasia among patients with terminal illness.

Palliative care, initiated in the face of a life-threatening illness, is an interdisciplinary collaboration that focuses on patient-defined goals of care and relief of the patient's and family's distress. Given the scope of the palliative care needs that arise in patients with advanced illness, optimal care requires a unique evaluative approach. While palliative care used to be seen as care that was provided for people who were not receiving any active treatment for cancer and were in fact dying of their disease, the principles of palliative care are equally applicable to early stage, potentially curable disease, and to the terminal stages of a life-threatening disease. It also extends to the bereavement period [21] following the patient's death. Palliative care can and should be provided alongside disease modifying treatment.

References

1. World Health Organization (WHO) definition of palliative care. http://www.who.int/cancer/palliative/definition/en. Accessed 7 Jan 2011.
2. Steinhauser KE, Alexander SC, Byock IR, et al. Do preparation and life completion discussions improve functioning and quality of life in seriously ill patients? Pilot randomized control trial. J Palliat Med. 2008;11:1234.
3. Barazzetti G, Borreani C, Miccinesi G, Toscani F. What "best practice" could be in Palliative Care: an analysis of statements on practice and ethics expressed by the main Health Organizations. BMC Palliat Care. 2010;9:1.
4. Weissman DE, Meier DE. Identifying patients in need of a palliative care assessment in the hospital setting: a consensus report from the center to advance palliative care. J Palliat Med. 2011;14(1):17.
5. http://www.fda.gov/SiteIndex/ucm148521.htm. Page last updated 05/04/2010.
6. MacIntyre NR, Cook DJ, Ely Jr EW, Epstein SK, Fink JB, Heffner JE, Hess D, Hubmayer RD, Scheinhorn DJ, American College of Chest Physicians, American Association for Respiratory Care, American College of Critical Care Medicine. Evidence-based guidelines for weaning and discontinuing ventilatory support: a collective task force facilitated by the American College of Chest Physicians; the American Association for Respiratory Care; and the American College of Critical Care Medicine. Chest. 2001;120(6 Suppl):375S.
7. Yale New Haven Hospital. Clinical practice manual, care of the patient with a tracheostomy. Revised 4/2010.
8. Yale New Haven Hospital. Clinical practice manual, endotracheal or tracheostomy suctioning of the adult. Revised 12/2011.
9. Yale New Haven Hospital. Clinical practice manual, enteral feeding-care of the adult patient. Revised 1/2012.
10. Vasilevsky C, Gordon P. Gastrointestinal cancers: surgical management. In: Colwell J, Goldberg M, Carmel J, editors. Fecal and urinary diversions: management principles. St. Louis: Mosby; 2004. p. 126.

11. Güenaga KF, Lustosa SA, Saad SS, et al. Ileostomy or colostomy for temporary decompression of colorectal anastomosis. Cochrane Database Syst Rev. 2007;(1):CD004647.
12. Erwin-Toth P, Doughty D. Principles and procedures of stomal management. In: Hampton B, Bryant R, editors. Ostomies and continent diversions: nursing management. St. Louis: Mosby; 1992. p. 29.
13. Colwell J. Principles of stoma management. In: Colwell J, Goldberg M, Carmel J, editors. Fecal and urinary diversions: management principles. St. Louis: Mosby; 2004. p. 240.
14. Yale New Haven Hospital. Clinical practice manual, colostomy/ileostomy: care of the patient with a fecal diversion. Revised 5/2009.
15. Demmy TL, Gu L, Burkhalter EM, et al. Comparison of in-dwelling catheters and talc pleurodesis in the management of malignant pleural effusions (abstract 9031). J Clin Oncol. 2010;28:643s.
16. Yale New Haven Hospital. Clinical practice manual, care of the patient with a chest tube. Revised 7/2010.
17. Leclercq C, Cazeau S, Le Breton H, Ritter P, Mabo P, Gras D, Pavin D, Lazarus A, Daubert JC. Acute hemodynamic effects of biventricular DDD pacing in patients with end-stage heart failure. J Am Coll Cardiol. 1998;32(7):1825.
18. Slaughter MS, Rogers JG, Milano CA, Russell SD, Conte JV, Feldman D, Sun B, Tatooles AJ, Delgado 3rd RM, Long JW, Wozniak TC, Ghumman W, Farrar DJ, Frazier OH, HeartMate II Investigators. Advanced heart failure treated with continuous-flow left ventricular assist device. N Engl J Med. 2009;361(23):2241.
19. Vatta M, Stetson SJ, Perez-Verdia A, Entman ML, Noon GP, Torre-Amione G, Bowles NE, Towbin JA. Molecular remodelling of dystrophin in patients with end-stage cardiomyopathies and reversal in patients on assistance-device therapy. Lancet. 2002;359(9310):936.
20. Heyland DK, Dodek P, Rocker G, et al. What matters most in end-of-life care: perceptions of seriously ill patients and their family members. CMAJ. 2006;174:627.
21. Wright AA, Zhang B, Ray A, et al. Associations between end-of-life discussions, patient mental health, medical care near death, and caregiver bereavement adjustment. JAMA. 2008;300:1665.

Review Questions

1. Palliative care is an interdisciplinary collaboration focusing on patient-defined goals of care

   (a) True
   (b) False

2. Hospital palliative care programs are for nonterminal patients and hospice patients

   (a) True
   (b) False

3. Of all the symptoms experienced, pain is the most common and most feared

   (a) True
   (b) False

4. When using opioid analgesia, dosing is prescribed as only when needed

   (a) True
   (b) False

5. Failure to be weaned from the ventilator leads to:

   (a) Lengthy intubation
   (b) Be in an intensive care unit
   (c) Erosion of the trachea and/or vocal cord injury
   (d) All of the above

6. Esophageal and head and neck patients suffer from:

   (a) Anorexia and malnutrition
   (b) Oral candida, mucositis
   (c) Dehydration
   (d) All the above

7. Fecal and urinary diversions are always reversible

   (a) True
   (b) False

8. Patients who experience acute and chronic heart failure and are refractory to treatment are considered for left ventricular assist device implantation

   (a) True
   (b) False

9. Left ventricular assist device patient education must emphasize infection control and anticoagulation therapy

    (a) True
    (b) False

10. Recurrent pleural effusions are caused by malignancies

    (a) True
    (b) False

11. Psychological distress will worsen if the patient is informed about their advanced disease

    (a) True
    (b) False

Answers

1. (a)
2. (a)
3. (a)
4. (b)
5. (d)
6. (d)
7. (b)
8. (a)
9. (a)
10. (b)
11. (b)

Chapter 14
Drug Formulary

Angèle Ryan

Patients with advanced disease requiring symptom management are frequently prescribed a complex regimen of therapies that includes pharmacologic agents. Avoiding the pitfalls of polypharmacy is a universal goal in the practice of medicine. In palliative medicine this is of vital importance as these patients are already compromised by the burdens of the disease, without the added complications of drug adverse effects. To this end, medications should be carefully chosen to achieve the maximum benefit with minimum use of drugs. A unique application of the term "portmanteau" has been used in palliative medicine to describe this philosophy of using medications with multiple effects in order to minimize pharmacologic assault [1]. This is a French word meaning "a large suitcase" which carries numerous objects. When applied to pharmacotherapy, this concept suggests an aggressive use of medications beyond the labeled uses, and exploration of effects typically considered adverse but potentially beneficial in end of life care. An example is the preferential use of sedating drugs if insomnia accompanies other symptoms. Rediscovery of older medications adds to this pharmacological armamentarium. To this end, practitioners have come to rely on published lists of commonly used medications that fulfill these requirements. The International Association of Hospice and Palliative Care (IAHPC) has published a list of essential palliative care drugs based on the most common symptoms encountered in palliative care (see Table 14.1) as an incentive for other countries to develop lists based on need and resources [2]. The World Health Organization (WHO) also includes a section of palliative care drugs in their model list of essential medicines (see Table 14.2) [3, 4]. An independent

A. Ryan, M.D. (✉)
Department of Anesthesiology, Keck School of Medicine,
University of Southern California, Los Angeles, CA, USA
e-mail: angel@ix.netcom.com

N. Vadivelu et al. (eds.), *Essentials of Palliative Care*,
DOI 10.1007/978-1-4614-5164-8_14,
© Springer Science+Business Media New York 2013

Table 14.1 Most common symptoms in palliative care according to IAHPC [2]

Pain	Dyspnea
Terminal respiratory congestion	Dry mouth
Hiccups	Anorexia/cachexia
Constipation	Diarrhea
Nausea	Vomiting
Fatigue	Anxiety
Depression	Delirium
Insomnia	Terminal restlessness
Sweating	

Table 14.2 Essential drugs in palliative care [5]

Drug	Symptom
Morphine[a,b]	Pain, cough, dyspnea
Fentanyl (transdermal)[b]	Pain
Methadone[a,b]	Pain
Dexamethasone[a,b]	Pain, nausea, cough, dyspnea, anorexia
Amitriptyline[a,b]	Pain, insomnia, depression
Carbamazepine[a,b]	Pain
Gabapentin[a]	Pain, insomnia
Haloperidol[a,b]	Delirium, nausea, hiccups
Metoclopamide[a,b]	Nausea, vomiting
Midazolam[a]	Anxiety, terminal restlessness
Lactulose	Constipation, hepatic encephalopathy
Acetaminophen	Pain, fever
Hyoscamine[a] (glycopyrrolate in the USA)	Nausea, bowel obstruction, drooling
Senna[a,b]	Constipation
Diclofenac[a]	Pain
Clonazepam	Anxiety, depression, pain, insomnia, myoclonus
Megestrol acetate[a]	Anorexia, cachexia
Diazepam[a,b]	Anxiety, insomnia
Codeine[a,b]	Diarrhea, pain mild to moderate
Nystatin	Candida
Tramadol[a]	Pain

[a]World Health Organization essential medicines [3]
[b]International Association of Hospice and Palliative Care list of essential medicines for palliative care [2]

global survey of international palliative medicine practitioners produced a list of 20 essential drugs [5]. The most common symptoms encountered in advanced disease have defined these lists. Patients receiving care in the home may also be supplied with a specific "kit" containing common medications for anticipated symptoms [6, 7]. As novel new agents become available, the pharmacological toolkit continues to evolve, and lists of the most popular palliative care drugs will grow [1, 8]. A significant number of the widely beneficial medications are categorized in the classes of analgesics and adjuvants, antipsychotics, antiemetics, and laxatives paralleling the common symptoms treated in palliative medicine. Thus, a collection of medications that is particularly suitable for the most common symptoms seen in advanced disease will likely provide a creative medicine bag for treating these patients.

Medications Used for Analgesia (Opioids and Non-Opioids)

Acetaminophen is a synthetic centrally active non-opioid analgesic, a step one drug on the WHO stepladder guidelines, commonly available over the counter and indicated for treatment of mild pain and fever. Although it is an antipyretic drug, the mechanism of action is the inhibition of cyclooxogenase enzyme and formation of prostaglandins in the central nervous system, therefore does not share the peripheral anti inflammatory actions of NSAID's. It has the advantage of lacking the cardiac, renal, and gastrointestinal untoward effects of the anti-inflammatory drugs. The onset of analgesia is approximately 11 min after oral administration of acetaminophen [9], reaching peak serum concentration in 45–60 min in tablet form, and 30 min after liquid form. Bioavailability after oral administration is 60–85%, but more variable after rectal administration ranging from 24 to 98% [10] and its half-life is 1–4 h. Metabolism occurs in the liver, producing mostly inactive compounds that are excreted by kidneys. One minor but liver toxic intermediate metabolite is *N*-acetyl-benzoquinone imine (NAPQI), and is formed by a mechanism mediated by the cytochrome system. Under normal circumstances, this metabolite is rapidly conjugated by glutathione to a non-toxic byproduct, and subsequently safely excreted by the kidneys. Toxicity results when acute administration of acetaminophen beyond recommended doses brings about a rapid rate of production of this metabolite that exceeds the rate of deactivation. This results in accumulation of NAPQI. Despite common use and benefit of acetaminophen, this drug has gained attention as a result of this hepatotoxicity.

With appropriate use, however, acetaminophen has an important role for monotherapy in treatment of mild pain. For treatment of moderate to severe pain, it provides synergistic opioid-sparing benefit when combined with the stronger drugs. Single doses must be limited to less than 1,000 mg every 4–6 h, as it reaches a therapeutic ceiling effect at this level in adults. Maximum dose in 24 h is 4,000 mg. Acetaminophen is a safe drug in appropriate doses and offers an effective alternative for elderly patients and patients with renal, cardiac, or gastrointestinal disease.

Morphine is the prototype opioid, a hydrophilic alkaloid, originally derived from the juice of the opium poppy and has been used in medical practice for 200 years [11]. It exerts its analgesic effect by binding to opioid receptors, most notably μ receptors, in the nervous system and peripheral tissues. This inhibits neurotransmitters in the pain pathways. Morphine provides effective analgesic in nociceptive pain

Table 14.3 Opioid side effects

Opioid-naïve patient	Opioid-tolerant patient
• Nausea and vomiting	• Constipation
• Clouding of sensorium, delirium	• Nausea and vomiting, with dose escalation
• Respiratory depression	• Myoclonus (high doses)
• Pruritis	• Urinary retention
• Urinary retention (with neuraxial route)	• Xerostomia
• Constipation	• Pruritis

conditions that result from injury in peripheral tissues. In recent decades it has been widely utilized for medical indications to become the gold standard against which all other opioids are compared. There are many reasons why morphine enjoys this status. It is effective and well tolerated in most patients, is manufactured in various sustained release and immediate acting formulations and may be administered via several routes. This flexibility allows administration via the gastrointestinal tract, parenterally, and neuroaxial routes. Despite recent developments of newer opioid preparations, morphine remains the drug of choice when a strong opioid is indicated. Onset of action with immediate acting oral preparations occurs in 30 min, reaching peak serum concentrations in one. Duration of action is 3–4 h. It is metabolized in the liver by glucuronization, forming active metabolites, morphine-3-glucuronide (M3G) and morphine-6-glucuronide (M6G), which are, in turn, excreted by the kidneys. The half-life of the M6G metabolite is greater than the parent compound [12, 13] and may result in accumulation in the presence of renal compromise. Caution is advised when renal insufficiency is present.

In contrast, M3G is not analgesic and is felt to possess neuroexcitatory actions resulting in adverse effects such as hyperalgesia, myoclonus, and delirium. Accumulation of toxic metabolites should be suspected in patients receiving high doses of morphine who exhibit these symptoms.

Morphine, like all opioids, has no organ toxicity. There are, however. physiologic side effects (see Table 14.3) that include mental clouding, nausea, vomiting, respiratory depression, constipation, urinary retention, pruritis, and myoclonus. It is associated with histamine release and should be used with caution in asthmatics. Morphine is available in several formulations of immediate release tablets, liquid, and rectal suppositories. Coated, sustained release preparations allow convenient dosing schedules for patients with chronic pain. These tablets may not be crushed as this breaks the coated seal releasing large boluses of medication into the circulation in a short period of time. A unique dose form of encapsulated pellets allows for use with percutaneous feeding tubes in patients who are unable to swallow the intact sustained release pills.

Although analgesic effect is the main feature of morphine, it has a history of benefit for treatment of dyspnea and is a potent cough suppressor. The constipating effect of opioids has been exploited historically for treatment of diarrhea.

Unconventional routes are frequently used for control of symptoms. The use of sublingual morphine is common when patients have limited oral swallowing ability, but it is likely that absorption is achieved by a slow swallow [14]. Concentrated oral solution is combined with saliva, and eventually swallowed. Nebulized morphine is frequently offered for treatment of dyspnea, but evidence is lacking to justify use of this route over the systemic route. The required apparatus of mask and tubing may be intrusive and obstructive for the patient, adding little benefit. There is also the risk of inducing bronchospasm.

With the discovery of peripheral opioid receptors in inflammatory tissue sites, there has been an interest in the use of topical morphine in ulcers [15].

Fentanyl is a purely synthetic opioid, the result of efforts to develop newer opioids with more favorable profiles, specifically for use in anesthesia and analgesia during surgical procedures. It is a low molecular weight, high potency lipophilic agent with short duration of action making it useful as an anesthetic agent. After intravenous injection, it has an almost immediate onset of action, and duration of action between 30 and 60 min. This short duration of action and lack of histamine release provide hemodynamic advantage over morphine, and produces no active metabolites.

The popularity of this agent in palliative medicine is a result of the development of the transdermal formulation, a unique skin patch delivery system that allows high-dose opioids to be administered noninvasively. The low molecular size and the lipophilic nature of this drug make this delivery system feasible. The drug is initially deposited in the skin layer and slowly diffuses to the blood stream approximating a continuous intravenous infusion. Side effects are similar to those associated with other opioids. There is some indication that risk of constipation is reduced [16], allowing for decreased use of laxatives [17]. The disadvantage is the cumbersome timeline that does not allow for rapid titration during sudden changes in pain levels. Stable steady state is reached at 48–72 h after initial application or dose change.

This formulation allows high-dose opioid therapy for patients with compromised gastrointestinal function and allows a lifestyle unencumbered by invasive drug delivery apparatus. Transdermal formulations are available in 12, 25, 50, 75, and 100 mcg doses.

In intensive care settings, fentanyl is favored for intravenous use over other opioids due to its lack of histamine release and short action, which allows rapid dose changes in hemodynamically unstable patients. Newer formulations administered by transbuccal [18], intranasal [19], and nebulized [20] route offer promise as rescue medication for patients lacking swallow ability. The rapid absorption and quick clinical response via these routes provides safe and effective treatment of breakthrough pain. The development of the fentanyl iontophoretic transdermal system (ITS) offers an additional option for patients lacking oral route. This self-contained patient-activated system delivers a preprogrammed dose on demand similar to an intravenous patient-controlled analgesia device, using electric current to drive ionized drug molecules across the skin to the circulation [21]. This active transport system provides a rapid delivery of drug in contrast to the traditional passive transdermal system currently in use.

Methadone is a pure synthetic lipophilic opioid indicated for the treatment of heroin abuse. It exerts its action in a manner similar to morphine at μ-opioid receptors with the added action of antagonism at NMDA receptors. It is a racemic mixture of L and D isomers, with L-methadone providing most of the analgesic effect [22]. Methadone has potency several times that of morphine, no known toxic metabolites and is readily absorbed via multiple routes with a high oral bioavailability of approximately 80%. After oral administration, methadone is rapidly absorbed, reaching peak plasma concentrations at 2.5–4 h [23]. It is metabolized by hepatic cytochrome system and elimination is by redistribution from the blood stream. This creates a whole-body reservoir and accumulation over time. Along with high degree of protein binding, this makes for an unpredictable and variable long half-life ranging from 10 to 75 h [24]. Clinically, this translates to delay in reaching steady state following initial treatment or dose change, and increased risk of delayed toxicity. Drug interactions are numerous due to the involvement of the hepatic cytochrome system in metabolism of the drug. Examples include some selective serotonin reuptake inhibitors, antiviral, and antifungal agents. There are recent concerns regarding the occurrence of cardiac arrhythmias with use of methadone, as it may cause prolongation of the QT interval, particularly in doses higher than 200 mg daily [23]. Cardiac monitoring is recommended when prescribing methadone.

Despite the complexities of dosing and titration, methadone has emerged as a viable option for treating patients who experience a neuropathic component of pain, making it a cost-effective rising star in the treatment of cancer pain. It is an opioid that provides long-acting analgesia approximately 6–8 h, without requiring special formulation such as sustained release morphine or oxycodone. The blockade of the NMDA receptors in the spinal cord gives this drug the distinguishing feature as a broad-spectrum opioid . The NMDA receptors are responsible for development of opioid-resistant neuropathic and is also believed to be involved in development of tolerance.

These features allow noninvasive dosing options in patients who require high-dose opioids. The potent conversion ratio in highly tolerant patients makes for convenient administration of high-level analgesia with use of convenient lower dose formulation. The longer duration of action is not dependent on specialized coated formulation, therefore, tablets may be crushed in small amounts of liquid for ease of swallowing. Rapid onset of action occurs within 30 min after oral route [22]. Sublingual and rectal routes offers additional flexibility as a result of the lipid solubility of this drug [25]. Alternatively, liquid formulation provides the flexibility of administration via G-tubes. The rapid onset of action also makes it suitable for use as a rescue medication. The lack of active metabolites makes it an excellent choice for patients with impaired hepatic and renal function.

The robust opioid agonist coupled with anti-NMDA action that makes this an effective analgesic in highly opioid-tolerant patients also brings pitfalls. The action on NMDA receptors and reversal of tolerance result in a significant and nonlinear conversion ratio when rotating from a different μ-receptor agonist. Skilled prescribing is required when attempting an opioid rotation, particularly in highly tolerant patients. Conventional conversion tables are based on single doses, and not reliable when rotating to methadone in an opioid-tolerant individual. Several methods of rotation have been described [26, 27] with all methods sharing

Table 14.4 Methadone conversion ratios [28]

Pre conversion morphine equivalent daily dose	Conversion ratio
Less than 90 mg	5:1
90–300 mg	8:1
300 mg or greater	12:1

the common themes of incremental conversion, conservative ratios, and intervals of several days between dose escalation. A guide to conversion ratios is suggested (see Table 14.4) [28]. As with any conversion tables, this is merely a guide for initial dosing. Ongoing individualized titration according to clinical response will provide optimal results.

Diclofenac as a representative of the general class of non-steroidal anti-inflammatory agents (NSAID) is a non-opioid and is indicated for the treatment of pain, fever, and inflammation. It merits a place on all three steps of the WHO step-ladder. Like other NSAID's it exerts its action by nonselective inhibition of the cyclooxygenase enzymes (COX) that converts arachidonic acid to prostaglandins. This enzyme consists of two forms, COX-I and COX-II. Effect is on both isoforms of COX I and COX II.

After oral ingestion it has fast onset of action within 30 min, with approximately 60% bioavailability, a half-life of 2 h, and long action of approximately 8 h. It is readily absorbed after rectal and intramuscular injection. Metabolism is by hepatic glucuronidation with subsequent elimination in urine and bile. Daily oral dose of 75–150 mg has been shown to be well tolerated and effective in acute and chronic pain conditions, with no dose adjustments needed for the elderly or patients with renal or hepatic impairment. COX-I is associated with physiologic regulation of gastrointestinal mucosa, renal perfusion, and platelet function, whereas COX-II is responsible for formation of inflammatory products. The therapeutic effect is a result of the blockade of COX-II, and adverse effects occur from disruption of the physiologic benefit conveyed by the COX I isoform on the target organs. This results in compromise of renal perfusion, gastrointestinal integrity, and increased bleeding risk. The NSAIDs differ widely in their relative effect on each COX isoform, which accounts for the variable benefit to risk ratio that exists within this drug category. Diclofenac appears to have a favorable COX-II selectivity. It is well tolerated in a wide variety of patients. Patients should be monitored for dose-dependent adverse effects common to all drugs in this category, which include gastrointestinal irritation or bleeding, fluid retention and cardiac failure, coagulation disorder, and renal toxicity. When an NSAID is required, the efficacy and favorable side effect profile makes this agent a suitable first-line therapy or a reasonable alternate option when patient in unable to tolerate other NSAIDs [29].

Topical preparations in gel, solution, and transdermal formulations are available with reduced systemic effects, thus providing additional improvement in the benefits/burdens ratio [30], targeting specific sites for analgesic action while minimizing the load on metabolic systems. Adverse effects of topical preparations are generally limited to localized skin reactions.

Tramadol is a unique synthetic analgesic with the dual actions of opioid and non-opioid mechanisms and is indicated for the treatment of mild to moderate pain. It exhibits a weak to moderate affinity for opioid receptors and also acts on the transmission of noradrenaline and serotonin [31]. It has an oral bioavailability of 75%, is rapidly absorbed, reaching peak serum levels within 2 h. It has a half-life of 6–8 h, producing an active metabolite O-desmethyltramadol (M1), which has a greater affinity than the parent compound for μ opioid receptors and a longer half-life of about 8 h [32]. Half-life is prolonged in the elderly or in patients with hepatic or renal impairment [33]. It is metabolized by the cytochrome enzyme system in the liver and excreted by the kidneys. Dose given is 25–50 mg every 4–6 h with titration up to a maximum of 400 mg/daily.

The benefit of tramadol is the low incidence of typical opioid side effects on gastrointestinal function and respiration, and may be considered for patients with low tolerance to stronger opioids. The action on noradrenaline adds anti-neuropathic mechanism. The most common adverse effects attributed to tramadol are nausea, vomiting, dizziness, and sedation.

Tapentadol, a newer agent, is a centrally acting oral analgesic similar to tramadol sharing the dual action as a weak μ agonist and a norepinephrine reuptake inhibitor, thus exhibiting both opioid and non-opioid analgesia. The potency of tapentadol is between tramadol and morphine [34] and has a lower risk of gastrointestinal adverse effects [35]. It is indicated for acute pain of moderate to severe intensity.

Codeine is a weak opioid, used for treatment of pain, cough, and diarrhea. Although it is a naturally occurring compound, originally isolated from the opium poppy, it is most commonly a manufactured drug, and one of the most commonly prescribed opioids worldwide. Most of the activity of codeine is believed to be due to conversion to morphine, its most active metabolite, by the CYP2D6 enzyme [36]. CYP2D6 function is genetically determined and accounts for variable metabolism of codeine among individuals, affecting analgesic response. Codeine can be administered orally, subcutaneously, intramuscularly, and rectally. It is rapidly absorbed after oral administration reaching peak levels in 1–2 h, providing analgesic onset after 30–60 min.

In palliative medicine it may be of benefit in patients with mild to moderate pain. Despite the historical use as an antitussive, validation in controlled studies has been inconsistent [37], efficacy possibly linked to typically low doses used in most cough preparations. The constipating effect of codeine is used therapeutically to treat patients experiencing diarrhea.

Amitriptyline is a tricyclic antidepressant (TCA) drug indicated for the treatment of depression. After oral ingestion, time to peak concentration in serum is approximately 4 h, with an average half-life of 15 h. The onset of antidepressant action, however, requires 4–6 weeks. Amitriptyline is metabolized by the liver producing the active metabolite of nortriptyline. Excretion is by the kidneys with 18% of drug excreted unchanged.

It has particular application in palliative medicine in that it is the most studied antidepressant for the treatment of a wide variety of pain syndromes, specifically neuropathic conditions such as diabetic neuropathy and post-herpetic neuralgia. The analgesic benefit is independent of the antidepressant effect [38]. Amitriptyline exerts action via the inhibition of the reuptake of serotonin and norepinephrine in the nervous system, with the norepinephrine being responsible for the majority of the analgesic result, and serotonin playing a lesser role [39]. Side effects are a result of anticholinergic action, and include dry mouth, sedation, urinary retention, and cardiac conduction abnormalities. The sedative effect is desirable for patients who may be sleep deprived as a result of previously unrelieved pain. Initial analgesic dose of amitriptyline is 10–25 mg orally at bedtime with escalation every 3–5 days. Antidepressive doses may reach 150 mg daily, but this is rarely necessary for treatment of pain. Parenteral route for intramuscular injection is available but should be avoided as the use of intramuscular injections is painful. Other TCAs may be considered if a patient does not tolerate amitriptyline.

Carbamazepine is a first-generation anticonvulsant. It is also used as a mood stabilizer and has demonstrated proven efficacy for treatment of trigeminal neuralgia [40, 41]. As with other traditional anticonvulsants, its use has been supplanted by newer agents that have the advantage of fewer drug interactions, better tolerability, and broader spectrum of activity.

Gabapentin is a gamma-aminobutyric acid (GABA) analog, with indications for treatment of epilepsy and post-herpetic neuralgia. Bioavailability varies with dose, approximately 80% at lower doses (300 mg daily) and decreasing as low as 27% with higher doses (3,600 mg daily) [42]. Absorption is relatively slow, and the drug reaches peak plasma concentrations after 3 h. Elimination half-life is 5–7 h. Metabolism is negligible and the drug is excreted essentially unchanged in the urine, thus elimination from circulation is dependent on renal function. The relatively short half-life requires multiple daily doses. Gabapentin has several mechanisms of action with resultant increased GABA activity in the central nervous system and decreased excitation of neurons [43]. The unique mechanisms of action of gabapentin result in multiple uses. Indeed, more than 80% of prescriptions for this agent initially involved off-label indications such as nonspecific neuropathic pain, migraine headaches, spasticity, and bipolar disorder [44]. Gabapentin is also rapidly becoming the first-line therapy for neuropathic pain of numerous origins [45, 46]. Classic studies have demonstrated benefit in the treatment of post-herpetic neuralgia [47] and diabetic neuropathy [48]. The favorable side effect profile offers an alternative to the traditional tricyclics and older anticonvulsants. Since it lacks hepatic metabolism, drug interactions is not a concern, as with the older agents in this category. The most common side effects of gabapentin are somnolence, fatigue, dizziness, and weight gain, which generally resolve within the first 2 weeks of therapy. Slow, gradual titration allows identification of optimal dose to achieve analgesia while minimizing side effects. Dose adjustment is required in patients with renal compromise.

Medications Used for the Treatment of Symptoms Other Than Pain

Haloperidol is an dopamine antagonist classified as an antipsychotic and prescribed for treatment of Schizophrenia/Psychosis, Tourette Syndrome. It has a half-life of 10–20 h, onset in 30–60 min, reaching peak plasma levels at 2–6 h orally, 10–20 min parenterally. It is extensively metabolized in the liver producing active and inactive metabolites most significantly a toxic pyridium metabolite. It is believed that this compound is responsible for the extrapyramidal side effects (EPS) of haloperidol. The intravenous route, however, is associated with fewer EPS even when high doses are administered [49], presumably due to lack of first-pass metabolism.

There are several applications in palliative medicine. It is a first-line drug in the treatment of delirium, as it is effective, lends itself well to rapid titration, has few anticholinergic, sedative, Autonomic, or hypotensive effects [49]. Doses of 0.5–1 mg hourly can be given orally, intravenously, intramuscularly, or subcutaneously until symptoms abate. Generally, doses of 1–10 mg daily are adequate to control symptoms [50], but doses as high as 240 mg in 24 h have been reported [51] without adverse effect.

The potent antidopamine action also makes this an excellent drug for treatment of nausea/vomiting, generally in doses of 1–2 mg daily [52]. It plays a role as part of a classic triad of drugs used for treatment of symptoms associated with inoperable bowel obstruction [53, 54].

Labeled warnings of prolonged QT interval and risk of torsade de pointes with the use of intravenous haloperidol suggest that patients require cardiac monitoring in such a setting. Evidence indicates, however, that in the absence of underlying cardiac disease, electrolyte abnormalities, or other proarrhythmic drugs, the risk of this is low when cumulative haloperidol doses less than 2 mg are used [55].

Metaclopramide is a prokinetic antiemetic indicated for symptomatic treatment of diabetic gastroparesis and gastroesophageal reflux. The mechanism of action is by the blockade of dopamine receptors. After oral ingestion, absorption is rapid, producing an onset of action within 30–60 min, therapeutic duration of action is 1–2 h. Half-life is 5–6 h. The usual dose is 10 mg orally or intravenously, typically given before meals and at bedtime.

In palliative medicine, it holds particular appeal not only as an antiemetic but also for the positive effect on GI motility, a desired benefit for patients who frequently receive medications that adversely affect GI motility.

Side effects may include extrapyramidal reactions including akathisia and dystonia. Caution is advised when using metaclopramide in patients receiving other dopamine antagonists.

Glycopyrrolate is an quaternary amine with anticholinergic actions and is representative of anti-secretory class of drugs. It has the advantage that it does not cross the blood brain barrier as do the tertiary amines, atropine, and scopolamine.

This agent was initially used for treatment of gastrointestinal disorders, and later became widely used in the anesthetic setting [56]. The anti-secretory action provides adjuvant antiemetic benefit in patients requiring multiple agents to control nausea and vomiting. This action is particularly suitable in management of inoperative bowel obstruction. In the terminal phase of illness, the drying effect prevents drooling and spares family members from the distress associated with "death rattle."

Senna is classified as a contact cathartic, a plant-derived glycoside that passes through the small intestine unabsorbed and subsequently activated by bacterial action in the large intestine. Active metabolites are produced that exert mechanical and secretory action directly on intestinal mucosa to promote bowel activity. The relatively gentle action of this vegetable-based compound makes it attractive to many patients. It is a safe first-line therapy, usually in conjunction with a stool softener or emollient, for regular use for management of constipation.

Lactulose is categorized as an osmotic laxative, a synthetic, non-digestible disaccharide composed of galactose and fructose. It is indicated for the treatment of constipation and hepatic encephalopathy. Metabolism occurs in the colon, producing acidic byproducts. Laxation of bowels occurs as a result of osmotic absorption of large amounts of water into the bowel, formation of intraluminal gas from fermentation, and increased peristalsis produced by the acidic environment created. It is this reduced pH that inhibits ammonia production. The laxative effect also clears ammonia forming flora in the gut and makes lactulose a viable treatment in hepatic encephalopathy. Doses of 30–45 ml up to four times daily are generally effective in promoting gut motility, and may be titrated to effect. Adverse effects include bloating, cramping, and diarrhea. This agent is generally well tolerated as it does not rely solely on osmotic action for effect.

Megestrol acetate is a progestational agent, used in the treatment of breast cancer. It is well absorbed orally, metabolized in the liver to free steroids and glucuronide conjugates. Half-life is 13–105 h, time to peak serum levels is 1–3 h. The undesirable weight gain effect [57] produced by that indication has attracted attention to the potential use of this drug for treatment of cachexia. This perceived adverse effect may be used creatively in palliative medicine as a positive benefit. It is considered one of the most effective appetite stimulants in patients suffering from cancer anorexia/cachexia syndrome, and associated with weight gain and caloric intake in patients with some cancers and autoimmune deficiency syndromes [58–61]. The impact on survival in not clear but if the goal is symptom management, quality of life, and patient well-being, the effect is satisfactory. An initial dose of 80 mg bid has been shown to be effective, with increased efficacy with higher doses [62, 63]. Titration to desired effect is suggested in order to obtain maximal clinical result and minimize side effects.

Dexamethasone is a potent synthetic corticosteroid with potent anti-inflammatory effects used for multiple indications in curative medicine. This diverse therapeutic value makes it suitable in palliative medicine as a broad-spectrum drug. It shares the common side effects of all corticosteroids, but lacks the mineralocorticoid properties of other adrenal hormones.

In patients with advanced disease, it provides relief from a myriad of symptoms including inflammatory and neuropathic pain, nausea and vomiting, anorexia, and fatigue, with improved sense of well-being. Although the adverse effects of corticosteroids are troublesome, they are not a concern when urgent control of symptoms takes precedence and life expectancy is short. Beneficial effects are short lived, but highly effective for the treatment of patients experiencing severe symptoms and having limited prognosis of less than 1 month.

In patients with less advanced disease, constant vigilance for adverse effects mandates low doses of corticosteroids and limits usefulness. Short courses of higher doses up to 16 mg daily are prescribed as temporary measures for emergency treatment of spinal cord compression, cerebral edema, or superior vena cava syndrome pending definitive disease-modifying treatments. The comfort level for most practitioners, however, is to remain with low doses in the range of 4–8 mg dexamethasone, or equivalent dose of alternate corticosteroid daily [64]. The use of doses in the range of 16–24 mg of dexamethasone up to four times daily with low incidence of adverse effects have been reported for terminal patients [65].

Benzodiazepines are a class of drugs with the common pharmacological effects of anxiolysis, muscle relaxation, sedation, and anticonvulsant. In palliative medicine, they are often indicated for the treatment of anxiety. In general practice, pharmacology alone is not the optimal treatment for this disorder, and psychotherapy is the preferred first-line therapy, but when treating distressing symptoms in severely ill patients, time urgency mandates the early use of pharmacologic intervention. The time constraints associated with short prognosis may not allow the fine tuning of medications versus psychotherapy. The standard concerns regarding dependence with the use of benzodiazepines in curative medicine are less relevant in patients with limited prognosis, particularly in light of the effectiveness of benzodiazepines for short-term treatment of acute symptoms. Instead, the cautions are focused on the immediate side effects of mental clouding and impaired function that may affect safety and quality of life. Specific characteristics of the individual agents will dictate their use for the other indications in end of life care. The international list of essential drugs in palliative care lists two agents in this class.

Midazolam is a short-acting water-soluble benzodiazepine formulated in injectable form and used to provide sedation during medical procedures and induction of anesthesia. It shares the actions of other benzodiazepines of anxiolysis, sedation, muscle relaxant, and anticonvulsant properties. The cardiovascular stability that it provides makes it suitable for the intensive care setting. Water solubility allows for painfree injection and use of subcutaneous route for continuous or intermittent administration.

The drug provides benefits during use of palliative sedation for treatment of agitation and restlessness or for the palliation of intractable symptoms. As oral route is compromised during this state, the intravenous or subcutaneous [66] route is preferred and is well tolerated. Onset of action is rapid within minutes. Coupled with the short half-life and absence of any significant metabolites, it is an ideal agent extended use, but also applicable for titration and short term respite sedation. It is a useful tool in the home setting empowering family to provide rapid unconsciousness during urgent and catastrophic events, such as uncontrolled hemorrhage. A subcutaneous small gauge butterfly needle may be quickly placed to administer a premeasured dose of medication, stored at room temperature, for immediate use.

Clonazepam, an anti-epileptic drug used for certain types of seizures, is a benzodiazepine. It has been used for a variety of disorders such as panic attacks [67], anxiety [68], spasticity [69], mania [70], and depression [71]. Clonazepam is rapidly absorbed after oral administration with bioavailablity of 90% and peak serum concentration achieved after 1–4 h. Half-life is approximately 19–60 h [72], establishing it as a long-acting agent. It is completely metabolized by liver and inactive metabolites excreted in urine. Doses range from 0.25 to 1 mg twice a day.

As a multipurpose medication, clonazepam plays a role in treating a myriad of symptoms encountered on a palliative care practice. The antidepressant action is a bonus for patients who may be treated with this medication for treatment of anxiety, a common occurrence in patients suffering with advanced disease. The anxiolytic effect is rapid, a clear advantage in patients with tenuous prognosis, allowing use as needed [68]. It also offers a long-acting alternative in patients who require frequent dosing of short-acting agents. In patients receiving high doses of opioids, accumulation of metabolites may result in myoclonus [73], a condition that responds to treatment with clonazepam [74]. Since myoclonus is frequently associated with a high-dose opioid regimen, and high probability of neuropathic pain, clonazepam will target both symptoms [75–77]. The sedating effect coupled with the relief of myoclonus provides a dual mechanism for treatment of insomnia. An available rapidly dissolving tablet is a benefit for patients with limited swallowing ability.

Nystatin is a traditional representative of a group of antibiotics, polyenes, used to prevent and treat a broad spectrum of fungal infections, particularly candidiasis. Nystatin exerts its antifungal action by binding and compromising the integrity of ergosterol, a component of cell membranes unique to fungi. Nystatin has the unique trait of not being absorbed from mucosal tissue, therefore passes through the gastrointestinal system unchanged. The direct topical effect on organisms prevents the spread and development of generalized infections. As parenteral administration is toxic, treatment is limited to topical application. Coupled with low absorption, this produces a safe and effective therapy with essentially no systemic adverse effects. When high doses are ingested orally, gastrointestinal symptoms include anorexia, nausea, and diarrhea, but these are mild and transient. Oral suspension or tablet is administered in doses of 0.5–1 million units four times a day.

Candida albicans is a common opportunistic organism in the oral cavity, present in 50–60% of humans [78]. Patients on a palliative care service have multiple risk factors for developing candidiasis including compromised immune status, malignancy, drug therapies, hyperalimentation, advanced age, and often require antifungal therapy. Newer systemic antifungal agents in the azole category suggest improvement over the traditional polyenes, but the azoles mechanism of action on the cytochrome P450 enzymes introduces the additional risk of numerous drug interactions. . In contrast to the azole agents, development of resistance remains low with nystatin [79, 80]. In balancing risk/benefits, nystatin remains a readily available option for pre-emptive treatment of candidiasis in severely ill patients.

New Directions

Depression

Depression is a frequent symptom in advanced disease [81] and antidepressant agents are frequently prescribed in the practice of palliative medicine. ***Mirtazepine*** is a newer antidepressant with dual noradrenergic and specific serotonergic mechanisms that enhance norepinephrine and serotonin neurotransmission (NaSSA). This is the result of presynaptic adrenergic receptors which in turn facilitates serotonergic transmission by action on adrenoreceptors on serotonergic nerve terminals. Mirazepine has high affinity for histamine receptors. It is administered orally, with peak levels occurring after 2 h, with a half-life of approximately 24 h allowing for once daily use. Unlike first-generation antidepressants such as tricyclics, therapeutic effects may be seen within 1 week, an advantage in patients with limited prognosis. Metabolism is via multiple pathways of demethylation, hydroxylation, oxidation, and flucuronidation, with resultant few drug interactions [82]. Mirazepine lacks the adverse anticholinergic and cardiac effects of the tricyclic antidepressants and the potential for extrapyramidal reaction and insomnia associated with the selective serotonin reuptake inhibitors. It is effective for treating multiple symptoms, including anorexia, nausea, insomnia, anxiety and depression [1]. The listed side effects of mirtazepine of increased appetite, weight gain, and sedation are embraced as positive effects as is common in the practice of palliative medicine. Effects vary with dosage. Low doses of 15 mg are sufficient for desired sedation to treat insomnia. The histamine effect that accounts for this is negated by increased adrenergic effects at higher doses of 30–45 mg. An orally disintegrating tablet is available for ease of swallowing.

Olanzepine is an atypical antipsychotic indicated for the treatment of Schizophrenia. It is formulated for oral administration, reaching peak blood levels within 5–8 h. The long half-life of 27–38 h provides convenient once daily dosing. It has selectively higher serotonin receptor activity compared to dopamine receptors and reduced incidence of extrapyramidal symptoms associated with older agents. The unique binding profile at dopamine, serotonin, achetylcholine, and histamine receptors also makes it a promising antiemetic for treatment of intractable nausea [83]. Metabolism by multiple pathways makes for few drug interactions, and no dose adjustments are required in patients with renal or hepatic compromise. The side effects of sedation and weight gain, generally considered undesirable, can be welcome effect in the terminally ill patient with multiple symptoms. Caution should be exercised when prescribing for patients at risk for seizures as olanzepine reduces seizure threshold. Initial dose is 2.5–5–10 mg orally daily, and may be increased up to 20 mg daily. A dissolvable disk formulation allows for ease of ingestion for patients with difficulty in swallowing.

Despite the higher costs of this agent compared to older medications, the value of this medication for use in caring for patients with advanced disease lies in the benefit for multiple symptoms of delirium, nausea, and cachexia [84], with reduced adverse effects. This drug has also gained attention as a potential tool in pain management [84].

Levorphenol is a synthetic agent with similar action but longer half-life than morphine. The sustained action was an advantage prior to the introduction of the coated sustained release opioids. The non-opioid mechanisms that it shares with methadone make it a potential tool in treatment of cancer pain [85]. In addition to its affinity for the opioid receptors, it is also an NMDA antagonist and inhibits the uptake of serotonin and norepinephrine. After oral administration, levorphanol is absorbed and produces peak plasma concentrations after 1 h, is metabolized by the liver to produce a glucuronide metabolite with no involvement of cytochrome oxidase enzymes, and excreted by kidneys. Duration of analgesia is 6–15 h. Like methadone, the long half-life requires that several days be allowed to establish steady state, approximately 72 h [86].

The non-opioid mechanisms of this drug make it a potential tool in the treatment of neuropathic pain and a logical choice for opioid rotation when standard opioids fail. Side effects are similar to those of other opioids.

Buprenorphine is a strong opioid with unique classification as a partial μ opioid receptor agonist. It also exhibits additional affinity for an opioid receptor-like (ORL-I) receptor, and antagonism to the kappa and delta receptors. It is administered in parenteral, sublingual, and transdermal routes. The oral bioavailability is low, about 10%, due to first-pass hepatic metabolism, dictating alternative modes of administration. Since it is a partial agonist, the effect will be reduced when compared to full μ receptor and this is believed to account for ceiling effect of analgesia. Binding to receptors is slow to dissociate resulting in sustained duration of action and lower risk of withdrawal symptoms if the drug is discontinued. The drug is highly protein bound. Sublingual route is currently used for treatment of substance abuse, and a newer transdermal preparation offers promise for treatment of pain. The highly potent, highly lipophilic nature, and low molecular weight of this drug makes it a suitable candidate for transdermal application offering specific benefit for patients receiving palliative care. This formulation allows for continuous absorption of the drug with effect starting in 12–24 h and reaching steady state in 24–48 h [87].

The non-opioid mechanisms and unique receptor affinities may result in blockade of central sensitization, and suggest a potential as an opioid with additional anti-neuropathic action [88]. Although this agent duplicates the non-oral and noninvasive advantages of the more widely used fentanyl patch, it adds specific targeting of the more difficult neuropathic components of pain.

Modafinil is a psychostimulant approved for use in the treatment of narcolepsy. Non-labeled uses applicable to the palliative care patient include depression [89] and opioid-induced sedation [90]. Since sedation and fatigue are common complaints encountered in the practice of palliative medicine, psychostimulants have played a role in the treatment of these symptoms in patients with advanced disease, not only for promoting wakefulness and cognitive function, but also as adjuvants for pain management [91]. Modafinil represents the new arrival in this category. Although the precise mechanism of action is unknown, modafinil appears to exert a unique action in the hypothalamus [92] unlike the other commonly used stimulants such as methylphenidate or amphetamine. This selective action on arousal systems is not associated with adverse effects such as hypertension, appetite suppression, anxiety, or abuse potential that is typical of older stimulants [90]. Modafinil reaches peak plasma levels approximately 2–3 h after oral administration, half-life is approximately 10–12 h. It is metabolized in the liver and inactive metabolites are excreted in urine. Dose used is typically 200 mg daily given as a single morning dose or divided in two doses in the morning. There is involvement of the cytochrome system, and thus some drug interactions. Reported side effects are generally mild, and include headache, nausea, diarrhea, xerostomia, and nervousness [93]. This agent offers promise as a beneficial tool in the treatment of multiple symptoms such as fatigue, sedation, and depression with less adverse effect than the traditional psychostimulants.

Octreotide is a somatostantin analog, a synthetic drug that exerts action by inhibiting various hormones in the body. The synthesized drug has a longer duration of action with a half-life of approximately 1½ h, completely absorbed after subcutaneous injection, but also well tolerated via intravenous injections or infusion. It is indicated for the treatment of excessive hormonal states such as hormone-secreting tumors. Its use for treatment of acromegaly is due to inhibition of growth hormone. In the gastrointestinal tract, it inhibits the release of peptides resulting in decrease peristalsis, splanchnic blood flow, and secretions. This provides effective treatment for conditions such as gastrointestinal hemorrhage, management of fistulas, and diarrhea. In oncology practice, its antitumor effect presents a treatment option for patients for various neuroendocrine hepatic tumors [94, 95]

In palliative care, its use in the symptomatic treatment of inoperable bowel obstruction has been frequently reported . The actions on the gastrointestinal result in reduced secretions and peristalsis which quiets colic, pain, and nausea/vomiting, the usual symptoms of inoperable bowel obstruction [54, 96–99]. Octreotide is typically administered subcutaneously. About 600–800 µg daily in divided doses is generally effective [100], although the intravenous route may be used for rapid results. An intramuscular depot formulation is available for monthly injections, and may be feasible in the home setting.

More recently, an increased role of octreotide in end of life symptom management has been suggested. Many patients with carcinomatosis often present with severe ascites, causing numerous symptoms of pain, pressure, peripheral edema, and respiratory compromise. The use of this agent in the treatment of ascites has been suggested through several postulated mechanism, including enhancement of diuretic efficacy, direct tumor antisecretory effect, and reduction of splanchnic blood flow [101]. When consideration is given to the burden of frequent paracentesis that are required to alleviate discomfort in the presence of ascites, a trial with octreotide with aggressive use of diuretics is justified.

Octreotide may be considered in patients who have gastrointestinal fistulas. The inhibitory action on copious secretions may provide relief from fluid and electolyte depletions. This mechanism offers benefit in patients suffering from loperamide-resistant diarrhea, as well [102].

In low doses, the drug is generally well tolerated. Mild transient gastrointestinal symptoms of abdominal pain, dry mouth, flatulence, and steatorrhea may be minimized with timing of doses between meals.

Although this is an expensive drug, the effectiveness, low side effect profile, and multiple uses of this agent make evidently justifies its place in the palliative medicine toolchest.

PRN as Needed Dosing

The prescribing of medications often is accompanied by specific instructions, as patients rely on the healthcare provider's expertise to guide him. In the management of symptoms, this control if often shifted to the patient and care giver, as in the case of taking medications "as needed." As the goal of symptom management is comfort, this is an endpoint that can only be determined by the patient himself, thus the burden of titration to the desired outcome requires vigilant assessment and judicious medicating. Obstacles to this include fear of medication and ignorance regarding appropriate use for a given medication, as in the case of rescue drugs for breakthrough pain. It is essential that patients and care givers are empowered to self-titrate and receive education about the value of pharmacologic tools prescribed for comfort and quality of life, and encouraged to optimize the use of symptom-relieving therapies. This will allow maximal comfort while reducing the feared side effects.

Routes

In the general patient population, there are few obstacles in taking prescribed medications as ordered. In the patient receiving palliative care, the availability of oral route is not routinely guaranteed, and the ongoing quest for alternate routes is fundamental in providing drugs for these patients. The astute prescriber continually assesses for factors that may compromise the oral route, such as disease status, GI obstruction, or presence of nausea.

Loss of oral route is common in advanced disease. Thus, alternative and creative methods for administering medications must be considered. In the hospital setting, parenteral routes are readily available and taken for granted, but in transitioning to other settings, the least invasive route is most compatible with normal activity and quality of life. In the desire to maintain noninvasive administration, sublingual route is often an optimistic route used in patients unable to swallow. There is little evidence to support this practice when using hydrophilic agents such as morphine, oxycodone, or hydromorphone, but more promising results with use of lipophilic drugs such as methadone, fentanyl, and possibly buprenorphine [103, 104]. In addition to offering simplicity of administration and avoiding the more cumbersome invasive techniques, sublingual route offers the potential advantage over the oral route of rapid onset and avoiding the first-pass metabolism. Currently transmucosal formulations for fentanyl are available. Some patients find the exercise of transmucosal administration, such as fentanyl lozenges, unpalatable, and cumbersome compared to a simple swallow, and may not use these medications appropriately resulting in diminished results. There are medications that are formulated with convenient oral dissolving properties such as olanzepine orally disintegrating disk, ondansetron orally dissolving wafers, and clonazepam disintegrating tablets, but these features offer ease of swallow and not intended for absorption other than via oral ingestion. Therefore, it is important to bear in mind that, although noninvasive routes are preferred, reliability of absorption takes precedence.

Transdermal route has become very accepted and desirable since the advent of Fentanyl in this formulation. There are other medications that are introduced with this convenient method. The topical lidocaine patch offers a local anesthetic that is effective without systemic absorption. Since most anti-neuropathic medications are limited to oral route, a lidocaine patch offers a unique advantage. NSAID's as in the diclofenac patch may also be given transdermally.

Rectal route is an age-old method of providing medication, and provides a noninvasive advantage over injections. What is generally considered unappealing in general use, may provide a creative means of treating symptoms when oral or parenteral routes become difficult. Limited availability of rectal formulations require inventive use of other formulations, particularly in emergency situations outside of an acute care setting. Crushing tablets in small amounts of water or use of liquid formulations provide impromptu medications. Benzodiazepines are a class of medications that are readily absorbed rectally and provide prompt treatment of common symptoms that arise in advanced disease such as agitation or seizures. Absorption is influenced by drug properties, formulation and volume, and rectal health [105].

Subcutaneous route is frequently used for continuous infusions in the home setting. Painful intramuscular injections are to be avoided as alternative parenteral options are available.

It is our goal to utilize the most effective and efficient pharmacologic tools to treat our patients and provide optimal quality of life with minimal polypharmacy. The quest for the ideal formulary is a continual process as we make use of time-tested agents, accept the conventionally defined "side effects" as desired benefit, and learn from established mechanisms to develop newer agents for the best treatment of our patients.

References

1. Davis MP, Dickerson ED, Pappagallo M, et al. Mirtazapine: heir apparent to amitriptyline? Am J Hosp Palliat Care. 2001;18(1):42–6.
2. IAHPC issues list of essential palliative care drugs. J Support Oncol. 2006;4(8):409.
3. http://www.who.int/medicines/publications/essentialmedicines.
4. Davis MP, Dickerson ED, Pappagallo M, Benedetti C, Grauer PA, Lycan J. Mirtazepine: heir apparent to amitriptyline? Am J Hosp Palliat Care. 2001;18(1):42–6.
5. Dickerson ED. The 20 essential drugs in palliative care. Eur J Palliat Care. 1999;6(4):130–5.
6. Wowchuk SM, Wilson AE, Embleton L, Garcia M, Harlos M, Chochinov HM. The palliative medication kit: an effective way of extending care in the home for patients nearing death. J Palliat Med. 2009;12(9):797–803.

7. Snapp J, Kelley D, Gutgsell TL. Creating a hospice pharmacy and therapeutics committee. Am J Hosp Palliat Care. 2002;19(2):129–34.

8. Nauck F, Ostgathe C, Klaschik E, Bausewein C, Fuchs M, Lindena G, Neuwöhner K, Schulenberg D, Radbruch L. Drugs in palliative care: results from a representative survey in Germany. Palliat Med. 2004;18:100–7.

9. Moller PL, Sindet-Pedersen S, Petersen C, Juhl GI, Dillenschneider A, Skoglund LA. Onset of acetaminophen analgesia: comparison of oral and intravenous routes after third molar surgery. Br J Anaesth. 2005;94(5):642–8.

10. Bertolini A, Ferrari A, Alessandra O, Guerzoni S, Tacchi R, Leone S. Paracetamol: new vistas of an old drug. CNS Drug Rev. 2006;12(3 4):250 75.

11. Hamilton GR, Baskett TF. History of anesthesia in the arms of Morpheus: the development of morphine for postoperative pain relief. Can J Anesth. 2000;47(4):367–74.

12. Portenoy RK, Khan E, Layman M, et al. Chronic morphine therapy for cancer pain: plasma and cerebrospinal fluid morphine and morphine-6-glucuronide concentrations. Neurology. 1991;41:1457–61.

13. Hanna MH, Peat SJ, Knibb AA, Fung C. Disposition of morphine-6-glucuronide and morphine in healthy volunteers. Br J Anaesth. 1991;66:103–7.

14. Coluzzi PH. Sublingual morphine: efficacy reviewed. J Pain Symptom Manage. 1998;16:184–92.

15. LeBon B, Zeppetella G, Higginson IJ. Effectiveness of topical administration of opioids in palliative care: a systematic review. J Pain Symptom Manage. 2009;37(5):913–7.

16. Staats PS, Markowitz J, Schein J. Incidence of constipation associated with long-acting opioid therapy: a comparative study. South Med J. 2004;97(2):129–34.

17. Radbruch L, Sabatowski R, Loick G, Kulbe C, Kasper M, Grond S, Lehmann KA. Constipation and the use of laxatives: a comparison between transdermal fentanyl and oral morphine. Palliat Med. 2000;14(2):111–9.

18. Zeppetella G, Messina J, Xie F, Slatkin NE. Consistent and clinically relevant effects with fentanyl buccal tablet in the treatment of patients receiving maintenance opioid therapy and experiencing cancer-related breakthrough pain. Pain Pract. 2010;10(4):287–93.

19. Zeppetella G. An assessment of the safety, efficacy, and acceptability of intranasal fentanyl citrate in the management of cancer-related breakthrough pain: a pilot study. J Pain Symptom Manage. 2000;20(4):253–8.

20. Zeppetella G. Nebulized and intranasal fentanyl in the management of cancer-related breakthrough pain. Palliat Med. 2000;14(1):57–8.

21. Power I. Fentanyl HCl iontophoretic transdermal system (ITS): clinical application of iontophoretic technology in the management of acute postoperative pain. Br J Anaesth. 2007;98(1):4–11.

22. Wheeler WL, Dickerson ED. Clinical applications of methadone. Am J Hosp Palliat Care. 2000;17(3):196–203.

23. Chhabra S, Bull J. Methadone. Am J Hosp Palliat Med. 2008;25(2):146–50.

24. Eap CB, Curndet C, Baumann P. Binding of D-methadone, L-methadone and DL-methadone to proteins in plasma of healthy volunteers: role of variants of X1-acid glycoprotein. Clin Pharmacol Ther. 1990;47:338–46.

25. Hagen NA, Fisher K, Stiles C. Sublingual methadone for the management of cancer-related breakthrough pain: a pilot study. J Palliat Med. 2007;10(2):331–7.

26. Morley JS, Makin MK. The use of methadone in cancer pain poorly responsive to other opioids. Pain Rev. 1998;5:51–8.

27. Ripamonti C, Groff L, Brunelli C, et al. Switching from morphine to oral methadone in treateing cancer pain: what is the equianalgesic dose ratio? J Clin Oncol. 1998;16:3216–21.

28. Bruera E, Sweeney C. Methadone use in cancer patients with pain: a review. J Palliat Med. 2002;5:127–38.

29. Gan TJ. Diclofenac: an update on its mechanism of action and safety profile. Curr Med Res Opin. 2010;26(7):1715–31.

30. Galer BS, Rowbotham M, Perander J, Devers A, Friedman E. Topical diclofenac patch relieves minor sports injury pain: results of a multicenter controlled clinical trial. J Pain Symptom Manage. 2000;19(4):287–94.

31. Raffia RB, Friderichs E, Reimann W, Shank RP, Codd EE, Vault JL. Opioid and nonopioid components independently contribute to the mechanism of action of tramadol, an 'atypical' opioid analgesic. J Pharmacol Exp Ther. 1992;260(1):275–85.
32. Cleary JF. The pharmacologic management of cancer pain. J Palliat Med. 2007;10(6):1369–94.
33. Leppert W. Tramadol as an analgesic for mild to moderate cancer pain. Pharmacol Rep. 2009;61:978–92.
34. Tschentke TM, de Vry J, Terlinden R, Hennies H-H, Lange C, Strassburger W, Haurand M, Kolb J, Schneider J, Buschmann H, Finkam M, Jahnel U, Friedrichs E. Tapentadol hydrochloride. Drugs Fut. 2006;31(12):1053.
35. Hale M, Upmalis D, Okamoto A, Langec C, Rauschkolb C. Tolerability of tapentadol immediate release in patients with lower back pain or osteoarthritis of the hip or knee over 90 days: a randomized, double-blind study. Curr Med Res Opin. 2009;25(50300–7995):1095–104.
36. Sindrup SH, Brosen K. The pharmacogenetics of codeine hypoalgesia. Pharmacogenetics. 1995;5:335–46.
37. Smith SM, Schroeder K, Fahey T. Over the counter medications for acute cough in children and adults in ambulatory settings. Cochrane database Syst Rev. (4):CD001831.
38. Dworkin RH, Backonja M, Rowbotham MC, et al. Advances in neuropathic pain: diagnosis, mechanisms, and treatment recommendations. Arch Neurol. 2003;60:1524–34.
39. Atkinson JH, Slater MA, Wahlgren DR, Williams RA, Zisook S, Pruitt SD, Epping-Jordan JE, Patterson TL, Grant I, Abramson I, Garfin SR. Effects of noradrenergic and serotonergic antidepressants on chronic low back pain intensity. Pain. 1999;83(2):137–45.
40. Killian JM, Fromm GH. Carbamazepine in the treatment of Neuralgia:Use and Side Effects. Arch Neurol. 1968;19:129–36.
41. Blom S. Tic douloureaux treated with new anticonvulsant. Arch Neurol. 1963;9:285–90.
42. Stewart BH, Kugler AR, Thompson PR, et al. A saturable transport mechanism in the intestinal absorption of gabapentin is the underlying cause of the lack of proportionality between increasing dose and drug levels in plasma. Pharm Res. 1993;10(2):276–81.
43. Stefan H, Feuerstein TJ. Novel anticonvulsant drugs. Pharmacol Ther. 2007;113:165–83.
44. LaRoche SM, Helmers SL. The new antiepileptic drugs. JAMA. 2004;291(5):605–14.
45. Mellick GA, Mellick LB. Gabapentin in the management of reflex sympathetic dystrophy. J Pain Symptom Manage. 1995;10:265–6.
46. Rosenberg JM, Harrell C, Ristic H, Werner RA, de Rosayro AM. The effect of gabapentin on neuropathic pain. Clin J Pain. 1997;13:251–5.
47. Rowbotham M, Harden N, Stacey B, et al. Gabapentin for the treatment of postherpetic neuralgia: a randomized controlled trial. JAMA. 1998;280:1837–42.
48. Rice AS, Maton S, For the Postherpetic Neuralgia Study Group. Gabapentin in postherpetic neuralgia: a randomized, double blind, placebo controlled study. Pain. 2001;94:215–24.
49. Vella-Brincat J, Macleod AD. Haloperidol in palliative care. Palliat Med. 2004;18:195–201.
50. Han C, Kim Y. A double-blind trial of risperidone and haloperidol for the treatment of delirium. Psychosomatics. 2004;45:297–301.
51. Adams F. Emergency intravenous sedation of the delirious, medically ill patient. J Clin Psychiatry. 1988;49(Suppl):22–7.
52. O'Brien C. Nausea and vomiting. Can Fam Physician. 2008;54:861–3.
53. Baines MJ. ABC of palliative care: nausea, vomiting, and intestinal obstruction. BMJ. 1997;315:1148.
54. Ripamonti C, Twycross R, Baines M, Bozzetti F, Capri S, De Conno F, Gemlo B, Hunt TM, Krebs HB, Mercadante S, Schaerer R, Wilkinson P. Clinical-practice recommendations for the management of bowel obstruction in patients with end-stage cancer. Support Care Cancer. 2001;9:223–33.
55. Meyer-Massetti C, Cheng CM, Sharpe BA, Meier CR, Guglielmo BJ. The FDA extended warning for intravenous haloperidol and torsades de pointes: how should institutions respond? J Hosp Med. 2010;5(4):E8–16.
56. Ramamurthy S, Shaker MH, Winnie AP. Glycopyrrolate as a substitute for atropine in neostigmine reversal of muscle relaxant drugs. Can Anaesth Soc J. 1972;19:399–411.

57. Tchekmedyian NS, Tait N, Moody M, et al. Appetite stimulation with megestrol acetate in cachectic cancer patients. Semin Oncol. 1986;13:37–43.

58. Loprinzi CL, Schaid DJ, Dose AN, et al. Body-composition changes in patients who gain weight while receiving megestrol acetate. J Clin Oncol. 1993;11:152–4.

59. Loprinzi CL, Ellison NM, Schaid DJ, Krook JE, Athmann LM, Dose AM, Mailliard JA, Johnson PS, Ebbert LP, Feeraerts LH. Controlled trial of megestrol acetate for the treatment of cancer anorexia and cachexia. J Natl Cancer Inst. 1990;82(13):1127–32.

60. Bruera E, Ernst S, Hagen N, Spachynski K, Belzile M, Hanson J, Summers N, Brown B, Dulude H, Gallant G. Effectiveness of megestrol acetate in patients with advanced cancer: a randomized, double-blind, crossover study. Cancer Prev Control. 1998;2(2):74–8.

61. Von Roenn JH, Murphy RL, Weber KM, et al. Megestrol acetate for treatment of cachexia associated with human immunodeficiency virus (HIV) infection. Ann Intern Med. 1988;109:840–1.

62. Loprinzi CL, Michalak JC, Schaid DJ, Mailliard JA, Athmann LM, Goldberg RM, Tschetter LK, Hatfield AK, Morton RF. Phase III evaluation of four doses of megestrol acetate as therapy for patients with cancer anorexia and/or cachexia. J Clin Oncol. 1993;11(4):762–7.

63. Nelson KA, Walsh D, Hussein M. A phase II study of low-dose megestrol acetate using twice daily dosing for anorexia in nonhormonally dependent cancer. Am J Hosp Palliat Care. 2002;19(3):206–10.

64. Needham PR, Daley AG, Lennard RF. Steroids in advanced cancer: survey of current practice. BMJ. 1992;305(6860):969–70.

65. Rousseau P. The palliative use of high-dose corticosteroids in three terminally ill patients with pain. Am J Hosp Palliat Care. 2001;18(5):343–6.

66. Bottomley DM, Hanks GW. Subcutaneous midazolam infusion in palliative care. J Pain Symptom Manage. 1990;5(4):259–61.

67. Cloos J. The treatment of panic disorder. Curr Opin Psychiatry. 2005;18(1):45–50.

68. Cascade E, Kalali AH, Weisler RH. Varying uses of anticonvulsant medications. Psychiatry. 2008;5(6):31–3.

69. Cendrowski W, Sobczyk W. Clonazepam, baclofen and placebo in the treatment of spasticity. Eur Neurol. 1977;16:257–62.

70. Chouinard G. The search for new off-label indications for antidepressant, antianxiety, antipsychotic and anticonvulsant drugs. J Psychiatry Neurosci. 2006;31(3):168–76.

71. Morishita S. Clonazepam as a therapeutic adjunct to improve the management of depression: a brief review. Hum Psychopharmacol Clin Exp. 2009;24:191–8.

72. Riss J, Cloyd J, Gates J, Collins S. Benzodiazepines in epilepsy: pharmacology and pharmacokinetics. Acta Neurol Scand. 2008;118:69–86.

73. Mercadante S. Pathophysiology and treatment of opioid-related myoclonus in cancer patients. Pain. 1998;74(1):5–9.

74. Eisele Jr JH, Grigsby EJ, Dea G. Clonazepam treatment of myoclonic contractions associated with high-dose opioids: case report. Pain. 1992;49:231–2.

75. Bouckoms AJ, Litman RE. Clonazepam in the treatment of neuralgic pain syndrome. Psychosomatics. 1985;26(12):933–6.

76. Bartusch SL, Sanders BJ, D'Alessio JG, Jernigan JR. Clonazepam for the treatment of lancinating phantom limb pain. Clin J Pain. 1996;12(10):59–62.

77. Reddy S, Patt RB. The benzodiazepines as adjuvant analgesics. J Pain Symptom Manage. 1994;9:510–4.

78. Ellpoial ANB, Samaranayakel LP. Oral candidal infections and antimycotics. Crit Rev Oral Biol Med. 2000;11(2):172–98.

79. Schafer-Korting M, Blechschmidt J, Korting HC. Clinical use of oral nystatin in the prevention of systemic candidosis in patients at particular risk. Mycoses. 1996;39(9–10):329–39.

80. Davies A, Brailsford S, Broadley K, Beighton D. Resistance amongst yeasts isolated from the oral cavities of patients with advanced cancer. Palliat Med. 2002;16:527–31.

81. Hotopf M, Chidgey J, Addington-Hall J, Ly KL. Depression in advanced disease: a systematic review part 1. Prevalence and case finding. Palliat Med. 2002;16:81–97.

82. Davis MP, Khawam E, Posuelo L, Lagman R. Management of symptoms associated with advanced cancer: olanzepine and mirtazepine. Expert Rev Anticancer Ther. 2002;2(4):365–76.
83. Jackson WC, Tavernier L. Olanzapine for intractable nausea in palliative care patients. J Palliat Med. 2003;6(2):251–5.
84. Khojainova N, Santiago-Palma J, Kornick C, Breitbart W, Gonzales GR. Olanzapine in the management of cancer pain. J Pain Symptom Manage. 2002;23(4):346–50.
85. McNulty JP. Can levophanol be used like methadone for intractable refractory pain? J Palliat Med. 2007;10(2):293–6.
86. Prommer E. Levorphanol: the forgotten opioid. Support Care Cancer. 2007;15:259–64.
87. Johnson RE, Fudala PJ, Payne R. Buprenorphine: considerations for pain management. J Pain Symptom Manage. 2005;29(3):297–326.
88. Induru RR, Davis MP. Buprenorphine for neuropathic pain – targeting hyperalgesia. Am J Hosp Palliat Med. 2009;26(6):470–3.
89. DeBattista C, Lembke A, Solvason HB, Ghebremichael R, Poirier J. A prospective trial of modafinil as an adjunctive treatment of major depression. J Clin Psychopharmacol. 2004;24(1):87–90.
90. Webster L, Andrews M, Stoddard G. Modafinil treatment of opioid-induced sedation. Pain Med. 2003;4(2):135–40.
91. Bruera E, Brenneis C, Patterson A, et al. Use of methylphenidate as an adjuvant to narcotic analgesics in patients with advanced cancer. J Pain Symptom Manage. 1989;4:3–6.
92. Scammell TE, Estabrooke IV, McCarthy MT, et al. Hypothalamic arousal regions are activated during modafinil-induced wakefulness. J Neurosci. 2000;20:8620–8.
93. Pappagallo M. Modafinil: a gift to portmanteau. Am J Hosp Palliat Care. 2001;18:408–10.
94. Schoniger-Hekele M, Kettenbach J, Peck-Radosavljevic M, Muller C. Octreotide treatment of patients with hepatocellular carcinoma – a retrospective single centre controlled study. J Exp Clin Cancer Res. 2009;28:142–9.
95. Saijo F, Naito H, Funayama Y, Fukushima K, Shibata C, Hashimoto A, Kitayama T, Nagao M, Matsuno S, Sasaki I. Octreotide in control of multiple liver metastases from gastrinoma. J Gastroenterol. 2003;38(9):905–8.
96. Mangili G, Aletti G, Frigerio L, Franchi M, Panacci N, Vigano R, De Marzi P, Zanetto F, Ferrari A. Palliative care for intestinal obstruction in recurrent ovarian cancer: a multivariate analysis. Int J Gynecol Cancer. 2005;15:830–5.
97. Mercadante S, Ferrera P, Villari P, Marrazzo A. Aggressive pharmacological treatment for reversing malignant bowel obstruction. J Pain Symptom Manage. 2004;28(4):412–6.
98. Mercadante S, Ripamonti C, Casuccio A, Zecca E, Groff L. Comparison of octreotide and hyoscine butylbromide in controlling gastrointestinal symptoms due to malignant inoperable bowel obstruction. Support Care Cancer. 2000;8:188–91.
99. Khoo D, Hall E, Motson R, et al. Palliation of malignant intestinal obstruction using octreotide. Eur J Cancer. 1994;30A:28–30.
100. Jatoi A, Podratz KC, Gill P, Hartmann LC. Pathophysiology and palliation of inoperable bowel obstruction in patients with ovarian. Cancer Support Oncol. 2004;2:323–37.
101. Murphy E, Prommer EE, Mihalyo M, Wilcock A. Octreotide. J Pain Symptom Manage. 2010;40(1):142–8.
102. Mercadante S. The role of octreotide in palliative care. J Pain Symptom Manage. 1994;9(6):406–11.
103. Weinberg DS, Inturrisi CE, Reidenberg B, Moulin DE, Nip TJ, Wallenstein S, Houde RW, Foley KM. Sublingual absorption of selected opioid analgesics. Clin Pharmacol Ther. 1988;44:335–42.
104. Reisfield GM, Wilson GR. Rational use of sublingual opioids in palliative medicine. J Palliat Med. 2007;10:465–75.
105. Davis MP, Walsh D, LeGrand SB, Naughton M. Symptom control in cancer patients: the clinical pharmacology and therapeutic role of suppositories and rectal preparations. Support Care Cancer. 2002;10:117–38.

Review Questions

1. Advantages of methadone use in palliative medicine include all the following except:

   (a) High-potency opioid-tolerant patients
   (b) Anti-neuropathic mechanism via N-methyl-d-aspartate (NMDA) receptor antagonism
   (c) Short half-life
   (d) No active metabolites
   (e) Ease of administration

2. Which of the following medications are effectively administered by transmucosal route:

   (a) Olanzepine
   (b) Morphine
   (c) Fentanyl
   (d) Tramadol
   (e) Amitriptyline

3. All of the following medications offer benefit for the treatment of neuropathic pain with the exception of

   (a) Gabapentin
   (b) Buprenorphine
   (c) Carbamazepine
   (d) Codeine
   (e) Amitriptyline

4. Drug interactions are most likely with which of the following drugs

   (a) Acetaminophen
   (b) Diclofenac
   (c) Gabapentin
   (d) Haloperidol
   (e) Methadone

5. Which of the following benefits is not provided by octreotide in the care of terminally ill patients

   (a) Reduction of secretions and gut motility in inoperable bowel obstruction
   (b) Cost effective
   (c) Management of fistulas
   (d) Enhancement of diuretic therapy in treatment of ascites
   (e) Treatment of diarrhea

Answers

1. (c). A disadvantage of methadone is the prolonged and variable half-life which limits rapid titration. It remains a viable opioid option for patients who are highly tolerant or exhibit a neuropathic component of pain. Liquid formulation allows for creative administration in patients with compromised swallowing.
2. (c). Fentanyl has high lipid solubility making it an excellent choice for transdermal absorption. Although morphine, in concentrated liquid formulation, is often placed sublingually for patients with impaired swallowing, it is essentially swallowed with saliva. Similarly, an orally dissolving olanzepine disk is formulated for ease of swallowing. Tramadol is rapidly absorbed by oral route.
3. (d). The common classes of medication for treatment of neuropathic pain are anticonvulsants and antidepressants. Codeine is a weak opioid without antineuropathic effect. Buprenorphine has unique non-opioid mechanisms of action suggesting a role in treating neuropathic pain.
4. (e). Methadone is involved in numerous drug interactions as a result of metabolism via the cytochrome system.
5. (b). Despite the effectiveness of octreotide in symptom management, the cost remains an impediment to its use.

Chapter 15
Interventional Radiology in Palliative Care

Oliver Hulson, Neal Larkman, and Sreekumar Kunnumpurath

Introduction

Interventional radiological procedures have expanded greatly over the past decade. What was once a small aspect of clinical care is now available to provide a significant input in a variety of patients. A number of retractable and troublesome symptoms in end-of-life care may be improved or abated by procedures. Many of which are performed under local anaesthetic or sedation. In addition, many of these procedures are performed percutaneously, through a single, small skin incision, thereby improving recovery time and reducing hospital stay, imperative at a time when aiming to return a patient home to rest is paramount [1].

A description of a selection of these procedures follows, along with the indications, contraindications and a brief description of what the procedure entails. Whilst this is not an attempt to train the reader in becoming competent at these procedures, it is hoped that this will aid the palliative care team and the patient in making a fully informed decision when considering such treatment options.

O. Hulson, M.B.Ch.B. (Hons.) (✉) • N. Larkman, M.B.B.S., M.P.H.
Leeds and Bradford Radiology Training Scheme, Leeds General Infirmary,
Leeds, UK
e-mail: ohulson@doctors.org.uk

S. Kunnumpurath, M.B.B.S., M.D., F.F.P.M.R.C.A., F.R.C.A., F.C.A.R.C.S.I.
Department of Anaesthetics, Epsom and St Helier University Hospitals NHS Trust,
Carshalton, Surrey, UK

N. Vadivelu et al. (eds.), *Essentials of Palliative Care*,
DOI 10.1007/978-1-4614-5164-8_15,
© Springer Science+Business Media New York 2013

Angiography

Indications

Even with the advent and advances in CT and MR imaging techniques, conventional angiography remains an essential adjunct in the assessment and imaging of the vascular system, and is the basis of many more complex and technically difficult procedures. The benefits of this technique over others is that, whilst invasive, it can be both diagnostic and therapeutic, improving blood flow at the same time as identifying the cause of a critically ischaemic limb.

In the palliative care setting, angiography may be employed in order to treat symptoms related to the patients' terminal illness, for example embolisation in haemoptysis secondary to lung carcinoma, or for a condition independent of this, such as limb ischaemia. Specific indications such as embolisation and cerebral angiography will be discussed later in this chapter.

Contraindications

The only truly "absolute" contraindication to angiography is the unstable patient with multisystem failure [2]. Other relative contraindications are listed below. Those perhaps most relevant to a palliative patient are highlighted in bold:

Recent myocardial infarction

- **Electrolyte abnormalities**
- **Impaired renal function** (due to the administration of contrast)
- Confused or uncooperative patient (may require general anaesthesia)
- **Coagulopathy**
- **Inability to lie flat on operative table** (due to congestive cardiac failure or poor respiratory reserve)
- Pregnancy

While it may be felt that "pregnancy" is as an absolute contraindication to exposure to any ionising radiation, in reality if it is felt that harm will come to the mother by circumventing a study such as a CT or angiography examination, then the study should not be ruled out [3]. Unfortunately, it is a simple fact of life that if harm should come to the mother, then the risk of harm to the unborn foetus is likely to be greater than the risk from radiation exposure. In practice, if and when this scenario arises, a fully informed discussion between the patient, a consultant radiologist and consultant obstetrician is likely to occur, and steps taken to reduce the radiation exposure to the foetus.

Procedural Method

There are a wide variety of techniques, sheaths and catheters employed by specialist vascular interventional radiologists, but the basic principles remain largely the same. This relates to the Seldinger technique employed elsewhere in chest drain or central line insertion, and involves three steps:

1. **Vessel puncture** (Fig. 15.1a): Performed under direct vision using anatomical landmarks or under ultrasound or fluoroscopic guidance. The liberal use of local anaesthetic agents from skin down to artery will increase patient comfort and subsequently improve outcome. A "give" will be felt once the cannula passes through the arterial wall, and pulsatile blood flow will confirm that the needle tip lies within the lumen of the artery.

2. **Guide wire passage** (Fig. 15.1b): Once intraluminal access is confirmed, a dilator or small incision adjacent to the puncture site may be needed to ensure smooth introduction of the guide wire and catheter. A wide variety of guide wires are available depending on indication and operator preference. The wire is introduced and positioned ready for the insertion of the catheter.

3. **Catheter insertion** (Fig. 15.1c): Great care is taken when introducing the catheter over the guide wire, to ensure that the guide wire is not advanced into the artery in its entirety. Again, a variety of catheters are available from a variety of manufacturers, varying in size, shape and flexibility (see Fig. 15.2). The catheter and wire are then manipulated along the arterial system to the region of interest (for example the aortic arch or lower limb vessels). At this point, the wire may be removed, contrast medium injected and angiography performed, for an instantaneous, detailed image of the area in question. If a stenosis or occlusion is found, intervention may be attempted.

Angioplasty

Angioplasty is the process of mechanically widening the lumen of a vessel, usually due to a stenosis from atheroma, or an occlusion due to acute thromboembolism. The interventional options are numerous and outside the scope of this text, but a brief overview of treatment options is likely to be beneficial when considering such treatment or caring for the patient post-operatively. In order to succeed in intervention, the blockage or occlusion must first be traversed by the guide wire, which can be difficult and take time.

Once the occlusion or stenosis has been successfully traversed, a balloon catheter can be introduced over the wire, to the site of the occlusion, and inflated to reopen the vessel. The balloon exerts a high pressure upon the vessel wall, stretching the vessel to an appropriate size. A contrast run is then likely to be performed, to both assess the degree of remaining stenosis, and also check for distal run-off (a recognised complication is distal embolisation due to plaque dislodgment).

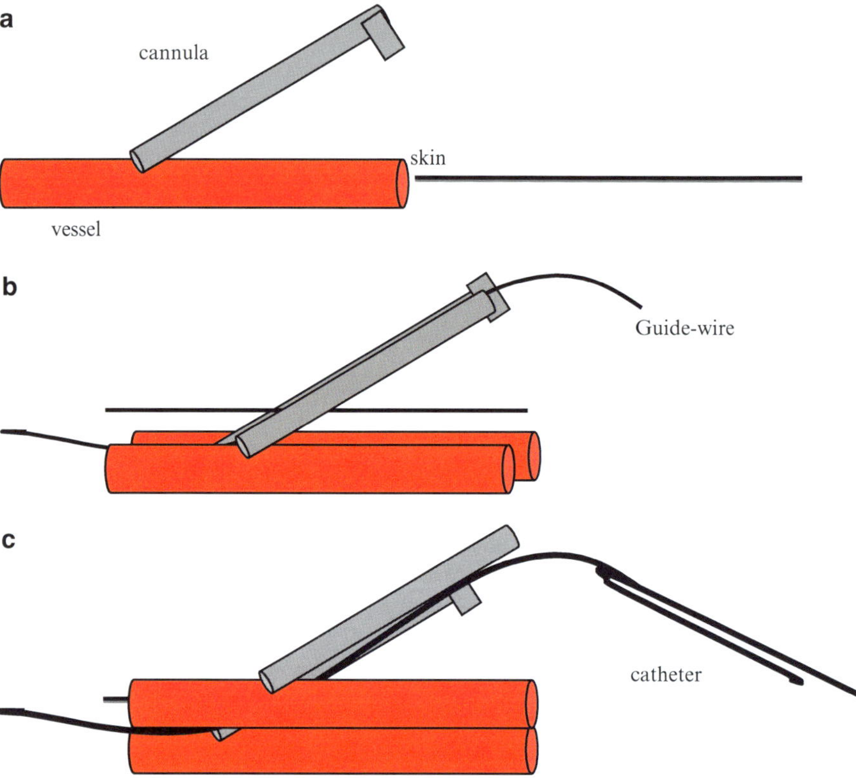

Fig. 15.1 (**a**) The cannula is introduced percutaneously, into the artery or vein. (**b**) A guide-wire is introduced through the cannula and sits within the vessel lumen. (**c**) The catheter is introduced over the guide wire into the vessel lumen, through which interventions such as angiography can take place

If the vessel does not maintain an adequate lumen size post-angioplasty, a stent may be introduced, aiming to mechanically maintain luminal diameter. However, introduction of a stent in an artery with relatively sluggish blood flow may precipitate further thrombus formation, and although drug-eluting stents counteract this to some degree, it may not always be in the patient's best interest to have a stent inserted.

Complications

As with any procedure, post-operative complications can occur, and it is useful for healthcare staff to be aware of such complications, to ensure early detection and resolution. The Society for Cardiac Angiography and Interventions (SCAI) cite an incidence of

Fig. 15.2 Diagram
showing variety of catheters
available [4]

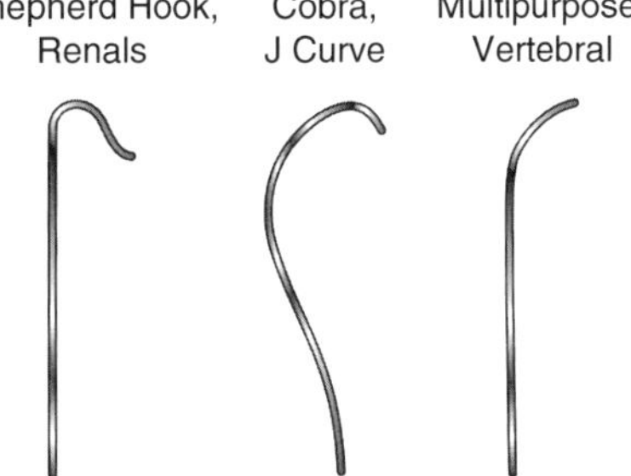

0.5 % for local vascular complications; these include thrombosis of the punctured vessel, dissection, retroperitoneal haemorrhage, haematoma, distal embolisation and false aneurysm formation [4].

Embolisation Procedures

Indications

Deliberate embolisation of a vein or artery may be indicated in a variety of settings, for instance in the acute setting in uncontrolled bleeding in pelvic or abdominal trauma, and also electively in the treatment of subfertility by the selective embolisation of a testicular varicocele [5]. Of relevance in the palliative care setting, selective chemoembolisation of hepatic metastases or indeed other tumours is a relatively new venture utilising this technology [6]. Whilst the techniques describing the procedure have been around for some time, as technology and embolic agents advance and become more refined, the procedures attempted by the interventional radiologist become increasingly diverse and complex.

Contraindications

Again however, it is a procedure not without risks, and correct patient choice is fundamental in achieving a successful outcome. The absolute and relative contraindications of such a procedure are the same as for angiography discussed previously. In addition, there are considerations to be made when embarking on such a procedure, to minimise the chance of a futile intervention, and maximise the chance of success. Patients who are severely shocked due to presumed intra-abdominal bleeding are unlikely to benefit from such a procedure, and exploratory laparotomy is often the only option.

Splenic trauma in the relatively stable patient however may be managed in this way, with selective embolisation of the culprit branch of the splenic artery aiming to

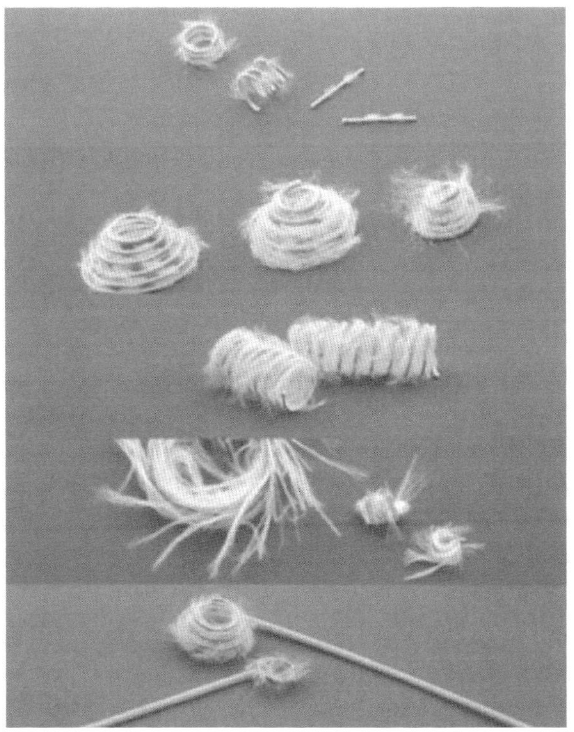

Fig. 15.3 Intravascular coils, displaying the fibrous, thrombogenic surface ([1]; reproduced with permission)

contain the bleeding sufficiently to avoid laparotomy and splenectomy [7]. Also, the treatment of uterine fibroids (or leiomyomata), once the bread and butter of the gynaecological surgeon's operating list, has been transformed by selective embolisation of the vessels supplying these benign tumours [8].

Embolic agents can be mechanical, including "coils" (so-called as they coil in the target vessel, occluding flow) which are often made of stainless steel or platinum, with a fibrous thrombogenic surface (see Fig. 15.3). Particulate or liquid agents including polyvinyl alcohol (PVA), sclerosants and glues are also available, and can be either temporary or permanent depending on the indication.

The initial procedure is the same as for angiography and angioplasty discussed previously, as adequate pre-embolisation angiography is vital in isolating the target vessel and selecting the appropriate embolic agent. A catheter with a single end-hole is used to ensure optimum position of the deployed embolic agent, and care is taken to ensure that the embolic agent is delivered only to the target vessel.

Once successful embolisation has been achieved, close post-procedure monitoring is vital, both for signs of further bleeding, and also infarction or ischaemia of the target area. Post-embolisation syndrome and tissue necrosis are recognised complications from such a procedure [7].

Chemoembolisation and Radioembolisation

Two specific embolisation procedures employed in the oncology setting include chemoembolisation and radioembolisation. These two novel techniques can be utilised in the treatment of hepatocellular carcinoma (HCC) as a bridging therapy prior to transplantation [9], and also in the treatment of unresectable liver metastases in colorectal carcinoma for example [10].

Chemoembolisation, as the name suggests, is a targeted embolisation procedure as described previously, but in this instance, the target vessel is one supplying the lesion of interest. Chemotherapeutic agents are first instilled locally, providing localised, targeted therapy to the lesion, before releasing a traditional embolic agent to severe the blood supply. Radioembolisation differs in that radioactive beads are used as the emboli, providing localised radiotherapy whilst again aiming to reduce blood supply to the lesion.

Points to Consider

Not all embolisation coils are safe to use in magnetic resonance imaging (MRI) and so if it is known that a patient has undergone an embolisation procedure for a berry aneurysm following a subarachnoid haemorrhage for example, it is imperative that the radiologist is informed of this before requesting the examination, and ideally, the surgical notes for the procedure interrogated to ascertain what material was used.

Cerebral Angiogram and Coiling for Brain Aneurysms

Indications

Cerebral angiography is most commonly implemented for the investigation of suspected intracranial aneurysms (in the management of subarachnoid or intracerebral haemorrhage for example) or arteriovenous malformations (AVM). It may also be employed in the investigation of cerebrovascular disease, and in the preoperative work-up for space-occupying intracranial lesions, but has largely been superseded in these areas by computed tomography (CT) and magnetic resonance (MR) angiography. It is by no means a routine procedure, and usually only performed by a select number of individual interventional neuroradiologists in a specialist or tertiary-referral centre.

In the context of palliative care, it is difficult to envisage many scenarios where such a procedure may be indicated, except perhaps if debulking surgery of a space occupying lesion were to be considered, or a similar procedure attempted in the endovascular treatment of impending carotid blowout in patients suffering from head and neck cancers [11]. It is important to acknowledge that the procedure is not without its risks, and if such an intervention is to take place, a full and frank discussion should occur between the patient (and significant others) in order to ensure that they are fully aware of the potential benefits and risks, and confirm that the treatment is in harmony with the ethos of good palliative care.

Contraindications

In patients who have recently suffered a stroke or cerebral haemorrhage, time should be taken to ensure that their neurology has stabilised. Other general contraindications are the same as that for angiography discussed previously. Discussion with a specialist interventional neuroradiologist is advised before requesting such a procedure. Local guidelines should also be adhered to regarding anticoagulation, and appropriate anticoagulant cover initiated whilst drugs such as warfarin are stopped.

Procedural Method

Depending on the indication, the procedure may be performed under mild sedation or general anaesthesia (with adequate anaesthetic cover). If general anaesthesia is to be used, local policies regarding preoperative starvation should be adhered to.

A Seldinger percutaneous catheter introduction technique is used, often puncturing the right common femoral artery. Selective catheterisation of the internal carotid artery is achieved by advancing the catheter (over a guide-wire) through the arterial system and into the cerebral circulation. A number of "runs" are performed when the catheter is in place. Contrast medium is injected into the catheter under fluoroscopy, while ensuring that the vascular area in question is adequately interrogated. Digital subtraction angiography (DSA) may be implemented to provide adequate spatial contrast.

Again depending on the indication, an intervention may be attempted during the same procedure. For example, the introduction of coils for cerebral aneurysms or a carotid stent deployed in the prevention of carotid blowout discussed previously. Strict monitoring of the patient post-operatively is mandatory, to ensure that any complications or sequelae from the procedure (such as distal embolisation causing cerebral infarct) are identified promptly and dealt with appropriately.

In cases of coiling following a subarachnoid haemorrhage, "triple-H therapy" (hypervolaemia, hypertension and haemodilution) may be implemented in an attempt to reduce the likelihood of cerebral vasospasm (and it is associated complications), aiming to maintain cerebral perfusion [12]

Tissue Plasminogen Activator in Acute Ischaemic Stroke

Though not strictly an interventional procedure, the use of tPA in the treatment of ischaemic stroke has gained some ground in recent years, due to a number of high-profile health promotion campaigns, and the utilisation of early CT imaging to distinguish between ischaemic and haemorrhagic stroke. A recent review article concluded that tPA can be effective when administered up to 4.5 h after symptom onset, but time is key, and early administration of this thrombolytic agent.

Indications

The use of tPA in stroke has been shown to improve clinical outcomes at 3 months despite the increased incidence of intracerebral haemorrhage [13]. That said, as touched upon above, time is of the essence; Cronin, for the Journal of Emergency Medicine concluded that, "the benefits of thrombolysis with tPA outweigh the risks up to 4.5 h from symptom onset", but that careful patient selection and strict criteria should be applied before treatment. Thus the most obvious indications are that the patient has suffered an ischaemic stroke, and that he/she has presented within the treatment window. Hospital policy may vary internationally, but the timeframe is likely to be similar to that discussed above. For UK practice, the *National Institute of Clinical Excellence (NICE)* state that tPA should be commenced within 3 h of symptom onset [14].

Immediate brain imaging is essential, in order to distinguish from haemorrhagic and ischaemic stroke, and treatment commenced as soon as possible. *NICE* also stipulate that treatment should only be initiated in those centres where there are staff trained in delivering thrombolysis and in monitoring for any associated complications; and immediate access to imaging and re-imaging is essential.

Contraindications

The narrow timeframe for patient presentation is currently the major limiting factor in the initiation of thrombolysis in acute ischaemic stroke, and an area in which health promotion is aiming to improve public awareness. Haemorrhagic stroke is also another absolute contraindication, and necessitates the utilisation of immediate brain imaging.

Other contraindications stated by *Boehringher Ingelheim* (the manufacturers of *Actilyse*, the fibrinolytic agent licensed for use in the UK for the treatment of stroke) are listed below. Those that may have increased relevance to the palliative patient are highlighted in bold:

- **Major surgery within 14 days of the stroke**
- **Haemorrhagic diathesis**
- **The use of oral anticoagulants**
- Documented ulcerative gastrointestinal disease during the last 3 months
- **Oesophageal varices**
- **Neoplasm with increased bleeding risk**
- **Severe liver disease**, including hepatic failure, cirrhosis, portal hypertension and active hepatitis
- **Major surgery** or significant trauma in **past 3 months**
- **Platelet count <100,000/mm^3**
- Systolic blood pressure greater than 185 or diastolic greater than 110 mmHg (or aggressive management necessary to reduce BP to these limits)
- Blood glucose <50 or >400 mg/dl

Procedural Method

Once the diagnosis of an acute ischaemic stroke has been made, haemorrhage has been ruled out and the patient is within the appropriate time window, the tPA dose is calculated. For *Actilyse* (used within the UK), the dose is weight related and thus is calculated individually. Part of the dose is often given as initial intravenous bolus, with the remainder infused over a set time period. Monitoring by nursing staff trained in the usage of thrombolysis is vital, as the commonest side-effect is an increased risk of bleeding. Reimaging may be necessary if the patient's neurology progresses at any point during or after treatment, as this may suggest the development of concurrent intracerebral haemorrhage.

Intra-arterial Thrombolysis

Indications

Intra-arterial thrombolysis (IAT) is indicated in acute or acute-on-chronic limb ischaemia, or in thrombosis or embolisation following an interventional or surgical procedure (for example an occluded bypass graft). The degree of critical limb ischaemia is important, and often dictates both initial and subsequent management. Table 15.1 outlines the categorisation of an acute ischaemic episode, along with clinical signs and brief management.

A recent review article in the European Journal of Vascular and Endovascular Surgery surveyed 22 of the 24 UK centres who contribute to the "Thrombolysis Study Group" and generated some interesting trends [16]. A decline in the use of IAT was seen in 19/22 centres, with no centres reporting in an increased use. The main reasons cited for this decline were due to the concern regarding possible complications (including major haemorrhage) and regarding the efficacy of the treatment. Related to the above categorisation, the study found that the most popular use of AIT in limb ischaemia was in category I—no sensory loss.

In everyday practice, IAT is likely to be considered as a useful adjunct to either surgical or angioplasty intervention, and management choice is likely to be formed between radiologist, clinician and surgeon on an individual case basis.

Contraindications

As suggested in the above review article, IAT is not without risk, and appears to be the co-contributor to its demise. The contraindications are the same as that for thrombolysis in stroke and PE discussed previously.

Procedural Method

Once diagnosis of acute, reversible, critical limb ischaemia has been made and confirmed by appropriate imaging, the decision for IAT, surgery or endovascular intervention needs to be addressed. As stated previously, this often a multidisciplinary discussion, taking into account the patient's comorbidities, clinical condition and site of the occlusion for example. If it is agreed that IAT is the most appropriate treatment option, a single arterial puncture is ideal (as multiple puncture sites increase the risk of bleeding complications). Arterial puncture close to the site of occlusion is best, and puncture directly into a graft itself may even be indicated. The catheter used to deliver the thrombolytic agent is introduced and embedded in the thrombus, in order to maximise efficacy. Unfractionated heparin may be infused concomitantly to reduce the risk of catheter-site thrombosis. The exact infusion regimen will depend on operator and centre preference, but angiography is often carried out at regular intervals and the catheter tip repositioned as necessary.

Peri-procedural monitoring must take place in a dedicated vascular or high dependency unit, as the risk of bleeding complications has been quoted as high as 10 %. Regular arterial site checks and observations including blood pressure and urine output are required, and interval assessment of the threatened limb, to ensure resolution of the thrombus.

Table 15.1 Assessment of limb viability and subsequent management

Category	Description	Capillary return	Muscle paralysis	Sensory loss	Arterial Doppler signal	Venous Doppler signal
I Viable	Not immediately threatened	Intact	None	None	+	+
IIa Threatened	Salvageable if treatment commenced promptly	Intact/slow	None	Partial	–	+
IIb Threatened	Salvageable if treatment commenced immediately	Slow/absent	Partial	Partial	–	+
III Irreversible	Amputation regardless of treatment	Absent	Complete	Complete	–	–

(Adapted from the Consensus report on thrombolysis, J Intern Med, 1996 [15])

Thrombolysis in Venous Thromboembolism

Indications

Intravenous thrombolysis may be considered in the treatment of pulmonary emboli (PE) and associated deep vein thrombosis (DVT), which are often referred to under the umbrella term of "venous thromboembolism" (VTE). The most recent guidelines from the British Thoracic Society (BTS) date back to 2003; NICE guidelines on the treatment of VTE are awaited.

The BTS guidelines state that thrombolysis is indicated as first line treatment in "massive PE" (defined as one severe enough to cause circulatory collapse) diagnosed on computed tomographic pulmonary angiography (CTPA) or transthoracic echocardiography (TTE). However, the guidelines do state that *alteplase* can be administered on clinical grounds alone if it is felt that cardiac arrest is imminent [17].

In non-massive PE, the guidance becomes more limited, and there is a relative paucity of convincing data in favour of thrombolysis. A study undertaken in the USA in 2002 found that there was no survival advantage in those patients with "sub-massive PE" given thrombolysis compared to a control group [18]. The risk of haemorrhage is stated to be twice that with heparin; the consensus view is that thrombolysis should be reserved for those patients described above [19].

As for thrombolysis in stroke, treatment protocols may vary between centres. The BTS guidelines state that in the case of impending arrest, a 50 mg intravenous bolus of alteplase can be given. This is likely to be followed by an intravenous infusion, either of tPA or unfractionated heparin. The contraindications for thrombolysis in VTE is as described previously, and again, staff trained to look after patients receiving thrombolytic agents is vital, to monitor for complications associated with bleeding.

Inferior Vena Cava filters

Inferior vena cava (IVC) filters are an alternative treatment option in venous thromboembolic disease, in cases where anticoagulation therapy is contraindicated or has failed, or as a temporary device whilst anticoagulant therapy is ceased to allow a procedure to be undertaken. It is likely therefore that the palliative care team may come across such a patient, as both contraindications to anticoagulant or thrombolytic therapy are more common in this patient subgroup, and the increased thrombogenicity seen in patients with malignancy may increase the risk of recurrent venous thromboembolism. The filter may either be permanent or temporary depending on the indication, but filter thrombosis is a serious and recognised side-effect; figures vary but have been quoted as high as 10 % within 5 years, and so this must be considered if survival is expected beyond this.

Procedural Method

An internal jugular vein puncture is commonly used for access to the IVC. Once the catheter has traversed the venous into the IVC, angiography is performed to assess the size, patency and confirm position of the renal veins. Once this has been imaged and necessary measurements recorded, placement of the filter can be decided by the radiologist. It is preferable to place the filter below the renal veins, aiming to spare these should filter become thrombosed at a later date. Once placement is decided, the filter can be deployed, and further angiography may be indicated to ensure stability and patency. Ideally the patient will receive concurrent anticoagulation to minimise the risk of filter thrombosis.

Temporary filters can be retrieved within two weeks of placement, beyond this the filter begins to embed in the vein wall. Specialist retrieval devices are often manufactured by the company providing the filter, and the retrieval procedure often involves a jugular or femoral puncture (depending on insertion) and manipulating the filter into a sheath before removal.

Tunnelled Central Venous Access

Peripherally introduced central catheters (PICC or PIC lines) or tunnelled central venous catheters (CVCs) are utilised when long-term intravenous access is desirable for the patient, for example for chemotherapy or total parenteral nutrition (TPN). Hospitals increasingly provide a nurse or anaesthetist led "PICC service" but this may also be the remit of the radiology department. Advantages of placement under radiological guidance are in the accurate positioning afforded to the patient, hopefully minimising complications due to incorrect siting. A variety of lines are available depending on the indication, including Hickman and Groshong to name two, and it is important to know what line the patient has, as it may have a bearing on which lumen is used for medication infusion (in the case of multi-lumen catheters) and also in the removal of the line.

Asepsis is mandatory, as septicaemia secondary to an infected central line can have devastating consequences for a patient who may already be immunocompromised due to chemotherapeutic agents or associated comorbidity. An article published in *Cancer* cited the incidence of catheter-related infection as 18 % in a cohort of 71 patients with cancer and a tunnelled CVC in situ [20]. This perhaps gives greater credence to the insertion of such lines in an arguable cleaner environment such as the operating theatre or the radiology interventional suite, as opposed to insertion at the patient's bedside on a ward.

Procedural Method

The major steps in the insertion of any tunnelled CVCs are venous puncture, subcutaneous tunnelling and finally line positioning and securing; the order of the first two steps may vary depending on which device is being inserted. Venous access is nowadays likely to be achieved under ultrasound guidance, into the right internal jugular vein (IJV), although the left IJV and subclavian veins can also be used. Whilst it is possible to successfully cannulate these vessels using anatomical reference points, the risk of inadvertent arterial puncture is reduced with the implementation of ultrasound [21].

Once venous access has been confirmed, a small skin incision is often made to aid in the insertion of initially one or two dilators, to create a sufficient hole in the vessel wall through which to introduce the catheter. Subcutaneous tunnelling can then be commenced, with a tunnelling device usually included in the procedural pack. A subcutaneous passage should be made with relative ease, and a considered chosen exit site for the device is important to ensure ease of use and comfort the patient.

Finally, the line is introduced over a guide wire, with the tip advanced under fluoroscopic guidance to lie adjacent to the right atrium within the superior vena cava (SVC). The line is then sutured in place, and, depending on manufacturer, may have a locking device in place to secure the line whilst fibrosis around the cuff takes place.

Possible post-procedural complications include inadvertent arterial puncture (hopefully recognised at the time of the procedure), pneumothorax (necessitating the requesting of a post-procedure chest radiograph both to exclude this, and to confirm line position), infection as discussed previously, and line thrombosis. For this reason, regular line flushes with saline or heparinised saline may be indicated.

Percutaneous Vertebroplasty and Kyphoplasty

Percutaneous vertebroplasty and kyphoplasty are both bone augmentation techniques that involve inserting a small amount of cement into a collapsed vertebral body.

The first percutaneous vertebroplasty were conducted in France in the early 1980s. The aim of this percutaneous treatment is to obtain an analgesic effect by vertebral stabilisation in patients complaining of back pain related to lesions weakening the spine [22].

Percutaneous kyphoplasty was first used in America in the early 1990s. It differs from vertebroplasty as it uses an inflatable balloon prior to cement insertion with the idea of restoring vertebral body height and reducing kyphotic deformity as well as relieving pain.

The superiority of each technique has been debated and whilst both do restore vertebral height, kyphoplasty has been shown to increase it more but does cost significantly more [23].

Non-blinded studies into both techniques have demonstrated better pain control compared to medication[24, 25]. However a blinded study showed no significant difference in pain improvement when comparing bone augmentation to sham procedure control groups [26].

The indications for vertebroplasty and kyphoplasty are for treatment of painful vertebral compression fractures secondary to osteoporosis or osteolytic tumour infiltration that are refractory to conservative management.

The absolute contraindications include active infection within the bone, uncontrolled bleeding disorders and unstable fractures involving the posterior cortex of the vertebral body.

Both procedures use an aseptic technique and a local anaesthetic for analgesia and pre-procedural antibiotic cover. A spinal surgeon is required on standby in case of any complication requiring surgical intervention. Depending on the vertebrae involved a transpedicular or anterolateral approach is used for insertion of varying gauge biopsy needles. The position of the needle and introduction of cement is monitored under fluoroscopic or CT guidance to ensure correct placement and to avoid excessive cement migration.

Kyphoplasty differs as a balloon catheter is introduced and inflated to improve vertebral height. It is then deflated and the cement is introduced. The bone cement used in both techniques is methylmethacrylate based.

Complications include infection, neurological problems such as loss of sensation in the lower limbs, no improvement or worsening of pain and a risk of venous thromboembolism secondary to cement entering the local venous system.

Coeliac Plexus and Superior Hypogastric Plexus Blocks

The coeliac plexus consists mainly of two coeliac ganglia connected by a large network of fibres that include pre-ganglionic and post-ganglionic sympathetic fibres, pre-ganglionic parasympathetic fibres and visceral afferent fibres. It is located around the origins of the coeliac artery. It innervates much of the upper abdomen including the pancreas, stomach, liver, gallbladder and bowel proximal to the transverse colon.

The Superior hypogastric plexus is similarly a network of mainly sympathetic nerve fibres but is located around the bifurcation of the aorta. It innervates the lower abdominal and pelvic organs such as the descending colon, rectum and male and female reproductive organs [27].

Indication

If pain from organs innervated by these plexuses is not being controlled by conventional analgesia then these interventions have been shown to be effective in stopping pain or reducing pain and the amount of opiate analgesia required [27]. Its use is not limited to cancer related pain, for example coeliac plexus blocks can be used for chronic pancreatitis. Its efficacy depends on the ability to adequately access the plexus which may be prevented by scar tissue, fibrosis or tumour infiltration even with good procedural technique.

Procedural Method

There are both anterior and posterior approaches used to block the coeliac plexus. No one approach is superior to the other in effectiveness but they have different merits. One or two needles (depending on technique) are inserted under radiological guidance in the region of the coeliac plexus.

Several posterior approaches under fluoroscopic guidance exist. These require the patient to lie prone. The needles in the retrocrural approach remain behind the diaphragms whilst the needles in the transcrural approach goes through the diaphragm. In the trans-aortic approach one needle passes through the aorta and the splanchnic approach is one vertebra higher at T12 and targets the splanchnic nerves.

The anterior approaches use ultrasound or CT guidance. These approaches are useful for patients who could not tolerate lying prone. In can be done relatively rapidly and has less chance of neurologic complications [28].

As with a coeliac plexus block, several approaches exist for the superior hypogastric plexus block, with the classical approach again being a bilateral posterolateral approach (and anterior approaches using CT guidance also possible).

When the needles are in position a diagnostic blockade using a local anaesthetic block can be performed; however in up to 28 % of cases this will not correlate with the effect of a neurolytic agent [29]. The neurolytic agent is an alcohol or phenol based solution.

Contraindications

The relative contraindications include uncontrolled bleeding disorders, infections, large aortic aneurysms, severe atherosclerotic disease and invasion of the tumour into anterior body wall as nerve supply is different.

Complications

For coeliac plexus blocks, complications include back pain, orthostatic hypotension and transient diarrhoea secondary to the loss of sympathetic innervation to the bowel and vascular supply. The approach used relates to the side effects experienced [30]. Other complications include retroperitoneal haemorrhage, abdominal aortic dissection due to direct trauma to the aorta, paraplegia and transient motor paralysis.

The complications for a hypogastric block include back pain, bleeding, haematoma and renal or ureteric puncture.

Biliary Interventions

Percutaneous cholecystostomy is indicated as management of both acalculous and calculous acute cholecystitis. It can be used as a definitive or temporary measure if a patient is expected to improve sufficiently for elective surgery. The decision to use it as a definitive or temporary measure will depend on a patient's response and multi-disciplinary clinical discussion. It can also be used as an access to the biliary tract; however, it is not the preferred method.

With regard to palliative care, this treatment may be considered in empyema of the gallbladder that has not responded to antibiotics and where biliary duct stenting has not improved the clinical picture [31]. Coagulopathy is a relative contraindication and should be corrected or improved prior to the procedure.

Procedural Method

Prior to the procedure, antibiotic cover and duration should be considered. Under fluoroscopic and ultrasound guidance the gallbladder is punctured and a catheter inserted via a transhepatic or transperitoneal approach using a trocar-needle catheter or Seldinger technique. If fluoroscopy is used, contrast can be injected to confirm position. The cholecystostomy catheter has to be left in to allow tract maturation and reduce the risk of bile leakage into the peritoneum. The time it is left in will vary and the tract may be injected with contrast under fluoroscopy to check tract maturation prior to catheter removal

The major complications of the procedure include peritonitis and abscess (2.9 %) , sepsis (2.5 %), bleeding (2.2 %), transgression of adjacent structures (1.6 %) and death (2.5 %) [32]. A later complication can be the displacement of the catheter.

Biliary Catheter insertion

Under the auspices of biliary catheter insertion are several procedures. A percutaneous transhepatic cholangiography (PTC) is performed first and is indicated as a way of demonstrating the level of obstruction in a dilated biliary tract. The PTC is rarely used just for diagnostic purposes and is usually followed by a therapeutic intervention such as balloon dilatation of benign strictures, stent insertion for malignant strictures and drains for infected systems or difficult to pass strictures.

Contraindications

Coagulopathy is a relative contraindication for biliary interventional procedures and should be corrected or improved prior to the procedure. Local guidelines should be consulted and adhered to. Biliary tract sepsis is a relative contraindication but in some cases may be the indication for the procedure.

Procedural Method

Prior to the procedure, antibiotic cover and duration should be considered, again in line with local guidelines. Using ultrasound and fluoroscopic guidance, local anaesthesia and an aseptic technique, a chiba needle is inserted into the left or right lobe of the liver. Contrast medium is injected to assess whether the needle is correctly sited, and images outlining the biliary tree are taken.

At this point the needle can be removed, or if an intervention is to be conducted then a guide wire is introduced, followed by a sheath through which catheters and stents can be introduced over the wire. Post-procedural care includes monitoring the patient for 6 h, antibiotics and regularly flushing of the external drains.

The complications of PTC include a 2 % risk of sepsis, cholangitis, bile leak, haemorrhage or pneumothorax. The major complications of a therapeutic intervention include a 2.5 % risk of sepsis or haemorrhage, 1.2 % risk of infection or inflammation (abscess, peritonitis, cholecystitis or pancreatitis) and a 1.7 % mortality rate [32].

Percutaneous Gastrostomy

Gastrostomy can be performed surgically, endoscopically or radiologically. The two percutaneous procedures were introduced in the last 30 years and the endoscopic technique is the commonest method used today. Radiological inserted gastrostomy has comparable mortality and morbidity rates to endoscopic insertion [33, 34]. In the palliative setting its main advantage is that it can be done with minimal sedation compared to endoscopic or surgical gastrostomy, however a smaller calibre tube is inserted.

It is indicated, as with the other direct enteral methods, in patients who will be requiring enteral feeding for a prolonged period and particularly in patients unable to undergo an endoscopic procedure. The decision should be made using a multi-disciplinary approach.

Contraindications

Uncontrolled coagulopathy is an absolute contraindication to the procedure. Difficult approaches due to a high lying stomach or colon overlying the anterior stomach wall are also contraindications if no safe approach is found. Other relative contraindications include gastric varices and neoplasm.

Procedural Method

The patient should be fasted prior to the procedure for 6 h if possible. Prophylactic antibiotic coverage is not usually necessary unless patients are immunocompromised. There are several catheter types available including loop, balloon and mushroom catheters. They have differing benefits and limitations and should be chosen based on patient and physician requirements. The catheters are inserted by either a push (Sacks–Vine) or pull (Ponsky–Gauderer) technique. In radiological gastrostomy the push technique is more commonly used but the pull technique can be performed. Gastropexy, where the stomach is fastened to the anterior abdominal wall, can be used particularly in patients with ascites [35].

Complications

The major complications of gastrostomy include peritonitis, haemorrhage and external catheter leaks. Nursing staff caring for and using PEG tubes in patients should be trained to be aware of the signs of any of these complications.

Transjugular Intrahepatic Portosystemic Shunt for End Stage Liver Diseases

A Transjugular intrahepatic portosystemic shunt (TIPS) is a percutaneously inserted stent between the portal and systemic venous systems within the liver. The aim of the stent is to reduce the complications associated with portal hypertension. It allows the abnormally high pressure within the portal system to decrease by shunting blood directly from the portal veins into the hepatic veins.

Indications for TIPS include variceal haemorrhage refractory to other medical treatment, refractory ascites, portal hypertensive gastropathy, Budd–Chiari syndrome and hepatic hydrothorax [36].

Contraindications

Contraindications include uncontrolled coagulopathy, elevated heart pressures, heart failure, unrelieved biliary obstruction, extensive metastatic or primary hepatic malignancy, rapidly progressive liver failure, sepsis, severe hepatic encephalopathy and polycystic liver disease.

Procedural Method

Prophylactic antibiotic cover should be considered prior to the procedure. A catheter is inserted via the jugular vein into the hepatic veins and a hepatic venogram is performed. Under fluoroscopic guidance a long curved needle is passed from the hepatic vein through the liver into an intrahepatic portal vein; measures of the portal and systemic pressures are taken, the passage is balloon dilated and a stent is passed. The reduction of the portal:systemic gradient is assessed and the stent is dilated as required.

Complications

Important complications to be aware of include encephalopathy (which is common and usually transient and medically manageable through can be severe and contribute to death in some cases). Other major complications include shunt occlusion, haemoperitoneum (0.5 %), gallbladder puncture (1 %), haemobilia (2 %), hepatic infarction (1 %) and hepatic artery injury (1 %), renal failure, accelerated liver failure and cardiac failure [36].

References

 1. Cope L, Wynne H. The role of interventional radiology in palliative care of malignant disease. Rev Clin Gerontol. 2009;18(02):129. doi:10.1017/S0959259809002780.
 2. Kandarpa K, Machan L. Handbook of interventional radiologic procedures. Chapter 9. 2011.
 3. Health Protection Agency, The Royal College of Radiologists, & The College of Radiographers. Protection of pregnant patients during diagnostic medical exposures to ionising radiation. Environ Hazards. 2009.
 4. Dieter R. Peripheral arterial disease. McGraw-Hill: New York; 2009. p. 351.
 5. Kuroiwa T, Hasuo K, Yasumori K, Mizushima A, Yoshida K, Hirakata R, Komatsu K, et al. Transcatheter embolization of testicular vein for varicocele testis. Acta Radiol. 1991;32(4):311–4.
 6. Gee M, Soulen MC. Chemoembolization for hepatic metastases. Tech Vasc Interv Radiol. 2002;5(3):132–40. Retrieved from http://ovidsp.ovid.com/ovidweb.cgi?T=JS&CSC=Y&NEWS=N&PAGE=fulltext&D=med4&AN=12524644.
 7. Ekeh AP, McCarthy MC, Woods RJ, Haley E. Complications arising from splenic embolization after blunt splenic trauma. Am J Surg. 2005;189(3):335–9. Retrieved from http://www.ncbi.nlm.nih.gov/pubmed/15792763.
 8. Weintraub JL, Romano WJ, Kirsch MJ, Sampaleanu DM, Madrazo BL. Uterine artery embolization: sonographic imaging findings. J Ultrasound Med. 2002;21(6):633–7. Quiz 639–40. Retrieved from http://www.ncbi.nlm.nih.gov/pubmed/12054299.
 9. Lewandowski RJ, Kulik LM, Riaz A, Senthilnathan S, Mulcahy MF, Ryu RK, Ibrahim SM, et al. A comparative analysis of transarterial downstaging for hepatocellular carcinoma: chemoembolization versus radioembolization. Am J Transplant. 2009;9(8):1920–8. doi:10.1111/j.1600-6143.2009.02695.x.
10. Hong K, McBride JD, Georgiades CS, Reyes DK, Herman JM, Kamel IR, Geschwind J-FH. Salvage therapy for liver-dominant colorectal metastatic adenocarcinoma: comparison between

transcatheter arterial chemoembolization versus yttrium-90 radioembolization. J Vasc Interv Radiol. 2009;20(3):360–7. doi:10.1016/j.jvir.2008.11.019.

11. Koutsimpelas D, Pitton M, Külkens C, Lippert BM, Mann WJ. Endovascular carotid reconstruction in palliative head and neck cancer patients with threatened carotid blowout presents a beneficial supportive care measure. J Palliat Med. 2008;11(5):784–9.

12. Lee KH, Lukovits T, Friedman JA. "Triple-H" therapy for cerebral vasospasm following subarachnoid hemorrhage. Neurocrit Care. 2006;4(1):68–76. Retrieved from http://www.springerlink.com/index/A033Q3425424X202.pdf.

13. Troke STS, Roup STG. Tissue plasminogen activator for acute ischemic stroke. N Engl J Med. 1995;333(24):1581–7. doi:10.1056/NEJM199512143332401.

14. Jones ML, Holmes M. Alteplase for the treatment of acute ischaemic stroke: a single technology appraisal. Health Technol Assess. 2009;13 Suppl 2:15–21. doi:10.3310/hta13supp12/03.

15. Thrombolysis in the management of limb arterial occlusion. Towards a consensus interim report. J Intern Med. 1996;240(6):343–55. doi:10.1046/j.1365-2796.1996.82882000.x.

16. Richards T, Pittathankal AA, Magee TR, Galland RB. The current role of intra-arterial thrombolysis. Eur J Vasc Endovasc Surg. 2003;26(2):166–9. doi:10.1053/ejvs.2002.1915.

17. British Thoracic Society. British Thoracic Society guidelines for the management of suspected acute pulmonary embolism. Thorax. 2003;58(6):470–83. Retrieved from http://www.ncbi.nlm.nih.gov/pubmed/12775856.

18. Konstantinides S, Geibel A, Heusel G, Heinrich F, Kasper W. Heparin plus alteplase compared with heparin alone in patients with submassive pulmonary embolism. N Engl J Med. 2002;2:1143–50. Retrieved from http://www.ncbi.nlm.nih.gov/pubmed/12932312.

19. Perlroth DJ, Sanders GD, Gould MK. Effectiveness and cost-effectiveness of thrombolysis in submassive pulmonary embolism. Arch Intern Med. 2007;167(1):74–80. Retrieved from http://www.ncbi.nlm.nih.gov/pubmed/18664972.

20. Howell PB, Walters PE, Donowitz GR, Farr BM. Risk factors for infection of adult patients with cancer who have tunnelled central venous catheters. Cancer. 1995;75(6):1367–75. doi:10.1002/1097-0142(19950315)75:6<1367::AID-CNCR2820750620>3.0.CO;2-Z.

21. Keenan SP. Use of ultrasound to place central lines. J Crit Care. 2002;17(2):126–37.

22. Deramond H, Depriester C, Galibert P, Le Gars D. Percutaneous vertebroplasty with polymethylmethacrylate. Technique, indications, and results. Radiol Clin North Am. 1998;36(3):533–46. Retrieved from http://www.ncbi.nlm.nih.gov/pubmed/9597071.

23. Hiwatashi A, Sidhu R, Lee RK, deGuzman RR, Piekut DT, Westesson P-LA. Kyphoplasty versus vertebroplasty to increase vertebral body height: a cadaveric study. Radiology. 2005;237(3):1115–9. doi:10.1148/radiol.2373041654.

24. Klazen CAH, Lohle PNM, de Vries J, Jansen FH, Tielbeek AV, Blonk MC, Venmans A, et al. Vertebroplasty versus conservative treatment in acute osteoporotic vertebral compression fractures (Vertos II): an open-label randomised trial. Lancet. 2010;376(9746):1085–92. doi:10.1016/S0140-6736(10)60954-3.

25. Wardlaw D, Cummings SR, Van Meirhaeghe J, Bastian L, Tillman JB, Ranstam J, Eastell R, et al. Efficacy and safety of balloon kyphoplasty compared with non-surgical care for vertebral compression fracture (FREE): a randomised controlled trial. Lancet. 2009;373(9668):1016–24. doi:10.1016/S0140-6736(09)60010-6.

26. Buchbinder R, Osborne RH, Ebeling PR, Wark JD, Mitchell P, Wriedt C, Graves S, et al. A randomized trial of vertebroplasty for painful osteoporotic vertebral fractures. N Engl J Med. 2009;361(6):557–68. Retrieved from http://www.nejm.org/doi/full/10.1056/NEJMoa0900429.

27. Plancarte R, de Leon-Casasola OA, El-Helaly M, Allende S, Lema MJ. Neurolytic superior hypogastric plexus block for chronic pelvic pain associated with cancer. Reg Anesth. 1997;22(6):562–8. Retrieved from http://www.ncbi.nlm.nih.gov/pubmed/9425974.

28. Romanelli D, Beckmann C, Heiss F. Celiac plexus block: efficacy and safety of the anterior approach. Am J Roentgenol. 1993;160(3):497–500. Retrieved from http://www.ajronline.org/cgi/content/abstract/160/3/497.

29. Fugère F, Lewis G. Coeliac plexus block for chronic pain syndromes. Can J Anaesth. 1993;40(10):954–63. doi:10.1007/BF03010099.
30. Ischia S, Ischia A, Polati E, Finco G. Three posterior percutaneous celiac plexus block techniques. A prospective, randomized study in 61 patients with pancreatic cancer pain. Anesthesiology. 1992;76(4):534–40. Retrieved from http://www.ncbi.nlm.nih.gov/pubmed/1550278.
31. Ainley CC, Williams SJ, Smith AC, Hatfield ARW, Russell RCG, Lees WR. Gallbladder sepsis after stent insertion for bile duct obstruction: management by percutaneous cholecystostomy. Br J Surg. 1991;78(8):961–3. doi:10.1002/bjs.1800780822.
32. Saad WEA, Wallace MJ, Wojak JC, Kundu S, Cardella JF. Quality improvement guidelines for percutaneous transhepatic cholangiography, biliary drainage, and percutaneous cholecystostomy. J Vasc Interv Radiol. 2010;21(6):789–95. doi:10.1016/j.jvir.2010.01.012.
33. Grant DG, Bradley PT, Pothier DD, Bailey D, Caldera S, Baldwin DL, Birchall MA. Complications following gastrostomy tube insertion in patients with head and neck cancer: a prospective multi-institution study, systematic review and meta-analysis. Clin Otolaryngol. 2009;34(2):103–12. doi:10.1111/j.1749-4486.2009.01889.x.
34. Wollman B, D'Agostino HB. Percutaneous radiologic and endoscopic gastrostomy: a 3-year institutional analysis of procedure performance. AJR Am J Roentgenol. 1997;169(6):1551–3. Retrieved from http://www.ncbi.nlm.nih.gov/pubmed/9393163.
35. Ryan JM, Hahn PF, Mueller PR. Performing radiologic gastrostomy or gastrojejunostomy in patients with malignant ascites. AJR Am J Roentgenol. 1998;171(4):1003–6. Retrieved from http://www.ncbi.nlm.nih.gov/pubmed/9762985.
36. Haskal ZJ, Martin L, Cardella JF, Cole PE, Drooz A, Grassi CJ, Mccowan TC, et al. Quality improvement guidelines for transjugular intrahepatic portosystemic shunts. J Vasc Interv Radiol. 2003;14(9 Pt 2):S265–70. doi:10.1097/01.RVI.0000094596.83406.19.

Review Questions

1. Absolute contraindications to interventional procedures include:

    (a) Pregnancy
    (b) Renal impairment
    (c) Coagulopathy
    (d) Significant haemodynamic instability

2. Regarding percutaneous interventional procedures:

    (a) The Seldinger technique is rarely utilised
    (b) Complications include retroperitoneal haematoma, pseudoaneurysm formation and vessel thrombosis
    (c) Angioplasty is the process of inserting a stent into a vessel to maintain luminal diameter
    (d) The usual order to gain vascular access is vessel puncture, catheter insertion, guide wire insertion

3. Regarding specific interventional procedures:

    (a) Chemoembolisation and radioembolisation are new procedures that can only be utilised in the treatment of unresectable liver metastases
    (b) Cerebral angiography is a relatively risk-free procedure that is available in most district general hospitals
    (c) Computed tomography (CT) and magnetic resonance (MR) angiography are useful alternatives to conventional cerebral angiography
    (d) Triple-A therapy is often implemented in the management of patients who have suffered a subarachnoid haemorrhage (SAH)

4. Regarding specific procedures:

    (a) In ischaemic stroke, the benefits of tissue plasminogen activator (tPA) outweigh the risks for up to 4½ h following symptom onset
    (b) If ischaemic stroke is suspected out-of-hours, tPA should be commenced as soon as possible, and imaging undertaken the following working day
    (c) In stage III ischaemia, intra-arterial thrombolysis, amputation of the affected limb may be prevented if intra-arterial thrombolysis (IAT) is commenced promptly
    (d) It is desirable that peripherally inserted central catheters (PICC) lines are inserted on the ward by appropriately trained staff, to avoid any patient disruption

5. Regarding specific interventional procedures:

    (a) Potential complications in vertebroplasty and kyphoplasty include infection, neurological sequelae and worsening of pain and/or symptoms
    (b) Percutaneous cholecystostomy is indicated as the first-line treatment in the management of the empyema of the gallbladder
    (c) Radiological inserted gastrostomy is advantageous in comparison to surgical and endoscopic methods as a larger tube can be inserted
    (d) TIPS procedure in the treatment of portal hypertension involves diverting the portal venous blood to the adjacent hepatic artery

Answers

1. (d) is true. Whilst pregnancy, renal impairment and coagulopathy may all discourage the radiologist from undertaking the procedure, if it is felt that the potential benefits outweigh the risks, it may be undertaken. In reality, the only truly "absolute" contraindication is haemodynamic instability such that the procedure cannot be undertaken without further patient compromise. A full and frank discussion should take place between the clinical team, the consultant radiologist and the patient and his or her family.

2. (b) is true. The usual order of vascular access is vessel puncture, guide wire insertion, catheter insertion. Angioplasty is the process of "ballooning" a vessel lumen open, which may then proceed to stent insertion to maintain luminal diameter. The Seldinger technique is standard procedure.

3. (c) is true. Chemoembolisation and radioembolisation are a possible treatment option in the management of hepatocellular carcinoma (HCC). Cerebral angiography is a procedure with significant risk attached, including stroke and death, and is provided only in specialist centres. Triple-H therapy (hypervolaemia, hypertension, and haemodilution) is implemented in the management of patients with SAH.

4. (a) is true. Out-of-hours imaging is now available in the vast majority of hospitals, and if stroke is suspected, CT imaging should be organised as soon as possible. Stage III ischaemia, is by definition, irreversible, and amputation is inevitable. PICC lines or tunnelled central venous catheters (CVCs) can be inserted on the ward by trained staff, but insertion in a dedicated theatre or imaging suite is advantageous as sterility can be ensured, and image-guidance available.

5. (a) is true. Percutaneous cholecystostomy is indicated when antibiotic treatment has failed in the management of empyema of the gallbladder. Radiological inserted gastrostomy is advantageous as it may be done under light sedation, but the disadvantage is that a smaller tube is employed. Transjugular intrahepatic portosystemic shunt (TIPS) procedure involves diverting the portal venous blood to the adjacent hepatic venous system, to treat associated portal hypertension.

Chapter 16
Stroke, Epilepsy, and Neurological Diseases

María Gudín

Palliative care addresses the physical and psychological aspects of end of life. The World Health Organization defines palliative care as: "an approach that improves quality of life of patients and their families facing the problem associated with life-threatening illness, through the prevention and relief of sufferings by means of early identification and impeccable assessment and treatment of pain and other problems, physical, psychosocial, and spiritual. Palliative care: provides relief either for pain and other distressing symptoms; affirms life and regards dying as a normal process; intends neither to hasten nor to postpone death; integrates the psychosocial and spiritual aspects of patient care; offers a support system to help patient live as active as possible until death; offers a system to help the family cope during the patient illness and in their own bereavement, counseling, if indicated; will enhance quality of life, and may also positively influence the course of the illness; is applicable early in the course of the illness, in conjunction with other therapies that are intended to prolong life, such as chemotherapy and radiation therapy and includes those investigations needed to better understand and manage distressing clinical complications" [1].

Even though palliative care was developed around terminal cancer care, nowadays palliative care principles are applicable to neurology illnesses. Given the chronic course of the neurological life-threatening diseases, some authors support incorporing palliative care in neurology in early stages of the disease. Current opinion in neurology is to integrate palliative aid before the final stage of neurological disease (i.e., approximately the final 2 week of life) [2].

M. Gudín, Ph.D. (⊠)
Neurology Department, Ciudad Real General University Hospital,
Ciudad Real, Castilla–La Mancha, Spain
e-mail: mariagudinrm@gmail.com; mgudin@sescam.jccm.es

N. Vadivelu et al. (eds.), *Essentials of Palliative Care*,
DOI 10.1007/978-1-4614-5164-8_16,
© Springer Science+Business Media New York 2013

Stroke

Neurologist care for many patients who die because cerebrovascular disease is the third leading cause of death in the USA [3]. The incidence of stroke continues to rise [4] despite prevention strategies such as blood pressure control, treatment on atrial fibrillation, smoking dishabituation, weight control, instituting a modest exercise regimen [5], and aggressive treatment with thrombolytic agents [6, 7]. Stroke results in high levels of mortality and morbidity, yet very little is known about the nature and extent of palliative care services that are available to this patient group, and the ways in which such services could be delivered. A critical review of the international literature found only seven papers that attempted to identify the palliative care needs of patients diagnosed with stroke [8]. The results of the review showed that the preferences of stroke patients and their families in relation to palliative care services are largely unknown. The review also indicated the paucity of data in regard to the distinction between provision of palliative care services for patients who die in the acute phase of stroke and for those patients who die later. Establishing reliable assessments of need are central to designing and implementing effective interventions and further research is required in this area. Further data on how the input of palliative care experts and expertise could be of benefit to patients, and the most effective ways these inputs could be targeted and delivered are required.

After the acute initial period in which the patient may die [9], stroke patients tend to be chronically ill patients that need multidisciplinary support. In this sense, for most stroke patients, palliative care is not related to end-of-life support, but it refers to the measures that reduce disability and impairment. Most treatment techniques focus on disability reduction, patients must learn new strategies to solve common problems of daily life.

The particular combination of impairments increases disability and reduces the possibility to reach independence [10].

Initial Attention of Stroke: Medical Care

First weeks after acute stroke, altered cognition and sensorimotor function contributes to distorted communication, immobility, pain, and depression.

Nutritional Needs and Access

Initially care must focus on the vegetative needs of the stroke patient; particularly on feeding and excretional function. The patient must receive adequate nutritional, fluids, and airways projection. Following stroke, the swallowing reflex is altered. Oral feeding must begin as soon as the patient has recovered this reflex. If oral intake seems to be dangerous, or ineffective, the nutrition can be delivered by tube feeding. Nasogastric tube feeding must be replaced by gastrostomy within 2 weeks. In order to implant the gastrostomy tube, the severity of stroke and the potential duration of tube feeding must be taken in consideration. Percutaneous endoscopic gastrostomy is a minimally invasive gastrostomy method with low morbidity and mortality rates, and is easy to follow-up and to replace when blockage occurs [11].

Although it is necessary to indicate other factors, such as the physical status to establish better rehabilitation networks, clinical assessment of swallowing in acute stroke is very important to determine whether the patients can go home directly or not [12].

Urinary incontinence following acute stroke is common, affecting between 40 and 60 % of people in hospital after a stroke. Bladder dysfunction is provoked because the lesion interferes with the detrusor reflex. Conservative interventions (e.g., bladder training, pelvic floor muscle training, and prompted voiding) are very important to prevent urine retentions, and infections [13]. An integrated qualitative evaluation must be conducted to ameliorate stroke survival. It has been confirmed that post-stroke urinary incontinence is a predictor of greater mortality at 1 week, 6 months, and 12 months after stroke. However, patients who regain normal bladder control in the first week have a comparable prognosis as the patients who do not have micturition disturbances following stroke [14].

Care of Common Complications of Stroke

Venous Thrombosis

Neurological disorders are often associated with immobilization, thus placing patients at increased risk for venous thromboembolism (VTE) and pulmonary thromboembolism. This risk is very high in patients with acute ischemic stroke. Nearly 10 % of post-stroke deaths are due to pulmonary embolism [15]. The benefit of prophylactic strategies remains in discussion. After a comprehensive and systematic review of the literature, a panel of experts formulated recommendations for the prevention of VTE in stroke and other neurological diseases. Patients with acute ischemic stroke should routinely receive pharmacological prophylaxis to be started within 48 h and continued for approximately 14 days; patients with acute hemorrhagic stroke should routinely receive mechanical prophylaxis, pharmacological prophylaxis should be considered once the patient is stable; patients with neuromuscular degenerative diseases and with other major risk factors for venous thrombosis should be considered for the administration of pharmacological or mechanical prophylaxis [16].

Pressure Sores

The motor deficit leads to immobility and a constantly stressed skin tends to breakdown. The stroke patient frequently suffers urinary incontinence. Once skin breakdown occurs, pressure, friction, and maceration related to incontinence must be prevented with appropriate measures. In some cases plastic surgery may be required. To help prevent pressure ulcers in stroke patient is important that healthcare providers assess activity, moisture, nutrition, friction, and shearing, as well as psychological assessment for depression [17].

Shoulder-Hand Syndrome

The hemiparetic stroke patient is most susceptible to shoulder trauma. To avoid shoulder damage, the caregiver must have notions of how to move the patients in bed or how to change patient from the chair wheel to other position. The shoulder-hand syndrome (SHS) occurs in 20–30 % of patients despite optimal rehabilitation programs [18].

The onset and severity of SHS appears to be related with the etiology of the stroke, the severity and recovery of motor deficit, spasticity and sensory disturbances [19]. Based on systematic analysis of the literature, the following conclusions seem justified (1) the shoulder is involved in only half of the cases with painful swelling of wrist and hand, suggesting a "wrist-hand syndrome" between simple hand edema and SHS; (2) hand edema is not lymph edema; (3) SHS usually coincides with increased arterial blood flow; (4) trauma causes aseptic joint inflammations in SHS; (5) no specific treatment has yet proven its advantage over other physical methods for reducing hand edema; and (6) oral corticosteroids are the most effective treatment for SHS [20].

Palliative Care of Stroke Patients: Reduce Disability and Impairment

There is evidence to support rehabilitation in well coordinated multidisciplinary stroke units or through provision of early supported provision of discharge teams. Potentially beneficial treatment options for motor recovery of the arm include constraint-induced movement therapy and robotics. Promising interventions that could be beneficial to improve aspects of gait include fitness training, high-intensity therapy, and repetitive-task training. Repetitive-task training might also improve transfer functions. Occupational therapy can improve activities of daily living; however, information about the clinical effect of various strategies of cognitive rehabilitation and strategies for aphasia and dysarthria is scarce. Several large trials of rehabilitation practice and of novel therapies (e.g., stem-cell therapy, repetitive transcranial magnetic stimulation, virtual reality, robotic therapies, and drug augmentation) are underway to inform future practice.

Language and Perceptual Impairment

In general, improvement in auditory comprehension is significantly better than improvement in language [21]. There is no standard therapy for aphasia, but actually the notion that more practice leads to more improvement is widely extended and provides good results. Some reports suggest that specific speech therapy program is only modestly better than sustained conversation or stimulation by trained nurses [22, 23].

The main conclusion of this review is that speech and language therapy treatment for people with aphasia after a stroke has not been shown either to be clearly effective or clearly ineffective within a RCT. Decisions about the management of patients must therefore be based on other forms of evidence. Further research is required to find out if effectiveness of speech and language therapy for aphasic patients is effective. If researchers choose to do a trial, this must be large enough to have adequate statistical power, and be clearly reported [24].

This study was repeated in 2010, the authors found out some evidence that aphasia treatment may be beneficial for patients [25].

Disturbances in visual perception show a prompt recovery from left neglect, anosognosia, prosopagnosia and unilateral neglect. When the neglect also includes hemianopia, hemiparesis, motor impersistence, or extinction recovery is slowed. Patients with executive problems, such as constructional apraxia and dressing apraxia, have only moderate recovery [26]. There is no consensus about what type of therapy may be developed for recovery of these functions [27].

Sensorimotor Training

Cortical plasticity underlies post-stroke motor recovery of the impaired extremity. Motor skill learning in neurologically intact individuals is thought to involve the primary motor cortex, and the majority of studies in the animal literature have studied changes in the primary sensorimotor cortex with motor rehabilitation. Whether changes in engagement in the sensorimotor cortex occur in humans after stroke currently is an area of much interest. Twenty-eight studies investigating upper extremity neural representations (e.g., TMS, fMRI, PET, or SPECT) were identified and 13 met inclusion criteria as upper extremity intervention training studies [28]. The results of this meta-analysis indicate that neural changes in the sensorimotor cortex of the damaged hemisphere accompany functional paretic upper extremity motor gains achieved with targeted rehabilitation interventions.

Patients exposed to more training decreased impairment and in some studies also reduced disability [29–31]. Some investigators have employed neuromuscular stimulation [32], and transcranial magnetic stimulation to improve recovery [33]. Robotic devices have been designed to enhance sensorimotor training. Robotic rehabilitation techniques have emerged to provide a repetitive, activity-based therapy at potentially lower cost than conventional methods. Many patients exhibit intrinsic resistance to hand extension in the form of spasticity and/or hypertonia. A robotic device that is capable of compensating for tone to assist patients in opening the paretic hand [34, 35].

Spasticity

Over the weeks flaccidity in paralyzed limbs is replaced by enhanced reflex responses and increased muscle tone to passive and active movements.

Spasticity treatment must be considered in relation to other impairments with functional goals defined prior to intervention. The effects of muscle co-contraction and involuntary limb movement associated with exaggerated cutaneous reflexes or efforts as well as stretch reflex hyperexcitability need to be considered. Exacerbating factors such as pain must be identified. Physical therapy and conventional orthoses are the mainstays of spasticity management during acute rehabilitation. Botulinum toxin shows promise but needs further evaluation in the context of acute rehabilitation. Phenol chemodenervation can produce good results in spasticity refractory to standard treatments. Muscle strengthening exercises may be appropriate in chronic hemiparesis without adversely affecting tone. Electrical stimulation may be a useful adjunct to other spasticity treatments [36].

Depression

Depression is a common mental health problem in palliative medicine, but it is poorly understood, sometimes it is underdiagnosed, and not properly treated [37]. Post-stroke depression is difficult to quantify due to methodologic differences in studies, but the prevalence appears to range from 17 to 61 % [38]. Stroke severity, physical disability, and cognitive impairment have been consistently associated with depression after stroke [39].

The theory that depression is more commonly associated with left than with right hemisphere strokes and with lesions of the left anterior brain than with other regions [40] is not supported by the data. In a systematic review of 48 studies, the relative risk of depression after a left versus right hemisphere stroke was 0.95 (95 % CI 0.83–1.10) [41]. Similarly, the risk of depression after a left anterior lesion compared with all other brain lesions was 1.17 (0.87–1.62). Restriction of the analyses to reports from high-quality studies or major depressive disorder did not substantially change the results.

Depression at 3 months is correlated with a poor outcome at 1 year, although causation cannot be inferred from this [38]. Nonetheless, when patients are matched for initial functional outcome, remission of depression is associated with a better functional outcome at 3 and 6 months than continued depression [42, 70]. There appears to be a relationship between depression and 12 and 24 months mortality, but confounders likely exist [43].

At the end of the chapter, it will review the possibilities of treatment.

Epilepsy

Patients with epilepsy whose seizures do not successfully respond to antiepileptic drug (AED) therapy are considered to have drug-resistant epilepsy (DRE). This condition is also referred to as intractable, medically refractory, or pharmacoresistant epilepsy. As many as 20–40 % of patients with epilepsy are likely to have refractory epilepsy [44].

Individuals with DRE have an increased mortality rate: community-based studies and reports from more selected epilepsy populations consistently reveal persons with epilepsy to have a mortality rate two to three times that of the general population [45]. The higher mortality is partly related to the underlying disorder causing epilepsy rather than a direct consequence of the seizures. For example, mortality in cerebrovascular diseases is increased, deaths due to neoplasms, and in particular brain tumors are also increased among patients with epilepsy. But, other causes directly related to epilepsy are also important: accidents, status epilepticus, and sudden unexpected death (SUD). The risk of SUD is closely related to seizure frequency, being 40 times higher in patients who continue to have seizures than in those who are seizure-free. In this sense, individuals who become seizure free have no increased mortality [46].

Palliative Treatment

When a patient does not respond to medical or conventional surgical treatment, there are some options of palliative care; such as non-conventional surgical treatments, ketogenic diet, and vagus nerve stimulation.

Other Surgical Palliative Treatment

Hemispherectomy, corpus callosotomy, multiple subpial transections are sometimes employed for palliative treatment in children and sometimes adults with catastrophic epilepsy syndromes.

Hemispherectomy

Hemispherectomy is performed in children whose seizures are associated with a disease that diffusely affects one cerebral hemisphere. The largest reported series of pediatric hemispherectomy evaluated the post-operative outcomes of 115 children with different pathologic substrates for seizures, including 16 children with hemimegalencephaly, 39 with hemispheric cortical dysplasia, 21 with Rasmussen encephalitis, 27 with infarct/ischemia, and 12 classified as other/miscellaneous [47]. The median age at surgery was 3.5 years.

The results of this study support early surgical intervention in children who have severe refractory seizures. A shorter seizure duration before surgery was associated with a better outcome regardless of the underlying pathology [48]. The post-surgical developmental gains reported in these and other hemispherectomy studies are generally modest, but development is often limited by severe preexisting brain damage that may involve the non-operated hemisphere [49].

Corpus Callosotomy

In a corpus callosotomy, the fibers of the corpus callosum are surgically divided. Typically, an anterior two-thirds callosotomy is performed first, with completion of the callosotomy done only if seizures persist after the first procedure. The only seizure type that has clearly been shown to benefit from this surgery is atonic seizures, which are most commonly seen in epileptic encephalopathies such as Lennox-Gastaut syndrome [50]. However, many reports suggest that a substantive reduction in generalized tonic–clonic seizures and other seizure types can result after corpus callosotomy, and that improvements in behavior, IQ, and overall quality of life are also possible [51].

Multiple Subpial Transections

Multiple subpial transection (MST) is a surgical technique mainly used when epileptiform activity arises from eloquent or functional brain cortex. Neuroanatomic studies show that the basic functional cortical unit is arranged vertically, and epileptic activity spreads horizontally. Minimal cortical unit is essential for maintenance of cortical activity. Vertical incisions in the cortex interrupt transverse synaptic connections, preventing seizure propagation while preserving the vertical column subserving neuronal function. In the past, it has been difficult to assess the efficacy of MSTs per se, as they have usually been performed together with cortical resection or lesionectomy. After MSTs, studies show that 33–46 % of treated children are in Engel class I or II [52]. The permanent complication rate is low with no permanent language or motor disabilities.

Vagus Nerve Stimulation

Ketogenic Diet

The ketogenic diet (high-fat, low protein) diet has demonstrated efficacy in children with IE, with more than one-third experiencing a 50 % or greater reduction in seizures

In two small case series of adult patients, the traditional ketogenic diet and a modified Atkins diet reduced seizure frequency by 50 % or more in half of the patients with DRE [55, 56].

Palliative Care in Terminal Stage of Other Neurological Disease

More than 15 years ago, the American Academy of Neurology has declared that neurologist have a duty to provide adequate palliative care of their terminal patients instead of assisted suicide or active euthanasia and avoid the euthanasia practice

[57, 58]. In the Netherlands in 1996 the euthanasia rate for Amyotrophic Lateral Sclerosis was 4.1 % [59], 6 years later in the same country Veldink and coworkers published the proportion of euthanasia in a cohort of ALS patient was 17 %, 3 % of the patients in that study died as a result of physician-assisted suicide. An additional 48 patients (24 %) received palliative treatment, which probably shortened their lives [60].

Neurological disease at terminal stage shows a high rate both of euthanasia and medical-assisted suicide. In palliative care management of a disease is management of symptoms, independently of the diagnosis. Subsequently, this article will focus on the symptoms of neurological disease that may be ameliorated by palliative care in terminal sate.

General Aspects

Communication

The firs aspect to deal with is how to communicate an awful diagnosis to a patient. Patient and health care system benefits when clinicians engage in end-of-life conversations with patients diagnosed with life-limiting illnesses, yet most clinicians focus on life-preserving treatments and avoid conversations about end-of-life care. It is not ready to standardize the way to communicate such news; each case should be individualized. The diagnosis must be revealed to the patient and relatives gradually. All questions must be answered honestly but always avoiding provoking a hopelessness state on the patient.

Advance Care Planning

The Patient Self Determination Act of 1990 mandates healthcare providers to speak with patients about end-of-life preferences and advance directives. Individuals from differing ethnic backgrounds are likely to turn to their traditional norms of practice when ill or treatment choices must be made. Healthcare provider must be aware of cultural differences in the current era of increased globalization. Education on cultural differences and how to lead discussions promotes advance care planning. Initiating conversations about advance care planning can be facilitated by using open-ended questions that respect the values and beliefs of various cultures [61].

Depending on diagnosis many future situations may be foreseeing and discussed. Aspects such as refusal of terminal intubation in ALS patients should be spoken. The conversations with patients and family must be noted in medical records. It is very important to designate proxy decision makers to guide medical care after a patient has become incompetent [62].

Routes of Drug Administration

The most useful route in palliative care is the oral route [63]. Intravenous routes reduce the mobility of patient and are a source of infections [64]. Since most patients will develop difficulty in swallowing alternative routes may be rectal or subcutaneous. Parenteral routes—in necessary—may be sublingual or intravenous but using a syringe driver to avoid multiple injections.

Management of Symptoms

Dyspnea

Dyspnea is a common symptom experienced by many patients with neurological disease, above all the ones that affect muscle strength and contraction (myopathies, motorneurone disease, and polyneuropathies). Its significance is amplified due to its impact on family and caregivers.

The antidyspneic medication must ameliorate the respiratory awareness, but preserving the ventilatory drive. A respiratory rate of 15–20/min must be attempted. Opioids in modest doses have been demonstrated to give effective relief of dyspnea, whether or not identifiable reversible causes exist [65]. A dose of 5 mg diazepam has a positive effect on improving sleep duration without worsening nocturnal hypoxemia [66]. Medical management of dyspnea can be directed at the underlying cause when the potential benefits outweigh the burdens of such treatment. In rare cases where symptomatic treatment is unable to control dyspnea to the patient's satisfaction, sedation is an effective, ethical option.

Death Rattle

Noisy breathing (death rattle) occurs in 23–92 % of people who are dying. The cause of death rattle remains unproven but is presumed to be due to an accumulation of secretions in the airways. It is therefore managed physically (repositioning and clearing the upper airways of fluid with a mechanical sucker) or pharmacologically (with anticholinergic drugs) [67]. Anticholinergic stop the production of new secretions, there are no significant differences in effectiveness or survival time among atropine, hyoscine butylbromide, and scopolamine in the treatment of death rattle [68].

But it is important to aspirate secretions in order to avoid the noise that sometimes must be associated to patient perceived dyspnea.

Terminal Restlessness

Dying patients frequently experience that, which is known as terminal restlessness, this phenomenon must be accurately diagnosed as myoclonus, delirium, or pure motor restlessness. There are treatable causes of restlessness such as pain, a distended bladder or rectum, cerebral anoxia or dyspnea, a paradoxical reaction to benzodiazepines, or a response to anticholinergic drugs [69].

Findings suggest the need for comprehensive treatment plans to meet the special supportive and information needs of these families, specific supportive strategies for the professional caregivers and further studies to develop ethical criteria and evidence-based guidelines for the use of sedation in the management of terminal restlessness [70].

Delirium

Delirium is a common neuropsychiatric complication experienced by patients with advanced illness, occurring in up to 85 % of patients in the last weeks of life. Although some studies have identified agitation as a central feature of delirium in 13–46 % of patients, other studies have found up to 80 % of patients near the end of life develop a hypoactive, non-agitated delirium. Both the agitated (hyperactive) and non-agitated (hypoactive) forms of delirium are associated with increased morbidity in patients who are terminally ill, causing distress for patients, family members, and staff. Delirium is a sign of significant physiological disturbance, usually involving multiple causes, including infection, organ failure, and medication adverse effects. Often these causes of delirium are not reversible in the dying patient, and this influences the outcomes of its management. Delirium can also significantly interfere with the recognition and control of other physical and psychological symptoms, such as pain. Unfortunately, delirium is often misdiagnosed or unrecognized and thus inappropriately treated or untreated in terminally ill patients. To manage delirium in terminally ill patients, clinicians must be able to diagnose it accurately, undertake appropriate assessment of underlying causes, and understand the benefits and risks of the available pharmacological and no pharmacological interventions [71].

Standard management of delirium requires an investigation of the etiologies, correction of the contributing factors, and management of symptoms. Symptomatic and supportive therapies, including numerous pharmacologic approaches, are important, but several aspects of the use of neuroleptics and other agents in the management of delirium in the dying patient remain controversial [72].

Starting treatment with neuroleptics may lead to extrapyramidal movement disorder, seizures, and drop in blood pressure. Symptomatic treatment of these conditions may be provided, using antiepileptic drugs, saline fluids, and anticholinergic drugs.

Drowsiness

Depending on the underlying pathology some patient will lose consciousness long before death while other remains lucid until the end. Fainsinger and coworkers in a huge cohort find out that the level of consciousness by the day of death was alert (2 %), drowsy (41 %), unresponsive (57 %) [73].

There are many causes of drowsiness in terminal neurologic patients: raise in intracranial pressure, seizures, hypoxia, infections, drug side effects, etc. The drug regimen must be reorganized and treatable causes must be looked for.

Epileptic Seizures

Epilepsy in terminal stages of neurological diseases is a frequent condition, and must be considered if a sudden change in the level of consciousness occurs. EEG must be performed and often is the only way to diagnose a non-convulsive status epilepticus. If the patient presents a generalized tonic–clonic seizure 10 mg of diazepam, immediate therapy consists of diazepam 10 mg rectally or midazolam 10 mg parenterally. Sometimes antiepileptic drug medication with phenytoin or valproic acid intravenously must begin.

Refractory status epilepticus (RSE) is defined as status epilepticus that continues despite treatment with benzodiazepines and one antiepileptic drug. Focal RSE without impairment of consciousness might initially be approached conservatively; conversely, early induction of pharmacological coma is advisable in generalized convulsive forms of the disorder. At this stage, midazolam, propofol, or barbiturates are the most commonly used drugs. Several other treatments, such as additional anaesthetics, other antiepileptic or immunomodulatory compounds, or non-pharmacological approaches (e.g., electroconvulsive treatment or hypothermia), have been used in protracted RSE [74].

Myoclonus

In terminal stage it is very frequent myoclonic movements, the causes for terminal myoclonus include hypoxia, hypoglycemia, and secondary effects of drugs; such as opioids and anticholinergic agents or terminal multiorganic failure. Pirazetam, clonazepam, and valproic acid are election treatment in terminal myoclonus in which a treatable cause has been excluded.

Pain

Pain occurs less frequently in end stage of neurological disease than in cancer. Nevertheless, chronic pain is a frequent component of many neurological disorders, affecting 20–40 % of patients for many primary neurological diseases. Neurological pain results from a wide range of pathophysiologies including traumatic injury to the central nervous system, neurodegeneration, and neuroinflammation. Whether pain originates in the central or peripheral nervous system, it frequently becomes centralized through maladaptive responses within the central nervous system that can profoundly alter brain systems and thereby behavior (e.g., depression). The treatment of pain in neurological patients is greatly complicated by the lack of objective measures; often it is sometimes difficult to obtain even a subjective evaluation of pain, as is the case for patients in a vegetative state or end-stage Alzheimer's disease [75].

Opioids are commonly prescribed for chronic non-cancer pain and may be effective for short-term pain relief. However, long-term effectiveness of 6 months or longer is variable with evidence ranging from moderate for transdermal fentanyl and sustained-release morphine to limited for oxycodone and indeterminate for hydrocodone and methadone [76].

In terminal stages of neurological diseases it is frequent to find altered states of consciousness. Patients with stuporous or comatose pose a huge dilemma in diagnosis and treatment of pain, in this state pain is misdiagnosed in 43 % of cases, in this terminal stage is very difficult to determinate whether a patient is experiencing pain and suffering [77].

Different therapies applied to treat neurological chronic pain [78, 79] are also used to treat pain associated to neurological diseases. The most notably successful are the anti-epilepsy drugs, but antidepressants, membrane stabilizers, and opioids have also been used to treat chronic pain, with varying levels of success.

Headache due to raised intracranial pressure is a frequent symptom in terminal neurological patients. Corticoid therapy is well known to treat elevated pressure due to brain trauma [80] or metastasis [81]; but, glucocorticoids are not considered to be useful in the management of cerebral infarction or intracranial hemorrhage.

Nausea and Vomiting

Nausea, the unpleasant sensation of being about to vomit, can occur alone or can accompany vomiting (the forceful expulsion of gastric contents), dyspepsia, or other gastrointestinal symptoms [82].

Nausea and vomiting are mediated primarily by visceral stimulation through dopamine and serotonin, by vestibular and central nervous system causes through histamine and acetylcholine, and by chemoreceptor triggers zone stimulation through dopamine and serotonin. Treatment is directed at these pathways. Antihistamines and anticholinergic agents are most effective in patients with nausea resulting from vestibular and central nervous system causes [83].

Depression

Diagnosing and treating depression in terminally ill patients involve unique challenges. Evidence of hopelessness, helplessness, worthlessness, guilt, and suicidal ideation are better indicators of depression in this context than neurovegetative symptoms.

Depression is highly correlated with a reduced quality of life, greater difficulty in managing the course of the patient's illness, decreased adherence to treatment, and earlier admission to inpatient or hospice care [84]. Depression also impairs the patient's capacity for pleasure, meaning, connection, and doing the emotional work of separating and saying goodbye; it amplifies pain and other symptoms, and causes anguish and worry in family members and friends [85].

Although terminally ill patients often have suicidal thoughts, they are usually fleeting [86]. Sustained suicidal ideation should prompt a comprehensive evaluation. Clinicians should have a low threshold for treating depression in terminally ill patients. Psychostimulants, because of their rapid onset of action, are useful agents and are generally well tolerated. Selective serotonin reuptake inhibitors and tricyclic antidepressants may also be used. Psychological interventions—including eliciting concerns and conveying the potential for connection, meaning, reconciliation, and closure in the dying process—can also facilitate coping.

References

1. WHO. www.who.int/cancer/palliative/definition/en/.
2. Gofton TE, Jog MS, Schulz V. A palliative approach to neurological care: a literature review. Can J Neurol Sci. 2009;36(3):296–302.
3. Foley KM, Carver AC. Palliative care in neurology. Neurol Clin. 2001;19(4):789–99.
4. Kleindorfer DO, Khoury J, Moomaw CJ, Alwell K, Woo D, Flaherty ML, Khatri P, Adeoye O, Ferioli S, Broderick JP, Kissela BM. Stroke incidence is decreasing in whites but not in blacks: a population-based estimate of temporal trends in stroke incidence from the Greater Cincinnati/ Northern Kentucky Stroke Study. Stroke. 2010;41(7):1326–31.
5. Futtrell L, Millikan CH. Stroke in emergency. Dis Month. 1996;42:199–264.
6. Bott T. Bogousslavsky: treatment of acute ischemic stroke. N Engl J Med. 2000;334:710–22.
7. Frankel MR, Morgensen LB, Kwiatowski T, et al. Early stroke treatment associated with better outcome: the NINDS rt-PA study. Neurology. 2000;55:952–9.
8. Stevens T, Payne SA, Burton C, Addington-Hall J, Jones A. Palliative care in stroke: a critical review of the literature. Palliat Med. 2007;21(4):323–31.
9. Collins TC, Petersen NJ, Menke TJ, Souchek J, Foster W, Ashton CM. Short-team, intermediate-term, and long-term mortality in patients hospitalized for stroke. J Clin Epidemiol. 2003;56(1):81–7.
10. Alexander LD, Pettersen JA, Hopyan JJ, Sahlas DJ, Black SE. Long-term prediction of functional outcome after stroke using the Alberta Stroke Program Early Computed Tomography Score in the subacute stage. J Stroke Cerebrovasc Dis. 2011. doi:10.1016/j.strokecerebrovasdis.2011.03.010
11. Hossein SM, Leili M, Hossein AM. Acceptability and outcomes of percutaneous endoscopic gastrostomy (PEG) tube placement and patient quality of life. Turk J Gastroenterol. 2011;22(2):128–33.
12. Maeshima S, Osawa A, Miyazaki Y, Seki Y, Miura C, Tazawa Y, Tanahashi N. Influence of dysphagia on short-term outcome in patients with acute stroke. Am J Phys Med Rehabil. 2011;90(4):316–20.
13. Thomas LH, Watkins CL, French B, Sutton C, Forshaw D, Cheater F, Roe B, Leathley MJ, Burton C, McColl E, Booth J. Study protocol: ICONS: identifying continence options after stroke: a randomised trial. Trials. 2011;12:131.
14. Rotar M, Blagus R, Jeromel M, Skrbec M, Tršinar B, Vodušek DB. Stroke patients who regain urinary continence in the first week after acute first-ever stroke have better prognosis than

patients with persistent lower urinary tract dysfunction. Neurourol Urodyn. 2011;30(7):1315–8. doi:10.1002/nau.21013.

15. Sato Y, Kuno H, Kaji M, Etoh K, Oizumi K. Influence of immobilization upon calcium metabolism in the week following hemiplegic stroke. J Neurol Sci. 2000;175(2):135–9.

16. Ageno W, Agnelli G, Checchia G, Cimminiello C, Paciaroni M, Palareti G, Pini M, Piovella F, Pogliani E, Testa S. Prevention of venous thromboembolism in immobilized neurological patients: guidelines of the Italian Society for Haemostasis and Thrombosis (SISET). Thromb Res. 2009;124(5):e26–31.

17. Suttipong C, Sindhu S. Predicting factors of pressure ulcers in older Thai stroke patients living in urban communities. J Clin Nurs. 2012;21(3–4):372–9. doi:10.1111/j.1365-2702.2011.03889.x.

18. Braus DF, Krauss JK, Strobel J. The shoulder-hand syndrome after stroke: a prospective clinical trial. Ann Neurol. 1994;36(5):728–33.

19. Pertoldi S, Di Benedetto P. Shoulder-hand syndrome after stroke. A complex regional pain syndrome. Eura Medicophys. 2005;41(4):283–92.

20. Geurts AC, Visschers BA, van Limbeek J, Ribbers GM. Systematic review of aetiology and treatment of post-stroke hand oedema and shoulder-hand syndrome. Scand J Rehabil Med. 2000;32(1):4–10.

21. Damasio AR. Aphasia. N Engl J Med. 1992;326(8):531–9.

22. Hartman J, Landau WM. Comparison of formal language therapy with supportive counseling for aphasia due to acute vascular accident. Arch Neurol. 1987;44(6):646–9.

23. Shewan CM, Kertesz A. Effects of speech and language treatment on recovery from aphasia. Brain Lang. 1984;23(2):272–99.

24. Greener J, Enderby P, Whurr R. Speech and language therapy for aphasia following stroke. Cochrane Database Syst Rev. 2000;(2):CD000425.

25. Kelly H, Brady MC, Enderby P. Speech and language therapy for aphasia following stroke. Cochrane Database Syst Rev. 2010;(5):CD000425.

26. Hier DB, Mondlock J, Caplan LR. Recovery of behavioral abnormalities after right hemisphere stroke. Neurology. 1983;33(3):345–50.

27. Cooke DM, McKenna K, Fleming J. Development of a standardized occupational therapy screening tool for visual perception in adults. J Scand J Occup Ther. 2005;12(2):59–71.

28. Richards LG, Stewart KC, Woodbury ML, Senesac C, Cauraugh JH. Movement-dependent stroke recovery: a systematic review and meta-analysis of TMS and fMRI evidence. Neuropsychologia. 2008;46(1):3–11.

29. Feys HM, De Weerdt WJ, Selz BE, Cox Steck GA, Spichiger R, Vereeck LE, Putman KD, Van Hoydonck GA. Effect of a therapeutic intervention for the hemiplegic upper limb in the acute phase after stroke: a single-blind, randomized, controlled multicenter trial. Stroke. 1998;29(4):785–92.

30. Kwakkel G, Wagenaar RC, Twisk JW, Lankhorst GJ, Koetsier JC. Intensity of leg and arm training after primary middle-cerebral-artery stroke: a randomised trial. Lancet. 1999;354(9174):191–6.

31. Sunderland A, Fletcher D, Bradley L, Tinson D, Hewer RL, Wade DT. Enhanced physical therapy for arm function after stroke: a one year follow up study. J Neurol Neurosurg Psychiatry. 1994;57(7):856–8.

32. Powell J, Pandyan AD, Granat M, Cameron M, Stott DJ. Electrical stimulation of wrist extensors in poststroke hemiplegia. Stroke. 1999;30(7):1384–9.

33. Hoyer EH, Celnik PA. Understanding and enhancing motor recovery after stroke using transcranial magnetic stimulation. Restor Neurol Neurosci. 2011;29(6):395–409.

34. Godfrey SB, Schabowsky CN, Holley RJ, Lum PS. Hand function recovery in chronic stroke with HEXORR robotic training: a case series. Conf Proc IEEE Eng Med Biol Soc. 2010;2010:4485–8.

35. Krebs HI, Hogan N, Aisen ML, Volpe BT. Robot-aided neurorehabilitation. IEEE Trans Rehabil Eng. 1998;6(1):75–87.

36. Bhakta BB. Management of spasticity in stroke. Br Med Bull. 2000;56(2):476–85.

37. Lloyd-Williams M, Friedman T, Rudd N. A survey of antidepressant prescribing in the terminally ill. Palliat Med. 1999;13(3):243.

38. Herrmann N, Black SE, Lawrence J, Szekely C, Szalai J. The Sunnybrook Stroke Study: a prospective study of depressive symptoms and functional outcome. Stroke. 1998;29(3):618.
39. Dennis M, O'Rourke S, Lewis S, Sharpe M, Warlow C. Emotional outcomes after stroke: factors associated with poor outcome. J Neurol Neurosurg Psychiatry. 2000;68(1):47.
40. Robinson RG, Price T. Post-stroke depressive disorders: a follow-up study of 103 patients. Stroke. 1982;13(5):635.
41. Carson AJ, MacHale S, Allen K, Lawrie SM, Dennis M, House A, Sharpe M. Depression after stroke and lesion location: a systematic review. Lancet. 2000;356(9224):122.
42. Chemerinski E, Robinson RG, Kosier JT. Improved recovery in activities of daily living associated with remission of poststroke depression. Stroke. 2001;32(1):113.
43. House A, Knapp P, Bamford J, Vail A. Mortality at 12 and 24 months after stroke may be associated with depressive symptoms at 1 month. Stroke. 2001;32(3):696.
44. Kwan P, Schachter SC, Brodie MJ. Drug-resistant epilepsy. N Engl J Med. 2011;365:919.
45. Shackleton DP, Westendorp RG, Kasteleijn-Nolst Trenité DG, et al. Survival of patients with epilepsy: an estimate of the mortality risk. Epilepsia. 2002;43:445.
46. Mohanraj R, Norrie J, Stephen LJ, et al. Mortality in adults with newly diagnosed and chronic epilepsy: a retrospective comparative study. Lancet Neurol. 2006;5:481.
47. Jonas R, Nguyen S, Hu B, et al. Cerebral hemispherectomy: hospital course, seizure, developmental, language, and motor outcomes. Neurology. 2004;62:1712.
48. Duchowny M. Hemispherectomy for epilepsy: when is one half better than two? Neurology. 2004;62:1664.
49. Basheer SN, Connolly MB, Lautzenhiser A, et al. Hemispheric surgery in children with refractory epilepsy: seizure outcome, complications, and adaptive function. Epilepsia. 2007;48:133.
50. Asadi-Pooya AA, Sharan A, Nei M, Sperling MR. Corpus callosotomy. Epilepsy Behav. 2008;13:271.
51. Cukiert A, Burattini JA, Mariani PP, et al. Outcome after extended callosal section in patients with primary idiopathic generalized epilepsy. Epilepsia. 2009;50:1377.
52. Benifla M, Otsubo H, Ochi A, Snead 3rd OC, Rutka JT. Multiple subpial transections in pediatric epilepsy: indications and outcomes. Childs Nerv Syst. 2006;22(8):992–8.
53. A randomized controlled trial of chronic vagus nerve stimulation for treatment of medically intractable seizures. The Vagus Nerve Stimulation Study Group. Neurology. 1995;45:224.
54. DeGiorgio CM, Schachter SC, Handforth A, et al. Prospective long-term study of vagus nerve stimulation for the treatment of refractory seizures. Epilepsia. 2000;41:1195.
55. Sirven J, Whedon B, Caplan D, et al. The ketogenic diet for intractable epilepsy in adults: preliminary results. Epilepsia. 1999;40:1721.
56. Kossoff EH, Rowley H, Sinha SR, Vining EP. A prospective study of the modified Atkins diet for intractable epilepsy in adults. Epilepsia. 2008;49:316.
57. The American Academy of Neurology Ethics and Humanities Subcomité. Palliative Care in neurology. Neurology. 1996;46:870–2.
58. Bernat JL, Goldstein ML, Viste Jr KM. The neurologist and the dying patient. Neurology. 1996;46(3):598–9.
59. van der Wal G, Onwuteaka-Philipsen BD. Cases of euthanasia and assisted suicide reported to the public prosecutor in North Holland over 10 years. BMJ. 1996;312(7031):612–3.
60. Veldink JH, Wokke JH, van der Wal G, de Jong JM V, van den Berg LH. Euthanasia and physician-assisted suicide among patients with amyotrophic lateral sclerosis in the Netherlands. N Engl J Med. 2002;346(21):1638–44.
61. Zager BS, Yancy M. A call to improve practice concerning cultural sensitivity in advance directives: a review of the literature. Worldviews Evid Based Nurs. 2011;8(4):202–11. doi:10.1111/j.1741-6787.2011.00222.x.
62. Miles SH, Koepp R, Weber EP. Advance end-of-life treatment planning. A research review. Arch Intern Med. 1996;156(10):1062–8.
63. O'Neill WM. Subcutaneous infusions – a medical last rite. Palliat Med. 1994;8(2):91–3.
64. Safdar N, Maki DG. Risk of catheter-related bloodstream infection with peripherally inserted central venous catheters used in hospitalized patients. Chest. 2005;128(2):489–95.

65. Thomas JR, von Gunten CF. Management of dyspnea. J Support Oncol. 2003;1(1):23–32.
66. Woodcock AA, Gross ER, Geddes DM. Drug treatment of breathlessness: contrasting effects of diazepam and promethazine in pink puffers. Br Med J (Clin Res Ed). 1981;283(6287):343–6.
67. Wee B, Hillier R. Interventions for noisy breathing in patients near to death. Cochrane Database Syst Rev. 2008;(1):CD005177.
68. Wildiers H, Dhaenekint C, Demeulenaere P, Clement PM, Desmet M, Van Nuffelen R, Gielen J, Van Droogenbroeck E, Geurs F, Lobelle JP, Menten J. Atropine, hyoscine butylbromide, or scopolamine are equally effective for the treatment of death rattle in terminal care. J Pain Symptom Manage. 2009;38(1):124–33.
69. Mazzarino-Willett A. Deathbed phenomena: its role in peaceful death and terminal restlessness. Am J Hosp Palliat Care. 2010;27(2):127–33.
70. Brajtman S. Terminal restlessness: perspectives of an interdisciplinary palliative care team. Int J Palliat Nurs. 2005;11(4):170, 172–8.
71. Breitbart W, Alici Y. Agitation and delirium at the end of life: "We couldn't manage him". JAMA. 2008;300(24):2898–910.
72. Friedlander MM, Brayman Y, Breitbart WS. Delirium in palliative care. Oncology. 2004;18(12):1541–50.
73. Fainsinger R, Miller MJ, Bruera E, Hanson J, Maceachern T. Symptom control during the last week of life on a palliative care unit. J Palliat Care. 1991;7(1):5–11.
74. Rossetti AO, Lowenstein DH. Management of refractory status epilepticus in adults: still more questions than answers. Lancet Neurol. 2011;10(10):922–30.
75. Borsook D. Neurological diseases and pain. Brain. 2012;135(Pt 2):320–44.
76. Trescot AM, Helm S, Hansen H, Benyamin R, Glaser SE, Adlaka R, Patel S, Manchikanti L. Opioids in the management of chronic non-cancer pain: an update of American Society of the Interventional Pain Physicians' (ASIPP) Guidelines. Pain Physician. 2008;11(2 Suppl):S5–62.
77. Coleman MR, Davis MH, Rodd JM, Robson T, Ali A, Owen AM, et al. Towards the routine use of brain imaging to aid the clinical diagnosis of disorders of consciousness. Brain. 2009;132:2541–52.
78. Finnerup NB, Sindrup SH, Jensen TS. The evidence for pharmacological treatment of neuropathic pain. Pain. 2010;150:573–81.
79. Haanpaa M, Attal N, Backonja M, Baron R, Bennett M, Bouhassira D, et al. NeuPSIG guidelines on neuropathic pain assessment. Pain. 2011;152:14–27.
80. Roberts I, Yates D, Sandercock P, Farrell B, Wasserberg J, Lomas G, Cottingham R, Svoboda P, Brayley N, Mazairac G, Laloë V, Muñoz-Sánchez A, Arango M, Hartzenberg B, Khamis H, Yutthakasemsunt S, Komolafe E, Olldashi F, Yadav Y, Murillo-Cabezas F, Shakur H, Edwards P, CRASH Trial Collaborators. Effect of intravenous corticosteroids on death within 14 days in 10008 adults with clinically significant head injury (MRC CRASH trial): randomised placebo-controlled trial. Lancet. 2004;364(9442):1321.
81. Koehler PJ. Use of corticosteroids in neuro-oncology. Anticancer Drugs. 1995;6(1):19.
82. Hasler WL, Chey WD. Nausea and vomiting. Gastroenterology. 2003;125(6):1860.
83. Flake ZA, Scalley RD, Bailey AG. Practical selection of antiemetics. Am Fam Physician. 2004;69(5):1169.
84. Christakis NA. Timing of referral of terminally ill patients to an outpatient hospice. J Gen Intern Med. 1994;9(6):314.
85. Pelletier G, Verhoef MJ, Khatri N, Hagen N. Quality of life in brain tumor patients: the relative contributions of depression, fatigue, emotional distress, and existential issues. J Neurooncol. 2002;57(1):41.
86. Chochinov HM, Tataryn D, Clinch JJ, Dudgeon D. Will to live in the terminally ill. Lancet. 1999;354(9181):816.

Review Questions

1. Current opinion in neurology is to integrate palliative aid before the final stage of neurological disease. Please, mark the correct answer:

   (a) The last 6 months
   (b) The last 2 weeks
   (c) The last hours
   (d) When a permanent deficit is established that will short the patient life

2. Initially care of stroke must focus on:

   (a) Feeding
   (b) Excretional function
   (c) Airways projection
   (d) All of the above

3. Patients with stroke should routinely receive pharmacological venous thromboembolism (VTE) prophylaxis. Mark wrong answer:

   (a) The VTE prophylaxis must be started within 48 h in patients with acute ischemic stroke
   (b) The VTE prophylaxis must be continued for approximately 14 days in patients with acute ischemic stroke
   (c) Patients with acute hemorrhagic stroke should routinely receive mechanical prophylaxis
   (d) Pharmacological prophylaxis is never used in acute hemorrhagic stroke
   (e) Patients with neuromuscular degenerative diseases and with other major risk factors for venous thrombosis should be considered for the administration of pharmacological or mechanical prophylaxis

4. Patients with epilepsy whose seizures do not successfully respond to antiepileptic drug (AED) therapy are considered to have drug-resistant epilepsy (DRE). Mark the wrong statement:

   (a) This condition is also referred to as intractable, medically refractory, or pharmacoresistant epilepsy
   (b) As many as 20–40 % of patients with epilepsy are likely to have refractory epilepsy
   (c) Individuals with DRE do not have an increased mortality rate
   (d) The risk of sudden unexpected death (SUD) is closely related to seizure frequency

5. When a drug-resistant epilepsy patient does not respond to medical or conventional surgical treatment, there are some options of palliative care, such as:

   (a) Hemispherectomy
   (b) Corpus callosotomy

   (c) Multiple subpial transections
   (d) Ketogenic diet
   (e) Vagus nerve stimulation
   (f) All of the above

6. About dyspnea, say which of the answers is wrong:

   (a) The antidyspneic medication must ameliorate the respiratory awareness, but preserving the ventilatory drive
   (b) A respiratory rate of 15–20/min must be attempted
   (c) Opioids in modest doses have been demonstrated to give effective relief of dyspnea, whether or not identifiable reversible causes exist
   (d) A dose of 50 mg diazepam has a positive effect on improving sleep duration without worsening nocturnal hypoxemia
   (e) In rare cases where symptomatic treatment is unable to control dyspnea to the patient's satisfaction, sedation is an effective, ethical option

7. There are treatable causes of terminal restlessness such as:

   (a) Pain
   (b) A distended bladder or rectum
   (c) Cerebral anoxia
   (d) Dyspnea
   (e) A paradoxical reaction to benzodiazepines
   (f) A response to anticholinergic drugs
   (g) All of the previous answers are treatable causes of terminal restlessness

Answers

1. (d) When a permanent deficit is established that will short the patient life
2. (d) All of the above
3. (d) Pharmacological prophylaxis is never used in acute hemorrhagic stroke
4. (c) Individuals with DRE do not have an increased mortality rate
5. (f) All of the above
6. (d) A dose of 50 mg diazepam has a positive effect on improving sleep duration without worsening nocturnal hypoxemia
7. (g) All of the previous answers are treatable causes of terminal restlessness

Chapter 17
Interventional Techniques in Palliative Care

Rinoo V. Shah, Alan David Kaye, Christopher K. Merritt, and Lien B. Tran

Introduction

Minimally invasive and percutaneous procedures play a role in multimodal palliative care. The concept is that a painful structure may be targeted under image guidance. Then, depending on the type of pathology, the structure can be ablated (nerve, tumor) or stabilized (bone). Targeted therapy complements systemic palliative care with analgesics.

Neurolysis

Neurolysis is the destruction of neural tissue that subserves a painful tumor. The neural tissue may be embedded within the tumor or may be remote from the tumor [1]. The direct targeting of soft tissue tumors is beyond the scope of this book. This chapter will focus on neural structures remote from the tumor. The neurobiology of pain is extremely complex, but the actual practice of neurolysis relies on knowing neural topography. Roughly, the nervous system is anatomically divided into central and peripheral components. The peripheral may be divided into somatic and sympathetic components.

R.V. Shah, M.D., M.B.A. (✉)
Department of Anesthesiology, Guthrie Clinic-Big Flats,
Horseheads, NY, USA
e-mail: rinooshah@yahoo.com

A.D. Kaye, M.D., Ph.D. • C.K. Merritt, M.D. • L.B. Tran, M.D.
Department of Anesthesiology, Louisiana State University School of Medicine,
New Orleans, LA, USA
email: alankaye44@hotmail.com; cmerr2@lsuhsc.edu; lngo@lsuhsc.edu

N. Vadivelu et al. (eds.), *Essentials of Palliative Care*,
DOI 10.1007/978-1-4614-5164-8_17,
© Springer Science+Business Media New York 2013

Destruction of neural structures occurs through the direct action of a chemical or thermal agent. Injury is followed by the release of vasoactive substances and thereafter, intraneural edema. Rising intraneural pressure leads to ischemia and permanent interruption of neural impulses [1].

Agent

Alcohol

Ethyl alcohol is a clear and hypobaric (relative to water) solution. Direct application leads to tissue dehydration. Neural components are extracted and precipitated. Axonal destruction is followed by Wallerian degeneration. The Schwann cell sheath/conduit is preserved, which allows for nerve regrowth. Sympathetic ganglia, however, are permanently destroyed. Higher concentrations of alcohol produce more complete destruction. Commonly used concentrations vary between 50 and 97%. A burning pain is followed by a warmth-type sensation, along the distribution of the nerve. Local anesthetic, hence, should be placed prior to injecting alcohol [1].

Since alcohol readily solubilizes and disperses, a large volume is required. This may collaterally injure other tissues. Neuropathic pain, following the injection, may last several weeks or months. Alcohol is rapidly metabolized by the liver, principally alcohol dehydrogenase. There is a low risk in reaching the legal limit for alcohol intoxication. Alcohol neurolysis is most commonly used for the celiac plexus, sympathetic ganglia, and spinal cord.

Phenol

Phenol is a chemical composite that is poorly soluble and colorless. Exposure to light may cause a red tinge. Phenol is hyperbaric. The maximum concentration in an aqueous medium is 6.7%. Since phenol is soluble in organic solvents, e.g., glycerol, alcohol, and nonionic contrast, admixture with these agents can raise the phenol concentration to 15%. Higher concentrations of phenol permit more complete neural destruction, but the risk of vascular injury is increased. When phenol is mixed with glycerol, diffusion is slowed and spread is limited. This enables more precise targeting, as compared to aqueous phenol [1].

Phenol is a nonselective neurolytic, acting via protein denaturation. Full degeneration may take a few weeks. Nerve cell body destruction is less successful with phenol, as compared to alcohol. Lower concentration phenol, e.g., 3%, acts as a local anesthetic. For this reason, phenol is less painful than alcohol neurolysis. On the other hand, the quality of neurolysis cannot be evaluated at 24–48 h due to the persistency of this local anesthetic effect. A full evaluation should be conducted at 3–7 days. If inadequate, repeat neurolysis may be performed. Due to disruption of the neural sheath conduit, nerve regeneration is more difficult; neuromas may form. Phenol is used for peripheral, sympathetic, and central neurolysis [1].

Side effects may include nervous system stimulation, including seizures, hemodynamic variability, nausea, and vomiting. Doses in the neurolytic range, e.g., 100–300 mg, should not cause serious side effects [1].

Glycerol

Glycerol is a milder neurolytic and is used for trigeminal ganglion blocks. The milder quality preserves facial sensation and V3 branch motor function. Usually, small aliquots of 1–2 ml of 100% are used. A perineural injection damages myelinated nerves [1].

Radiofrequency Thermocoagulation

A generator produces a high frequency (>250 kHz), alternating electrical current. The current passes through an attached electrode and exits out of the tip of an insulated needle. The current then passes through the body toward a grounding pad. In the process, local molecular oscillations occur. Heat is generated and protein denaturation occurs at the tip. Radiofrequency thermocoagulation affords very discrete neural ablation, while sparing collateral structures. Lesion shape is typically cocoon-like. However, ablation is nonselective and neuromas may form with somatic nerve targeting. Neural destruction occurs at temperatures of 45°C. So, radiofrequency generator temperatures are set at 60–80°C. Higher temperatures risk tissue boiling and tissue fragmentation. Typically, lesioning is continued for 60–90 s [2].

Patient-safety strategies include sensory stimulation (50 Hz, 0–1 mA) and motor stimulation (2 Hz, 3–5 mA), prior to neurolysis. During this testing, patients must be alert enough to communicate what they feel and what they can move during testing. Although the procedure may be performed under conscious sedation, these safety monitoring steps are essential. This will reduce the risk of inadvertent neural injury. This should be communicated during the informed consent process [2].

Cryoablation

Extreme cold is analgesic. One advantage of this, over other methods, is the relative absence of neuritis or neuroma formation. Nerve regrowth occurs, which makes this effect "reversible." Systemic side effects are absent. Pain relief could last for weeks or months. Disadvantages include lack of access to cryoablation equipment, large probe sizes (14–18 gauge), and the risk of frostbite [1, 2].

Cryolesioning occurs by freezing a small, 2–4 mm, segment of nerve tissue. Pressurized nitrous oxide rapidly expands at the probe tip and cools to temperatures of –60°C. The probe is left in place for 60–90 s. This is followed by a thaw period of 60 s, prior to removal. An ice ball of 2–4 mm forms near the nerve. Intraneural pressure rises over the next few hours and reduces after a day. This pressure oscillates and then stabilizes after 1 week. This leads to Wallerian degeneration and neurolysis [1, 2].

Complications

Chemical neurolysis is associated with some complications. Tissue necrosis and skin sloughing may occur, secondary to ischemia. Neuritis and neuromas may occur. Pain, allodynia, and hypersensitivity may be present. Some authors argue that nerve cell body destruction is imperative to reduce the risk of this complication. Anesthesia dolorosa or "painful numbness" may occur. Motor paralysis, along with bladder and bowel dysfunction, is worrisome complication. Systemic complications include impairment of the cardiovascular and central nervous systems [1, 2].

Radiofrequency neurolysis and cryoablation are safer, but require more precise targeting.

Techniques

General Considerations

Informed consent is essential.
Staff members may include a physician, nurse, radiological technologist, and surgical technologist.

Equipment

Procedure room for sterile procedures with C-Arm fluoroscopy
Needles: 25 g for skin infiltration, 22 g spinal needle 6–8 , angiocatheter introducer, 20 g curve blunt needle, 18–22 g insulated radiofrequency needle (sharp or blunt)
Emergency resuscitation equipment and drugs
Lidocaine 1–2%
Nonionic contrast, e.g., iohexol or isovue
Bupivacaine 0.25% or Ropivacaine 0.25%
Phenol 6–10%
Radiofrequency generator and electrode
Cryoablation equipment

Intrathecal Neurolysis

This is performed for segmental pain syndromes [1]. The baricity of the agent must be taken into account when performing this procedure. Alcohol is hypobaric and rises. So, a patient with severe pelvic pain due to a primary tumor or metastasis could undergo a subarachnoid injection of 50–99% alcohol, in the lower lumbar spine. The patient would then have to be positioned so that injection site is lower than the nerve roots selected for ablation. The alcohol would rise. An ongoing sensory examination would inform the practitioner when the block is complete. Phenol is hyperbaric and the opposite positional approach is needed. If a patient has a chest wall tumor, the patient should be placed in a decubitus position with the dependent side down. The phenol injection should be carried in the mid-thoracic levels. After the injection is complete, the patient should be rotated slightly posterior toward the practitioner. The phenol should settle down on the dependent side and with a dorsal positioning, the phenol should target the dorsal columns, sensory nerve rootlets, dorsal root ganglia, and spinothalamic tract. There should be sparing of the motor rootlets. The opposite strategy would be used with alcohol.

Peripheral Nerve Neurolysis

Peripheral nerve neurolysis is more commonly indicated for spasticity and not for cancer-related pain. However, some practitioners may perform intra-operative neurolysis as an adjunct to surgery, e.g., rib resection, thoracic surgery, and limb amputation. The methods employed are similar in strategy to those for peripheral nerve block, with use of electrical stimulation and ultrasound guidance. Phenol may then be injected; this agent is preferable to alcohol, secondary to the local anesthetic effect [1].

Celiac Plexus Neurolysis (Fig. 17.1)

Abdominal pain is the primary indication for celiac plexus neurolysis. The origin may be due to primary tumors, secondary extension, or metastases involving the following structures: stomach, liver, gall bladder, kidney, spleen, pancreas, descending aorta, lymph nodes, omentum, and retro peritoneum [1].

Intravenous access and volume preloading is imperative, e.g., 500–1,000 ml of lactated ringers. Patient is placed in a prone position. Special consideration must be given to increased pain in this position. Specific views under fluoroscopy are needed for optimal visualization. A posterior anterior view is followed by cephalocaudad angulation to "square off" the endplates. The C-arm is slowly rotated until the tip of transverse process is flush with edge of L1 vertebral body. The skin entry point will be the intersection of the inferior border of the T12 rib, paraspinal

Fig. 17.1 Celiac plexus neurolysis

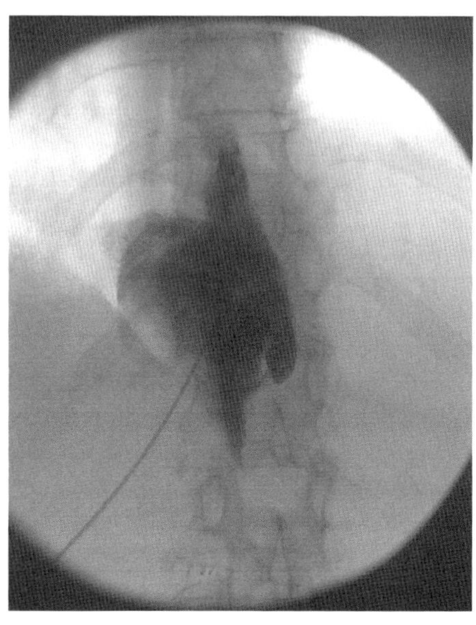

musculature, and horizontal extension of L2 transverse process/L1–2 intervertebral disc. Skin entry will be approximately 6–8 cm lateral from midline. This will be repeated on the contralateral side. With a 45° angulation, relative to the skin, the needle should be aimed cephalad toward the L1 vertebral body. The needle should pass just lateral to the vertebral body and advanced anterior to the L1 vertebral body. The needle tip should be aimed 1–2 cm anterior to the L1 vertebral body. After negative aspiration, nonionic contrast should be instilled. A relatively fixed prevertebral pattern (anterior to the aorta), with a vacuolated appearance will appear.

With serial aspiration, 20–25 ml of 1% lidocaine or 0.25% bupivacaine that is admixed (1:1) with 50% ethyl alcohol is instilled. Alternatively, 5–10 ml of 6% phenol may be instilled.

Sympathetic Neurolysis

Lumbar

Lumbar sympathetic neurolysis may be useful in patients with peripheral vascular disorders and tumors involving the lower extremities and urogenital structures [1].

The patient is placed in a prone position. Specific views under fluoroscopy are needed for optimal visualization. A posterior anterior view is followed by cephalocaudad angulation to "square off" the endplates. The C-arm is slowly rotated until the tip of transverse process is flush with edge of lumbar vertebral body.

A local anesthetic skin wheal is made, about 6–8 in. off of midline. Under fluoroscopy, the needle is advanced inferior to the tip of the transverse process and just lateral to the edge of the vertebral body. The needle should be close to the inferior endplate of the corresponding vertebral body (L2, L3, and L4); avoid the midline of the vertebral body, due to vascular (arterial) feeder vessels.

On a lateral fluoroscopic view, the needle is advanced just anterior to the vertebral body. A "loss of resistance" or tactile pop may be felt, once the anterior psoas fascia is penetrated. Aspiration should be negative for blood.

Contrast instillation should demonstrate a prevertebral filling pattern. The contrast should not demonstrate spread along the psoas or the vascular structures. An A-P view will demonstrate a vacuolated contrast pattern that remains fixed in position with respirations.

The procedure may be repeated at other lumbar levels.

Then slowly instill 5–7 ml of 3–6% phenol. Radiofrequency thermocoagulation is an alternate approach. Typically, insulated needles with 10–15 mm exposed tip may be placed. Discrete lesioning may be commenced at three levels (L2–4) to enhance efficacy. The location of the sympathetic ganglia is variable from patient to patient, but usually located near the endplates. Sensory stimulation is mandatory with radiofrequency thermocoagulation to reduce the risk of genitofemoral neuralgia. Arguably, chemical neurolytics should be instilled through an insulated needle to carry out sensory stimulation, as well. Sympatholysis may be demonstrated by lower limb venodilation and a skin temperature increase.

The needles should be flushed with local anesthetic, prior to removal.

Routine postprocedural care is necessary to ensure stable neurological and hemodynamic functioning.

Complications include genitofemoral neuralgia, intravascular injection, bleeding, and hypotension.

Thoracic

Thoracic sympathetic neurolysis may be useful in patients with peripheral vascular disorders, and tumors involving the chest wall and visceral structures and upper extremities. This procedure may help patients with chronic angina, upper extremity lymphedema, vascular diseases, and dyscrasias.

The patient is placed in a prone position, with a pillow under the chest to augment thoracic kyphosis. Specific views under fluoroscopy are needed for optimal visualization. A posterior anterior view is followed by cephalo-caudad angulation to maximize the space between ribs. The C-arm is slowly rotated so that separation of costo-transverse joint and facet articulation are visualized [1].

A local anesthetic skin wheal is made, about 4–5 cm off of midline. Under fluoroscopy, the needle is advanced inferior to the tip of the transverse process/ proximal rib head and just lateral to the edge of the vertebral body. The needle should be close to the inferior endplate of the corresponding thoracic vertebral body; avoid the midline of the vertebral body, due to vascular (arterial) feeder vessels. A single needle may be used for chemical neurolysis. Two to three needles may be used for radiofrequency neurolysis.

The needle should be advanced anterior to the thoracic foramina. The needle tip should be approximately at the anterior 2/3 / posterior 1/3 margin. There is no psoas muscle equivalent in the thoracic spine, i.e., a muscle that separates the sympathetic ganglia and nerve roots. So, needle placement is critical. The needle tip should be located near the endplates.

A blunt needle should be considered for this procedure, in order to reduce the risk of a pneumothorax. Aspiration should be negative for blood. Contrast instillation should demonstrate a "clamshell" type spread, which hugs the lateral margin of the vertebral body. This spread should not dissipate with respirations and vascular uptake should be negative. The procedure may be repeated at other thoracic levels.

Ten to fifteen milliliters of local anesthetic may be instilled. Sympatholysis may be demonstrated venodilation in the hands, reduction in palmo-plantar hidrosis, and a skin temperature increase. Then slowly instill 5–7 ml of phenol. Radiofrequency thermocoagulation is an alternate approach. Typically, insulated needles with 10–15 mm exposed tip may be placed. Discrete lesioning may be commenced at three levels, for instance, T2–T4, in order to enhance efficacy. The choice of level depends on the location of the pathology. The needles should be flushed with local anesthetic, prior to removal.

Routine postprocedural care is necessary to ensure stable neurological and hemodynamic functioning. Complications include thoracic radiculopathy, pneumothorax, intravascular injection, bleeding, and hypotension.

Trigeminal Ganglion

The trigeminal ganglion is an important neural relay for pain originating in face, brain (meninges), head, and upper neck. This structure is accessible through the foramen ovale, which transmits the mandibular branch (V3). This is an advanced procedure [1].

The patient is placed in a supine position, with the neck slightly extended and the jaw recessed. Fluoroscopy is used to identify the foramen ovale, which is located medial to the upper portion of the mandible. The C-arm is positioned, so the image intensifier is almost touching the chest (submental view).

A local anesthetic skin wheal, typically 2 cm lateral to the labial commissure. An angiocatheter introducer typically advanced to the upper portion of the mandible, inferior to the skull base. Direct palpation in the oral mucosa will determine if the buccal mucosa is violated. Thereafter, a curved blunt needle is advanced into the foramen ovale. The patient may feel pain due to dysesthesia along the V3 distribution. The needle is then advanced 3–5 mm further. Sensory stimulation should produce paresthesias in the distribution of V2 and V3. It is more difficult to get paresthesias in the V1 distribution. Actually, the yield of sensory stimulation is limited since many of these patients are sedated. Motor stimulation will lead to unilateral jaw contractions. Care must be taken to protect the lips, tongue, mucosa, and other oral structures. Neurolysis may be initiated. With radiofrequency thermocoagulation, temperatures of 60°C for about 60 s are ideal. The corneal reflex should be monitored during the procedure. With chemical neurolysis, glycerol may be used past the foramen ovale. Glycerol is less likely to spread and damage motor fibers (V3), as compared to phenol and alcohol. A curved, blunt needle is advised to do this procedure.

Intercostal Neurolysis

Tumors that invade the chest wall or surgery that transects ribs and associated neural structures can lead to severe neuropathic pain. The intercostal nerves may be interrupted with neurolysis, typically with cryoablation or phenol. The procedure is performed similarly to an intercostal nerve block [1].

After local anesthetic infiltration, a spinal needle is advanced 4–6 cm lateral to the thoracic midline toward the rib. Once bone contact occurs, the depth is noted. The needle is pulled back and advanced off the inferior margin of the rib to a depth of a few millimeters. Aspiration should be negative for air and blood. Contrast should demonstrate spread along the intercostal muscles and no spread proximally into the spinal canal. There should be no vascular washout of contrast. Contrast should not disperse with respirations. Thereafter, phenol 3–4 ml is instilled slowly with intermittent aspiration. In the case of cryoablation, a double-needle technique is utilized. Since the probe is large and since the ice ball will form at the distal tip, the technique should be modified. The angiocatheter should be advanced to the superior margin of the rib. The cryoprobe should be advanced through the angiocatheter toward the cephalad rib. The probe should be passed under this superior rib. Cryoneurolysis should be carried out. Despite greater invasiveness, cryoablation may reduce the risk of neuroma pain.

Complications include pneumothorax, paralysis, hematoma, and infection.

Skeletal Metastases

Skeletal metastases may cause significant morbidity. Direct palliation, with radiofrequency ablation and surgical removal, has been tried. These attempts may lead to protracted improvement and significant morbidity respectively. Vertebral augmentation and osteoplasty are viable alternatives. Cement produces an exothermic reaction that results in neurolysis. Cement stabilizes bone metastases and fractures. Vertebroplasty and kyphoplasty (Fig. 17.2) are two such procedures [1, 3, 4].

Fig. 17.2 Kyphoplasty

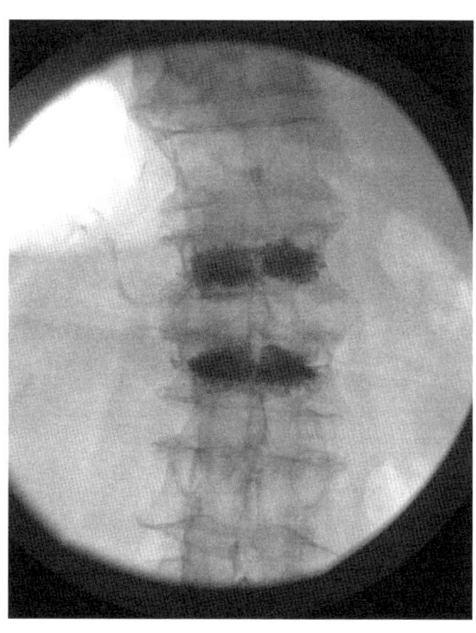

After preprocedural planning, the patient is placed in a prone position. Cannulas are advanced through the pedicle of the vertebral body. A unilateral approach is used for vertebroplasty and bilateral for kyphoplasty. A balloon or curette may be placed through the cannula into the vertebral body. These tools permit the creation of a cavity. The balloon and curette are removed. Other manufacturers have advocated implantation of biocompatible wafers to permit height restoration. Thereafter, a cement, typically poly methyl methacrylate is prepared. Once a very viscous consistency is reached, the cement is delivered in 0.1–0.5 ml aliquots under live fluoroscopy. Careful monitoring is imperative to ensure that the cement does not extravasate. Cement volumes may range between 3 and 7 ml. Degree of fill on fluoroscopy will determine when to stop. Cement should not extravasate outside the margins of the vertebral body. Sacral metastases may be targeted, as well as flat bones such as the sternum. The latter have demonstrated efficacy and safety.

Complications include cement extravasation, cement emboli, neural damage, spinal cord injury, morbidities of the patients, anesthesia, and pressure-related injuries (eyes, bony surfaces, and peripheral nerves).

Neurosurgical ablative approaches are not commonly performed, but they include neurectomy, sympathectomy, cordotomy, commissurotomy, mesencephalotomy, thalamotomy, and cingulotomy. In reality, these procedures are extremely rare and reserved for the most debilitated patients. These patients have very limited life expectancies and the safety of performing these procedures in this population is questioned.

Alternative options include neuromodulation with implantable devices. Intrathecal opioid pumps are more common in this population, as compared to spinal cord stimulation.

Fig. 17.3 Spinal cord stimulation

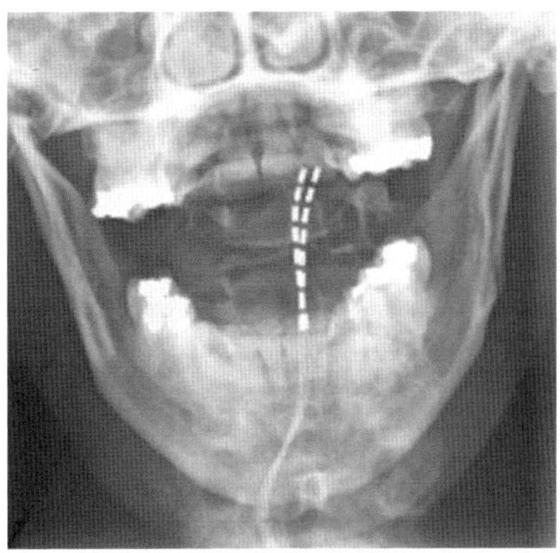

An intrathecal pump involves placing a catheter into the spinal canal. This catheter is tunneled subcutaneously toward the anterior abdomen. A programmable reservoir is placed subcutaneously in the anterior abdominal lower quadrant and connected to the catheter. The pump reservoir holds the drug and the pump delivers small aliquots of drug into the spinal canal. Typically, a preimplantation trial via a subarachnoid injection of morphine, 0.25–1 mg is used. The pump then delivers the drug continuously for pain relief. In some countries, patients can self-administer the drug as a periodic bolus.

Interventional Procedures in Noncancer Palliative Care

Spinal cord stimulation (Fig. 17.3) is a neuromodulatory device that has demonstrable efficacy in chronic angina and peripheral vascular disease. A special type of electrode is placed in the cervical or thoracic epidural space. A small electrical current passed to the spinal cord through the dura can help with pain control. These patients have a visceral and somatic component to their pain. Spinal cord stimulation may help with both of these types. Spinal cord stimulation does not block the pain to such an extent, wherein a life-threatening ischemic episode is not noticed [5].

Thoracic and lumbar epidural catheters may be used as a short-term strategy for acute or subacute pain syndromes. A catheter that is silastic and is cuffed may be useful for longer periods, e.g., weeks. This may play an important role in patients that are immunocompromised and have a short life expectancy.

The practicality of these procedures in patients with vascular disease is limited by anticoagulation and immune status [5–8].

Future areas of investigation include the role of spinal cord stimulation in patients with co-morbidities that are adversely affected by opioids or sedatives, e.g., sleep apnea, pulmonary disease.

Intrathecal pumps may be a better option for some patients on anticoagulants. However, this procedure will primarily benefit patients with thoracic, chest wall, abdominal, pelvic, and lower extremity pain syndromes [5–8]. Some neurosurgeons have reported direct cisternal or upper cervical catheter implantations for cranio-cervical disorders.

HIV patients have a host of associated neurological disorders that may be amenable to neuromodulation. Infection is an important consideration and the risks should be carefully weighed with the benefits.

Neurolytic procedures, e.g., lumbar sympathectomy, may be of use in patients with lower extremity vascular disease. Thoracic sympathectomy may be of use in patients with chronic upper extremity insufficiency or Raynaud's disease.

Conclusion

Palliative care specialists should be aware that the pain and fear of inadequate pain relief are of major concern to patients. Since many analgesics have untoward side effects or adverse events, consideration should be given to the above procedures. Close consultation with an interventional pain specialist is advised.

References

1. Gehdoo R. Neurolytic agents and neurodestructive techniques. In: Baheti D, editor. Interventional pain management: a practical approach. New Delhi: Jaypee; 2008. p. 27–35.
2. Sharma A. Radiofrequency thermocoagulation. In: Baheti D, editor. Interventional pain management: a practical approach. New Delhi: Jaypee; 2008. p. 308–26.
3. Shah RV. Sacral kyphoplasty for the treatment of painful sacral insufficiency fractures and metastases. Spine J. 2012;12(2):113–20.
4. Shah RV. Sternal kyphoplasty for metastatic lung cancer: image-guided palliative care, utilizing fluoroscopy and sonography. Pain Med. 2012;13(2):198–203.
5. Longnecker DE. Anesthesiology. 2nd ed. New York: McGraw-Hill; 2012.
6. Gayle JA, et al. Anticoagulants: newer ones, mechanisms, and perioperative updates. Anesthesiol Clin. 2010;28(4):667–79.
7. Raj PP, et al. Bleeding risk in interventional pain practice: assessment, management, and review of the literature. Pain Physician. 2004;7(1):3–51.
8. Shah RV, Kaye AD. Bleeding risk and interventional pain management. Curr Opin Anaesthesiol. 2008;21(4):433–8.

Review Questions

1. Which of the following agents can be used for neurolysis techniques:

   (a) Alcohol.
   (b) Phenol.
   (c) Glycerol.
   (d) All of the above.
   (e) None of the above.

2. Which is false regarding RFTC:

   (a) A generator produces a high frequency (<1 kHz), alternating electrical current in RFTC.
   (b) The current passes through an attached electrode and exits out of the tip of an insulated needle.
   (c) Heat is generated and protein denaturation occurs at the tip. Radiofrequency thermocoagulation affords very discrete neural ablation, while sparing collateral structures.
   (d) Lesion shape is typically cocoon-like.
   (e) However, ablation is nonselective and neuromas may form with somatic nerve targeting. Neural destruction occurs at temperatures of 45°C. So, radiofrequency generator temperatures are set at 60–80°C.

3. Which is false:

   (a) Ethyl alcohol is a clear and hypobaric (relative to water) solution.
   (b) Direct application leads to tissue dehydration.
   (c) Neural components are extracted and precipitated. Axonal destruction is followed by Wallerian degeneration.
   (d) The Schwann cell sheath/conduit is preserved, which allows for nerve regrowth. Sympathetic ganglia, however, are permanently destroyed.
   (e) Lower concentrations of alcohol produce more complete destruction. Commonly used concentrations vary between 50 and 97%. Alcohol neurolysis is most commonly used for the celiac plexus, sympathetic ganglia, and spinal cord.

4. Which is true regarding metastasis and pain techniques

   (a) Cement produces an exothermic reaction that results in neurolysis. Cement stabilizes bone metastases and fractures. Vertebroplasty and kyphoplasty are two such procedures.
   (b) A cement, typically poly methyl methacrylate is prepared. Once a very viscous consistency is reached, the cement is delivered in 0.1–0.5 ml aliquots under live fluoroscopy. Careful monitoring is imperative to ensure that the cement does not extravasate. Cement volumes may range between 3 and 7 ml.

   (c) Degree of fill on fluoroscopy will determine when to stop. Cement should not extravasate outside the margins of the vertebral body. Sacral metastases may be targeted, as well as flat bones such as the sternum. The latter have demonstrated efficacy and safety.
   (d) Complications include cement extravasation, cement emboli, neural damage, spinal cord injury, vascular uptake, hematoma, and infection. Other complications may be due to the medical co-morbidities of the patients, anesthesia, and pressure-related injuries (eyes, bony surfaces, and peripheral nerves).
   (e) All are true.

5. Which is false:

   (a) Spinal cord stimulation is a neuromodulatory device that has demonstrable efficacy in chronic angina and peripheral vascular disease. A special type of electrode is placed in the cervical or thoracic epidural space.
   (b) Spinal cord stimulation does not block the pain to such an extent, wherein a life-threatening ischemic episode is not noticed.
   (c) Thoracic and lumbar epidural catheters may be used as a short-term strategy for acute or subacute pain syndromes.
   (d) A catheter that is silastic and is cuffed may be useful for longer periods, e.g., weeks. This may play an important role in patients that are immunocompromised and have a short life expectancy.
   (e) All are true.

6. Which is a false statement

   (a) There is no role for neurolytic procedures in Palliative Care.
   (b) Strict sterile technique is required for all interventional pain procedures.
   (c) Significant side effects can occur in interventional pain medicine procedures.
   (d) Cryoablative procedures are indicated in certain pain states.
   (e) Monitoring patients for interventional pain procedures is important, as patients may require procedural sedation, and complications such as local anesthetic toxicity, pneumothorax, nerve injury, vascular puncture, and bleeding can occur.

7. Examples of interventional pain blocks include:

   (a) Intercostal block.
   (b) Celiac block.
   (c) Transforaminal nerve root block.
   (d) Lumbar facet block.
   (e) All of the above.

8. Regarding spinal cord modulation:

   (a) Options include neuromodulation with implantable devices.
   (b) Intrathecal opioid pumps are more common in this population, as compared to spinal cord stimulation.

   (c) An intrathecal pump involves placing a catheter into the spinal canal. This catheter is tunneled subcutaneously toward the anterior abdomen.

   (d) A programmable reservoir is placed subcutaneously in the anterior abdominal lower quadrant and connected to the catheter. The pump reservoir holds the drug and the pump delivers small aliquots of drug into the spinal canal. Typically, a preimplantation trial via a subarachnoid injection of morphine, 0.25–1 mg is used. The pump then delivers the drug continuously for pain relief. In some countries, patients can self-administer the drug as a periodic bolus.

   (e) All are true.

9. Regarding peripheral neurolysis:

   (a) Peripheral nerve neurolysis is more commonly indicated for spasticity and not for cancer-related pain.

   (b) Some practitioners may perform intra-operative neurolysis as an adjunct to surgery, e.g., rib resection, thoracic surgery, and limb amputation.

   (c) The methods employed are similar in strategy to those for peripheral nerve block, with use of electrical stimulation and ultrasound guidance. Phenol may then be injected; this agent is preferable to alcohol, secondary to the local anesthetic effect.

   (d) All are true.

   (e) All arc false.

10. Regarding trigeminal ganglion procedures:

   (a) The trigeminal ganglion is an important neural relay for pain originating in face, brain (meninges), head, and upper neck. This structure is accessible through the foramen ovale, which transmits the mandibular branch (V3).

   (b) The patient is placed in a supine position, with the neck slightly extended and the jaw recessed. Fluoroscopy is used to identify the foramen ovale, which is located medial to the upper portion of the mandible.

   (c) The yield of sensory stimulation is limited since many of these patients are sedated. Motor stimulation will lead to unilateral jaw contractions. Care must be taken to protect the lips, tongue, mucosa, and other oral structures. With radiofrequency thermocoagulation, temperatures of 60°C for about 60 s are ideal.

   (d) All are false.

   (e) All are true.

Answers

1. (d)
2. (a). It is >250 kHz
3. (e). Higher concentrations of alcohol produce more complete destruction
4. (e)
5. (e)
6. (a)
7. (e)
8. (e)
9. (d)
10. (e)

Chapter 18
Headache in Palliative Care

Nicholas Connolly, Matthew Peña, and Tara M. Sheridan

Introduction

Headaches comprise a relatively common pain condition with etiologies ranging from benign to life-threatening. The International Headache Society categorizes headaches into primary, such as migraine, cluster or tension headaches, and secondary, such as due to an underlying infection, neoplasm or other disease process. Many patients experience headaches of a chronic nature, which are refractory to standard treatments, and which require more intensive and/or invasive care. These patients include those who are suffering from secondary headaches associated with potentially terminal conditions, such as HIV encephalitis or intracranial tumor burden, but also include patients suffering from more common, yet severe forms of benign primary headache disorders. It is crucial to recognize life-threatening causes of headache, as well as to identify benign but incapacitating etiologies. Here, we focus on the differential diagnosis to consider in patients presenting to pain clinic with refractory headaches, including appropriate work up and treatment options. As migraine and cluster headache are two of the most common and disabling headache disorders in the chronic pain patient population, this chapter highlights considerations for these patients in particular.

N. Connolly, M.D. • M. Peña, M.D.
Department of Anesthesiology, Naval Medical Center San Diego,
San Diego, CA, USA

T.M. Sheridan, M.D. (✉)
Department of Anesthesiology, Naval Medical Center San Diego,
Bethesda, MD, USA
e-mail: tara.sheridan@med.navy.mil

N. Vadivelu et al. (eds.), *Essentials of Palliative Care*,
DOI 10.1007/978-1-4614-5164-8_18,
© Springer Science+Business Media New York 2013

Migraines

Migraine afflicts approximately 6% of men, 18% of women, and 4% of children in Europe and the USA [1]. Cases are most frequent in women of child-bearing years, the gender difference beginning at the age of menarche, and falling off after age 60. Peak prevalence occurs during the second and third decades of life, traditionally periods of high productivity, and over half of migraine patients report significant impact on their daily lives, such as requiring bed rest and missing school or work. The risk of having migraines is 50% higher in relatives of migraineurs than in relatives of controls. The majority of people who suffer from migraines do not seek professional advice from primary care physicians, but instead self-medicate with over-the-counter medications. However, surveys suggest that 5% of Emergency Department patients present with migraine headaches, and that greater than 90% of those patients who do see their primary care doctor with a chief complaint of headache are diagnosed with migraine [2]. The fiscal impact of medical cost and lost worker productivity is estimated to be in the range of $15 billion annually in this country [3].

Definition and Classification

Migraine is a paroxysmal primary disease occurring in otherwise healthy individuals. It is characterized by distinct periods of severe head pain, lasting from several hours to days, often accompanied by photophobia (light sensitivity), phonophobia (sound sensitivity), nausea, and vomiting.

Migraine is divided into four specific phases: prodrome, aura, headache, and postdrome. The prodrome is a premonitory phase which occurs in about 20–60% of migraine patients and consists of symptoms such as mood changes, food cravings, yawning, fatigue, and increased urination. Patient may recognize these symptoms as being indicative of impending headache pain.

About 20% of migraine patients experience aura prior to onset of headache pain. Aura is a temporary, reversible change that causes focal neurologic findings. Visual auras are most common, but sensory, memory, or speech changes may occur. Typically, visual auras manifest as colored spots, flashing lights, or bright shapes moving slowly across the visual field. Auras usually last 5–60 min and resolve completely, with headache following within an hour of onset. To be diagnosed as migraine with aura, the patient must experience at least two such headaches [1].

The third phase of the migraine is the headache itself, characterized by unilateral, moderate to severe throbbing pains, lasting 4–72 h. Migraines extending past 72 h, regardless of therapy, are considered "status migrainosus." Acute treatments are partially or completely ineffective for status migrainosus, as the pain is only transiently relieved by abortive medications.

The second edition of the *International Headache Classification (ICHD-2)* defines diagnostic criteria for both migraines with aura ("classic") and migraines without aura ("common") [4]. The criteria stipulate the following rules:

1. At least five headaches lasting 4–72 h in duration, with no or unsuccessful treatment

2. At least two of the following characteristics

    (a) Unilateral location
    (b) Throbbing quality
    (c) Moderate to severe intensity
    (d) Worse with routine activity

3. In addition, at least one of the following features

    (a) Nausea/vomiting
    (b) Photophobia
    (c) Phonophobia

4. Normal neurologic examination, without evidence of another attributable disorder

The fourth and final migraine phase is the postdrome, which occurs in approximately 65% of migraineurs. Patients notice symptoms such as fatigue, weakness, irritability, depression, and scalp tenderness for several hours to days after resolution of the headache pain.

Etiology and Pathophysiology

From the 1940s to the 1990s migraine was defined as strictly a vascular anomaly, whereas it is now considered a more complex neurovascular disorder, involving multiple genetic, environmental, and neurohormonal factors [5].

According to a theory postulated by Dr. Harold Wolffe in the 1940s, cranial vascular constriction leads to decreased cerebral blood flow and subsequent vascular vasodilation, causing migraine pain. However, in the 1990s Jes Olsen's blood flow studies demonstrated that cerebral blood flow does not correlate with the symptoms of migraine [5]. More current research suggests that cortical spreading depression (CSD) is the basis of migraine aura, and is a trigger for headache pain [6]. CSD is a regenerative wave of neuronal and glial depolarization that propagates slowly across the neocortex, causing extracellular efflux of potassium ions, at a rate of approximately 2–3 mm/min [7]. It was first described by Dr. Aristes Leao, as he studied animal models of epilepsy [5]. The relationship between CSD and migraine aura was made by observing the similar rates of progression between the two phenomena, as described by Dr. Milner et al. in the 1958 paper entitled, "Note on a possible correspondence between the scotomas of migraine and spreading depression of Leao." These transient scintillations and flashes track across the visual field just prior to the onset of headache pain, moving peripherally over the course of 10–15 min at a rate of 2–3 mm/min. Ongoing human neuroimaging studies (i.e., functional MRI/PET scan) [8] lend further support to the correlation between neocortical spreading depression and migraine aura. CSD causes plasma protein extravasation from the dura mater, triggering trigeminal ganglion-mediated pain pathways and activating parasympathetic nervous system-mediated nausea and fatigue. More specifically, activation of the trigeminovascular system's nerves and vessels stimulates meningeal secretion of such neurotransmitters as substance P, serotonin and calcitonin gene-related peptide, resulting in cranial vessel dilation and inflammation [9].

Neuronal hyperactivity in the hippocampus may stimulate nociceptive activation of the trigeminal nucleus caudalis, and be the initiating factor in nonaural (common) migraines [7].

Diagnosis

Headache evaluation should include a thorough history, with special attention paid to the character and pattern of head pain, associated symptoms, triggering factors, and medication history. A physical examination to rule out systemic causes of headache as well as a neurologic examination should be performed. High-risk features of headache that should prompt neuroimaging include age greater than 50, sudden onset of symptoms, history of trauma, accelerating pattern of headache, altered mental status, and systemic features, such as fever, rash, or occipitonuchal rigidity [10]. Neurologic deficits in patients with cancer or human immunodeficiency virus (HIV) infection may signify increased intracranial pressure due to edema or growth of a space-occupying lesion [11]. Headaches may also be associated with chronic opioid use. Opioids can trigger migraine, tension or rebound headaches, particularly when a patient is overusing short-acting opioids [12]. Headache is reported by 40–50% of patients with HIV, especially in the later stages of disease. The differential diagnosis includes HIV encephalitis, atypical aseptic meningitis, opportunistic infections of the central nervous system (CNS), acquired immune system deficiency syndrome (AIDS)-related CNS neoplasms, sinusitis, tension, migraine, and zidovudine-induced headache [11].

As for what studies to order, computerized tomography (CT) detects the majority of significant conditions that may cause headaches, such as acute head trauma, subarachnoid hemorrhage, or osseous defects. These images are quick to obtain but do expose the patient to relatively high radiation levels and are not ideal for identifying vascular, infectious, or neoplastic lesions, particularly in cervicomedullar region or the posterior fossa. Magnetic resonance tomography (MRI) is more sensitive that CT in detecting posterior fossa, cervicomedullary or pituitary pathology, white matter changes, central venous thrombosis, subdural and epidural hematomas, and meningeal disease. MRI does not expose patients to radiation and is safe during pregnancy, although a small percentage of patients may have an allergic reaction to iodinated or gadolinium contrast agents, or may not be able to tolerate the claustrophobia associated with obtaining this longer scan.

EEG is not useful in the routine assessment of headache pain, for either adult or pediatric populations. However, it is notable that migraine and epilepsy share many commonalities. Both are chronic, paroxysmal neurologic conditions with distinct, sporadic episodes, and no appreciable symptoms after attack resolution. Both have complex heritable components and are triggered by abnormal neuronal hyperexcitability. In fact, antiepileptic drugs such as topiramate, valproate, and gabapentin are successfully utilized as migraine prophylactic agents [5]. They may belong within a common disorder spectrum, and additional findings suggestive of seizure disorder, such as atypical aura, lapses in consciousness, or tonic–clonic movements should prompt EEG evaluation in migraine patients [13].

Lumbar puncture is reserved for cases in which there is a high suspicion for such diseases as meningitis, encephalitis, meningeal carcinomatosis, or lymphomatosis, subarachnoid hemorrhage, and pseudotumor cerebra. MRI or CT is routinely performed prior to lumbar puncture, to evaluate for risk of herniation, and platelet count should be verified as being at least 50,000 prior to needle placement. Recording the opening pressure is helpful in working up headache etiology. In order to reduce the risk of causing a postdural puncture headache, which is a common complication and may certainly confound diagnosis of the original, presenting headache, the practitioner should use a small gauge (25 g) Sprotte or Whitacre pencil needle for the procedure.

Serum studies are not usually indicated in the evaluation of headache. However, certain exceptions may be warranted, such as an erythrocyte sedimentation rate (ESR) or C-reactive protein (CRP) level in potentially inflammatory etiologies, such as temporal arteritis in an older patient presenting with new onset migraine. ESR, CRP, rheumatoid factor, and antinuclear antibody titers may be obtained to rule out other inflammatory, autoimmune diseases, or collagen vascular diseases associated with headaches, such as rheumatoid arthritis or systemic lupus erythematosis. In teenagers with headache, arthralgia, and cervical lymphadenopathy, a monospot assay may rule out mononucleosis. For immunocompromised patients, complete blood count, liver function, HIV test, or Lyme antibody may be indicated. Hypothyroidism may be associated with headache presentation, so a thyroid-stimulating hormone level can be ordered in patients additionally complaining of fatigue, weight gain, cold intolerance, dry skin, and hair loss. Endocrine studies are warranted in patients with concern for a pituitary tumor. Symptoms vary depending on the pituitary tumor type, size, location, and hormones secreted, if any. The most common pituitary tumor, prolactinoma, is associated with headaches and changes in menstruation, vision, and libido. Other tumor types may be associated with changes in weight and blood pressure, as well as headache.

Patients determined to have migraines should be interviewed about the onset, severity, and quality of their headaches, including exacerbating and relieving factors, identifiable "triggers" and other risk factors, such as head trauma or family medical history of migraines. There are no specific laboratory abnormalities associated with migraines, and neuroimaging is not recommended for patients with migraine presentation and a normal physical examination [13].

Headache triggers consist of a wide array of influences which make the patient more vulnerable to, or actually precipitate migraine onset. Common factors include alterations in sleep or meal patterns, emotional stress, physical exertion, and illness [14].

Other triggers may include bright or fluorescent lighting, elevated altitude, barometric pressure or weather changes, and such odors as household cleaning products, car exhaust, or perfumes. Dietary triggers that affect some migraineurs include monosodium glutamate, aspartame, chocolate, citrus fruits, and tyramine containing foods, such as aged cheeses and red wine. Other types of alcohol most frequently implicated as migraine triggers include whisky, beer, and champagne. Nitrate or nitrite food preservatives are associated with causing cerebral vessel dilation and triggering migraines also. Of note, caffeine may be used as a treatment for migraines, speeding the onset and effectiveness of other pain relievers by up to 40%. However, caffeine overuse makes migraineurs particularly vulnerable to rebound headaches, and its use should be otherwise curtailed in this population. In 60% of women of reproductive age who experience migraines, normal cyclical fluctuations precipitate migraines, the fall in estrogen levels prior to menses onset thought to be the causative factor [15]. A subset of migrainous women experience catamenial (menstrual) migraines, which are defined as attacks of migraine without aura that occur regularly on day 1 of menstruation, ±2 days, and at no other time [15]. Comorbidities frequently associated with migraine headaches include obesity, depression and/or anxiety disorders, epilepsy, diabetes mellitus, obstructive sleep apnea, and tension-type headaches [16].

A headache diary is a critically useful tool in helping to identify patterns in the patient's migraines, and to determine what factors trigger, aggravate, or alleviate the process. Medication use and other treatment strategies should also be documented, to track compliance, efficacy and side effects [17].

Previous observational studies suggested a possible relationship between patent foramen ovale (PFO) and migraine [18]. However, further investigation has shown no association, and screening transthoracic echocardiograms (TTEs) are not indicated in the evaluation of migraines [18].

Treatment Options

In addition to alternative and complementary nonpharmacologic strategies, there are two broad categories of medication therapy for migraines: acute/abortive and preventative/prophylactic. Exclusive acute care migraine treatment is not enough for those patients who suffer from frequent migraine attacks or who experience severe disability despite appropriate abortive therapy. In fact, excessive use of acute medications can result in decreased efficacy, increased head frequency, medication-induced "rebound" headaches, and the development of chronic daily headaches [19].

Abortive therapy targets acute head pain and associated symptoms, such as nausea and vomiting. Preventative therapy aims to reduce the frequency and/or intensity of attacks, to improve daily functioning and quality of life. Prophylaxis is suitable for patients with frequent or severe migraines, considerable disability or resistance to acute therapy. Neither type of therapy can substitute for appropriate lifestyle changes or the avoidance of identifiable migraine triggers.

Table 18.1 Indications for migraine prophylaxis

1. 3–7 headaches/month (8 or more may be indicative of overuse headache)
2. Lasting longer than 2 days
3. Causing severe disability, including hemiplegia
4. Refractory to abortive therapy
5. For which standard therapy is intolerable, overused or contraindicated
6. With a predictable pattern of occurrence (such as menstrual migraines)

Nonpharmocologic Treatments

Some patients prefer nonpharmacologic strategies in lieu of, or in addition to medications. A multimodal approach that incorporates both may include behavioral treatments (relaxation training, biofeedback, cognitive therapy for stress management) as well as pharmacologic prevention. Evidence-based recommendations for the use of hypnosis, acupuncture, transcutaneous electrical nerve stimulation (TENS), chiropractic or osteopathic cervical manipulation in reducing migraine frequency and severity are quite variable [20]. Acupuncture has some success with chronic headache treatment, and its effects are thought to be due to the release of endogenous opiates, as well as activation of descending inhibitory pain pathways. However, there may also be a significant placebo effect [21].

Prophylaxis

Although migraine prophylaxis cannot substitute for adhering to lifestyle improvements and avoidance of known triggers, it can certainly benefit a large number of chronic migraineurs, perhaps as many as 25% by some estimates, and studies suggest that preemptive therapies are currently underutilized. Prophylaxis should be considered in patients who experience two or more headaches per week, whose headaches cause significant impact on their lives despite appropriate use of medication or who require abortive medication treatment on 2 or more days per week, potentially putting them at risk for chronic daily headaches (see Table 18.1). Prophylaxis is considered effective if it decreases migraine frequency by at least 50% within 3 months [22]. The goals of prophylaxis include a reduction in the frequency and severity of migraine symptoms, improved functionality and quality of life, decreased reliance on, and improved responsiveness to, abortive therapies, and prevention of migraine progression. Patients need to be educated about the potential risks and benefits of any preventative medications that are prescribed, and advised that most medications take 2–3 months to show full effect. Patients should be further encouraged to keep a daily headache journal during the trial of their prophylaxis, in order to help in evaluating adherence, efficacy, and any adverse effects. For most medications, the lowest possible dose should be selected initially, and titrated up over several weeks or months, as needed. Prophylactic medications are chosen based on the patient's headache characteristics, patient preference, side effect tolerability, and any coexisting diseases. Efficacy of medications may be limited by poor compliance from intolerable side effects, inadequate results, or need for daily administration.

There are several medications demonstrated to be effective in decreasing the number of migraines experienced monthly by half. These include antidepressants, beta-adrenergic blockers, calcium channel blockers, nonsteroidal anti-inflammatories, anticonvulsants, and botulinum toxin type A [23]. Patients with underlying hypertension are often trialed on beta blockers or calcium channel blockers. Patients with mood disorders such as anxiety or depression may be prescribed tricyclic antidepressants, serotonin antagonists, or venlafaxine [24, 25]. Obese patients, for whom weight gain may be a particularly intolerable side effect, may prefer topiramate, which can actually facilitate weight loss. Patients with concurrent seizure disorders may benefit from treatment with antiepileptics, such as topiramate, gabapentin, or valproate. Nonprescription prophylactic medications may include magnesium, riboflavin (B2), Coenzyme Q-10, and butterbur. Other options include botulinum toxin type A, occipital nerve blocks, and acupuncture [26, 27]. Refer to Table 18.2 for a synopsis of prophylactic medications.

- Botulinum toxin type A (Botox)
- Botulinum toxin type A is a focally acting protein that blocks the release of acetylcholine from presynaptic nerve endings and the release of pro-inflammatory nociceptive mediators such as substance P, glutamate, bradykinin, cytokines, prostaglandins, and calcitonin gene-related peptide. Reducing these peripheral nociceptive mediators decreases central sensitization and its attendant effects of inflammation, vasodilation, and edema. Botox has been shown to be effective in decreasing headache frequency in patients with refractory migraines, and the effect lasts for approximately 3 months. Total doses of 100 units of Botox can be injected into five sites (glabella, temporal, frontal, suboccipital, and trapezius) with high safety and tolerability. Treatment efficacy is associated with a high incidence of unilateral headaches and scalp allodynia—apparent predictors of responsiveness to Botox therapy. Adverse effects include injection site pain, blepharoptosis, diplopia, and atrophy of injected muscles, particularly the temporalis muscle ("hourglass" concavity) [28, 29].
- Fluoxetine (Prozac)
- Fluoxetine is a selective serotonin receptor inhibitor that downregulates serotonin receptors, thereby increasing synaptic serotonin. It is a good option for those with comorbid depression as it has been shown to both decrease headache frequency and improve mood in this population.
- Amitriptyline (Elavil)
- Amitriptyline, a tricyclic antidepressant, downregulates serotonin receptors, increases the levels of synaptic amines (norepinephrine and serotonin), enhances endogenous opioid receptor action and facilitates descending modulation of nociception in the trigeminal nucleus caudalis. It is another good option for mood enhancement as well as migraine prevention.

Table 18.2 Migraine prophylaxis medications

Medication	Adverse effects	Notes
Beta blockers		
	Fatigue, postural symptoms, asthma exacerbation, depression, impotence	Caution with diabetes mellitus, chronic heart failure, asthma, cardiac conduction defects, depression or Rayaud's syndrome. Useful in patients with comorbid cardiovascular disease or anxiety disorder. Avoid abrupt discontinuation. Trial for 1 month
• Propranolol (Inderal) 20 mg BID (40–160 mg/day)		First-line agent
• Atenolol (Tenormin) 50–200 mg daily	Fewer side effects than propanolol	
• Metoprolol (Lopressor/Toprol) 100–200 mg daily		Use short acting formulation BID or longer acting QD
Calcium channel blockers		
• Verapamil (Calan, Covera) 40 mg TID (40–80 mg TID)	Constipation, hypotension, dizziness, dry mouth, peripheral edema, weight gain	Evidence is mixed as to efficacy in migraine prophylaxis
ACE inhibitor/ARB		
• Lisinopril (Prinivil, Zestril) 20 mg daily	Cough, teratogenic	Moderate benefit demonstrated
• Candesartan (Atacand) 16 mg daily	Dizziness, teratogenic	Angiotensin receptor blocker with benefit shown in limited studies
Anticonvulsants		
• Topiramate (Topamax) 25 mg qhs (25–200 mg/day)	Paresthesias, weight loss, fatigue, memory impairment	May be helpful in patients particularly concerned about weight gain as an intolerable side effect of migraine prevention
• Gabapentin (Neurontin) 300 mg BID (900–3,600 mg/day)	Sedation, dizziness, paresthesias, fetal anomalies	Limited data showing efficacy
• Valproic acid (Depakote) 250 mg BID (500–1,500 mg/day)	Drowsiness, tremor, nausea, dizziness, weight gain, hepatotoxicity. Neural tube teratogenicity	First-line agent but must be used cautiously with liver disease, thrombocytopenia or pregnancy. Indicated for atypical migraine aura and for comorbid epilepsy, mania, trigeminal neuralgia, tension type or cluster headache. Unclear mechanism of action for headache prevention

(continued)

Table 18.2 (continued)

Medication	Adverse effects	Notes
Antidepressants		
• Amitriptyline (Elavil) 10 mg qhs (10–75 mg qhs)	Drowsiness, dry mouth, weight gain	Tricyclic antidepressant (TCA). Successful in multiple studies, especially in patients with mixed migraine and tension type headache. One of the most commonly prescribed preventive drugs in the USA
• Nortriptyline (Pamelor) 10 mg qhs (10–150 mg qhs)	Less sedating TCA	
• Venlafaxine (Effexor) 75–225 mg daily	GI upset, sedation, constipation	Selective serotonin–norepinephrine reuptake inhibitor. Useful in comorbid anxiety disorder or tension type headache
• Fluoxetine (Prozac) 10 mg daily (10–80 mg/day)	GI upset, somnolence, tremor, impotence	Selective serotonin reuptake inhibitor (SSRI) of unclear benefit in migraine prevention
Miscellaneous		
• Naproxen (Aleve) 500–1,000 PO QD	GI upset, peptic ulcers, coagulopathy, renal dysfunction	Short course therapy may be helpful for menstrual migraines: daily $\times$ 1 week
• Butterbur 75 mg BID	GI upset	Good response after 4 months of treatment shown in studies
• Coenzyme Q 100 mg TID	Well tolerated	Potential benefit demonstrated in multiple studies. Three months to full effect. Improves mitochondrial function
• Riboflavin (Vitamin B2) 400 mg daily	Few side effects	Improves mitochondrial energy metabolism. Studied in pediatric populations also. Low cost
• Feverfew 6.25 mg TID (6.25–18.75 mg TID)	Potential ill effects from long term COX-2 inhibition: i.e., GI, pulmonary, coagulation	Exact mechanism unclear, but thought to work by through inhibition of cyclooxygenase-2 (COX-2), interleukin-1 and tumor necrosis factor

(continued)

Table 18.2 (continued)

Medication	Adverse effects	Notes
• Magnesium 300 mg daily (300–600 mg/day)	Diarrhea, GI upset with higher doses	Shown to be effective in certain patients. May help in preventing aura
• Botulism Toxin Type A (Botox) 100 units	Few reports of ptosis, blurry vision, hematoma at injection site	Long duration of action, requiring injections every 3 months for continued effect. Good option for refractory migraine or in patients with poor compliance with, or tolerance for other preventative strategies
• Acupuncture	Rare. Patients must be tolerant of needles	Difficulty in conducting double-blind, randomized controlled trials to minimize sham, placebo or practitioner-specific effects confounds results. Nonetheless, considered by some to be extremely beneficial in migraine prevention when employed regularly. Effects may be due to release of endogenous opiates and to the serotonergic descending pain inhibitory pathway

- Topiramate (Topamax)
- Topiramate is an antiepileptic that blocks voltage-sensitive sodium and voltage-activated calcium channels, inhibits glutamate release, and increases gamma amino butyric acid (GABA) levels. It has been shown in several studies to be safe, effective, and well tolerated in migraine prevention. Side effects include paresthesias, anorexia, dizziness, and difficulty with word finding.

Abortive Medications

Using the patient's headache diary to determine migraine pattern, severity and frequency, and considering any other health conditions, a step-wise, individualized pharmacologic management plan should be formulated. For milder headaches, over-the-counter medications may be adequate.

- Nonsteroidal anti-inflammatory drugs (NSAIDS) and nonopiate analgesics
- The majority of migraine sufferers does not seek advice from their primary care physicians, but instead self-medicate with over-the-counter analgesics.

Interestingly, the addition of an antiemetic may significantly improve the efficacy of these regimens.

- A 2010 Cochrane analysis of ten recent studies showed that compared to placebo, 1,000 mg PO acetaminophen was effective in relieving migraine pain, nausea, photophobia, and phonophobia. When 10 mg PO metoclopramide was added to this acetaminophen dose, results were comparable to 100 mg PO sumitriptan [30]. Another 2010 Cochrane review of nine relevant studies showed that 200–400 mg PO ibuprofen was effective in relieving pain and associated migraine symptoms by 2 h in 26% of patients (versus 12% in the control groups). A separate Cochrane review showed that 400 mg PO ibuprofen was as effective as 1,000 mg PO aspirin. There was no information about adding anti-emetics. Adverse effects were rare, but caution should be employed in patients with impaired renal function or history of gastrointestinal ulcers or bleeding [31].
- Oral NSAIDS alone, or in combination with caffeine and/or an anti-emetic are a reasonable first-line choice for mild to moderate migraines. Ketorlac IM may be administered as a rescue agent in the hospital or emergency room, but the evidence for its efficacy is mixed.
- Antiemetics
- Oral antiemetics are a useful adjunct for the nausea and vomiting associated with migraine. Metoclopramide IM/IV is particularly effective, and has also been used as migraine monotherapy. Prochloperazine IV, IM and PR and chlorpromazine IV are similarly effective in many patients.
- Triptans
- Triptans are the first-line treatment for migraine, and are specifically approved by the Federal Drug Administration (FDA) for the treatment of migraines (see Table 18.3). They are high-affinity serotonin $(5\text{-HT})_{1B/1D}$ receptor agonists with several mechanisms of action, and with few pharmacodynamic differences between the different triptans available. They cause vasoconstriction of dilated meningeal, dural, extracerebral, and pial blood vessels via the 5HT 1B receptors, inhibit release of nociceptive neuropeptides (e.g., substance P, neurokinin) from trigeminal nerve terminals via presynaptic 5-HT 1D receptors , and inhibit ascending thalamic transmission of painful sensory afferents via 5-HT 1D receptors in the trigeminal nucleus caudalis region of the brainstem. This drug class is very effective in targeting migraine pain relief, but is neither preventative nor curative, requires a prescription, and is relatively expensive. Triptans are well tolerated with few side effects and a well-established safety record. They are available in oral, subcutaneous, parenteral, and intranasal preparations, although more than 80% of all triptan prescriptions are for the oral formations. However, because of their vasoconstrictive effect, they are contraindicated in patients with hypertension, cardiovascular, or peripheral vascular discase, arrhythmias, severe liver disease and in those patients concurrently prescribed monoamine oxidase (MAO) inhibitors. There have been reported associations with stroke and myocardial ischemia, but the overall risk appears to be minimal when prescribed

Table 18.3 Triptans

Medication	Dosing	Notes
• Sumatriptan (Imitrex)	25, 50, 100 mg PO 5, 10, 20 mg IN spray 4, 6 mg SC injection	Patients with nausea and vomiting, as well as pediatric populations, seem to benefit from the intranasal and subcutaneous forms. Half-life of 2.5 h
• Zolmitriptan (Zomig)	2.5, 5 mg PO 5 mg IN spray	2.5, 5 mg PO disintegrating tablets also available. Half-life of 3 h
• Naratriptan (Amerge)	1, 2.5 mg PO	Half-life of 6 h
• Rizatriptan (Maxalt)	5, 10 mg PO	Half-life of 2–3 h
• Eletriptan (Relpax)	20, 40, 80 mg PO	Half-life of 4 h
• Almotriptan (Axert)	6.25, 12.5 mg PO	12.5 mg dosing tends to be most effective. Half-life of 3–4 h
• Frovatriptan (Frova)	2.5 mg PO	Long half-life (26 h) makes this a good choice for longer migraines, such as menstrual migraines
• Sumatriptan + Naproxen (Treximet)	The recommended dose is one tablet (85 mg of sumatriptan and 500 mg of naproxen sodium)	Combination of a triptan with an NSAID. Contraindicated in third trimester of pregnancy and during lactation, and caution with asthma. Half life of 2 h (sumatriptan) and 12–17 h (naproxen). Do not take a second dose within 2 h of the first. Do not take more than two tablets in 24 h

to lower-risk patient populations. They are all FDA Pregnancy Category C. Although extremely successful as abortive medications, triptans must be used cautiously to guard against medication-overuse ("rebound" or "drug induced") migraines. Some practitioners recommend acute therapy no more than two headache days per week on a regular basis. Requiring more than this amount likely indicates that preventive therapy is required.

- Opioids and barbiturates
- Neither opioids nor barbiturates are FDA-approved migraine treatments. Opioids include morphine, codeine, and the opioid-containing drugs OxyContin (oxycodone), Percocet (acetaminophen and oxycodone), and Vicodin (acetaminophen and hydrocodone). Barbiturate-containing drugs include Fiorinal (aspirin, butalbital, and caffeine) and Fioricet (acetaminophen, butalbital, and caffeine). A 2007 survey by the National Headache Foundation found that neither opioids or barbiturates are regularly prescribed as first-line migraine treatments, but that when another first treatment fails, 25% of general practitioners—but only 7% of neurologists—prescribe these drugs as second-line treatments. There may still be a limited role for these opioids, such as for pregnant patients, or for patients with heart disease, hypertension, or stroke history, for whom triptans are not an option. However, opioids are clearly linked to causing rebound headaches [19].

Chronic ("Transformed") Migraine

Chronic migraine, previously known as transformed migraine, is defined by having 15 or more headache days per month for more than 3 months. Chronic migraines may be less intense, but more disabling and less responsive to treatment. There are multiple genetic and environmental risk factors for transformation from episodic to chronic migraine, including female gender, Caucasian race, lower socioeconomic status, obesity, depression, sleep disorders, frequent life stressors, and the overuse of caffeine and acute-headache medications (analgesics, triptans, opioids, and ergotamine) [32]. The exact mechanisms of chronic migraine transformation are unclear, but physiologic alterations are demonstrable in chronic migraine patients. Magnetic resonance imaging and positron emission tomography reveal baseline hyperexcitability in the occipital cortex and neuronal changes within the periaqueductal gray matter, thalamus, and trigeminovascular system. Also, cerebrospinal fluid studies demonstrate increased levels of inflammatory neuropeptides, suggestive of persistent activation of nociceptive pathways. This "central sensitization," whereby the threshold for peripheral nociceptive input and central processing is reduced, seems to be the anatomic basis for chronic migraine pathology.

In regard to treatment options for chronic migraine, one of the most promising agents is topiramate (Topamax), a GABA agonist, because it reduces cortical hyperexcitability. Cutaneous allodynia is poorly responsive to triptan therapy, because triptans cannot block ongoing sensitization of trigeminovascular neurons, making successful headache treatment more challenging in these patients.

Refractory Migraines

There is a small but significant subgroup of migraine patients who do not respond to accepted therapies, and who are considered to have refractory migraines. Rarely, they may require care in-patient therapy, such as parenteral analgesics, antiemetics, steroid, fluid or possibly, hyperbaric oxygen therapy (HBOT). Refractory patients may also be offered preventative drug treatments with higher risks of side effects or toxicity.

- Transcranial magnetic stimulation
- Noninvasive transcranial magnetic stimulation for the acute treatment of migraine with aura has been shown in clinical trials to be effective in aborting headache pain and in providing sustained pain relief at 24 and 48 h after treatment, with minimal side effects. It may be a tool for certain patients in whom aura signals an impending migraine, to neutralize headache progression. Optimum dosing, appropriate patient populations and overall cost-effectiveness are yet to be fully elucidated for this therapy, however [33].
- Hyperbaric oxygen therapy (HBOT)
- A recent Cochrane review of nine trials showed that there is some weak evidence that hyperbaric oxygen therapy, the therapeutic administration of 100% oxygen at environmental pressures greater than one atmosphere, may be effective in the treatment of acute migraine attacks. Pooled data from three trials found evidence that 70% of study patients obtained noticeable relief within 40 min of initiating hyperbaric oxygen compared to a sham therapy. There is no evidence that it can reduce the incidence of nausea and vomiting or decrease requirements for rescue medication. As well, neither normobaric nor hyperbaric oxygen therapy has been shown to have any effect in preventing migraine episodes. No serious adverse effects have been recorded in studies to date on HBOT for migraine treatment. However, high-dose oxygen may increase oxidative stress through free radical species. Precautions against chamber fire in the oxygen rick environment must be followed. Also, HBOT may cause aural, sinus, or pulmonary barotrauma from supra-atmospheric pressures. Other risks include temporary worsening of short-sightedness and claustrophobia. HBOT is relatively expensive and requires complex equipment not readily available in many locations. It has not been specifically studied in refractory migraine populations and cannot be recommended as a routine therapy [34].
- Steroids
- For acute relief of severe, refractory headaches, such as patients who are withdrawing from overuse of acute care medications, IV corticosteroids may alleviate the severity of migraine pain. A British Medical Journal reviewed seven relevant randomized, control trials conducted in Emergency Departments from 1999 to 2008,

in which corticosteroids were compared to placebo for efficacy in acute migraine relief and prevention of recurrence at 72 h. Each trial, consisting of 55–205 participants, included a standard abortive migraine treatment plus the addition of 10–25 mg IV dexamethasone or a saline placebo. Dexamethasone and placebo were equally effective at acute pain reduction, but dexamethasone was more successful at reducing headache recurrence at 72 h [35]. No significant side effects were found. The reviewers did not have enough data to perform subgroup analysis to determine which migraine patients had most favorable results or to compare differences between abortive agents chosen.

- Migraine surgery
- Certain patients who experience severe migraines may be candidates for surgical decompression of peripheral nerves that act as migraine triggers. Surgical intervention is a novel alternative for those patients who do not respond adequately to traditional therapies or who cannot tolerate medication side effects. Dissection of the supraorbital, supratrochlear, greater occipital, and various trigeminal nerve branches have been described to deactivate frontal, temporal, and occipital trigger sites, with excellent outcomes [26]. Careful patient selection is extremely important, including a trial of injections with local anesthetic or botulinum toxin in the described trigger sites to determine potential effectiveness of surgical decompression. If trial with botulinum yields significant improvement (at least 50% reduction from baseline frequency and/or severity for at least 4 consecutive weeks), then surgical treatment of the peripheral nerve triggers can be considered [20].

Special Populations/Comorbidities

Pregnancy and Lactation

Migraine frequency tends to decrease during pregnancy, although some women have worse headaches early in pregnancy until their hormones levels stabilize. By the third trimester almost 90% of migraineurs report significant improvement [36]. The use of triptans, barbiturates, and aspirin-containing medications remain controversial. Of the seven triptans marketed in the USA, three have voluntary pregnancy registries. Animal studies conducted on each of the triptans suggest that these drugs are relatively safe, and may be used if benefits outweigh risks. One observational study suggested an increased risk of preterm delivery and low birth weight term newborns [37]. Acetaminophen, opioids, and appropriate antiemetics, such as prochlorperazine (Compazine) are the treatment options of choice for migraines during pregnancy. Ergot alkaloids are contraindicated [37]. For prophylaxis, beta blockers have been well studied in pregnancy, with few negative findings. Occipital nerve blocks may also be employed.

A rebound increase in migraine severity tends to occur after delivery unless the patient is breast feeding, in which case, this relapse may occur after cessation of lactation, and resumption of regular menstrual cycles. Triptans are detected in breast milk, but at very low levels unlikely to affect the infant.

Pediatric Populations

Migraine is a prevalent disease in children and adolescents, estimated to be up to 20% in the older age groups. Presentation is generally similar to adult patients, except that children may have migraines that are of shorter duration and with bilateral head pain. Also, in pediatric migraine clinical trials, there is noted to be a higher response to placebo interventions [38], making it more difficult to identify clinically helpful treatment strategies. There are not many randomized controlled trials published on pediatric migraine care.

With regard to the teenage population, inability to participate in sporting and social activities due to migraine headaches can be very distressing. As well, one study demonstrated a 4.6 times higher incidence of suicidal thoughts in teenagers who suffer from classic migraines headaches, compared to teenagers without migraines. Another independent factor noted in this study was headache frequency, with more than 7 days/month being significant. It was not clear from this research whether there was an associated increase in suicidal behaviors [39].

Medications found most consistently to be successful for pediatric patients include acetaminophen, ibuprofen, triptans (particularly 10–20 mg nasal sumitriptan), and intravenous prochlorperazine for emergency department rescue [40].

Prognosis

Migraine is a chronic disorder and its prognosis has not been well established in any given population of patients who suffer from this condition. There is wide variability in long-term outcomes, with some patients having complete remission, others partial remission, and still others a persistent, progressive course. In fact, a review from 2008 revealed that over a 1-year period, 84% of patient continued to have migraines, 10% had complete remission, 3% had partial remission, and another 3% developed chronic migraine. Risk factors associated with progression, such as obesity, depression, medication, and caffeine overuse, were confirmed in this study. Partial remission tends to increase with age, especially in postmenopausal females.

There are a number of studies suggesting an increased risk for ischemic stroke in patients with migraine, particularly women who experience migraine with aura. Fortunately, this association between migraine with aura and ischemic cerebrovascular events in otherwise healthy women also demonstrates good functional outcomes for these patients [16].

In summary, those patients who are effectively controlled with appropriate preemptive and abortive medications and lifestyle modifications (i.e., avoidance of known triggers) have a more optimistic chance of partial or complete remission from migraine than those patients who are incompletely or inadequately managed in the care of this serious condition.

Cluster Headache

Introduction

Cluster headache is a primary headache disorder characterized by attacks of excruciating unilateral pain with associated cranial parasympathetic symptoms and restlessness. These attacks are considered to be the most painful of any headache disorder, with some women sufferers comparing the pain as being worse than childbirth and others contemplating or attempting suicide during the attack as a way to end the pain. A hallmark of cluster headache is the regular periodicity of attacks. A cluster attack is a single instance of pain, whereas a cluster period, or cycle, is the period of weeks to months during which the attacks occur regularly. People of any age can be affected by cluster headache, with a mean onset of 29–35 years old. The prevalence of cluster headache is 0.1–0.2% of the population, based on European studies. Overall, the male:female ratio is 4.3:1. However, males are even more likely to have chronic cluster headache with a ratio of 15:1 compared to a male:female ratio of 3.8:1 for episodic cluster headaches [41, 42]. Epidemiological surveys indicate a genetic basis for cluster headache, with first-degree relatives being 5–18 times more likely to have cluster headache than the general population [43]. Cluster headache patients have a markedly decreased health-related quality of life and experience greater limitations in social function than patients with migraine. Greater than 75% of patients with cluster headache had restrictions in activities of daily living and 13% report activity inhibitions outside their cluster cycle [44].

Definition and Classification

Cluster headache belongs to the group of primary headache disorders referred to as trigeminal-autonomic cephalgias (TAC). This group is named for the distribution of pain in the first division of the trigeminal nerve and accompanying ipsilateral cranial autonomic symptoms.

Cluster headache is diagnosed clinically using the criteria defined by the *International Classification of Headache Disorders*, 2nd edition (Table 18.4) [45]. A cluster headache is strictly unilateral with pain usually occurring without warning and often being described as piercing, boring, or stabbing. The pain is associated with cranial parasympathetic symptoms on the same side as the pain, such as conjunctival injection or lacrimation, nasal congestion or rhinorrhea, eyelid edema, forehead or facial swelling, miosis or ptosis. Additionally, patients are usually

Table 18.4 Cluster Headache Criteria (The International Classification of Headache Disorders, 2nd edition)

(A) At least five attacks fulfilling B–D

(B) Severe unilateral orbital, supraorbital or temporal pain lasting 15–180 min if untreated. During part (but less than half) of the time course of cluster headache, attacks may be less severe or of shorter or longer duration

(C) Headache is associated with at least one of the following:

  1. Ipsilateral conjunctival injection or lacrimation

  2. Ipsilateral nasal congestion

  3. Ipsilateral eyelid edema

  4. Ipsilateral forehead and facial sweating

  5. Ipsilateral miosis or ptosis

  6. A sense of restlessness or agitation

(D) Attacks have a frequency from one every other day to eight per day. During part (but less than half) of the time course of cluster headache, attacks may be less frequent

(E) Not attributable to another disorder

Episodic cluster headache

(A) Attacks fulfilling the criteria for cluster headache

(B) At least two cluster periods lasting 7–365 days and separated by pain-free remission periods of greater than 1 month. Cluster periods generally last between 2 weeks and 3 months

Chronic cluster headache

(A) Attacks fulfilling the criteria for cluster headache

(B) Attacks recur for greater than 1 year without remission or remission periods less than 1 month

agitated, unable to lie down, and characteristically pace the floor during an attack. Cluster headaches have a frequency from one every other day to eight per day. However, the majority of subjects have one to two headaches daily for weeks to months at a time. To fulfill the criteria for cluster headache, one must have a history of at least five attacks that cannot be attributed to any other disorder. As many as 90% of cluster headaches are episodic, which is defined as having attacks for 7 days to 1 year with a break of at least a month between cycles for at least two cycles. In chronic cluster headache, attacks recur over 1 year without remission, or have remission periods less than 1 month.

Etiology and Pathophysiology

The pathophysiology of cluster headache is not fully understood and the disorder has been known by many names (Table 18.5). Major features of cluster headache are a trigeminal distribution of pain, cranial autonomic symptoms, and an episodic pattern of attacks [4]. Triggers of cluster headache include alcohol, nitroglycerine, exercise, and elevated environmental temperatures. Classically, cluster headache was referred to as a vascular headache based on an angiographic observation of localized narrow-

Table 18.5 Older terms for cluster headache

• Erythroprosalgia of Bing	• Petrosal neuralgia (Gardner)
• Ciliary neuralgia	• Vidian neuralgia
• Migrainous neuralgia	• Sluder's neuralgia
• Erythromelgia of the head	• Hemicrania angioparalytica
• Horton's headache	
• Histaminic cephalgia	

Modified from [46]

ing of the internal carotid artery in the region of the cavernous sinus made during an acute cluster headache. More recent theories implicate a neuronal discharge triggering vascular change. Pain afferents from the trigeminovascular system transmit signals from the cranial vessels and dura mater to the trigeminocervical complex, trigeminal nucleus caudalis, and dorsal horns of C1 and C2. This, ultimately leads to activation of the frontal and cingulated cortices, causing unilateral head pain. Reflex autonomic activation of the parasympathetic nervous system via the facial nerve (CN VII) acts in a positive feedback manner, causing lacrimation, eye reddening, nasal congestion, and a partial Horner's Syndrome. Neuropeptide release from central and peripheral synapses of trigeminal neurons, particular vasodilatory peptides substance P, calcitonin gene-related peptide, and vasoactive intestinal polypeptide, is a potential cause for cluster headache [46, 47].

Observations of the seasonal variation and circadian timing of cluster headaches suggest the hypothalamus, as a regulator of biological rhythms, plays a role in these attacks. Abnormalities in the serum levels of testosterone, cortisol, and growth hormone during cluster periods have been demonstrated, further implicating the hypothalamus as having a role in cluster headaches [48]. Positron emission tomography imaging of nitroglycerin induced and spontaneous cluster attacks have identified an activated area in the posterior hypothalamic gray area that is particular to cluster headache [49].

Diagnosis

Proper classification of the headache is important to identify potential secondary causes of headaches that may require investigation. Many individuals with headaches that have a typical history, clinical picture, and response to treatment have been found to have a secondary cause on neuroimaging [50]. Patients who present with a presumed diagnosis of cluster headache likely warrant a brain magnetic resonance imaging scan. Identifying the attacks as cluster headache gives clarity to the patient and focuses the treatments offered by the physician. Even among the headaches in the TAC group with similar features, patients can experience very different responses to treatments.

With cluster headache being a relatively rare primary headache disorder, a high index of clinical suspicion is required to make the diagnosis. Assessment includes a thorough history and physical, including a neurological examination. A detailed history of the patient's headaches should be sought, especially detailing the site of pain, associated symptoms, periodicity, duration of symptoms, and family history. Known triggers of cluster headache include alcohol ingestion and vasodilators, such as nitroglycerine and histamine; these triggers are known to only precipitate a cluster attack during a cluster period [51]. During a particular cluster cycle, headaches always occur on the same side of the head and have a similar severe intensity, although the attacks at the beginning and end of a cycle may be submaximal. Most headaches will remain unilateral on the same side throughout an individual's history. Less frequently, the attack may switch sides from one cluster cycle to another. The attacks often display great regularity. Commonly, a patient will have one to two headaches a day, each occurring at approximately the same time of day and may even display seasonal variation in the early course of the disorder. Approximately 50% of the attacks occur during the night, usually occurring 90 min after the onset of sleep.

Treatment Options

The pharmacologic treatments for cluster headache can be divided into three categories: abortive, transitional, and preventive. These treatments are discussed in detail below (see Table 18.6).

Abortive Treatment

Due to the sudden onset and short duration to peak intensity of cluster attacks, desirable characteristics of abortive treatments include fast onset, high bioavailability, reliable headache relief, and minimal side-effects, even with multiple doses daily. Subcutaneous sumatriptan, a 5-hydroxytryptamine receptor agonist, is the most effective self-administered abortive cluster headache treatment and the only pharmaceutical treatment that is FDA-approved specifically for cluster headache. In a placebo-controlled trial, subcutaneous sumatriptan 6 mg was significantly more effective than placebo at 15 min, with 74% of patients reporting complete relief compared to 26% of those taking the placebo [52, 53]. The maximum recommended dose of sumatriptan by injection is 12 mg/day. Contraindications to sumatriptan, as with other medications from this class, are uncontrolled hypertension or a history of myocardial infarction or stroke.

Intranasal sumatriptan has also been shown to be significantly more effective than placebo, although it is not as efficacious as the injectable route. In a randomized, placebo-controlled study comparing intranasal sumatriptan 20 mg to placebo, the 57% of patients taking the study medication reported an improvement in pain from severe or very severe to mild or moderate at 30 min and 42% were pain-free at

Table 18.6 Medications for cluster headache

Medication	Adverse effects/contraindications	Notes
Abortive treatment		
Sumatriptan 6 mg SC (up to 12 mg daily)	Injection site reaction, nausea/vomiting, dizziness, fatigue, paresthesias. Contraindicated in patients with coronary artery disease, uncontrolled hypertension	First-line treatment
Sumatriptan 20 mg IN	Bitter taste	
Zolmitriptan 5–10 mg PO	Paresthesias, nausea, dizziness	
Zolmitriptan 5 mg intranasal	Unpleasant taste, nasal discomfort, somnolence, dizziness, throat tightness	
Oxygen 7–15 L/min by nonrebreather mask for 15–20 min	Safety concerns with smoking	First-line treatment
Lidocaine 4% IN 1 spray every 10–15 min	Nasal congestion, unpleasant taste	
Olanzapine 2.5–10 mg PO	Sedation	Indicated for patients that do not respond to oxygen and have contraindications to triptans
Chlorpromazine 25–50 mg PR		
Indomethacin 50 mg PR every 30 min (max 150 mg daily)		
Octreotide 100 mcg SC	Nausea, abdominal bloating, injection site reaction, dull background headache, lethargy	
Transitional treatment		
Prednisone 60–80 mg PO, tapered over 12 days		First-line transitional therapy
Dexamethasone 4 mg PO BID for 2 weeks followed by 4 mg PO daily for 1 week		
Dihydroergotamine 1 mg IM/IV BID-TID for 1–7 days Or ergotamine tartrate 2–4 mg PO daily	Contraindicated in patients with peripheral vascular disease, uncontrolled hypertension, coronary artery disease or pregnancy. Contraindicated within 24 h of using a triptan medication	

Greater occipital nerve blockade with 0.5 cc of lidocaine 2% with a mixture of long and short acting betamethasone (2.5 mL)	Transient injection site pain	
Naratriptan 2.5 mg PO BID for 7 days or Frovatriptan 2.5–5 mg daily	Nausea/vomiting, dizziness, fatigue, paresthesias. Contraindicated in patients with coronary artery disease, uncontrolled hypertension	
Preventive treatment		
Verapamil 240–960 mg PO daily, in divided doses (TID recommended)	Constipation, hypotension, dizziness, dry mouth, peripheral edema, weight gain, risk of AV block increases with doses over 480 mg/day	First-line treatment
Lithium carbonate 300–900 mg PO daily	Tremor, diarrhea, polyuria	
Valproic acid 500 mg PO qhs, up to 3,000 mg daily	Nausea, weight gain, hair loss, tremor, lethargy. Possible pancreatitis, thrombocytopenia, or hepatic dysfunction	
Topiramate 25–200 mg PO daily	Paresthesias, fatigue, anorexia, nausea, cognitive impairment	
Gabapentin 100–300 mg PO TID	Sedation, dizziness, paresthesias, teratogenic	
Melatonin 9–10 mg qhs	None	
Civamide 25 mcg IN	Nasal burning, lacrimation, pharyngitis, rhinorrhea	
Baclofen 15–30 mg PO 3–4 times daily	Sedation	

this time, compared to 26% and 18%, respectively for placebo [54]. Similarly, intranasal zolmitriptan 5 and 10 mg have been shown to be effective in the treatment of cluster headache; patients with more frequent or less severe attacks may benefit more from the 5 mg dose compared to the 10 mg dose since this may be taken more frequently and possibly tolerated better [55, 56]. Triptans can be used up to three times daily when administered intranasally. Oral zolmitriptan has been shown to be more effective than placebo at alleviating episodic cluster headaches. In a double-blind, randomized, crossover study of 124 patients, headache response, defined as a 2-point reduction on a 5-point scale at 30 min, for patients taking placebo, 5 mg, and 10 mg PO zolmitriptan was 29%, 40%, and 47%, respectively; this was statistically significant for 10 mg zolmitriptan compared to placebo [57]. In the same study, there was no significant difference between the treatments in patients with chronic cluster headaches. At one time, cluster headache patients were thought to be free from the risk of medication overuse headaches. More recent studies, however, suggest some patients may experience increased frequency of their cluster headaches or a mild daily headache as a result of medication overuse [58, 59]. Many of the patients who have reported these symptoms had histories of migraine headaches or other frequent headache types.

Inhalation of 100% oxygen is an excellent abortive treatment for cluster headache. Doses of 7–15 L/min delivered by firm plastic nonrebreather mask for 15–20 min have been very effective. In a recent double-blind, randomized, placebo-controlled, crossover trial of 109 patients, oxygen, 12 L/min for 15 min rendered 78% of patients pain-free or with adequate pain relief compared to 20% of patients treated with high flow air [60]. There were no adverse effects associated with the use of oxygen and there is no limit to how many treatments can be used in a day. In a recent survey of 1,134 individuals with cluster headache in the USA, patients reported difficulties getting oxygen prescribed by their doctors, prescribed rates that are too low to be efficacious, a lack of proper training on use and safety and a significant expense in obtaining the medical grade oxygen [61]. There have been reports of an increased response to oxygen when used together with a triptan. While some patients may not experience significant headache relief from oxygen, a patient should not be considered refractory to oxygen treatment unless a trial of up to 15 L/min for 20 min has been completed.

Other possible abortive therapies for patients who have intractable cluster headache may be used on their own, but often are more effective when used to augment other abortive therapies. Intranasal 4% lidocaine, given as one spray to the ipsilateral nostril can be repeated every 10–15 min for a total of four doses per day [51, 62]. This therapy achieves a moderate reduction of pain in only one-third of patients. Olanzapine 2.5–10 mg administered orally is often very sedating, but may be useful in patients who cannot use triptans or who have failed oxygen therapy [63, 64]. Chlorpromazine suppository 25–50 mg can also be used for abortive treatment [63]. While not classically responsive to nonsteroidal anti-inflammatory drugs, indomethacin suppository 50 mg can be repeated every 30 min up to 150 mg/day to abort a headache [63]. Subcutaneous octreotide, 100 mcg, was significantly superior to placebo in the treatment of cluster headache attacks in a randomized, placebo-controlled, double-blind crossover study of 57 patients with cluster headache [65].

Transitional Treatment

Preventive therapies are indicated in cluster headache due to the frequency of the attacks, with many people experiencing more than one attack per day, and the duration of cluster periods, lasting from weeks to months to years. To use abortive treatments as monotherapy would be exhausting and risk toxicity from multiple daily medication doses. Many preventive treatments take days to weeks to reach therapeutic levels. Thus, a transitional therapy is indicated to provide headache relief and bridge the gap between cluster headache diagnosis and the time when prophylactic therapy is efficacious. Oral prednisone, 60–80 mg PO tapered over 12 days, and dexamethasone have both been effective at inducing remission of cluster headache, typically within 24–48 h. In an open label study, 77% of 77 patients with episodic cluster headache had substantial headache relief and another 12% had partial relief [51]. The treatment is less efficacious in chronic cluster headache. Although headaches may recur after the completion of the corticosteroid taper, the long-term use of these medications is not advocated.

Dihydroergotamine, either daily intramuscular injections (1 mg once or twice daily) or intravenous infusion (1 mg BID or TID), is typically effective at stopping cluster headaches within 1–2 days of treatment; this effect can last days to months [51]. This treatment often requires that the patient be admitted for 3–7 days of treatment or use an outpatient infusion center. Dihydroergotamine is contraindicated in patients with peripheral vascular disease, coronary artery disease, uncontrolled hypertension, and during pregnancy. The use of sumatriptan and other vasoconstrictive agents cannot be used concurrently with dihydroergotamine therapy.

Greater occipital nerve blockade with corticosteroids has been shown to be an effective office treatment. In a placebo-controlled trial of 23 cluster headache patients treated with a 2.5 mL mixture of short- and long-acting betamethasone mixed with 0.5 mL of 2% lidocaine, 85% of the patients were attack free at 1 week and 61% of steroid-injected patients were attack free from within 72 h of treatment and 4 weeks after compared to no patients treated with saline and lidocaine alone [66]. The use of 2.5 cc of 0.5% bupivicaine combined with 20 mg methylprednisolone has also been described.

Preventive Treatment

Preventive agents are started in conjunction with the transitional therapy and are continued throughout the anticipated duration of the cluster period before being taped off. Continuing to take the preventive agent between cluster periods does not seem to prevent a subsequent cluster cycle from starting. Medications are typically titrated rapidly at the onset of preventive therapy to get the desired therapeutic response. Treatments are generally the same for both episodic and chronic cluster headache. Medications may be used in much higher doses than those used for other disorders when treating cluster headache. Polypharmacy may be required to adequately control cluster headaches. If a patient gets partial relief with one agent, adding another preventive agent may be beneficial.

Verapamil is typically the first-line preventive agent and can be used along with sumatriptan, ergotomine, or corticosteroids. The initial starting dose of 80 mg TID can be titrated over 3–5 days. Doses are then increased by 80 mg every 3–7 days until the desired therapeutic effect is met. Cluster headache patients may require up to 1,200 mg daily for headache control [63]. Another strategy would be to start a patient at 60 mg daily and increase by 80 mg daily every second week with electrocardiogram control [67]. Electrocardiograms are necessary prior to each dose increase above 480 mg daily and every 3–6 months while on stable doses above this threshold to evaluate for atrioventricular conduction abnormalities. In a study of 108 patients, 19% had abnormalities in the AV conduction while on verapamil with one patient requiring a permanent pacemaker [68].

Lithium carbonate is considered to be a standard preventive therapy, but has a narrow therapeutic window and a high side-effect profile. In multiple studies, 78% of chronic cluster headache patients and 63% of episodic cluster headache patients have improved while on lithium [63]. Standard doses range from 300 to 900 mg daily. During the initial treatment phase, serum lithium concentrations should be checked repeatedly to prevent toxicity. Prior to treatment, renal and thyroid functions need to be checked. Adverse effects often relate to tremor, diarrhea, polyuria, thyroid and renal dysfunction and cognitive effects.

Several antiepileptic drugs have shown promise in the preventive treatment of cluster headache. In several open label and retrospective studies, valproic acid treatment demonstrated favorable cluster headache response rates from 54 to 73% [69]. Although a double-blind, placebo-controlled study of valproic acid published in 2002 failed to show a significant improvement in the number of patients showing a 50% reduction in headaches compared to placebo, it is still considered an effective treatment for cluster headache [70]. Suggested dosing is extended release divalproex sodium starting at 500 mg at bedtime, increasing by 500 mg daily every 5–7 days to a maximum of 3,000 mg [63]. Reported side effects include nausea, weight gain, hair loss, tremor, and lethargy. Pancreatitis, thrombocytopenia, and hepatic dysfunction have also been reported. There is also clinical evidence from open-label studies that topiramate is efficacious in cluster headache at doses ranging from 25 to 200 mg daily [69]. Adverse effects, such as paresthesia, fatigue, anorexia, nausea, and cognitive impairment have limited its use. Limited clinical data show gabapentin to be a potentially effective preventive treatment for cluster headache that has been refractory to other agents. In a pilot open-label study of 12 patients with otherwise medically refractory cluster headaches, gabapentin was initiated at 100 mg TID and increased to 300 mg TID after 3 days and all patients were rendered headache free within 8 days with only minor side-effects (drowsiness) reported [69].

Melatonin, which is under the regulatory control of the hypothalamus, is a sensitive marker of circadian rhythm in humans. Serum melatonin concentration is reduced in patients with cluster headache during a cluster headache period. Melatonin 10 mg was evaluated in a double-blind, placebo-controlled trial. Cluster headache remission within 3–5 days occurred in five of ten patients treated with melatonin, compared to none in the placebo group [63]. Studies using lower doses of melatonin have not shown significant efficacy. Melatonin 9–10 mg has also been shown to decrease the doses of more traditional preventive treatments necessary to treat cluster headaches [63].

Civamide, a synthetic isomer of capsaicin, is a vanilloid receptor agonist and a neuronal calcium channel blocker that inhibits the release of excitatory neurotransmitters, such as substance P and calcitonin gene-related peptide, and depletes neurons of their neurotransmitter content. In a randomized, double-blind vehicle-controlled pilot study of 28 patients with cluster headache, 100 µl of 0.025% civamide (25 mcg) intranasally was shown to significantly decrease the frequency of cluster headache during the first post-treatment week [47]. The most common reported side effect was nasal burning after the application of the nasal spray. Further study is needed to determine the efficacy of civamide for longer-term preventive treatment of cluster headache.

Surgical Treatment

Surgical treatment for cluster headache may be considered for headaches that are refractory to medication management or when a patient's history precludes the use of typical cluster headache abortive and preventive medications. It is estimated that 10–20% of cluster headaches will fail to respond to medical therapy. Bilateral procedure may need to be considered in the minority of patients that experience cluster attacks that alternate sides. Early procedures aimed at the cranial parasympathetic system, or sectioning the greater superficial petrosal nerve, the nervus intermedius, or the sphenopalatine ganglion have provided inconsistent pain relief and are associated with a high rate of headache recurrence [63]. Procedures directed toward the sensory trigeminal nerve have been the most successful treatments, but are associated with the possibility of severe adverse effects. These procedures include alcohol injection into supraorbittal and infraorbital nerves, alcohol injected into the Gasserian ganglion, avulsion of the infraorbital, supraorbital, or supratroclear nerves, retrogasserian glycerol injection, radiofrequency trigeminal gangliorhizolysis, and trigeminal root section. Radiofrequency thermocoagulation is the most commonly used surgical technique and provides one of the best options for pain relief. In a retrospective analysis of 66 patients with refractory cluster headache treated with radiofrequency treatment of the sphenopalatine gangion, this therapy was found to be more effective in episodic cluster headache than in chronic cluster headache. In this analysis, 60.7% of 56 patients with episodic cluster headache experienced complete pain relief from 12 to 70 months compared to only three of ten patients in the chronic cluster headache group [71]. In a more recent review of 15 patients with intractable chronic cluster headache, a significant improvement in mean attack frequency and intensity for up to 18 months following radiofrequency treatment of the sphenopalatine ganglion [72]. Epistaxis, cheek hematoma, and reflex bradycardia have been reported following radiofrequency treatment of the sphenopalatine ganglion [73]. Additionally, complications of radiofrequency treatments include moderate to severe facial dysesthesia, corneal sensory loss, and anesthesia dolorosa [63]. Pulsed radiofrequency of the spenopalatine ganglion may have an improved side-effect profile compared to ablative treatments, but so far descriptions of this technique are limited to few case reports [73].

Hypothalamic stimulation is a treatment that has come about after positron emission tomography (PET) studies of patient's during cluster headaches. These studies indicated a unique activation of the ipsilateral inferior posterior hypothalamic gray matter with cluster headaches [49, 74]. While it is unclear whether this hypothalamic activation is a cluster headache generator or modulator, stimulation of the ipsilateral posterior hypothalamus has been shown to be efficacious in the improvement of medically intractable cluster headache. A recent review of multiple case series of deep brain stimulation found that approximately 60% of patients had a greater than 50% reduction in frequency or intensity of the cluster attacks [75]. While effective for medically refractory cluster headaches, deep brain stimulation does have a small risk of fatal hemorrhage [75]. The postoperative and stimulation-related side effect of visual disturbance has limited the amplitude and voltage of the stimulation [49, 75].

Occipital nerve stimulation is a promising treatment for refractory cluster headaches that involves placement of electrodes implanted in suboccipital region. In several small studies, approximately 60% of patients with an occipital nerve stimulator have experienced a greater than 50% reduction in headache severity or frequency [76, 77]. There has been a significant latency period of 2 months or more between the time of lead implantation and clinical effect [78]. Relatively few side effects, mostly related to lead migration or battery depletion, have been reported with this procedure [63]. The leads and impulse generator may be placed with the patient under general anesthesia and ultrasound guidance may be used effectively [79]. Occipital nerve stimulation does not seem to have same potential risks as deep brain stimulation and trigeminal nerve destruction and should be considered prior to these more invasive or ablative therapies.

Prognosis

For patients diagnosed with episodic cluster headache at onset, 80.7% will remain episodic, 12.9% will develop chronic cluster headache and 6.4% will develop a combined form within a 10-year period. For those patients diagnosed with the chronic form at onset, 52.4% will remain chronic, 32.6% will revert to episodic and 14.3% will develop a combined form of cluster headache. Poor prognosis may be related to an older age at onset, male gender, or disease duration greater than 20 years [42].

References

1. Ashkenazi A, Silberstein S. Headache management for the pain specialist. Reg Anesth Pain Med. 2004;29(5):462–75.
2. Edlow J, Panagos P, Godwin S, Thomas T, Decker W. Clinical policy: critical issues in the evaluation and management of adults patients presenting to the emergency department with acute headache. J Emerg Nurs. 2009;35(3):e43–71.

3. McConaghy J. Headache in primary care. Prim Care. 2007;34:83–97.
4. Headache Classification Subcommittee of the International Headache Society. The International Classification of Headache Disorders, 2nd edition. Cephalgia. 2004;24 Suppl 1:1–160.
5. Rogawski MA. Common pathophysiologic mechanisms in migraine and epilepsy. Arch Neurol. 2008;65(6):709–14.
6. Sanchex M, Reuter U. Pathophysiology of headache. Curr Neurol Neurosci Rep. 2003;3:109–14.
7. Parsons A. Cortical spreading depression: its role in migraine pathogenesis and possible therapeutic intervention strategies. Curr Pain Headache Rep. 2004;8:410–6.
8. Aurora S. Spectrum of illness – understanding biological patterns and relationships in chronic migraine. Neurology. 2009;72 Suppl 1:S8–13.
9. Romero-Reyes M, Graff-Radford S. Is there hope for chronic pain and headache? Headache. 2007;47(8):1262–71.
10. Grayson S, Neher J. When is neuroimaging warranted for headache? J Fam Pract. 2005;54(11):988–91.
11. Loeser JD, Butler SH, Chapman CR, Turk DC, editors. Bonica's management of pain. 3rd ed. Philadelphia: Lippincott Williams and Wilkins; 2001.
12. Harris JD, Kotob F. Management of opioid-related side effects. In: De Leon-Casasola OA, editor. Cancer pain: pharmacological, interventional and palliative care approaches. Philadelphia: Saunders Elsevier; 2006.
13. Bigal ME, Lipton RB. Clinical course in migraine: conceptualizing migraine transformation. Neurology. 2008;71:848–54.
14. Silberstein S. Practice parameter: evidence-based guidelines for migraine headache (an evidence-based review). Evidence-based guidelines in the primary care setting: neuroimaging in patients with nonacute headache. American Academy of Neurology; 2000. p. 1–25.
15. Evans R. Diagnostic testing for migraine and other primary headaches. Neurol Clin. 2009;27:393–415.
16. Pringsheim T, Davenport WJ, Becker W. Prophylaxis of migraine headache. CMAJ. 2010;182(7):E269–76.
17. Pringsheim T, Davenport WJ, Dodick D. Acute treatment and prevention of menstrually related migraine headache: evidence based review. Neurology. 2008;70:1555–63.
18. Bigal ME, Lipton RB. Excessive acute migraine medication use and migraine progression. Neurology. 2008;71:1821–8.
19. Mathew NT. Dynamic optimization of chronic migraine treatment: current and future options. Neurology. 2009;72 Suppl 1:S14–20.
20. Dodick D. Chronic daily headache. N Engl J Med. 2006;354:158–65.
21. Silberstein S. Preventive migraine treatment. Neurol Clin. 2009;27:429–43.
22. Colombo B, Annovazzi POL, Comi G. Therapy of primary headaches: the role of antidepressants. Neurol Sci. 2004;25:S171–5.
23. Lin J, Chen W. Review: acupuncture analgesia in clinical trials. Am J Chin Med. 2009;37(1):1–18.
24. Ozyalcin S, Talu G, Kiziltan E, Yucel B, Ertas M, Disci R. The efficacy and safety of venlafaxine in the prophylaxis of migraine. Headache. 2005;45:144–52.
25. Ashkenazi A, Levin M. Greater occipital nerve block for migraine and other headaches: is it useful? Curr Pain Headache Rep. 2007;11:231–5.
26. Saranitzky E, White M, Baker E, Baker W, Coleman C. Feverfew for migraine prophylaxis: a systematic review. J Diet Suppl. 2009;6(2):91–103.
27. Cady R, Schreiber C. Botulinum toxin type A as migraine preventative treatment in patients previously failing oral prophylactic treatment due to compliance issues. Headache. 2008;48:900–13.
28. Ashkenazi A, Silberstein S. Botulinum toxin type A for the treatment of headache, why we say yes. Arch Neurol. 2008;65(1):146–9.
29. Vargas BB, Dodick DW. The face of chronic migraine: epidemiology, demographics, and treatment strategies. Neurol Clin. 2009;27:467–79.

30. Rabbie R, Derry S, Moore R, McQuay H. Ibuprofen with or without an antiemetic for acute migraine headaches in adults. The Cochrane Pain, Palliative and Support Care Group, Cochrane Collaboration. Cochrane Database Syst Rev. 2010;(10):CD008039.
31. Loder E. Triptan therapy in migraine. N Engl J Med. 2010;363:63–70.
32. Lipton RB. Tracing transformation: chronic migraine classification, progression, and epidemiology. Neurology. 2009;72 Suppl 1:S3–7.
33. Lipton R, Dodick D, Silberstein S, Saper J, Aurora A, Pearlman S, et al. Single-pulse transcranial magnetic stimulation for acute treatment of migraine with aura: a randomized, double-blind, parallel-group, sham-controlled trial. Lancet. 2010;9:373–9.
34. Trentman TL, Zimmerman RS, Dodick DW, Dormer CL, Vargas BB. Occipital nerve stimulator placement under general anesthesia: initial experience with 5 cases and review of the literature. J Neurosurg Anesthesiol. 2010;22:158–62.
35. Bennett MH, French C, Schnabel A, Wasiak J, Kranke P. Normobaric and hyperbaric oxygen therapy for migraine and cluster headache. Cochrane Database Syst Rev. 2008;(3):CD005219. doi:10.1002/14651858.CD005219.pub2.
36. Colman I, Friedman B, Brown M, Innes G, Grafstein E, Roberts R, Rower B. Parenteral dexamethasone for acute severe migraine headache: meta-analysis of randomized controlled trials for preventing recurrence. BMJ. 2008;336(7657):1359–61. http://www.bmj.com.
37. Goadsby PJ, Goldberg J, Silberstein SD. Pregnancy plus: migraines in pregnancy. BMJ. 2008;336:1502–4.
38. Soldin OP, Dahlin J, O'Mara DM. Triptans in pregnancy. Ther Drug Monit. 2008;30(1):5–9.
39. Fernandes R, Ferreira J, Sampaio C. The placebo response in studies of acute migraine. J Pediatr. 2008;152(4):527–33.
40. Hershey AD. Teens, migraine, suicide and suicidal thoughts. Neurology. 2009;72:e621–62.
41. Bailey B, McManus B. Treatment of children with migraine in the emergency department. Pediatr Emerg Care. 2008;24(5):321–30.
42. Fischera M, Marziniak M, Gralow I, Evers S. The incidence and prevalence of cluster headache: a meta-analysis of population based studies. Cephalgia. 2008;28:614–8.
43. Broner SW, Cohen JM. Epidemiology of cluster headache. Curr Pain Headache Rep. 2009;13:141–6.
44. Russell MB. Epidemiology and genetics of cluster headache. Lancet. 2004;3:279–83.
45. Jensen RM, Lynberg A, Jensen RH. Burden of cluster headache. Cephalgia. 2007;27:535–41.
46. Goadsby PJ. Pathophysiology of cluster headache: a trigeminal autonomic cephalgia. Lancet. 2002;1:251–7.
47. Sicuteri F, Fanciullacci M, Nicolodi M, et al. Substance P theory: a unique focus on the painful and painless phenomena of cluster headache. Headache. 1990;30(2):69–79.
48. Saper JR, Klapper J, Mathew NT, et al. Intranasal civamide for the treatment of episodic cluster headaches. Arch Neurol. 2002;59:990–4.
49. McGeeney BE. Cluster headache and related disorders. Tech Reg Anesth Pain Manage. 2009;13:38–41.
50. Sillay KA, Sani S, Starr PA. Deep brain stimulation for medically intractable cluster headache. Neurobiol Dis. 2010;38:361–8.
51. Wilbrink LA, Ferrari MD, Kruit MC, Haan J. Neuroimaging in trigeminal autonomic cephalgias: when, how, and of what? Curr Opin Neurol. 2009;22(3):247–53.
52. Halker R, Vargas B, Dodick DW. Cluster headache: diagnosis and treatment. Semin Neurol. 2010;30:175–85.
53. The Sumatriptan Cluster Headache Study Group. Treatment of acute cluster headache with sumatriptan. N Engl J Med. 1991;325:322–6.
54. Gobel H, Linder V, Heinze A, Ribbat M, Deuschl G. Acute therapy for cluster headache with sumatriptan: findings of a one-year long term study. Neurology. 1998;51:908–11.
55. Van Vliet JA, Bahra A, Martin V, et al. Intranasal sumatriptan is effective in the treatment of acute cluster headache – a double-blind placebo controlled crossover study. Cephalgia. 2001;21:267–72.
56. Rapoport AM, Mathew NT, Silberstein SD, Dodick D, Tepper SJ, Sheftell FD, et al. Zolmitriptan nasal spray in the acute treatment of cluster headache. Neurology. 2007;69:821–6.

57. Cittadini E, May A, Straube A, Evers S, Bussone G, Goadsby PJ. Effectiveness of intranasal zolmitriptan in acute cluster headache. Arch Neurol. 2006;63:1537–42.
58. Bahra A, Gawel MJ, Hardebo JE, Millson D, Breen SA, Goadsby PJ. Oral zolmitriptan is effective in the acute treatment of cluster headache. Neurology. 2000;54:1832–9.
59. Paemeleire K, Bahra A, Evers S, Matharu MS, Goadsby PJ. Medication-overuse headache in patients with cluster headache. Neurology. 2006;67:109–13.
60. Paemeleire K, Evers S, Goadsby PJ. Medication-overuse headache in patients with cluster headache. Curr Pain Headache Rep. 2008;12:122–7.
61. Cohen AS, Burns B, Goadsby PJ. High-flow oxygen for treatment of cluster headache. JAMA. 2009;302(22):2451–7.
62. Rozen TD, Fishman RS. Inhaled oxygen and cluster headache sufferers in Untied States: use, efficacy and economics: results from the United States Cluster Headache Survey. Headache. 2011;51:191–200.
63. Evers S. Pharmacotherapy of cluster headache. Expert Opin Pharmacother. 2010;11(13):2121–7.
64. Rozen TD. Trigeminal autonomic cephalgias. Neurol Clin. 2009;27:537–56.
65. Rozen TD. Olanzapine as an abortive agent for cluster headache. Headache. 2001;41:813–6.
66. Matharu MS, Levy MJ, Meeran K, Goadsby PJ. Subcutaneous octreotide in cluster headache: randomized placebo-controlled double-blind crossover study. Ann Neurol. 2004;56:488–94.
67. Ambrosini A, Vandenheede M, Rossi P, Aloj F, Sauli E, Pierelli F, Schoenen J. Suboccipital injection with a mixture of rapid- and long-acting steroids in cluster headache: a double-blind placebo-controlled study. Pain. 2005;118:92–6.
68. Tfelt-Hansen P, Tfelt-Hansen J. Verapamil for cluster headache. Clinical pharmacology and possible mode of action. Headache. 2009;49:117–25.
69. Cohen AS, Matharu MS, Goadsby PJ. Electrocardiographic abnormalities in patients with cluster headache on verapamil therapy. Neurology. 2007;69:668–75.
70. Pascual J, Lainez MJA, Dodick D, Hering-Hanit R. Antiepilectic drugs for the treatment of chronic and episodic cluster headache: a review. Headache. 2007;47:81–9.
71. El Amrani M, Massiou H, Bouser MG. A negative trial of sodium valproate in cluster headache: methodological issues. Cephalgia. 2002;22:205–8.
72. Sanders M, Zuurmond WW. Efficacy of sphenopalatine ganglion blockade in 66 patients suffering from cluster headache: a 12- to 70-month follow-up evaluation. J Neurosurg. 1997;87:876–80.
73. Narouze S, Kapural L, Casanova J, Mekhail N. Sphenopalatine ganglion radiofrequency ablation for the management of chronic cluster headache. Headache. 2009;49:571–9.
74. Narouze S. Role of sphenopalatine ganglion neuroablation in the management of cluster headache. Curr Pain Headache Rep. 2010;14:160–3.
75. May A, Bahra A, Buchel C, et al. Hypothalamic activation in cluster headache attacks. Lancet. 2001;351:275–8.
76. Franzini A, Messina G, Cordella R, Marras C, Broggi G. Deep brain stimulation of the posteromedial hypothalamus: indications, long-term results and neurophysiological considerations. Neurosurg Focus. 2010;29(2):E13.
77. Ashkenazi A, Schwedt T. Cluster headache – acute and prophylactic therapy. Headache. 2011;51:272–86.
78. Burns B, Watkins L, Goadsby PJ. Treatment of medically intractable cluster headache by occipital nerve stimulation: long-term follow-up of eight patients. Lancet. 2007;369:1099–106.
79. Van Kleef M, Lataster A, Narouze S, Mekhail N, Geurts JW, van Zundert J. Cluster headache. Pain Pract. 2009;9(6):435–42.
80. Parsekyam D. Migraine prophylaxis in adult patients. West J Med. 2000;173:341–5.
81. Gersony W, Gersony D. Migraine headache and the patent foramen ovale. Circulation. 2010;121:1377–8.
82. Derry S, Moore A, McQuay H. Paracetamol (acetaminophen) with or without an antiemetic for acute migraine headaches in adults. The Cochrane Pain, Palliative and Support Care Group. Cochrane Collaboration. Cochrane Database Syst Rev. 2010;(11):CD008040.

Review Questions

1. What percentage of migraineurs experience aura?

   (a) Less than 10%
   (b) 15–20%
   (c) 40–50%
   (d) More than 80%

2. Common migraine triggers include all of the following *except*

   (a) Abrupt changes in sleep patterns
   (b) Hormonal fluctuations associated with the menstrual cycle
   (c) Sinus congestion associated with seasonal allergies
   (d) Tyramine containing foods, such as aged cheese and red wine

3. Which of the following is *not* a phase of the common migraine?

   (a) Prodrome
   (b) Aura
   (c) Headache
   (d) Postdrome

4. Which of the following treatments would be the least effective abortive agent for a cluster headache attack?

   (a) Sumatriptan 6 mg subcutaneous
   (b) Oxygen 12 L/min via nonrebreather mask
   (c) Lidocaine 4% intranasal spray
   (d) Verapamil 300 mg PO

5. A 33-year-old male patient with a past medical history significant only for episodic cluster headaches has been taking sumatriptan 6 mg subcutaneously twice daily over the past 2 weeks with partial relief of cluster headaches that occur 4–6 times daily. Which of the following would be the most appropriate next step in his treatment?

   (a) Deep brain stimulation of the posterior hypothalamus
   (b) Start dihydroergonovine 1 mg IM BID in addition to continuing his current therapy
   (c) Increase frequency of subcutaneous sumatriptan to three or four times daily
   (d) PO prednisone taper in addition to his current therapy

Answers

1. (b)
2. (c)
3. (b)
4. (d)
5. (d)

Chapter 19
Endoscopic Therapies for Palliation of Gastrointestinal Malignancies

Henry C. Ho and Uzma D. Siddiqui

Introduction

Malignant diseases of the gastrointestinal tract are often diagnosed at advanced stages when surgical options are limited. Due to involvement of luminal structures, obstructive symptoms are frequent. From a gastrointestinal standpoint, there are numerous endoscopic therapies available for palliative purposes to improve quality of life and short-term survival. Our experience with these techniques has improved with time and has provided alternatives to surgical or interventional radiology procedures. Furthermore, advances in imaging have allowed for better localization and planning of procedures.

Esophagus

Esophageal cancer is often diagnosed at an inoperable stage. Palliation of dysphagia and swallowing can be achieved via nonoperative techniques, thereby restoring nutritional status. In general, endoscopic techniques include those that ablate or displace neoplastic tissue. The principal techniques utilized for tissue ablation include argon plasma coagulation (APC), photodynamic therapy (PDT), and laser photoablation. Dilation and stent placement are used for displacement of malignant disease.

H.C. Ho, M.D. (✉)
Section of Digestive Diseases, Department of Internal Medicine,
Yale University School of Medicine, 333 Cedar Street, 1080 LMP,
New Haven, CT 06520-8019, USA
e-mail: henry.ho@yale.edu

U.D. Siddiqui, M.D.
Department of Medicine, University of Chicago Pritzker School of Medicine,
Chicago, IL, USA

N. Vadivelu et al. (eds.), *Essentials of Palliative Care*,
DOI 10.1007/978-1-4614-5164-8_19,
© Springer Science+Business Media New York 2013

First, APC is monopolar, noncontact, high-frequency electrocautery that uses ionized argon gas to cause tissue coagulation. Unfortunately, success with APC for malignant dysphagia has been limited. In one randomized study, 93 patients were treated with APC every 2–4 days until dysphagia improved. Patients were then randomized to APC alone or treatment with brachytherapy or PDT. Patients who underwent combination therapy had improved dysphagia-free period and limited side effects [1]. Unfortunately, as the depth of tissue ablation with APC is shallow, this technique is typically ineffective in ablating large, bulky tumors causing luminal obstruction [2]. There may be a role, however, in controlling surface hemorrhage from friable tumor masses or treating tumor in-growth in esophageal metal stents [3].

PDT uses a photosensitizing agent in combination with endoscopic, low-power laser exposure. The photosensitizing agent accumulates in malignant tissue after intravenous injection and the area is then endoscopically exposed to a laser that initiates a photochemical reaction to produce tumor necrosis [4]. Although the photosensitizing agent is typically cleared from tissue within a few days, several organs including skin can retain it for longer periods. Therefore, skin photosensitivity can be debilitating and may persist for 4–6 weeks. In a prospective, multicenter trial including 110 patients treated with PDT, 19% of patients experienced sunburn [5].

Laser photoablation using neodymium:yttrium-aluminum-garnet (Nd:YAG), potassium titanyl phosphate (KTP), and argon lasers have been used extensively in the palliation of malignant dysphagia. The majority of experience has been with the Nd:YAG laser; though this technique is generally reserved for large centers with expertise. The goal, as with the aforementioned ablative therapies, is to obliterate neoplastic tissue in order to restore luminal patency. Exophytic masses in the mid or distal esophagus are more easily accessed; however those near the esophagogastric junction or near the cricopharyngeus are difficult [6]. Treatments are performed at 48–72-h intervals over three to four sessions. In a consecutive study of 30 patients, luminal patency was achieved at 97%; however, only 70% of patients were able to achieve improved nutritional status to leave the hospital. Relief of symptoms lasted from 4 to 14 weeks [7]. Chest pain, odynophagia, low-grade fevers may occur post-procedure. Disadvantages to this technique include high cost, frequency of treatment sessions, and difficulty in managing long segments of tumor.

The endoscopic techniques that provide displacement of neoplastic tissue in the esophagus include esophageal dilation and stent placement. Esophageal dilation, however, provides only temporary palliation of malignant dysphagia and is often used as an adjunct to other therapies. Most patients experience symptom improvement from dilation to a luminal diameter of 12 mm (liquid to soft diet). Unfortunately, dilation can be complicated by perforation in up to 10% of cases [8]. Blind passage of Maloney dilators is not recommended in a complex malignant stricture due to higher risk of perforation [9]. Esophageal dilation with through-the-scope balloon (Fig. 19.1) or wire-guided polyvinyl bougie dilation catheter is most commonly used. Again, the effects of dilation are typically transient, which has led to the increasing use of esophageal stenting.

Esophageal stent use has increased rapidly due to ease of use and comparable outcomes to other palliative therapies for malignant dysphagia. Rigid plastic stents

Fig. 19.1 Endoscopic view of esophageal balloon dilation

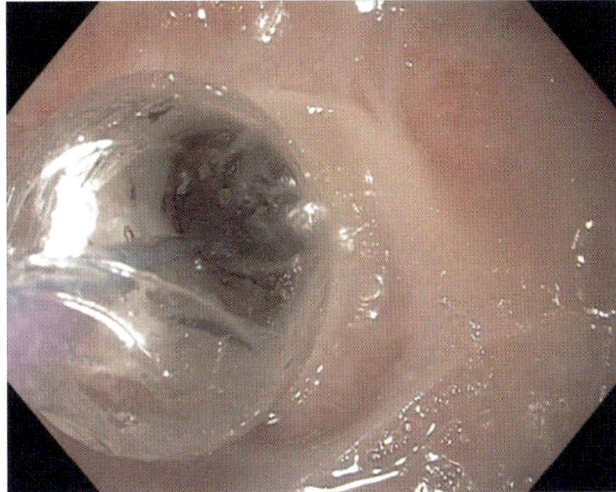

Fig. 19.2 Endoscopic view of esophageal stent

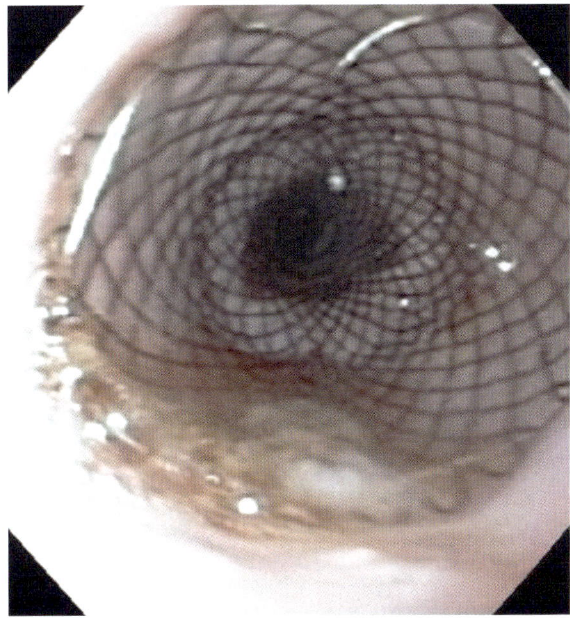

have been replaced by self-expanding metal stents (SEMS). Most SEMS are composed of nitinol, an alloy of titanium and nickel. SEMS are deployed over a guidewire under fluoroscopic guidance in cases where an endoscope cannot be passed beyond the obstructing tumor (Fig. 19.2). Oral contrast can be utilized with fluoroscopy to elucidate the lumen if the stricture is too narrow to accurately pass a guidewire. Accurate marking of the tumor margins (with recent contrast esophagram and initial endoscopic examination) in relation to the end of the SEMS is important. In addition,

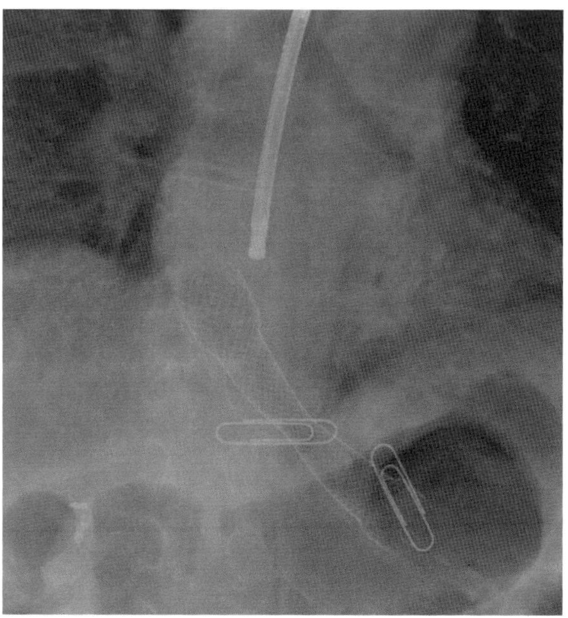

Fig. 19.3 Fluoroscopic view of esophageal stent

smaller caliber ultrathin endoscopes can often be passed beyond a tumor for passage of a guidewire and then placed alongside the guidewire allowing for stent deployment under both fluoroscopic and endoscopic guidance (Fig. 19.3).

Several variations in SEMS are available and include differences in coating (covered, partially covered, and uncovered/bare SEMS). The goal of fully covered stents is to prevent tumor in-growth and provide removability. However, they are associated with increased migration rates. Furthermore, fully covered metal stents are not approved by the Food and Drug Administration for removal (only self-expandable plastic stents are). Covered SEMS can be an effective treatment for management of esophagorespiratory fistula. SEMS vary in length from 7 to 19.5 cm. Due to high migration rates, more often completely uncovered or partially covered (ends are uncovered and body of stent is coated) SEMS are utilized for managing esophageal tumors. Uncovered metal stents cause tumor and tissue necrosis to occur and allow it to embed into the esophageal wall. There is little comparative information on different types of SEMS. Common complications of SEMS include migration, procedure-related perforation, food bolus impaction, reflux esophagitis, and aspiration (particularly when the stent is placed across the esophagogastric junction and patients are advised to not lie flat for 3–4 h after eating). In one study of 100 patients, 76 patients had covered SEMS and 14 patients had uncovered metal SEMS. Thirty percent of the patients had balloon dilation prior to SEMS insertion. Migration was noted in 5% of patients with an average time of 140 days; tumor in-growth through the stent and overgrowth at the stent ends was observed in less than 10% of cases [10]. Also of note, large proximal or mid-esophageal tumors should be evaluated

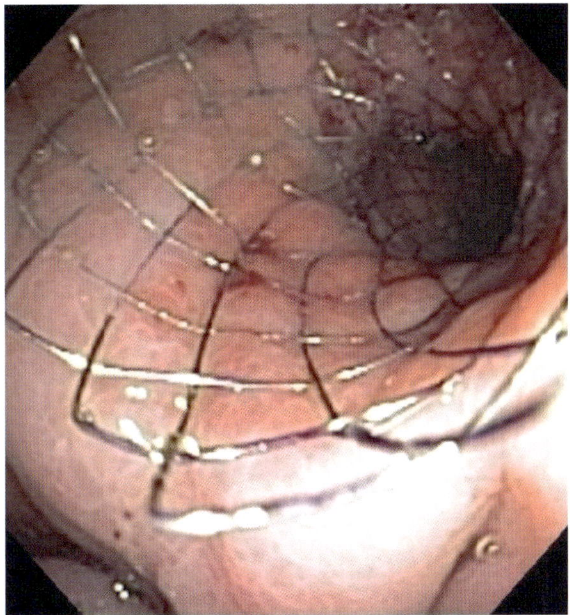

Fig. 19.4 Endoscopic view of enteral (duodenal) stent

for tracheal compression. Those patients may need airway stent placement prior to esophageal SEMS. Following stent placement, most patients should avoid dense and fibrous foods. SEMS placed across the esophagogastric junction allow constant flow of acid from the stomach and therefore patients are routinely placed on daily proton pump inhibitors. Though less effective, esophageal SEMS may also be placed for compression of the esophagus from extraesophageal malignancies.

Small and Large Intestines

Gastroduodenal obstruction most commonly occurs from pancreatic head cancer, gastric and duodenal cancers, and metastatic disease. Obstruction can lead to nausea, vomiting, malnutrition, and electrolyte imbalance. Traditionally, duodenal obstruction has been treated surgically with gastrojejunostomy. More recently, uncovered enteral stents have been developed. It should be noted, if there is known or impending malignant biliary obstruction, biliary stenting should be considered first since biliary access can be difficult after an enteral stent is placed into the duodenum.

There are dedicated duodenal or enteral stents that can be deployed through a therapeutic endoscope or colonoscope (Fig. 19.4). Often the diameter of the therapeutic endoscope (approximately 13 mm) is too large to pass through the point of obstruction.

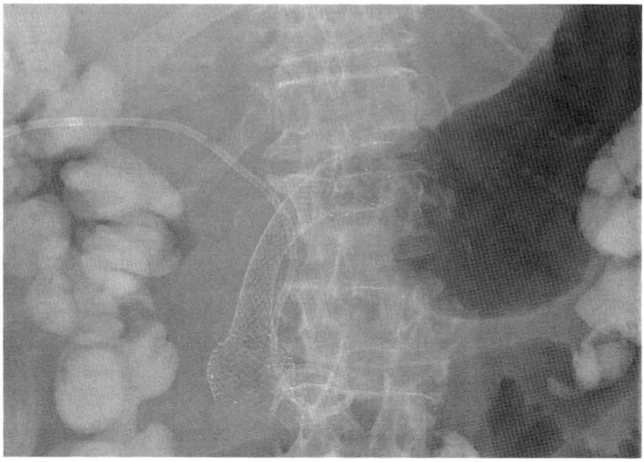

Fig. 19.5 Fluoroscopic view of enteral stent (with percutaneous biliary drain)

The length of the stricture can be assessed with injection of a radio-opaque contrast agent and passage of a guidewire under endoscopic and fluoroscopic guidance (Fig. 19.5). Complications related to the procedure include stent malposition, perforation and bleeding; later migration, fistula formation, perforation and bleeding can occur. While enteral stenting seems to have a similar success rate compared to surgical palliation, many patients require re-intervention. With the arrival of newer enteral stents, the levels of technical and clinical success are quite high. In a systematic review, stent insertion in 606 patients had 97% technical success in placement and 87% of patients achieved clinical success and were able to take a soft solids or a full diet within 4 days. Bleeding or perforation was noted in only 1.2%; and migration in 5%, which were mostly managed with additional stent placement. Stent obstruction did occur in 18%, mainly due to tumor infiltration or tumor overgrowth [11]. In another review of 44 publications on gastrojejunostomy and stent placement for palliation of gastric outlet obstruction, there were no major differences in technical success (96% versus 100%), early or late complications (7% versus 6% and 18% versus 17%), or persisting symptoms (8% versus 9%). Recurrent obstructive symptoms were more common after stent placement, however (18% versus 1%) [12].

Uncovered colonic SEMS have been proven to be effective in relieving malignant colonic obstruction before definitive resection or to palliate obstructive symptoms in advanced disease. In the first case, placement of a SEMS can allow optimization of a patient's medical status in order to avoid emergent surgery, which may be necessary if there is complete obstruction with signs of systemic toxicity. SEMS have also been used in proximal colon cancers, though most are treated with primary resection and anastomosis [13]. It can be helpful to obtain a rectal contrast CT or barium enema prior to colonic stent placement to assess anatomy. Some consider prophylaxtic antibiotics prior to stent placement, particularly if there is a significantly dilated colon due to the risk of microperforation and bacteremia. Since these SEMS can be deployed through the scope, it can be done under direct visualization (Fig. 19.6); fluoroscopic assistance can be helpful

Fig. 19.6 Endoscopic view of colonic stent

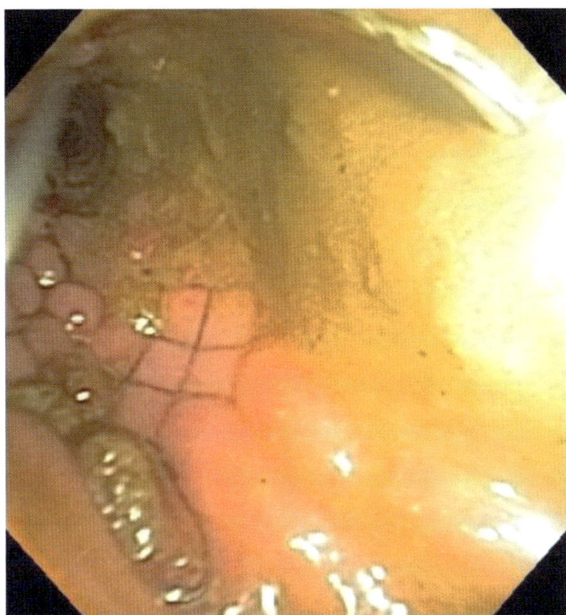

Fig. 19.7 Fluoroscopic view of colonic stent

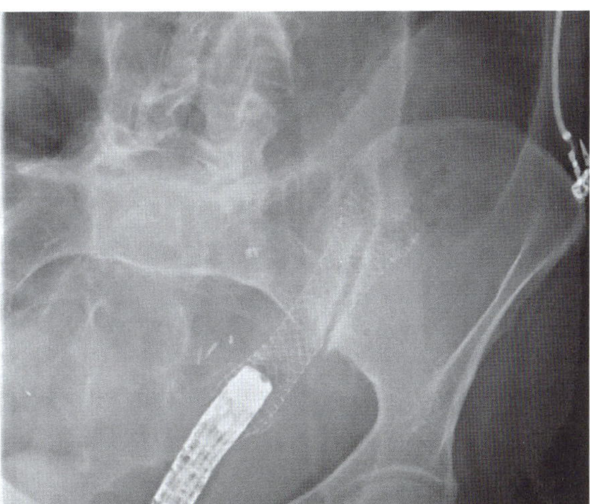

if the endoscope is unable to traverse the lesion (Fig. 19.7). Following stent deployment, patients should be advised to maintain soft stool consistency to avoid fecal impaction at the stent.

Complications include perforation, bleeding, abdominal pain, and migration. Perforation rates may be higher with antecedent radiation therapy or attempts at dilation at the time of stent placement. Failure to achieve decompression can be related to ineffective stent deployment across the lesion, extrinsic compression, early migration or fecal impaction. Stent failure could be managed with repeat stenting and APC or laser treatment of tumor ingrowth [14]. Post-procedure bleeding is typically minor and related to tumor friability. A randomized trial comparing stents versus surgery for palliation of malignant obstruction in the left colon was stopped prematurely due to a high rate of complications (including perforation rate of 13.7%) in the stent group on initial interim analysis [15]. Another study compared patency and complication rates between patients treated with stenting versus surgery over an 8-year follow-up. If patients were able to receive a second stent, similar late patency was achieved between surgical and stent groups. Regarding complications, however, in the stent group, two patients required emergent surgery for bowel perforation. Stent obstruction occurred in 7% requiring reintervention in all but one patient. In the surgical group, 4.1% patients died in the immediate postoperative period. Late complications appeared similar in frequency in both groups, requiring reintervention [16].

Pancreas and Biliary Tract

Multiple studies of patients with pancreatic cancer demonstrate that only 15–20% are resectable at the time of diagnosis [17]. Therefore, those with advanced disease commonly require palliation to relieve jaundice, duodenal obstruction, or pain. For malignant pancreaticobiliary obstruction, stents may be used as palliative measures for nonsurgical candidates in the setting of primary pancreaticobiliary malignancy, metastatic disease, or external biliary compression. Biliary decompression with endoscopically placed endoprosthesis via endoscopic retrograde cholangiopancreatography (ERCP) can prevent cholangitis and relieve jaundice and pruritis.

Endoscopic relief of malignant biliary obstruction can be achieved by placement of large-bore plastic or self-expanding metal stents (SEMS) across the malignant stricture. A key determination is the location of the stricture, whether distal to the bifurcation of the common hepatic duct or involving the bifurcation itself (hilar obstruction). Cross-sectional imaging is important prior to procedure to avoid attempts at drainage of an atrophic hepatic lobe or a lobe in which adequate drainage is not feasible due to significant metastatic disease. Injection of contrast during cholangiogram without subsequent drainage has increased risk of bacterial cholangitis.

The main limitation of plastic stents is the high rate of stent occlusion, but the advantage is easy removability. The median time for stent occlusion for standard large-bore plastic stents is approximately 3 months and patients need repeat ERCPs for stent change depending on their survival. Stent occlusion leads to cholestasis, recurrent jaundice, and usually cholangitis, which can be life-threatening (Figs. 19.8 and 19.9). SEMS, which can be uncovered or covered, have demonstrated superior patency due to the ability to resist bacterial biofilm coating on the stent. Uncovered SEMS are permanent and not typically removable endoscopically, whereas

Fig. 19.8 Endoscopic view of plastic biliary stent

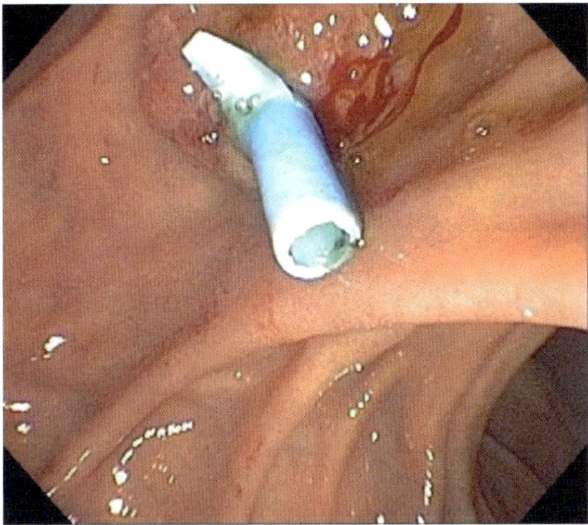

Fig. 19.9 Fluoroscopic view of plastic biliary stent

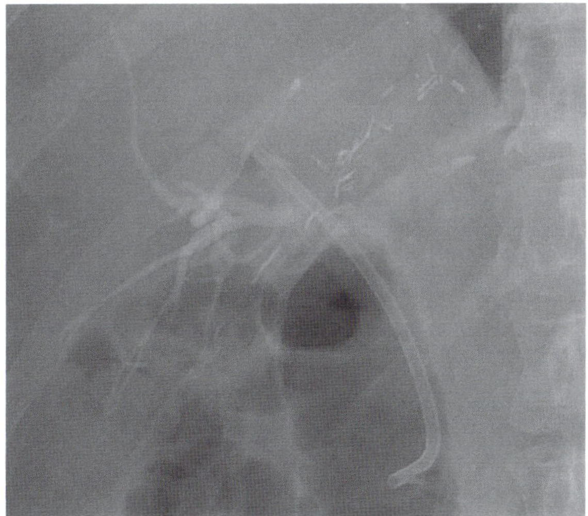

covered SEMS (CSEMS) can be removed endoscopically (Figs. 19.10 and 19.11). In a study comparing plastic to metal stents in advanced pancreatic cancer, stent occlusion was seen in 33% of patients with plastic stents after a median of 57 days; stent occlusion was only seen in 19% of metal stents after a median of 126 days [18]. Newer CSEMS have also been demonstrated to improve patency rates by resisting tumor overgrowth or tissue hyperplasia through the stent meshwork. In one study of unresectable distal biliary malignancies, stent occlusion was only 14% in the CSEMS group after a mean of 304 days compared to 38% after a mean of 166 days in the uncovered group [19]. Though in a meta-analysis comparing stent patency

Fig. 19.10 Endoscopic view of uncovered biliary SEMS

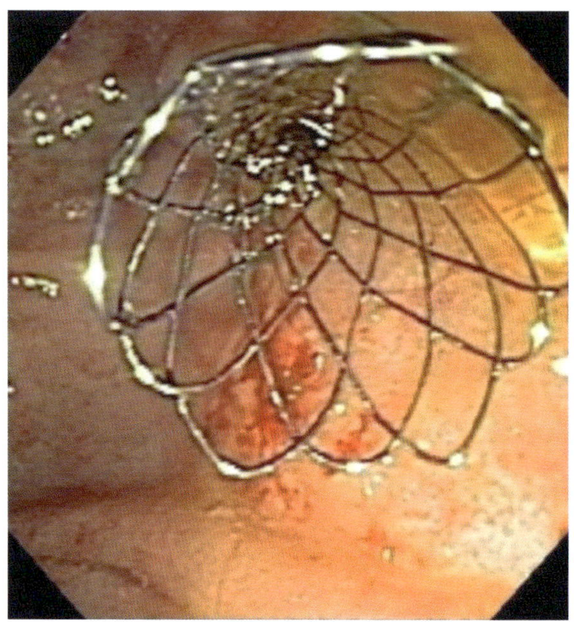

Fig. 19.11 Fluoroscopic view of uncovered biliary SEMS

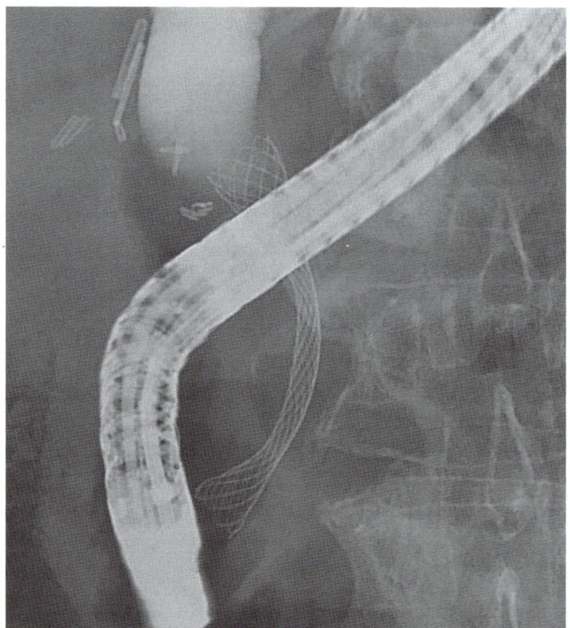

and survival of uncovered SEMS versus CSEMS, migration rates were higher in the CSEMS group in three different studies [20]. Because the cost of SEMS is much greater than plastic stents, placement of a SEMS is cost-effective generally if the patient survives longer than 3–6 months. Therefore, life expectancy is important when considering stent type. Furthermore, treatment of SEMS occlusion with further SEMS insertion can provide longer patency and survival and has been shown to be cost effective [21].

Pancreatic head cancer is the most common cause of malignant distal biliary obstruction. If resection is planned shortly after diagnosis, routine ERCP for biliary decompression may not be performed as complications may delay or prevent surgical resection. Indeed, a large, multicenter randomized study published in the *New England Journal of Medicine (NEJM) 2010* demonstrated that preoperative biliary drainage compared to surgery alone for patients with cancer of the head of the pancreas was associated with a higher rate of complications [22]. Patients were randomized to either preoperative biliary drainage for 4–6 weeks then surgery or surgery alone within 1 week of diagnosis. The rate of serious complication within 120 days was 39% in the early surgery group and 74% in the biliary drainage group. There has been criticism of this study, however, based on several issues including initial ERCP procedural failure rate of 25 and 46% of patients developing post-ERCP-related complications, both of which are quite high. Furthermore, stent occlusion accounted for the majority of cholangitis, which occurred in 26% of the stented group. If ERCP is performed, many endoscopists will favor placement of an SEMS for prolonged patency and then it can be resected along with tumor at the time of surgery or can be left in place for prolonged palliation if unresectable disease is found.

The indications for preoperative ERCP may therefore include acute cholangitis and severe pruritis. Stent placement is also indicated when neoadjuvant chemoradiation is administered because the time to surgical resection is usually prolonged. Studies have demonstrated improved outcomes for SEMS compared to plastic stents or surgical bypass in this clinical situation [23, 24]. However, the prior enthusiasm for preoperative stenting has been tempered by the aforementioned *NEJM* publication citing a high degree of complications.

Hilar strictures can be caused by cholangiocarcinoma or metastatic disease. The clinical success rate for achieving adequate palliation for hilar tumors is less than for distal lesions. Technical success rates for bilateral endoscopic stent placement are lower. Most patients with hilar obstruction can be palliated with only unilateral drainage. Patient whom have had both left and right biliary systems accessed during ERCP with contrast require stenting to prevent progressive cholangitis. It is not as clear that metal stents offer superior palliation compared to plastic stents for hilar tumors, as in the case of distal strictures. At this point, SEMS appear to offer improved palliation [25, 26]. From an endoscopic perspective, achieving successful drainage is more difficult technically for hilar tumors than for nonhilar tumors and a percutaneous approach may be necessary [27].

Photodynamic therapy (PDT) has been shown to be a feasible palliative treatment to reduce cholestasis. PDT involves systemic application of photosensitizing agent followed by localized illumination of the tumor at a specific wavelength [28]. PDT is not widely available, even in large tertiary care centers, and is only limited to endoscopists experienced in this technique. In addition, endobiliary bipolar radiofrequency ablation (RFA) has also been reported as a palliative treatment within the bile duct; though, published data are limited [29].

Pain Management

For patients with significant pain due to pancreatic adenocarcinoma, celiac plexus neurolysis can be offered and is discussed further in Chap. "Interventional Pain" of this book. Non-narcotic medical therapies are often inadequate for intense and refractory pain. Opioids commonly contribute to nausea and constipation, which can themselves be debilitating.

Celiac plexus neurolysis involves injection of absolute alcohol via CT-scan or endoscopic ultrasound (EUS)-guided techniques into the region of the celiac artery take-off from the aorta which is where the celiac ganglia are located. EUS guidance is usually safer and more long-lasting [30]. Potential complications, though rare, include severe postprocedural pain, and retroperitoneal abscess. Not uncommonly, there can also be transient diarrhea and hypotension due to sympathetic nerve block-ade and unopposed visceral, parasympathetic activity. Occasionally, altered anatomy from bulky lymphadenopathy or tumors may limit area of injection. While there are no large comparative studies to a percutaneous approach, the EUS-guided method has been proven to be safe and effective while also allowing for further tumor staging and tissue sampling if necessary. In a meta-analysis of eight studies, the pooled proportion of patients with pancreatic cancer who experienced pain relief was about 80%. Only a few patients developed self-limited diarrhea in the studies reviewed, and there were no neurological complications seen [31]. More recently, endosonographers have been able to identify the celiac ganglia and inject directly into them rather than the general area. A small study of 17 patients by Levy et al. demonstrated a high rate of pain relief (94%) in patients with directed celiac ganglion injection [32].

Nutrition

Most patients with malignant dysphagia need nutritional management for improvement of functional status potentially before and after surgery, during chemoradioation, or as an adjunct to palliative measures. Studies performed regarding percutaneous endoscopic gastrostomy (PEG) tube placement safety have demonstrated that the procedure is associated with low mortality and minimal significant complications (Fig. 19.12). In a prospective study of 128 patients followed after PEG placement for at least 31 days, there was 90% survival rate at 1 month. Major complications in 3% were seen including one aspiration pneumonia and two buried bumper syndromes [33]. Minor complications include peristomal leakage, wound infection, and tube dysfunction, which can generally be managed conservatively.

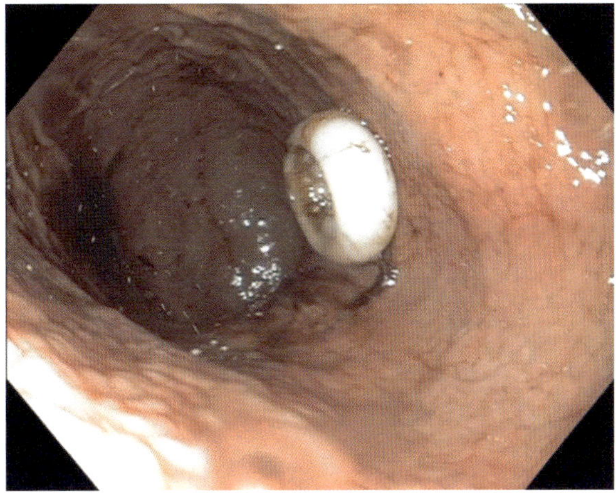

Fig. 19.12 Endoscopic view of internal bumper of PEG after placement

A surgical feeding jejunonstomy should be performed for patients undergoing esophagectomy. Percutaneous endoscopic gastrostomy (PEG) is contraindicated if gastric pull-up will be considered. In patients who have undergone esophagectomy, or those with a SEMS across the GE junction, feeding via a PEG may lead to recurrent aspiration and a PEG with jejunal feeding tube extension (PEG-J) or direct percutaneous endoscopic jejunostomy may be preferred. In a study of 38 patients randomized to either PEG or PEG-J, 2 patients in the PEG group developed nosocomial pneumonia compared to none in the jejunal feeding group [34]. PEG placement can also be considered for those with bowel obstruction and refractory symptoms for venting purposes [35]. Some of the barriers to PEG placement in a palliative population include difficulty in avoiding interposing bowel in a patient with prior abdominal surgery, or avoiding placement in a patient with ascites given the fear of fluid leakage and peritonitis.

Conclusion

Clearly there are numerous, endoscopic therapies available for palliation of patients with gastrointestinal malignancies. There is good evidence that many of the mentioned techniques are safe and effective. One must weigh the potential endoscopic complications and technical failures with the decision for surgical bypass or decompression. In general, patients with locally advanced disease and good performance status are candidates for surgical options; while those patients who are frail with more widespread, metastatic disease may be best palliated via endoscopic alternatives to minimize short-term complications, prolonged hospitalization and recovery. The options for endoscopic palliation are vast with increasing experience across centers and convincing published data to support their use. With technological improvements in endoscopic equipment and devices, there continues to be growing opportunities for more advanced therapies that can be provided for palliative treatments.

Conflicts of Interest The authors have no conflicts of interest to disclose.

References

1. Rupinski M, Zagorowicz E, Regula J, Fijuth J, Kraszewska E, Polkowski M, Wronska E, Butruk E. Randomized comparison of three palliative regimens including brachytherapy, photodynamic therapy, and APC in patients with malignant dysphagia (CONSORT 1a). Am J Gastroenterol. 2011. doi:10.1038/ajg.2011.178.
2. Akhtar K, Byrne JP, Bancewicz J, Attwood SE. Argon beam plasma coagulation in the management of cancer of the esophagus and stomach. Surg Endosc. 2000;14(12):1127–30.
3. Vanbiervliet G, Piche T, Caroli-Bosc FX, Dumas R, Peten EP, Huet PM, Tran A, Demarquay JF. Endoscopic argon plasma trimming of biliary and gastrointestinal metallic stents. Endoscopy. 2005;37(5):434–8.
4. Marcon NE. Photodynamic therapy and cancer of the esophagus. Semin Oncol. 1994;21 (6 Suppl 15):20.
5. Lightdale CJ, Heier SK, Marcon NE, McCaughan Jr JS, Gerdes H, Overholt BF, Sivak Jr MJ, Steigmann GV, Nava HR. Photodynamic therapy with porfimer sodium versus thermal ablation therapy with Nd:YAG laser for palliation of esophageal cancer: a multicenter randomized trial. Gastrointest Endosc. 1995;42(6):507.
6. Mellow MH, et al. Endoscopic laser therapy for malignancies affecting the esophagus and gastroesophageal junction. Analysis of technical and functional efficacy. Arch Intern Med. 1985;145(8):1443.
7. Haddad NG, et al. Endoscopic laser therapy for esophageal cancer. Gastrointest Endosc Clin N Am. 1994;4(4):863.
8. Boyce HW. Pallation of dysphagia of esophageal cancer by endoscopic lumen restoration techniques. Cancer Control. 1999;6(1):73.
9. Hernandez HW, et al. Comparison among the perforation rates of Maloney, balloon, and savary dilation of esophageal strictures. Gastrointest Endosc. 2000;51:460.
10. Dobrucali A, Caglar E. Palliation of malignant esophageal obstruction and fistulas with self expandable metallic stents. World J Gastroenterol. 2010;16(45):5739–45.
11. Dormann A, Meisner S, Verin N, Wenk Lang A. Self-expanding metal stents for gastroduodenal malignancies: systematic review of their clinical effectiveness. Endoscopy. 2004;36(6):543–50.
12. van Jeurnink SM, Eijck CH, Steyerberg EW, Kuipers EJ, Siersema PD. Stent versus gastrojejunostomy for the palliation of gastric outlet obstruction: a systematic review. BMC Gastroenterol. 2007;8(7):18.
13. Repici A, et al. Stenting of the proximal colon in patients with malignant large bowel obstruction: techniques and outcomes. Gastrointest Endosc. 2007;66(5):940.
14. Lo SK. Metallic stenting for colorectal obstruction. Gastrointest Endosc Clin N Am. 1999;9(3):459.
15. van Hooft JE, Fockens P, Marinelli AW, Timmer R, van Berkel AM, Bossuyt PM, Bemelman WA, Dutch Colorectal Stent Group. Early closure of a multicenter randomized clinical trial of

endoscopic stenting versus surgery for stage IV left-sided colorectal cancer. Endoscopy. 2008;40(3):184.

16. Lee HJ, Hong SP, Cheon JH, Kim TI, Min BS, Kim NK, Kim WH. Long-term outcome of palliative therapy for malignant colorectal obstruction in patients with unresectable metastatic colorectal cancers: endoscopic stenting versus surgery. Gastrointest Endosc. 2011;73(3):535–42.

17. Shaib YH, Davila JA, El-Serag HB. The epidemiology of pancreatic cancer in the United States: changes below the surface. Aliment Pharmacol Ther. 2006;24(1):87.

18. Weber A, Mittermeyer T, Wagenpfeil S, Schmid RM, Prinz C. Self-expanding metal stents versus polyethylenc stents for palliative treatment in patients with advanced pancreatic cancer. Pancreas. 2009;38(1):e7–12.

19. Isayama H, Komatsu Y, Tsujino T, Sasahira N, Hirano K, Toda N, Nakai Y, Yamamoto N, Tada M, Yoshida H, Shiratori Y, Kawabe T, Omata M. A prospective randomised study of "covered" versus "uncovered" diamond stents for the management of distal malignant biliary obstruction. Gut. 2004;53(5):729–34.

20. Saleem A, Leggett CL, Murad MH, Baron TH. Meta-analysis of randomized trials comparing the patency of covered and uncovered self-expandable metal stents for palliation of distal malignant bile duct obstruction. Gastrointest Endosc. 2011;74(2):321–7.

21. Rogart JN, Boghos A, Rossi F, Al-Hashem H, Siddiqui UD, Jamidar P, Aslanian H. Analysis of endoscopic management of occluded metal biliary stents at a single tertiary care center. Gastrointest Endosc. 2008;68(4):676–82.

22. van der Gaag NA, Rauws EA, van Eijck CH, Bruno MJ, van der Harst E, Kubben FJ, Gerritsen JJ, Greve JW, Gerhards MF, de Hingh IH, Klinkenbijl JH, Nio CY, de Castro SM, Busch OR, van Gulik TM, Bossuyt PM, Gouma DJ. Preoperative biliary drainage for cancer of the head of the pancreas. N Engl J Med. 2010;362(2):129–37.

23. Moss AC, Morris E, Leyden J, MacMathuna P. Malignant distal biliary obstruction: a systematic review and meta-analysis of endoscopic and surgical bypass results. Cancer Treat Rev. 2007;33(2):213.

24. Chen VK, Arguedas MR, Baron TH. Expandable metal biliary stents before pancreaticoduodenectomy for pancreatic cancer: a Monte-Carlo decision analysis. Clin Gastroenterol Hepatol. 2005;3(12):1229.

25. Raju RP, Jaganmohan SR, Ross WA, Davila ML, Javle M, Raju GS, Lee JH. Optimum palliation of inoperable hilary cholangiocarcinoma: comparative assessment of the efficacy of plastic and self-expanding metal stents. Dig Dis Sci. 2011;56(5):1557–64.

26. Perdue DG, Freeman ML, DiSario JA, Nelson DB, Fennerty MB, Lee JG, Overby CS, Ryan ME, Bochna GS, Snady HW, Moore JP, ERCP Outcome Study ERCOST Group. Plastic versus self-expandable metallic stents for malignant hilar biliary obstruction: a prospective multi-center observational cohort study. J Clin Gastroenterol. 2008;42(9):1040–6.

27. Larghi A, Tringali A, Lecca PG, Giordano M, Costamagna G. Management of hilar biliary strictures. Am J Gastroenterol. 2008;103(2):458.

28. Richter JA, Kahaleh M. Photodynamic therapy: palliation and endoscopic technique in cholangiocarcinoma. World J Gastrointest Endosc. 2010;2(11):357–61.

29. Steel AW, Postgate AJ, Khorsandi S, Nicholls J, Jiao L, Vlavianos P, Habib N, Westaby D. Endoscopically applied radiofrequency ablation appears to be safe in the treatment of malignant biliary obstruction. Gastrointest Endosc. 2011;73(1):149–53.

30. Levy MJ, Wiersema MJ. EUS-guided celiac plexus neurolysis and celiac plexus block. Gastrointest Endosc. 2003;57(7):923–30.

31. Puli SR, Reddy JB, Bechtold ML, Antillon MR, Brugge WR. EUS-guided celiac plexus neurolysis for pain due to chronic pancreatitis or pancreatic cancer pain: a meta-analysis and systematic review. Dig Dis Sci. 2009;54(11):2330.

32. Levy MJ, Topazian MD, Wiersema MJ, Clain JE, Rajan E, Wang KK, de la Mora JG, Gleeson FC, Pearson RK, Pelaez MC, Petersen BT, Vege SS, Chari ST. Initial evaluation of the efficacy and safety of endoscopic ultrasound-guided direct Ganglia neurolysis and block. Am J Gastroenterol. 2008;103(1):98–103.

33. Finocchiaro C, Galletti R, Rovera G, Ferrari A, Todros L, Vuolo A, Balzola F. Percutaneous endoscopic gastrostomy: a long-term follow-up. Nutrition. 1997;13(6):520–3.
34. Montecalvo MA, Steger KA, Farber HW, Smith BF, Dennis RC, Fitzpatrick GF, Pollack SD, Korsberg TZ, Birkett DH, Hirsch EF, et al. Nutritional outcome and pneumonia in critical care patients randomized to gastric versus jejunal tube feedings. The Critical Care Research Team. Crit Care Med. 1992;20(10):1377–87.
35. Holm AN, Baron TH. Palliative use of percutaneous endoscopic gastrostomy and percutaneous endoscopic cecostomy tubes. Gastrointest Endosc Clin N Am. 2007;17(4):795–803.

Review Questions

1. Photodynamic therapy (PDT) is sometimes used for tissue ablation to palliate obstructing esophageal cancers. Two potentially debilitating side effects which have limited the widespread use of PDT include:

   (a) Nephrotoxicity and tinnitus
   (b) Diarrhea and vomiting
   (c) Photosensitivity and stricture
   (d) Headache and diarrhea

2. All of the statements below are true regarding endoscopic dilation of obstruction due to esophageal cancer *except*:

   (a) Can be complicated by perforation
   (b) Usually done through the scope balloon
   (c) Typically provides long-lasting relief of dysphagia
   (d) Often does not provide palliation and patients require endoscopic stent placement

3. Self-expandable metal stents (SEMS) are used in the biliary tract for palliation of malignant obstruction. They can be covered, partially covered, or uncovered (bare). Covered SEMS are associated with:

   (a) Increased obstruction rates
   (b) Unacceptable rates of deployment failure
   (c) Increased perforation rates
   (d) Increased migration rates

4. Gastroduodenal obstruction (e.g., due to pancreatic head cancer) can be treated with enteral stent placement. The following should be considered prior to enteral stent placement:

   (a) Status of the biliary tract to assess need for biliary stenting
   (b) Helicobacter pylori status
   (c) PEG placement for tube feeds
   (d) Stent placement only if the endoscope can be passed beyond the duodenal obstruction

5. Several considerations should be made prior to plastic versus metal biliary stenting for malignant obstruction. All of the following would be included in the decision making process except:

   (a) Survival
   (b) Resectability
   (c) Location of stricture
   (d) Cost
   (e) Age of patient

6. In malignant colonic obstruction, one should always dilate the stricture prior to colonic metal stent placement

   (a) True
   (b) False

Answers

1. (c)
2. (c)
3. (d)
4. (a)
5. (e)
6. (b)

Chapter 20
The Role of Palliative Care in Cardiothoracic Surgery

Amit Banerjee

Cardiothoracic Surgery covers a very broad and at times ambiguous anatomical domain. Conflicting interpretations and controversial semantics often render the patient a victim of gaps and overlaps. Traditionally, surgical conditions involving anything within the thoracic cage viz., ribs, pleura, pericardium, heart, lungs, esophagus, great vessels, and other mediastinal contents, and additionally the entire vascular system, come within the jurisdiction of a cardiothoracic surgeon. However, in the process of diagnosis, treatment planning and crucial decision making, crucial roles may be played by cardiologists, pulmonologists, oncologists, etc. In many parts of the world, cardiothoracic surgery has branched out with the creation of cardiac surgeons, general thoracic surgeons, and vascular surgeons. An important anatomical component of the thorax, viz., the esophagus, has been taken over by gastrointestinal surgeons and several malignant conditions are treated by surgical oncologists.

As we discuss about palliative care in cardiothoracic surgery as a unified discipline, it needs to be pointed out that the connotation of the term palliation in cardiac surgery is a shade different from that applicable to advanced malignant thoracic conditions [1]. Palliative cardiac surgery comprises a subset of innovative, physiologically viable (without restoration of normal physiology) procedures usually performed in very early childhood. They allow the patient to stay alive in a reasonably satisfactory condition, as a stepping stone to more extensive and complex procedures at a later stage. This is in contradistinction to quality-improving or life-prolonging procedures in patients suffering from end-stage malignancies, dealt with in detail elsewhere.

A. Banerjee, M.S., M.Ch. (✉)
Department of Cardiothoracic Surgery,
Maulana Azad Medical College, New Delhi, India

Govind Ballabh Pant Hospital, University of Delhi,
New Delhi, India
e-mail: dramitbanerjee@gmail.com

N. Vadivelu et al. (eds.), *Essentials of Palliative Care*,
DOI 10.1007/978-1-4614-5164-8_20,
© Springer Science+Business Media New York 2013

Palliation in Cardiac Surgery

Among 'palliative' cardiac surgical procedures, systemic-to-pulmonary arterial shunts are by far the commonest. Conceived by Helen Taussig, a pediatric cardiologist at Johns Hopkins, and experimentally consummated by Vivien Thomas, a surgical technician, this path-breaking procedure was first performed on a 15-month-old cyanotic baby by Alfred Blalock, the Chief of surgery at the same university. Thus came into existent the Blalock–Taussig shunt, a procedure destined to bring succor to thousands of patients suffering from tetralogy of Fallot and other complex congenital cyanotic heart conditions [2]. The classic direct anastomosis between subclavian and pulmonary arteries was subsequently modified by Werner Klinner of Munich using an interposing vascular graft. Alternate techniques were subsequently devised and deployed by different surgeons. Notable among these were the Potts shunt (anastomosis of the left pulmonary artery to the descending aorta) and Waterston shunt between the ascending aorta and right pulmonary artery, later modified by Denton Cooley who recommended an intrapericardial anastomosis [3]. Currently a central shunt, wherein an expanded PTFE graft is interposed between the ascending aorta and the main pulmonary artery, is gaining in popularity [4].

William Glenn of Yale University designed a cavopulmonary shunt between the superior vena cava and the right pulmonary artery principally for right-sided cardiac anomalies like tricuspid atresia, Ebstein's anomaly, etc. Subsequently, the classic Glenn shunt underwent modifications like bidirectional Glenn procedure, and atriopulmonary connections such as fenestrated Fontan and complete Fontan circulation: all of them palliative options for the single ventricle. The Sano shunt revisits an option abandoned by Norwood. It connects the right ventricle to the pulmonary artery through an ePTFE conduit is found useful in specific situations.

Palliative surgery for hypoplastic left heart syndrome [5] comprises a series of essential components viz., atrial septectomy, anastomosis of the proximal pulmonary artery to the aorta with homograft augmentation of the aortic arch, and a suitable systemic–pulmonary connection. Application of this protocol is credited to Norwood and has undergone considerable fine-tuning over the years.

Pulmonary artery banding is another palliative option in cardiac surgery [6]. It is used as a stepping stone to definitive surgical corrections. Not too long ago, this served as an initial intervention for infants born with intracardiac defects causing severe left-to-right shunting and overloaded pulmonary circulation. Its primary goal is to restrict excessive pulmonary blood flow and protect the pulmonary vasculature from detrimental changes. Pulmonary artery banding has also been found to play a role in the preparation and "training" of the left ventricle in certain situations such as arterial switch procedure in older infants. Of late, good results following early definitive intracardiac repair has reduced the popularity of PA banding as a mode of palliation. Yet, it continues to find favor in certain subsets of very sick patients with congenital heart disease [7]. In fact, the development of a percutaneously adjustable pulmonary artery band which can be thoracoscopically implanted is underway. The dependence on shunts in many cyanotic cardiac conditions, especially tetralogy of Fallot, is also giving way to early intracardiac repair. However, it is too early to imagine that operative palliation in cardiac surgery is on its way out.

An extended form of palliation in cardiac surgery is the use of ventricular assist devices or artificial hearts in patients who are awaiting availability of suitable donors for cardiac transplantation. These 'bridges to transplant' are genuine life-sustainers before the patient gets a new lease of life following cardiac transplantation.

Palliation in Non-cardiac Thoracic Surgery

Surgical palliation in non-cardiac thoracic surgery has very limited but significant role to play. Large, inoperable, life-threatening mediastinal or pulmonary masses not amenable to surgical extirpation may need debulking to reduce compression on vital structures. Thoracoscopic pleurodesis with talc in patients with mesothelioma or pleural metastases may be adjunctive to biopsy.

One major avenue of palliation in thoracic surgery is pulmonary metastasectomy. The use of intraoperative laser technology minimizes parenchymal loss as lobectomy can be avoided in many instances. Nonsurgical interventional options including placement of expandable stents in the airways and use of laser to restore block airways are in the endoscopists' domain, but within the treating surgeon's circle of responsibility [8].

Chest wall tumors can be painful and may produce fungating ulcers. Their removal combined with reconstructive surgery of the chest wall defect might improve quality of life even in advanced stages.

Malignant masses in the thoracic esophagus may produce severe dysphagia and infiltrate the trachea creating a tracheoesophageal fistula. Various palliative intubation techniques have been available since long to re-create a passage for food to pass through or block a fistula. These include Souttar's tube, Celestin tube, Mousseau-Barbin tube, Atkinson's tube, etc. [9]. Currently, endoscopically implantable tubes such as self-expanding metallic stents, Wallstent, anti-reflux stents, etc., are available. The advancement in endoscopic armamentarium has now made palliation more satisfying through the dual approach of lumen restoration and wherever needed, placement of stent [10].

Although at times palliation for intrathoracic conditions may extend beyond the scope of a cardiothoracic surgeon, she/he is expected to take the lead, and not merely define boundaries of responsibility, in restoring a comfortable and dignified life to the patient.

References

1. Joffs C, Sade RM. Congenital Heart Surgery Nomenclature and Database Project: palliation, correction, or repair? Ann Thorac Surg. 2000;69:S369–72.
2. Blalock A, Taussig HB. The surgical treatment of malformations of the heart in which there is pulmonary stenosis or pulmonary atresia. JAMA. 1945;128:189–92.
3. Truccone NJ, Bowman FO, Malm JR, Gersony WM. Systemic-pulmonary arterial shunts in the first year of life. Circulation. 1974;49:508–11.
4. Amato JJ, Marbey ML, Bush C, Galdieri RJ, Cotroneo JV, Bushong J. Systemic-pulmonary polytetrafluoroethylene shunts in palliative operations for congenital heart disease. Revival of the central shunt. J Thorac Cardiovasc Surg. 1988;95:62–9.
5. Maxwell J, Pigott JD, Murphy JD, Barber G, Norwood WI. Palliative reconstructive surgery for hypoplastic left heart syndrome. Ann Thorac Surg. 1988;45:122–8.
6. Muller WH, Dammann JF. Treatment of certain congenital malformations of the heart by the creation of pulmonic stenosis to reduce pulmonary hypertension and excessive pulmonary blood flow: a preliminary report. Surg Gynecol Obstet. 1952;95:213.
7. Valente AS, Mesquita F, Mejia JA, Maia IC, Maior MS, Branco KC, Pinto Jr VC, Carvalho Jr W. Pulmonary artery banding: a simple procedure? A critical analysis at a tertiary center. Rev Bras Cir Cardiovasc. 2009;24(3):327–33.
8. Noppen N. Interventional palliative treatment options for lung cancer. Ann Oncol. 2002;13 Suppl 4:247–50.
9. Banerjee A, Shinghal RN, Singhal VS, Narayanan PS, Subbarao KS, Nair SK. Palliative surgical intubation for advanced oesophageal malignancy. Indian J Gastroenterol. 1985;4:221–3.
10. Boyce Jr HW. Palliation of dysphagia of esophageal cancer by endoscopic lumen restoration techniques. Cancer Control. 1999;6:73–83.

Review Questions

1. Systemic-to-pulmonary artery shunts as palliative cardiac procedures are performed in:

   (a) Children with coronary artery disease
   (b) Adults with valvular heart disease
   (c) Patients with acyanotic congenital heart disease
   (d) Children with cyanotic heart disease

2. Helen Taussig was a:

   (a) Cardiac anesthetist
   (b) Pediatric cardiac surgeon
   (c) Vascular Surgeon
   (d) Pediatric cardiologist

3. Glenn's original shunt was between:

   (a) Superior vena cava and the main pulmonary artery
   (b) Inferior vena cava and the right pulmonary artery
   (c) Superior vena cava and the right pulmonary artery
   (d) Superior vena cava and the left pulmonary artery

4. Indwelling stents are used for the palliation of:

   (a) Chest wall tumors
   (b) Pulmonary metastases
   (c) Advanced esophageal cancer
   (d) All of the above

5. All of the following are palliative surgical options *except*:

   (a) Metastasectomy
   (b) Pleurodesis
   (c) Debulking
   (d) Pneumonectomy

6. Palliation in cases of congenital heart disease is usually performed:

   (a) At school-going age
   (b) In early childhood
   (c) In the third decade of life
   (d) All of the above

Answers

1. (d)
2. (d)
3. (c)
4. (c)
5. (d)
6. (b)

Chapter 21
Management of Advanced Heart Failure Patients

Dominique Anwar and Asif Anwar

Introduction

The incidence of heart failure (HF) patients in the USA is estimated to be around six million, with half a million new cases adding each year [1, 2]. It is associated with high symptom burden, frequent hospital admissions, diminished quality of life, high costs, and remains the leading cause of death in the USA [3, 4]. It is expected that 70–80% of patients younger than age 65 will die within 8 years of their HF diagnosis, despite the availability of new medical and surgical options [2]. The evolution of HF in patients is typically characterized by acute crises or exacerbations followed by periods of stability lasting for months or even years. However, these patients are 6–9 times more likely to die of sudden cardiac death than the general population [2]. Several tools are available to help assess the prognosis in advanced HF patients: some are single-item predictors (such as the B-type natriuretic

D. Anwar, M.D. (✉)
Section of General Internal Medicine and Geriatrics,
Tulane University School of Medicine,
New Orleans, LA, USA
e-mail: danwar@tulane.edu

A. Anwar, M.D.
Heart and Vascular Institute, Department of Medicine,
Tulane University School of Medicine,
New Orleans, LA, USA

N. Vadivelu et al. (eds.), *Essentials of Palliative Care*,
DOI 10.1007/978-1-4614-5164-8_21,
© Springer Science+Business Media New York 2013

peptide [5], maximal oxygen consumption [6], creatinine level [7], other multivariable models (such as the Seattle Heart Failure Score [7] and the Acute Decompensated Heart Failure National Registry (ADHERE)) [8]. Similarly multiple prognostic factors are associated with increased likelihood of death in advanced HF, especially when coexistent: frequent emergency department visits or hospitalizations, symptoms at rest, dependency in activities of daily living, weight loss $\geq 10\%$, albumin 2.5 g/dL, ejection fraction $< 20\%$, symptomatic arrhythmia, prior cardiopulmonary resuscitation, prior syncope, and embolic stroke. However, even while using these algorithms and other tools, life expectancy remains difficult to predict in advanced HF [3], and this is probably one of the reasons why less than 12% of these patients benefit from hospice care [4].

The Role of Palliative Care and Hospice in the Management of Advanced HF Patients

An integrative model, with palliation occurring while life-prolonging therapies are administered, is currently considered as "the best available" option [9]. In their 2005 guidelines, the American College of Cardiology and American Heart Association recommended palliative/hospice care referrals for end-stage heart failure (stage D, level of Evidence 1A) [10]. The role of a palliative care consultation teaming with the cardiologists is, as for any other patient with advanced disease, to assure comfort, quality of life, and dignity. A palliative care team collaborating closely with the primary team may help not only for symptom management, but also support the medical decision-making process, allowing more regular reassessment of the goals of care. The addition of palliative care to cardiology expertise has been proved effective in regard not only to the patient's quality of life, but amazingly may also have an impact on survival, even at the late stages of the disease process when patients are referred to hospice. Indeed, a non-randomized study conducted by Connor et al. on hospice patients with advanced HF demonstrated a significant survival improvement of 81 days compared with those who did not receive hospice care [11]. The authors of the study postulate that this may be due to the avoidance of unnecessary procedures, less hospital stays, better focus on symptom relief, support for exhausted caregivers, as well as enhanced prevention of complications. Patient referral to hospice may also play a role in the overall medical cost reduction. Appropriate hospice referrals, whatever the diagnosis, can save up to 40% of healthcare costs during the last month of life and up to 17% during the last 6 months of life, with an average savings of $2,309 per hospice user [12]. Focusing on the advanced HF population only, Pyenson et al. demonstrated that hospice referral allowed a reduction in mean Medicare cost per patient from $53,528 to $46,792 [13].

Pharmacological/Nonpharmacological Treatments for Symptom Management

Pharmacological Treatment of HF

Patients with advanced HF usually receive a combination of several oral agents, usually ACE inhibitors or/and ARBs, diuretics (loop diuretics and spironolactone), and beta-blockers [14]. In the end-of-life period, it is important to plan which medications may be removed safely and in what time frame, in anticipation of the moment when patient's swallowing function may become compromised. There is a need to identify medications that should be ideally tapered (to avoid adverse discontinuation effects such as the risk of rebound tachycardia or hypertension with abrupt stop of beta-blockers). Thus beta-blockers and diuretic are probably the medications that should be maintained up to end to avoid worsening symptoms.

In regard to inotropic agents, even though they have not shown survival benefit, they may provide symptomatic relief for prolonged periods of time (Class IIB indication for end-stage heart failure) [15, 16].

Specific Pharmacological Approach of Dyspnea

Opioids

Even though only a few and small randomized controlled studies addressed specifically the HF population [17–19], there is evidence to support the use of short acting oral or parenteral opioids to palliate breathlessness, whichever its origin, while the use of nebulized opioids is not supported [20].

Benzodiazepines

The role of benzodiazepines has been studied mainly in the cancer and COPD population. Even though some studies, such as those from Navigante et al., have demonstrated an efficacy on the subjective sensation of dyspnea in patients with advanced cancer, especially coupled with an opioid [21, 22], a recent meta-analysis did not show evidence for a beneficial effect of benzodiazepines in the relief of breathlessness in patients with advanced cancer and COPD [23]. As discussed in this Cochrane review, studies focusing on HF-related dyspnea are urgently needed.

Nonpharmacological Approach of Dyspnea

No randomized controlled trials were identified addressing the specific issue of the efficacy of oxygen in reducing breathlessness in patients with advanced HF, whether hypoxemic or not [24]. Pursed-lip breathing, noninvasive positive pressure ventilation for sleep-disordered breathing, relaxation, and hypnosis may all be of interest, but there is little evidence-based data to support these approaches.

Management of Other Symptoms

Pain, related or not to the cardiac condition, should be addressed similarly as in other oncological/nononcological conditions. As advanced HF patients have very often compromised kidney function, they must often be monitored closely when receiving opioids with active metabolites, such as morphine or hydromorphone, to avoid side effects, especially opioid-related neurotoxicity. Fatigue and anorexia are distressing symptoms, which are frequent in advanced HF. Unfortunately resources to alleviate them are actually limited. Psychostimulants such as methylphenidate have not been studied in this population, and their potential cardiac side effects make them difficult to recommend in this population. Techniques, such as training in energy conservation and aerobic exercise, have been recommended. Sleep apnea may lead to fatigue and can be treated with noninvasive ventilation. Depression is very frequent in advanced HF, but the efficacy of antidepressant agents has once again never been assessed in the cardiac population.

Pacemakers

Many patients and families (as well sometimes team members) believe that the pacemaker (PM) will keep them alive or alternatively will prolong the period of agony. However, these are not resuscitative devices and will not keep a dying patient alive. They do not prolong survival as acidosis that develops at the end of life will not allow the myocardium to be depolarized by the PM stimulations [25]. In consequence, there is no medical indication to deactivate it. In addition, bradycardia symptoms will be alleviated by maintaining the PM function. Finally one must keep in mind that a pacemaker must be removed if the patient is cremated.

Implantable Cardioverter Defibrillator

There is an increasing use of implantable cardioverter defibrillator (ICD) for primary and secondary cardiac death prevention. This growing patient population requires a special attention in the terminal days. Indeed as heart failure worsens, patients are likely to receive more frequent shocks from ICDs, which not only cause significant pain and anxiety to the patient, but also tremendous distress to the family and medical team [26]. Of note repetitive ICD shocks also induce myocardial damage and are detrimental for the cardiac function. In light of these problems there is a general consensus to deactivate the ICD in the final days. This has been extensively addressed and reviewed by the American College of Cardiology, American Heart Association, and Heart Rhythm Society [27]. Therefore, the concept of future deactivation when approaching end of life should always be included in ICD pre-implantation discussions with the patient and family. Unfortunately, even nowadays, clinicians infrequently discuss ICD deactivation issues with patients and these devices may remain active until death [28]. Hospices usually require deactivation. In the unusual case where deactivation was not performed, hospices may use a magnet to avoid painful and distressing shocks at the end of life [29].

Left Ventricular Assist Devices as Destination Therapy

Left ventricular assist device (LVAD) function is to unload the failing heart and to provide an adequate forward cardiac output to maintain organ perfusion. Although they were originally used as a temporary bridge to recovery, then as a bridge to transplantation, they are increasingly used as a destination therapy. In the latter situation LVADs are used without any plan for transplantation. LVADs have been shown to improve quality of life and survival compared with inotropic agents, as well as exercise tolerance, end-organ function, and emotional well-being [30]. However, they are also associated with significant rates of long-term complications such as bleeding, infection, and neurologic events [31]. Some baseline symptoms may however remain or occur de novo after LVAD implantation. Longitudinal in- and outpatient care is therefore crucial for successful outcome and requires intensive involvement of patients and caregivers. Patients may have abrupt LVAD mechanical failure leading to a sudden decrease in cardiac output and fatal outcome. On the other hand, LVAD may continue to have adequate function while the patient develops other complications or pathologies (e.g., infectious, embolic, renal). They will continue to work after the patient is clinically brain dead, or they may prolong the dying process. Therefore, patients and physicians must carefully weigh potential risks and benefits in the patient's specific situation before implementing LVAD as destination therapy. In the follow-up they must also continue or initiate palliative care while implementing LVADs. It is also crucial to address not only the important issue of advanced directives, but to extend such directives to what is called a "preparedness plan," which adds to the usual directives the specific issues related to the LVAD [32].

Communication in Advanced HF Patients

Communicating with an advanced HF patient and the patient's loved ones can often present multifaceted barriers, so much so that Momen in a recent literature review called such communication the process of "addressing the elephant on the table" [33].

A survey conducted by McCarthy in 1997 among bereaved families of heart failure patients with no sudden cardiac death showed that 37% only were aware of a poor prognosis, 8% of patients and 44% of family members were told by a physician that time was short, and 36% of these patients died alone [34]. We may imagine that more emphasis is placed nowadays on accurate communication, but this is still a challenging issue.

Criteria for Hospice Referrals of Advanced HF Patients

In the USA, patients are eligible for hospice care reimbursement under Medicare regulations when they are likely to have a life expectancy of 6 months or less. Even though, as discussed previously, it is difficult to predict this life expectancy in patients with advanced HF, there are criteria to help the healthcare providers to confirm hospice eligibility [35]. The list of these criteria can be downloaded from several websites [36].

References

1. Tanner CE, Fromme EK, Goodlin SJ. Ethics in the treatment of advanced heart failure: palliative care and end-of-life issues. Congest Heart Fail. 2011;17(5):235–40.
2. Hupcey JE, Penrod J, Fenstermacher K. Review article: a model of palliative care for heart failure. Am J Hosp Palliat Care. 2009;26(5):399–404.
3. Teno JM, Weitzen S, Fennell ML, Mor V. Dying trajectory in the last year of life: does cancer trajectory fit other diseases?J. Palliat Med. 2001;4(4):457–64.
4. Davis MP. Palliation of heart failure. Am J Hosp Palliat Care. 2005;22:211–22.
5. Doust JA, Pietrzak E, Sanders S, Glasziou P. How well does B-type natriuretic peptide predict death and cardiac events in patients with heart failure: systematic review. BMJ. 2005;330(7492):625.
6. Mahon N, Blackstone E, Francis G, et al. The prognostic value of estimated creatinine clearance alongside functional capacity in ambulatory patients with chronic congestive heart failure. J Am Coll Cardiol. 2002;40:1106–13.
7. Levi WC, Mozaraffian D, Linker DT, et al. The Seattle Heart Failure Model: prediction of survival in heart failure. Circulation. 2006;113(11):1424–33.
8. Fonarow GC, Adamas Jr KF, Abraham WT, et al. Risk stratification for in-hospital mortality in acutely decompensated heart failure: classification and regression tree analysis. JAMA. 2005;293(5):572–80.
9. Adler ED, Goldfinger JZ, Kalman J, et al. Palliative care in the treatment of advanced heart failure. Circulation. 2009;120(25):2597–606.
10. Hunt SA, Abraham WT, Chin MH, et al. ACC/AHA 2005 Guideline Update for the Diagnosis and Management of Chronic Heart Failure in the Adult: a report of the American College of Cardiology/American Heart Association Task Force on Practice Guidelines (Writing Committee to Update the 2001 Guidelines for the Evaluation and Management of Heart Failure): developed in collaboration with the American College of Chest Physicians and the International Society for Heart and Lung Transplantation: endorsed by the Heart Rhythm Society. Circulation. 2005;112(12):e154–235.

11. Connor SR, Pyenson B, Fitch K, et al. Comparing hospice and nonhospice patient survival among patients who die within a three-year window. J Pain Symptom Manage. 2007;33(3):238–46.
12. Emanuel EJ. Cost savings at the end of life. What do the data show? JAMA. 1996;275(24):1907–14.
13. Pyenson B, Connors S, Fitch K, Kinzbrunner B. Medicare cost in matched hospice and non-hospice cohorts. J Pain Symptom Manage. 2004;28(3):200–10.
14. Goodlin SJ, Hauptman PJ, Arnold R, et al. Consensus statement: palliative and supportive care in advanced heart failure. J Card Fail. 2004;10(3):200–9.
15. Sindone AP, Keogh AM, Macdonald PS, et al. Continuous home ambulatory intravenous inotropic drug therapy in severe heart failure: safety and cost efficacy. Am Heart J. 1997;134(5 Pt 1):889–900.
16. Nauman DJ, Hershberger RE. The use of positive inotropes in end-of-life heart failure care. Curr Heart Fail Rep. 2007;4(3):158–63.
17. Chua TP, Harrington D, Ponikowski P, et al. Effects of dihydrocodeine on chemosensitivity and exercise tolerance in patients with chronic heart failure. J Am Coll Cardiol. 1997;29(1):147–52.
18. Johnson MJ, McDonagh TA, Harkness A, et al. Morphine for the relief of breathlessness in patients with chronic heart failure-a pilot study. Eur J Heart Fail. 2002;4:753–6.
19. Williams SG, Cooke GA, Wright DJ, et al. Peak exercise cardiac power output; a direct indicator of cardiac function strongly predictive of prognosis in chronic heart failure. Eur Heart J. 2001;22:1496–503.
20. Jennings AL, Davies AN, Higgins JP, Broadley K. Opioids for the palliation of breathlessness in terminal illness. Cochrane Database Syst Rev. 2001;(4):CD002066.
21. Navigante AH, Cerchietti LC, Castro MA, et al. Midazolam as adjunct therapy to morphine in the alleviation of severe dyspnea perception in patients with advanced cancer. J Pain Symptom Manage. 2006;31(1):38–47.
22. Navigante A, Castro MA, Cerchietti LC. Morphine versus midazolam as upfront therapy to control dyspnea perception in cancer patients while its underlying cause is sought or treated. J Pain Symptom Manage. 2010;39(5):820–30.
23. Simon ST, Higginson IJ, Booth S, Harding R, Bausewein C. Benzodiazepines for the relief of breathlessness in advanced malignant and non-malignant diseases in adults. Cochrane Database Syst Rev. 2010;(1):CD007354.
24. Mahler D, Selecki PA, Harrod CG. Management of dyspnea in patients with advanced lung or heart disease: practical guidance from the American college of chest physicians consensus statement. Pol Arch Med Wewn. 2010;120(5):160–6.
25. Mueller PS, Hook CC, Hayes DL. Ethical analysis of withdrawal of pacemaker or implantable cardioverter-defibrillator support at the end of life. Mayo Clin Proc. 2003;78(8):959–63.
26. Nohria A, Lewis E, Stevenson LW. Medical management of advanced heart failure. JAMA. 2002;287(5):628–40.
27. Ebstein AE, DiMarco JP, Ellenbogen KA, et al. ACC/AHA/HRS 2008 Guidelines for Device-Based Therapy of Cardiac Rhythm Abnormalities: a report of the American College of Cardiology/American Heart Association Task Force on Practice Guidelines (Writing Committee to Revise the ACC/AHA/NASPE 2002 Guideline Update for Implantation of Cardiac Pacemakers and Antiarrhythmia Devices) developed in collaboration with the American Association for Thoracic Surgery and Society of Thoracic Surgeons. J Am Coll Cardiol. 2008;51(21):e1–62.
28. Goldstein NE, Mehta D, Siddiqui S, et al. "That's like an act of suicide" patients' attitudes toward deactivation of implantable defibrillators. J Gen Intern Med. 2008;23(S1):7–12.
29. Fromme EK, Stewart TL, Jeppesen M, Tolle SW. Adverse experiences with implantable defibrillators in Oregon hospices. Am J Hosp Palliat Care. 2011;28(5):304–9.
30. Wilson SR, Givertz MM, Stewart GC, Mudge Jr GH. Ventricular assist devices the challenges of outpatient management. J Am Coll Cardiol. 2009;54(18):1647–59.

31. Lietz K, Long JW, Kfoury AG, et al. Outcomes of left ventricular assist device implantation as destination therapy in the post-REMATCH era: implications for patient selection. Circulation. 2007;116(5):497–505.
32. Swetz KM, Freeman MR, AbouEzzedine OF, et al. Palliative medicine consultation for preparedness planning in patients receiving left ventricular assist devices as destination therapy. Mayo Clin Proc. 2011;86(6):493–500.
33. Momen NC, Barclay SI. Addressing 'the elephant on the table': barriers to end of life care conversations in heart failure – a literature review and narrative synthesis. Curr Opin Support Palliat Care. 2011;5(4):312–6.
34. McCarthy M, Hall JA, Ley M. Communication and choice in dying from heart disease. J R Soc Med. 1997;90(3):128–31.
35. Stuart B, The NHO. Medical guidelines for non-cancer disease and local medical review policy: hospice access for patients with diseases other than cancer. Hosp J. 1999;14(3–4):139–54.
36. http://www.lmhpco.org/professionals/diseases/heart.shtml.

Review Questions

1. Which is the global leading cause of death in the USA nowadays?

   (a) Cancer
   (b) Heart failure
   (c) Suicide
   (d) End-stage pulmonary diseases

2. What is the best tool to determinate an advanced HF patient prognosis?

   (a) Single-item tools
   (b) Multivariate models
   (c) Prognosis factors
   (d) All and none of them: prognosis in advanced HF remains difficult

3. What is the role of opioids in advanced HF?

   (a) None, the risk of respiratory depression is too high
   (b) Pain management only
   (c) Pain management and dyspnea
   (d) For dyspnea, it works only if associated with benzodiazepines

4. PM, ICD in patients who are referred to hospice:

   (a) Both need to be discontinued
   (b) PM needs to be discontinued
   (c) ICD needs to be discontinued
   (d) Both can be maintain and will improve the patient's quality of life

5. LVAD as destination therapy:

   (a) Do not improve the quality of life
   (b) Do not present with severe complications
   (c) Are rather cheap
   (d) Can extend the duration of agony

Answers

1. (b)
2. (d)
3. (c)
4. (c)
5. (d)

Chapter 22
Palliative Care in Cardiac Electrophysiology

Eric Grubman

The field of clinical cardiac electrophysiology involves the management and prevention of cardiac rhythm disturbances. If untreated, many of these rhythm disturbances can rapidly prove fatal. Cardiac electrophysiology has grown dramatically over the past 20 years, fueled largely by the advances in cardiac pacing, implantable defibrillators, and cardiac ablation of arrhythmias. The results of this dramatic expansion have resulted in a field that can provide invasive therapy to improve the quality of life, as well as the duration of life.

Palliative care involves treatments designed to relieve or prevent suffering, rather than cure the disease process. Many of these patients suffer from chronic illness, or are nearing the end of life. Cardiac arrhythmias are far more common in these patients than in the general population. Modern treatment of cardiac rhythm disturbances can often relieve or prevent symptoms, and should be considered for patients undergoing palliative care.

This chapter first considers the treatment options available in cardiac electrophysiology, followed by a consideration of the specific arrhythmias, as well as palliative care decisions for each arrhythmia.

E. Grubman, M.D. (✉)
Department of Internal Medicine, Yale University School of Medicine,
New Haven, CT, USA
e-mail: grubman@sbcglobal.net

N. Vadivelu et al. (eds.), *Essentials of Palliative Care*,
DOI 10.1007/978-1-4614-5164-8_22,
© Springer Science+Business Media New York 2013

The Therapies

Devices

Cardiac Pacing

The modern era of cardiac pacing began in 1957, with the development of the implantable pacemaker [1]. Since that time, advances in cardiac pacing have resulted in a pacemaker that is smaller, lasts longer, and provides more physiologic heart rate control. Modern pacemakers can automatically change pacing rates, automatically change the pacing mode (i.e., both atria and ventricles or only one chamber), or pace both ventricles synchronously (biventricular pacing) in an attempt to improve functional status and survival.

Pacemakers are implanted for a variety of bradyarrhythmias, including potentially life-threatening arrhythmias (i.e., complete heart block), as well as arrhythmias that are symptomatic, but are not immediately life threatening (i.e., sinus node dysfunction). The implantation of cardiac pacemakers can be accomplished with minimal morbidity and mortality, and are frequently performed with minimal sedation. The recovery period following pacemaker implantation is short, and most patients require only a single overnight hospitalization.

After implantation, pacemaker function can be altered (reprogrammed) noninvasively, using a specialized transceiver, which can communicate with the pacemaker. Reprogramming of a pacemaker can activate, or deactivate, virtually any feature of the pacemaker.

Implantable Defibrillators (ICDs)

Implantable cardioverter-defibrillators (ICDs) first became available in 1970 [2], and have grown in clinical relevance since that time. Since their clinical introduction, ICDs have undergone multiple advances that have led to devices that are extremely efficient at detecting and terminating rhythms associated with sudden cardiac death (primarily ventricular fibrillation) [3]. In addition, currently available ICDs offer full pacemaker capability, including biventricular pacing, which has been shown to further improve both symptoms and survival in appropriate patients [4].

ICDs are implanted primarily to prevent sudden cardiac death in patients felt to be at high risk for this disorder. Similar to cardiac pacemakers, implantation can be accomplished with minimal morbidity and mortality, and are frequently performed with minimal sedation. The recovery period following implantation is similar to that of a cardiac pacemaker.

Reprogramming of an ICD can be accomplished noninvasively, much like that of a pacemaker. It is possible to activate or deactivate virtually any feature of the ICD in this manner. For example, it is possible to deactivate the therapies for ventricular tachycardia/ventricular fibrillation, which leaving the pacemaker functions (which treat bradyarrhythmias) intact.

If necessary, ICD therapy can be noninvasively deactivated. It is possible to "turn off" the therapies for ventricular tachycardia/ventricular fibrillation, while leaving pacing functions intact. It is also possible to deactivate pacing functions in these devices as well, via the same noninvasive strategy.

Catheter Ablation of Arrhythmias

Catheter ablation of cardiac arrhythmias using radiofrequency energy has been available since 1989 [5]. Since that time, it has been used to treat patients with a variety of tachyarrhythmias, including Wolff–Parkinson–White syndrome, AV nodal reentrant tachycardia, atrial tachycardia, and atrial flutter. It is associated with success rates that are generally greater than 90% [6]. The procedure is generally performed with minimal sedation, and, depending on the arrhythmia being treated, is associated with low morbidity and mortality. The recovery period following ablation is quite short, and an overnight hospital stay is the norm.

The Arrhythmias

Tachyarrhythmias

Supraventricular Tachyarrhythmias

Atrial Fibrillation

Atrial fibrillation is the most common arrhythmia, occurring in approximately 10% of patients over the age of 80 [7]. Although often asymptomatic, it can be associated with a variety of symptoms, including fatigue, palpitations, exercise intolerance, presyncope, and syncope. It is commonly associated with other chronic illnesses, and, as such, is often a target for palliative care.

Treatment of atrial fibrillation is either aimed at restoring normal sinus rhythm, or controlling the ventricular response to atrial fibrillation. Both of these strategies, if effective, will eliminate symptomatic atrial fibrillation. Either therapy can be quite intensive, involving complex medical regimens and invasive proceeders, including ablation.

Rhythm control strategies in atrial fibrillation are designed to maintain normal sinus rhythm. They frequently involve the use of antiarrhythmic drug therapy. These drugs have a relatively high side effect profile and require invasive monitoring. If palliative care is contemplated, it may be appropriate to change the focus of therapy toward rate control in atrial fibrillation. This strategy has not been shown to be inferior to a strategy of rhythm control [8].

In patients who are receiving a strategy of rate control, it is occasionally difficult to achieve adequate rate control. The resulting rapid ventricular response in atrial fibrillation can lead to worsening of symptoms, or in severe cases, exacerbations of congestive heart failure. In these cases, it is appropriate to consider an invasive strategy to provide palliative care. Radiofrequency ablation of the AV node (with concomitant permanent pacemaker implantation) will eliminate the need for rate control medications, and will guarantee adequate rate control in atrial fibrillation. Though invasive, this strategy is an appropriate palliative care in cases where rate control in atrial fibrillation is difficult to achieve.

Atrial fibrillation is associated with an increased risk of embolic stroke. This risk is increased in patients who are elderly, or patients with significant comorbidities (such as hypertension or diabetes mellitus). A strategy of intensive anticoagulation, typically with Coumadin, has been shown to decrease this risk dramatically. Coumadin therapy does require occasional blood work, which does involve some mild discomfort.

The goal of palliative care in patients with atrial fibrillation is to minimize the symptoms (palpitations, dizziness, syncope) as well as the risks (worsening congestive heart failure, stroke) that can accompany the arrhythmia. Palliative care decisions in atrial fibrillation may allow simplification of the medical regimen. Changing treatment strategy from a strategy designed to maintain sinus rhythm to one that allows atrial fibrillation, but provides adequate ventricular rate control, may simplify the medical regimen and limit the repeated hospitalizations which often occur in patients on antiarrhythmic drugs. Elimination of anticoagulation with coumadin will limit blood drawing, but at the expense of a dramatically increased risk of stroke.

Supraventricular Tachycardia

Supraventricular tachycardia (SVT) can be caused by a variety of mechanisms. They are not frequently life-threatening, but can be extremely symptomatic. They are often associated with palpitations, dizziness, fatigue, and, in rare cases, syncope.

SVT can often be prevented with medical therapy, including beta blockers, calcium channel blockade, or antiarrhythmic therapy. If these therapies fail, ablation has been very successful at eliminating these arrhythmias, with cure rates that are frequently greater than 90% [6]. Though successful at eliminating these arrhythmias, ablation is an invasive approach, which often requires some degree of sedation, a procedure which can last several hours, and, quite frequently, an overnight hospitalization.

Ventricular Tachycardia

Ventricular tachyarrhythmias are responsible for the majority of cases of sudden cardiac death. It is estimated that there are greater than 300,000 cases of sudden cardiac death annually in the USA [9]. These arrhythmias become more frequent as underlying structural heart disease worsens. Traditional treatment of these arrhythmias involved antiarrhythmic drug therapy, which was designed to prevent these arrhythmias. In the early 1990s, several seminal trials demonstrated the inferiority of antiarrhythmic drug therapy [10]. At the same time, the development of the implantable defibrillator proved to be a transformative event. Rather than preventing ventricular tachycardia/ventricular fibrillation, ICDs act rapidly to terminate these arrhythmias, before they can become fatal. The efficacy of these devices in terminating VT/VF is very high [3]. As a result, ICD implantation is extremely effective at preventing sudden death in patients at high risk, and has largely replaced the use of antiarrhythmic drug therapy in patients at high risk for ventricular arrhythmias and sudden death.

If untreated, ventricular fibrillation will almost invariably lead to rapid, painless death. Ventricular tachycardia is slightly less lethal, and can cause severe symptoms (extreme dizziness, palpitations, and/or syncope), or sudden death. If they occur in a patient with an ICD, the ICD will treat the arrhythmia, frequently by delivering a high energy defibrillation shock (up to 700 V). In patients with palliative care goals, it may be reasonable to deactivate ICD therapy, to eliminate the possibility of a painful shock. Patients and their surrogates have the right to refuse life-saving treatments, and deactivation of an ICD would fall directly into this category. Patients and caregivers should understand that any ventricular tachyarrhythmias which occur after the ICD has been deactivated, will likely prove fatal.

Bradyarrhythmias

Bradyarrhythmias are often associated with fatigue, dizziness, and syncope. Most cases of conduction system disease are caused by degeneration of the cardiac conduction system, which ultimately results in bradycardia, and symptoms. In some cases (i.e., complete heart block), the arrhythmia can prove rapidly fatal if untreated. Pacemaker implantation can be expected to relieve the symptoms associated with bradyarrhythmias entirely.

Whether patients with symptomatic bradyarrhythmias should undergo pacemaker implantation is a reasonable consideration when palliative care is being considered. The procedure, though minimal, is invasive, and requires a brief hospitalization and mild discomfort. It would be reasonable to consider pacemaker implantation as palliative care for patients with severe symptoms, such as syncope or dizziness, but it would also be reasonable to withhold pacemaker implantation in patients whose only symptom was fatigue.

In patients who already have pacemakers implanted, it is reasonable to consider deactivation of the pacemaker if requested by the patient or their surrogate. Patients have the right to refuse life-sustained treatments, and deactivation of a pacemaker (or ICD) would be considered to be refusal of a life-sustaining treatment. It is appropriate to do so in a palliative care situation, if requested by the patient or their surrogate [11].

Conclusion

Cardiac rhythm disturbances can be highly symptomatic, and are frequently associated with significant morbidity and mortality. They often occur in patients with other chronic illnesses. Treatments for the variety of cardiac rhythm disturbances has improved dramatically over the past 25 years, and now offers a variety of therapies for the vast majority of cardiac rhythm disturbances.

The field of palliative care is focused on the relief or prevention of suffering, rather than the cure of disease. Cardiac electrophysiologic procedures can be used to further these goals, and in many cases, is part of a palliative care strategy. However, these treatments are invasive. Though they often serve to prolong life, the treatments can lead to intermittent discomfort (i.e., ICD shocks). In these cases, it may be reasonable to limit, or reverse therapy in an attempt to achieve the goals of palliative care.

References

1. Weirich W, Gott V, Lillehei C. The treatment of complete heart block by the combined use of a myocardial electrode and an artificial pacemaker. Surg Forum. 1957;8:360–3.
2. Mirowski M, Mower MM, Staewen WS. Standby automatic defibrillator: an approach to prevention of sudden coronary death. Arch Intern Med. 1970;126:158–61.
3. Goldberger Z, Lampert R. Implantable cardioverter-defibrillators: expanding indications and technologies. JAMA. 2006;295(7):809–18.
4. Bristow MR, Saxon LA, Boehmer J. Cardiac-resynchronization therapy with or without an implantable defibrillator in advanced chronic heart failure. N Engl J Med. 2004;350(21):2140–50.
5. Jackman WM, Wang X, Friday KJ. Catheter ablation of accessory atrioventricular pathways (Wolff-Parkinson-White syndrome) by radiofrequency current. N Engl J Med. 1991;324:1605–11.
6. Calkins H, Yong P, Miller JM, Atakr Multicenter Investigators Group. Catheter ablation of accessory pathways, atrioventricular nodal reentrant tachycardia, and the atrioventricular junction: final results of a prospective, multicenter clinical trial. Circulation. 1999;99:262–70.
7. Go AS, Hylek EM, Phillips KA. Prevalence of diagnosed atrial fibrillation in adults. JAMA. 2001;285(18):2370–5.
8. The AFFIRM Investigators. A comparison of rate control and rhythm control in patients with atrial fibrillation. N Engl J Med. 2002;347:1825–33.
9. Mutchner L. The ABCs of CPR – again. Am J Nurs. 2007;107(1):60–9.
10. CAST Investigators. Preliminary report: effect on encainide and flecainide on mortality in a randomized trial of arrhythmia suppression after myocardial infarction. N Engl J Med. 1989;321:406–12.
11. Lampert R. HRS Expert Consensus Statement on the Management of Cardiovascular Implantable Electronic Devices (CIEDs) in patients nearing end of life or requesting withdrawal of therapy. Heart Rhythm. 2010;7(7):1008–26.

Review Questions

1. An 85-year-old woman with a previously implanted biventricular defibrillator is receiving palliative care, due to metastatic colon cancer. She is competent to make decisions regarding her care. She asks to have her ICD "turned off." You inform her that it would be appropriate to:

    (a) Deactivate the defibrillation features of the device only
    (b) Deactivation of biventricular pacing functions of the device only
    (c) Deactivation of rate responsive pacing functions of the device only
    (d) Deactivation of all pacing functions only
    (e) All of the above are appropriate

2. A 75-year-old man with ALS is receiving palliative care. He develops complete heart block, which results in recurrent syncope and severe dizziness. As his clinician, you inform him that:

    (a) Permanent pacemaker implantation is reasonable, given the symptomatic nature of his bradyarrhythmia
    (b) There is no role for pacemaker implantation in patients receiving palliative care
    (c) Temporary paccmaker implantation, which can be maintained for several days, is the most appropriate therapy for his arrhythmia
    (d) External pacing, though uncomfortable, is the most appropriate therapy for his arrhythmia

3. A 68-year-old woman has a previously implanted pacemaker, for the treatment of complete heart block. She would be asystolic without the pacemaker. She is receiving palliative care for metastatic pancreatic cancer. Her pacemaker battery has weakened to the point that the device should be changed. She is no longer making her medical decisions, but her daughter, who has assumed this role, asks that the pacemaker not be changed. She understands that this will likely lead to the patient's death. You should inform her that:

    (a) Pacemaker generator change is minimally invasive, and must be performed, as the therapy is vital
    (b) Pacemaker generator change must be performed, as it is considered "continuation of existing therapy" and is not part of palliative care decisions
    (c) It is appropriate not to replace the pacemaker, as long as the daughter understands the implications
    (d) Pacemaker generator change must be performed, as the decision not to replace the pacemaker can only be made by the patient, not her daughter

4. A 90-year-old man is receiving palliative care, due to severe, advanced dementia. He presents to the Emergency Room with newly a urinary tract infection. He is incidentally noted to have atrial fibrillation. He is hemodynamically stable. The most appropriate therapy for his atrial fibrillation would be:

   (a) Electrical cardioversion, followed by initiation of amiodarone therapy
   (b) Electrical cardioversion, without long-term antiarrhythmic drug therapy
   (c) Begin the patient on flecainide, with the hopes that it will restore normal sinus rhythm, without the use of electrical cardioversion
   (d) No further therapy is warranted, as the patient is asymptomatic

5. In patients receiving palliative care, ablation therapy for SVT:

   (a) Is not appropriate
   (b) Can be reasonable, if the arrhythmia is symptomatic and frequent
   (c) Can be reasonable, if they can be accomplished with minimal risk
   (d) Can be reasonable, only if they are likely to be life-saving

Answers

1. (e) All of the above are appropriate
2. (a) Permanent pacemaker implantation is reasonable, given the symptomatic nature of his bradyarrhythmia
3. (c) It is appropriate not to replace the pacemaker, as long as the daughter understands the implications
4. (d) No further therapy is warranted, as the patient is asymptomatic
5. (b) Can be reasonable, if the arrhythmia is symptomatic and frequent

Chapter 23
Palliation in Respiratory Disease

David R. Meek, Martin D. Knolle, and Thomas B. Pulimood

Introduction

Palliative care plays an important role in pulmonary disease; a common cause of acute and chronic terminal illness. Its role is well recognised in lung cancer but less so in other respiratory disease [1]. It can sometimes be difficult to differentiate between what is considered palliation and what is considered routine care. It is important therefore for the physician caring for patients with respiratory symptoms or disease to be able to integrate restorative/curative management and palliative measures as appropriate on an individual patient basis. This needs to be incorporated as part of their routine management plan. Similarly patients primarily receiving palliation benefit from curative and restorative measures such as treating pneumonia or wheeze in terminal care. Hence patients benefit from a holistic, multidisciplinary team approach to their management which focuses on the patient and their family's needs, wishes and expectations. The American Thoracic Society (ATS) have laid out a clinical policy statement related to palliative care for patients with respiratory diseases alluding to this in some detail [2]. This chapter outlines a symptom and disease-specific approach to palliation in respiratory disease.

D.R. Meek, M.R.C.P. (✉) • T.B. Pulimood, M.B.B.S., F.R.C.P.
Department of Respiratory and General Internal Medicine,
West Suffolk Hospital, University of Cambridge Teaching Hospital,
Bury St Edmunds, Suffolk, UK
e-mail: dr_meek@hotmail.com; Thomas.pulimood@wsh.nhs.uk

M.D. Knolle, M.B., B.Chir., M.R.C.P.
Department of Respiratory Medicine,
Lister Hospital, Stevenage, UK

N. Vadivelu et al. (eds.), *Essentials of Palliative Care*,
DOI 10.1007/978-1-4614-5164-8_23,
© Springer Science+Business Media New York 2013

Management of Symptoms

Breathlessness or Dyspnoea

Dyspnoea, a Greek word for "difficulty breathing", has been defined by the ATS as "a term used to characterize a subjective experience of breathing discomfort that is comprised of qualitatively distinct sensations that vary in intensity. The experience derives from interactions among multiple physiological, psychological, social, and environmental factors; and may induce secondary physiological and behavioural responses" [3].

Dyspnoea, together with pain, is one of the symptoms most common in and feared by patients with terminal illness requiring palliation [4, 5]. The physiological basis of the sensation of breathlessness is due to complex interactions between respiratory centres within the brain (medullary, pontine and cortical), peripheral and central chemoreceptor monitoring oxygen, carbon dioxide and pH levels, as well as, mechano and pain receptors in the lung.

Breathlessness is a symptom of numerous conditions, two thirds of which are primary respiratory or cardiac disease and in the other third it is multi-factorial [6]. Other causes include: anaemia, thyrotoxicosis, diabetic ketoacidosis, altitude sickness, anxiety and other neurological illness. Symptoms of breathlessness are not necessarily correlated to physiological parameters or underlying disease burden. It is important to bear in mind other contributory factors, such as anxiety and pain.

The assessment of dyspnoea should include an assessment of its severity. A commonly used scale for this is the modified BORG score [7], which ranks dyspnoea symptoms from 0 to 10. This provides an objective measure for comparison and monitoring symptoms. However, more importantly, the extent of disability caused by dyspnoea needs to be explored.

The first step in the treatment of dyspnoea is the diagnosis and treatment of any underlying cause. For example, treatment of pneumonia or pulmonary emboli in patients with terminal lung cancer might improve their symptoms sufficiently for the patient to be comfortable. Should patients remain short of breath despite appropriate or optimal management of their underlying respiratory disease, other non-pharmacological measures can be employed to help with dyspnoea [1]. Foremost is patient education by physicians and nurses. Patients and their families need to be aware of the level of dyspnoea and simple advice to control symptoms can go a long way. In addition, patients, particularly those with end-stage chronic obstructive pulmonary disease (COPD), may benefit from keeping physically active with pulmonary rehabilitation, which seeks to incorporate patient education, exercise training and nutritional advice [8]. A dietician may provide support for the latter, particularly if the labour of breathing increases calorie demands. Another simple measure may be a fan providing cold air to the face to relieve the feeling of dyspnoea. This provides facial cooling to the Vth cranial nerve region, i.e. mouth, nose and cheeks.

Table 23.1 Management of breathlessness

Non-pharmaceutical	Pharmaceutical
	Morphine[a]
Physical activity and pulmonary rehabilitation	Midazolam[b]
Breathing training	Lorazepam[b]
Relaxation and anxiety control techniques	Diazepam[b]
Symptom education	Phenothiazines[b]
Non-invasive ventilation	

[a]See ATS guideline [2]

[b]Evidence limited

In terms of medical management (see Table 23.1), opiate treatment is still considered the first line of treatment for palliation of breathlessness [9]. Opioids tend to be effective and have not been shown to have an adverse effect on length of life. These agents may be administered orally, subcutaneously, transdermally or intravenously. Unfortunately, opioids do have a side effect profile that includes: nausea, constipation and drowsiness. It is best to start with small doses of morphine 1–2.5 mg titrating up as required to a three times daily regime if needed. It can also be part of an emergency breathlessness plan.

Oxygen supplementation tends to be particularly helpful in patients with documented hypoxemia [10]; however, it does not tend to be effective in patients with adequate oxygen saturations [11]. Heliox, which is a mix of helium and oxygen (instead of nitrogen/oxygen in the normal atmosphere), is a less viscous gas, allows for a smoother flow of oxygen and has been shown to alleviate dyspnoea in patients with normal and low oxygen levels [12, 13]. This is particularly helpful with large airway obstruction.

Benzodiazepines, in particular midazolam, are also commonly used to combat terminal breathlessness. However, it should be noted that trial evidence does not support their effectiveness [14]. Nevertheless, these medications may be useful as adjuvant therapy [15] in combination with morphine. Midazolam is frequently used in conjunction with morphine as a continuous infusion at the end of life. Levomepromazine (previously known as methotrimeprazine), in a typical dose range of 6.25–12.5 mg, is helpful if anxiety, nausea and vomiting are significant associated symptoms.

Non-invasive ventilation (NIV) providing continuous positive airway pressure (CPAP) or bi-level positive airway pressure (BIPAP) in inspiration and expiration can also be employed in a palliative setting [16]. While some patients may not be able to tolerate NIV, most commonly related to a feeling of claustrophobia from the mask, it may relieve dyspnoea effectively without some of the undesirable effects of drug therapy, such as opiate-induced drowsiness. However, it is important to explore patient and family expectations before starting NIV and also outline clinical scenarios in which NIV may be discontinued.

Chest Pain

Chest pain is a common emergency and chronic presentation, and needs to be appropriately managed in patients with terminal illness. The initial assessment of patients suffering terminal disease who present with chest pain should aim to establish a diagnosis through history and investigations. However, investigations and management may vary in patients with terminal illness from those without, in accordance with the wishes of the patients and their families. If it is the patient's wish to be for active treatment of underlying causes of chest pain, this cause needs to be identified and treated appropriately. If on the other hand, patients do not wish to have active management of disease but rather symptom control, treatment of the latter should be sought. Treatment of pain in the palliative setting requires a multi-disciplinary, patient-centred approach. The palliative care team should be involved early if pain control proves difficult.

The World Health Organization (WHO) analgesic ladder provides good general guidance to pain control [17], starting with non-opioid analgesia such as acetaminophen/paracetamol or non-steroidal anti-inflammatory agents. This proceeds to further steps that include opioids, initially weak agents such as codeine and escalating to stronger medications, such as morphine or various alternatives. The exact choice of opioid may vary from patient to patient and needs to take into account the route of delivery. Different formulations are available and opioid analgesia is available in oral, subcutaneous, intravenous, transdermal or sublingual form. The right choice depends on the individual patient and their ability to take medications. The dose requirements again may vary greatly between patients. The starting doses of opioids should be equivalent to 2.5–10 mg of intravenous morphine and titrated up appropriately. Further discussion of opioid-related topics is described in Chap. 26 on "New Vistas in Pain Management". Constipation and nausea are common side effects of opioid treatment and should be pre-empted by considering laxatives and anti-emetics. A further side effect of opioids may be sedation. This should be frankly discussed with patients and family and may be taken into consideration when titrating opioid doses. However, overall it is felt that the treatment of pain is a priority, and that if sedation is a side effect, this may simply need to be accepted and explained to the patient [18].

Additional treatments can be considered for pain from specific causes. Primary or secondary tumours resulting in compression may be treated with high dose steroids (dexamethasone). Neuropathic pain caused by nerve compression, either secondary to tumours or pathological fractures may respond to treatment with gabapentin or amitriptyline. A new once daily formulation of gabapentin, Gralise, has similar efficacy with significant less side effects owing to its gastroretentive technology. Interventional procedures, described in Chap. 26, can provide significant relief to patients for a variety of pain states. Bone pain from bone metastasis may respond to treatment with bisphosphonate therapy and can be improved with single fraction radiotherapy. Other pain options are described throughout this book.

Cough

A chronic cough is an accompanying feature of many pathophysiological states affecting the airways, including diseases requiring palliative treatment such as lung cancer or end-stage COPD. It is easy to underestimate the disabling effect a cough may have on a patient's life, but a persistent cough is considered unacceptable in many social settings, such as movie theatres, concerts or restaurants. In addition, cough may result in syncope or urinary incontinence, which may cause major embarrassment and concerns for patients.

Cough is a symptom of different pathologies, which need to be explored. Cough in the context of terminal illness may accompany different conditions, such as neuromuscular pathologies, be a side effect of treatment such as chemotherapy or radiotherapy, or caused by a number of respiratory conditions such as tracheitis, acute bronchitis, chronic bronchitis, bronchiectasis, pneumonia, pulmonary fibrosis, lung cancer and pleural effusions amongst a wide range of respiratory pathology. Often, cough present in end-stage COPD or lung cancer is due to direct irritation of the airways and from accumulation of secretions in the airways. In order to relieve this, several treatment strategies may be helpful. It is worth noting that there is almost a dearth of credible evidence of management of cough in cancer patients [19]. This is an area that clearly requires further work. Pancoast tumours, which are tumours occurring in the lung apex can compress the recurrent laryngeal nerve, which results in incomplete apposition of the vocal cords, and subsequently a hoarse voice and a cough often described as a "bovine cough". Treatment of the cough caused by Pancoast tumours is through the treatment of the underlying malignancy.

Bronchodilation with inhaled or nebulised beta 2 agonists or muscarinic receptor antagonists may be particularly helpful in treating cough in end-stage COPD or in conditions with accompanying bronchospasm. In addition, inhaled or even oral glucocorticoids may help dampen down airway inflammation, as such reducing airway irritation and cough.

Secretions can be a problem in patients with terminal lung disease. For example, an obstructing lung lesion, such as either a primary lung tumour or distant metastasis can lead to accumulation of secretions behind the tumour and end-stage COPD can often be accompanied by a degree of traction bronchiectasis. Facilitating sputum clearance may alleviate the cough associated with these conditions. Methods include: positional drainage exercises, chest physiotherapy and cough machines. Treatments with mucolytic agents such as carbocysteine or nebulised saline to loosen secretions are effective. Benzonate (Tessalon perles, Zonatuss) anesthetises the stretch receptors and is effective in a number of cough states. Speech therapy and vocal hygiene strategies have also been helpful to treat cough. Manoeuvres such as pursed lip breathing, replacing cough with swallowing, avoiding smoking, avoiding mouth breathing, minimising alcohol consumption and caffeine or increasing water intake or steam inhalation are often simple measures used by these specialists in their cough rehabilitation sessions. Evidence for these strategies, however, is minimal but are worth considering when options are limited. With regards to symptom relief, drugs that act centrally can be used to suppress cough. These include opioids such as codeine and morphine, lidocaine and non-opioid agents such as dextromethorphan [20, 21]. It is important to note suppression of cough can result in pneumonia and therefore it is important to use cough suppressant drugs only after careful assessment of risks and benefits.

Wheeze and Stridor

Wheeze and stridor are terms that describe the physical signs produced by turbulent flow of air through narrowed airways. Stridor is a sign usually found in patients with upper respiratory tract narrowing or obstruction. It is described as a high-pitched, harsh, shrill, whistling or musical sound which can be present on inspiration and/or expiration. Inspiratory stridor can be indicative of serious airflow airway obstruction. It is therefore considered a medical emergency which necessitates urgent investigation and intervention. It should be noted that a fall in oxygen saturations is considered to be a late sign. Stridor can occasionally be intermittent if caused by a rapidly growing tumour that outgrows its blood supply resulting in repeated sloughing of necrotic tissue. It can also be present polypoid masses that case intermittent obstruction.

Wheeze is described as a high pitched, continuous, coarse whistling sound and can be present on inspiration, expiration or throughout the whole respiratory cycle. The site and timing of the wheeze and presence of a monophonic or polyphonic sound can help the examining physician differentiate between some pathologies. These characteristics can help guide further investigations and subsequent treatments. Examples of these would be a localised monophonic inspiratory and expiratory wheeze which can be associated with a discrete area of stenosis of the lower airways such as that caused by a malignant lesion. This can be contrasted with the diffuse polyphonic end expiratory wheeze heard in COPD or chronic asthma suggesting obstruction in multiple airways. In the typical case of wheeze seen with COPD, chronic asthma or lower respiratory tract infections, treatment should be given with bronchodilator therapy, such as salbutamol or ipatropium bromide in the nebulised or inhaled form and corticosteroids which help suppress inflammation within the airways. Intravenous or oral aminophylline or salbutamol could also be considered.

Emergency Management of Stridor

- Urgent assessment including concise history and examination
- Review of previous and current imaging for cause
- Attempt to ensure a calm and relaxing atmosphere in order to help relieve distress
- Constant reassurance and encouragement should be given

– High flow oxygen therapy to relieve respiratory distress and dyspnoea
– High dose corticosteroids such as dexamethasone 8 mg i.v./PO twice daily can be used to help reduce oedema although it should be remembered that this usually takes a number of hours to work
– Nebulised epinephrine can also help reduce airway oedema
– Heliox (mixed helium 70% and oxygen 30%) can be effective and occasionally provide an immediate benefit. The principle behind this treatment is that the low density and viscosity of helium reduces the turbulent flow through the airways, thus improving delivery of oxygen

Long-Term Management of Stridor

The long term management of patients with stridor secondary to malignancy includes pharmacological and physical interventions. Improvements in interventional bronchoscopic techniques as well as chemotherapy and radiotherapy regimes have meant that interventions can improve the patency of lumen of the airways, leading to an improvement in oxygen delivery to the lungs. These interventions include:

1. Tracheal and bronchial stenting.
   – Stents are deployed using the bronchoscope and are self-expanding.
   – Open up the airways and splint them open mechanically.
2. Cryotherapy "burns away" obstructing lesions and can lead to tumour necrosis by freezing the tissue locally.
3. Chemotherapy especially in the case of small cell lung cancer and lymphoma which are typically sensitive to current treatments.
4. Radiotherapy regimes leading to local tumour control and stopping further tumour growth and in some cases tumour regression. It should be noted that inflammation after radiotherapy can result in tissue expansion. A serious consequence if the obstruction is critical. It may be necessary to empirically stent or treat airways with other therapies prior to radiation therapy.
5. The consideration of tracheotomy in those patients with high tumours, e.g. at vocal cords.

In reality, these measures are not usually performed in isolation and combinations of therapies are typically used. To establish the most appropriate treatment, discussions with patients and their family are warranted and considerations made regarding the patients fitness to undergo invasive procedures or chemotherapy regimes. It would also be appropriate to adopt a multi-disciplinary approach taking into account the patient's prognosis and life expectancy.

List 23.1 Pulmonary causes of hemoptysis

- Malignancy
    - Bronchogenic carcinoma
    - Lung metastases
    - Kaposi's sarcoma
    - Carcinoid tumour
- Infections
    - Pneumonia
    - Lung abscess
    - Tuberculosis
    - Fungal infections
- Bronchiectasis
- Cystic fibrosis
- Vasculitis involving the lung
    - Wegner's granulomatosis
    - Goodpasture's syndrome
- Lung trauma/contusion
- Foreign body
- Pulmonary embolism

List 23.2 Non-pulmonary causes of "haemoptysis"

- Aspirated blood from nasal epistaxis or the upper respiratory tract. This could be precipitated by nasal oxygen therapy which leads to drying of the nasal mucosa or from any other cause for epistaxis
- Gastro-oesophageal reflux disease leading to irritation of the upper respiratory tract or leading to aspiration from an upper gastrointestinal (GI) bleed. In the case of palliative care, GI bleeds can be precipitated by the use of corticosteroid therapy as well as non-steroidal anti-inflammatory agents. The concurrent use of anti-coagulants or anti-platelet therapies can also worsen this process
- Trauma to the upper airways from, for example, following bronchoscopies or tracheostomies
- Congestive cardiac failure and mitral stenosis can lead to the production of the typical pink, frothy sputum described in textbooks although sputum in these diseases can often appear similar to hemoptysis

Hemoptysis

Hemoptysis is the expectoration (coughing up) of blood or of blood-stained sputum which is invariably a very distressing symptom for patients. It can range from minor blood streaking of sputum through to massive frank haemoptysis. Mild hemoptysis can usually be investigated as an outpatient providing the patient is otherwise well and haemodynamically stable with good respiratory function whereas massive haemoptysis is a medical emergency with a quoted mortality up to 80%. There is a possibility for patients to have a small "sentinel" or "herald" bleed prior to massive hemoptysis although this is a rare phenomenon.

The causes for haemoptysis are wide and a thorough history and examination should be performed in order to narrow down the likely aetiology (List 23.1). Decisions regarding appropriate use of imaging and invasive investigation techniques should then be guided by the differential diagnosis. It should be noted that some causes of hemoptysis may not be related to pulmonary pathology (List 23.2).

Investigations and Management

- Blood screening including: full blood count, coagulation and renal function tests. Further blood tests should be arranged as necessary.
- Chest X-ray (CXR) is usually easy to arrange and interpret. It can be performed quickly on the ward as a portable procedure, thus negating the need to transfer an unstable patient out of a controlled environment. Although the CXR does not give detailed information, it is usually required to plan further management. It can help look for signs suggestive of malignancy, infection or pulmonary emboli which are all potential causes of hemoptysis.
- Computer tomography (CT) imaging of the chest if the patient is stable allows a more detailed view of the thoracic anatomy. It is important to discuss the details of the clinical presentation so the radiologist can choose the right study protocol. Many units have a standard hemoptysis protocol. It is usually performed as a CT with contrast and contrast timings will vary depending on the main cause being considered. This investigation can give information on the cause of hemoptysis and also help exclude important negatives such as pulmonary emboli. The CT images can also help plan for further management including the need for therapeutic bronchoscopy or bronchial artery embolisation.
- Treatment should be guided by the underlying cause. If the CT imaging suggests infection, antibiotics or other therapeutic interventions should be given whereas pulmonary emboli should be treated with anti-coagulation.
- It is important to inspect the upper airway carefully especially if frank hemoptysis is present as this is often the cause of fresh bleeding. An ear, nose and throat specialist opinion is often helpful in this regard.
- Bronchial artery embolisation can be performed if the lesion/area bleeding is directly fed by a rich vascular supply with evidence of bleeding on bronchial angiography. The procedure is best performed in specialist centres due to the required expertise and risk of failure or the need to proceed to further definitive procedures if bleeding is not able to be controlled in this manner. The procedure involves the injection of glues or insertion of coils to "block" supplying arteries. It should be noted that the procedure carries a small risk of paraplegia (<1%) due to an anatomical variable where the anterior spinal artery originates from the bronchial arterial circulation [22, 23].
- Therapeutic bronchoscopy (as detailed below) [24].

– NB Hemoptysis of unknown cause is considered a contraindication to spirometry as the effort required to do the forced manoeuvres of the procedure can promote increased bleeding.

Massive Hemoptysis

A bleed of between 100 and 600 ml within a 24-h period is termed as massive hemoptysis and is a life-threatening emergency. It is usually extremely distressing for both the patient and their family or carers. As well as causing marked anxiety, it is associated with a mortality rate of up to 80% even with active treatment [25]. Due to the patient's general condition and hemodynamic and respiratory symptoms, investigations are usually difficult to perform and may be difficult to interpret.

Patients should be managed in the following way:

– High flow oxygen therapy.
– Cough suppressing agents such as opioids (oramorph, IM/IV morphine). If a patient has an ongoing cough, they may dislodge any clot that may have already formed.
– Tranexamic acid to aid coagulation.
– Intravenous access plus fluids (± blood) to maintain haemodynamic status.
– Positioning of patient in a lateral position with the affected side down. This prevents blood draining into the non-affected lung whilst "sacrificing" the diseased lung.
– Bronchoscopy—ideally rigid bronchoscopy where local treatment can be given directly to a bleeding lesion. Even flexible bronchoscopy can be beneficial with the application of iced saline or vasoconstrictors such as epinephrine/adrenaline or vasopressin onto a bleeding area to promote coagulation.
– In life-threatening cases, where appropriate, selective bronchial intubation can be used with the affected lung "blocked off" and single lung ventilation performed.
– Bronchial angiogram followed by bronchial artery embolisation can be performed by interventional radiologists if a specific bleeding area is identified.
– Surgical option is considered the last resort with lobectomy or pneumonectomy. This should obviously only be performed in selected cases where appropriate.

Infections

Lung infections can be the terminal event in many chronic lung conditions. In conditions such as cystic fibrosis, bronchiectasis and COPD, patients are particularly susceptible to developing recurrent lower respiratory tract infections, which can lead to progressive decline in lung function [26]. Recurrent infections can also lead to resistance to antibiotics due to repeated courses of antibiotics [27] and the presence of increasingly difficult to treat organisms such as *Pseudomonas aeruginosa*. Whereas these organisms are all treatable within the general population, the presence of nutritional deficiencies and relative immunodeficiency associated with some of these conditions leads to an increase in morbidity and mortality [28]. Furthermore, patients with malignancy can be more prone to lower respiratory tract infections due to partial/total obstruction of airways leading to post-obstructive pneumonias caused by an inability to clear out mucous. Combined with the immunosuppression caused by chemotherapy and radiotherapy, infections can be a major problem for these patients. As with the general population, it is important to review previous microbiological results in order to gain information on previously found organisms and their sensitivities. Many patients will already have sputum cultures or bronchoalveolar washing results available and antibiotic therapy should be targeted to these results. Further cultures should be sent prior to antibiotic therapy if possible and if the patient is stable enough to wait; otherwise, antibiotic therapy should be commenced as soon as possible. In the absence of previous positive cultures, broad spectrum antibiotics should be commenced which can be rationalised to targeted therapy depending on response and available results. In association with antibiotics, supportive therapy in the form of intravenous fluids should be given alongside sputum clearance techniques, which may include chest physiotherapy, humidified oxygen therapy or saline nebulisers and mucolytic therapy such as carbocysteine (mucodyne). Other treatments may include: steroid therapy and bronchodilator therapy plus prophylactic anti-coagulant therapy to prevent venous thromboembolic events. These should be decided on a case-by-case basis.

COPD

Chronic obstructive pulmonary disease (COPD) is a disease entity encompassing chronic bronchitis and/or emphysema, commonly caused by smoking and characterised by airflow limitation that is not fully reversible. The hallmark test for the diagnosis of COPD is spirometry and a forced expiratory volume in 1 second (FEV1) over a forced vital capacity (FVC) ratio of 0.7 or lower in the presence of symptoms or radiographic investigations suggestive of COPD and absence of an alternative explanation for the reduced FEV1/FVC ratio. COPD encompasses a spectrum that can range from a mild illness to a severe, life-threatening disease. However, as lung function declines with age COPD tends to get worse over time [29].

Globally, COPD is responsible for an increasing proportion of deaths. Cancer-based palliative care services are being extended to include non-malignant diseases such as COPD. About half of patients discharged from hospital after a COPD exacerbation will die within 2 years. In these patients with COPD, several indicators carry a poor prognosis. These include: poor nutritional status (low body-mass index), co-morbid heart disease, depression, continued smoking and older age. A low FEV1, poor exercise tolerance, frequent exacerbations and complications such as respiratory failure and cor pulmonale also affect prognosis [30]. Respiratory failure is defined as hypoxia with a $P_aO_2 < 60$ mmHg, while cor pulmonale is right-sided heart failure secondary to pulmonary disease. A combined tool to measure mortality in COPD is the BODE index, which combines measures of body-mass index, airway obstruction, dyspnoea and exercise capacity [31]. Accurate predictions, however, are extremely difficult and doctors familiar with these patients tending to overestimate survival. The only other condition where prognosis is less accurate is dementia. A policy focus on identifying a time point for transition to palliative care has little resonance from accounts of patients, professional and informal carers in a small qualitative study looking into this. COPD appears to be perceived as a way of life. A holistic assessment of needs could be linked with milestones such as hospital admission [32].

Treatment of patients with terminal COPD encompasses optimisation of their treatment. This employs inhaled or nebulised Beta-2 adrenergic agonists, inhaled or nebulised muscarinic antagonists, inhaled corticosteroids, oral theophylline or phospho-diesterase 4 inhibitors. In addition to medical therapy, smoking cessation therapy and vaccination (pneumococcal and influenza) should be offered to appropriate patients with COPD.

Additional therapy for COPD follows much along the same principles as treatment of dyspnoea, with a focus on patient education and pulmonary rehabilitation. Patients benefit from long-term oxygen therapy in terms of symptoms and survival if they develop hypoxemia (PaO_2 less than 55 mmHg, or PaO_2 less than 59 mmHg in the presence of pulmonary hypertension or polycythemia). Short burst oxygen therapy (2 h/day) may be beneficial in symptom control, as it may improve exertional dyspnoea and exercise tolerance. Patients suffering from hypercapnia may benefit from non-invasive ventilation, if tolerated. Please also see the sections above on "Cough", "Breathlessness or Dyspnea", and "Wheeze and Stridor."

Neurological Cases

Respiratory problems are commonly found in the neurological patient. More importantly, they are also a common cause of mortality within this patient population. From an increased risk of pulmonary embolism in the immobile patient, to recurrent aspiration, and ventilatory failure from bulbar and respiratory muscle weakness, the respiratory problems experienced within this patient subgroup are numerous. It should therefore be suggested that the respiratory physician should play a role in the management of patients suffering from long-term chronic neurological conditions.

Many neurological conditions are associated with bulbar weakness leading to dysfunction of swallow and the possibility of recurrent aspiration with repeated lower respiratory tract infections and aspiration pneumonia. These patients are usually further compromised by having a weak cough so limiting their ability to clear secretions from their chest. Management should therefore include active monitoring and aggressive treatment of the chest with involvement of a physiotherapist specialising

List 23.3 Causes of diaphragmatic weakness

- Brainstem CVAs and lesions
- Phrenic nerve injury/idiopathic dysfunction
- Guillan–Barre syndrome
- Lou Gehrig's disease (motor neurone disease)
- Muscular dystrophy
- Myotonic dystrophy

in chest conditions, a speech and language therapist and the respiratory physician. The patient's swallow should be examined and monitored for evidence of deterioration and the chest for evidence of aspiration. Infections should be treated early as the neurological patient tends to have a poor respiratory reserve and can decompensate quickly into ventilatory failure with a need for consideration for respiratory support.

A further problem with many neurological conditions is diaphragmatic weakness which can rapidly lead to ventilatory respiratory failure (List 23.3). The importance of the diaphragms is best seen during sleep, specifically the rapid eye movement (REM) stage of sleep. A feature of REM sleep is the presence of REM "paralysis" where the muscles, including the muscles of respiration become flaccid leading the body to rely on the diaphragms to maintain respiration. When the diaphragms are weak or paralysed the patient loses this respiratory mechanism leading to nocturnal hypoventilation which, with progression of the underlying disease leads to type II (hypercapnic, ventilatory) respiratory failure. It is very important to identify and prepare for this early particularly in patients with motor neurone disease as their progression to death is very rapid from the time of diagnosis of type II respiratory failure.

Where appropriate, early discussions should take place with the patient and their family or carers. The patient should be given information regarding their underlying condition and the likely future prognosis plus treatment options. Discussions should include the use of artificial nutrition and potential future need for respiratory support. Having an open discussion early in the disease process allows the patient to express their wishes for future treatment and also to express what they feel to be the limits of treatment that they would accept. In many neurological conditions with bulbar involvement, communication becomes progressively more difficult and it may become more difficult to appreciate a patient's decisions. It should be remembered that in many cases, neurological conditions are not curable and the role of artificial nutrition and respiratory support is to prolong life—thus, the decisions should involve what is considered by the patient to be an appropriate quality of life.

Treatment Options

Centres specialising in ventilatory failure in patients with neurological conditions are increasing. In early stages, oxygen therapy may be sufficient to control a patient's symptoms and respiratory difficulties. As the underlying disease progresses, neuromuscular function becomes further impaired and nocturnal hypoventilation can occur. This can be easily tested on simple overnight oximetry studies. Initially, these studies may show REM-related episodes of desaturation which typically occur every ~90 min through the night and become more frequent towards the end of the night where the proportion of REM sleep increases. Providing there is no evidence of ventilatory failure on arterial blood gas sampling or clinically (List 23.3), the patient can be followed up with serial overnight oximetry. If type II respiratory (ventilatory, hypercapnic) failure develops, non-invasive ventilation (NIV) can be commenced at night to improve oxygenation and carbon dioxide clearance [33]. As the muscles become weaker, NIV may be required for longer periods of time including daytime "top-ups". With further progression, tracheostomy and full-time invasive ventilation has been used. This is obviously a supportive measure with an aim to prolong a patient's life. It should therefore be established whether this is an acceptable quality of life for the patient and allow him or her to make up their own decisions regarding these treatments.

Lung Cancer

Lung cancer is the most common form of malignancy worldwide. It is by far the most common cause of cancer in male populations and although it is the fourth most common in females (behind breast, colorectal and cervix/uterus), its incidence is increasing with time. In 2008, the World Health Organisation via the International Agency for Research on Cancer released figures on the GLOBOCAN network with "the aim of providing estimates of the incidence of and mortality from major cancers, at national level, for all countries of the world". GLOBOCAN estimates that the annual incidence for all cancers in 2008 worldwide was 12.66 million. Of these, 1.6 million are thought to be from lung primary with 1.1 million cases being male and 500,000 females. Despite advances in the treatment of many forms of malignancy, lung cancer is still associated with a high mortality rate with 1.38 million deaths worldwide attributed to the disease. In 2008, GLOBOCAN estimates that there were 215,021 new diagnoses of lung cancer with 161,841 deaths in the USA. When compared with breast cancer (182,460 diagnoses and 40,481 deaths) and prostatic cancer (186,320 diagnoses and 28,660 deaths), it is clear that not only is lung cancer the most common malignancy, it also carries the worst prognosis.

The reason for the high mortality rate in lung cancer is usually seen as the late presentation. At present there are no national screening programmes in operation and the typical symptoms of lung cancer are usually fairly non-specific (List 23.4). Lung cancers are also typically aggressive with early local and metastatic spread often present at the time of diagnosis. Another factor is that patients are often found to have other co-morbidities such as ischemic heart disease and chronic obstructive pulmonary disease (COPD) due to their common risk factor of smoking. These underlying illnesses can mean that patients with cancer staged as being potentially resectable are not offered operative procedures due to the high risks associated with

List 23.4 Symptoms and signs in patients at risk of ventilatory failure

- Diaphragmatic weakness
  - Suggested by paradoxical (see-saw) respiration on lying supine
  - A decrease of 20% in FVC on supine spirometry as compared to erect spirometry
- FVC<1L
- Orthopnea
- Paroxysmal nocturnal dyspnoea
- Nocturnal hypoventilation as seen on overnight oximetry
- Early morning headaches, drowsiness, excessive daytime somnolence, worsening concentration levels

List 23.5 Symptoms of SVC obstruction

1. Facial oedema
2. Facial flushing
3. Headache
4. Distended veins in upper limb, upper body, head and neck
5. Dizziness
6. Inspiratory stridor
7. Dyspnoea

surgery. Poor lung function would also make radiotherapy to the chest difficult due to the likely damage to surrounding normal tissue, potentially further depleting an already limited physiological reserve. It should be noted that active treatments can be interwoven with palliative care strategies. This includes the use of radiotherapy to help with pain control from metastases and to help with symptoms from spinal cord compression. Radiotherapy and superior vena caval stenting can be performed to help with the symptoms of superior vena caval obstruction (List 23.5).

In summary, it is therefore important that respiratory physicians and palliative care teams work closely to ensure the best possible outcomes for patients. It is estimated that palliative care involvement can lead to relief from physical, psychosocial and spiritual problems in over 90% of patients with advanced cancer. It has also been shown that the early involvement of palliative care services in patients with advanced non-small lung cancer led to not only an improvement in quality of life, well-being and mood, but also showed that these patients had a longer survival even with less aggressive care at the end of life [34].

References

1. Johnson MJ, Booth S. Palliative and end-of-life care for patients with chronic heart failure and chronic lung disease. Clin Med. 2010;10(3):286–9.
2. Lanken PN, Terry PB, DeLisser HM, Fahy BF, Hansen-Flaschen J, Heffner JE, et al. An official American Thoracic Society clinical policy statement: palliative care for patients with respiratory diseases and critical illnesses. Am J Respir Crit Care Med. 2008;177(8):912–27.

3. Dyspnea. Mechanisms, assessment, and management: a consensus statement. Am J Respir Crit Care Med. 1999;159(1):321–40.

4. Grond S, Zech D, Diefenbach C, Bischoff A. Prevalence and pattern of symptoms in patients with cancer pain: a prospective evaluation of 1635 cancer patients referred to a pain clinic. J Pain Symptom Manage. 1994;9(6):372–82.

5. Stromgren AS, Sjogren P, Goldschmidt D, Petersen MA, Pedersen L, Groenvold M. Symptom priority and course of symptomatology in specialized palliative care. J Pain Symptom Manage. 2006;31(3):199–206.

6. Karnani NG, Reisfield GM, Wilson GR. Evaluation of chronic dyspnea. Am Fam Physician. 2005;71(8):1529–37.

7. Borg G. Perceived exertion as an indicator of somatic stress. Scand J Rehabil Med. 1970;2(2):92–8.

8. Ries AL, Bauldoff GS, Carlin BW, Casaburi R, Emery CF, Mahler DA, et al. Pulmonary rehabilitation. Chest. 2007;131(5 suppl):4S–2.

9. Light RW, Muro JR, Sato RI, Stansbury DW, Fischer CE, Brown SE. Effects of oral morphine on breathlessness and exercise tolerance in patients with chronic obstructive pulmonary disease. Am Rev Respir Dis. 1989;139(1):126–33.

10. Bruera E, de Stoutz N, Velasco-Leiva A, Schoeller T, Hanson J. Effects of oxygen on dyspnoea in hypoxaemic terminal-cancer patients. Lancet. 1993;342(8862):13–4.

11. Uronis HE, Currow DC, McCrory DC, Samsa GP, Abernethy AP. Oxygen for relief of dyspnoea in mildly- or non-hypoxaemic patients with cancer: a systematic review and meta-analysis. Br J Cancer. 2008;98(2):294–9.

12. Laude EA, Ahmedzai SH. Oxygen and helium gas mixtures for dyspnoea. Curr Opin Support Palliat Care. 2007;1(2):91–5.

13. Ahmedzai SH, Laude E, Robertson A, Troy G, Vora V. A double-blind, randomised, controlled Phase II trial of Heliox28 gas mixture in lung cancer patients with dyspnoea on exertion. Br J Cancer. 2004;90(2):366–71.

14. Simon ST, Higginson IJ, Booth S, Harding R, Bausewein C. Benzodiazepines for the relief of breathlessness in advanced malignant and non-malignant diseases in adults. Cochrane Database Syst Rev. 2010;(1):CD007354.

15. Navigante AH, Cerchietti LC, Castro MA, Lutteral MA, Cabalar ME. Midazolam as adjunct therapy to morphine in the alleviation of severe dyspnea perception in patients with advanced cancer. J Pain Symptom Manage. 2006;31(1):38–47.

16. Mercadante S, Villari P, David F, Agozzino C. Noninvasive ventilation for the treatment of dyspnea as a bridge from intensive to end-of-life care. J Pain Symptom Manage. 2009;38(3):e5–7.

17. Ventafridda V, Tamburini M, Caraceni A, De CF, Naldi F. A validation study of the WHO method for cancer pain relief. Cancer. 1987;59(4):850–6.

18. Quill TE, Lee BC, Nunn S. Palliative treatments of last resort: choosing the least harmful alternative. University of Pennsylvania Center for Bioethics Assisted Suicide Consensus Panel. Ann Intern Med. 2000;132(6):488–93.

19. Wee B, Browning J, Adams A, Benson D, Howard P, Klepping G, Molassiotis A, Taylor D. Management of chronic cough in patients receiving palliative care: review of evidence and recommendations by a task group of the Association for Palliative Medicine of Great Britain and Ireland. Palliat Med. 2012;26(6):780–7.

20. Molassiotis A, Bailey C, Caress A, Brunton L, Smith J. Interventions for cough in cancer. Cochrane Database Syst Rev. 2010;(9):CD007881.

21. Matthys H, Bleicher B, Bleicher U. Dextromethorphan and codeine: objective assessment of antitussive activity in patients with chronic cough. J Int Med Res. 1983;11(2):92–100.

22. Daliri A, Probst NH, Jobst B, Lepper PM, Kickuth R, Szucs-Farkas Z, et al. Bronchial artery embolization in patients with hemoptysis including follow-up. Acta Radiol. 2011;52(2):143–7.

23. Shin BS, Jeon GS, Lee SA, Park MH. Bronchial artery embolisation for the management of haemoptysis in patients with pulmonary tuberculosis. Int J Tuberc Lung Dis. 2011;15(8):1093–8.

24. Sakr L, Dutau H. Massive hemoptysis: an update on the role of bronchoscopy in diagnosis and management. Respiration. 2010;80(1):38–58.
25. Gollins SW, Ryder WD, Burt PA, Barber PV, Stout R. Massive haemoptysis death and other morbidity associated with high dose rate intraluminal radiotherapy for carcinoma of the bronchus. Radiother Oncol. 1996;39(2):105–16.
26. Zoumot Z, Wilson R. Respiratory infection in noncystic fibrosis bronchiectasis. Curr Opin Infect Dis. 2010;23(2):165–70.
27. Desai H, Richter S, Doern G, Heilmann K, Dohrn C, Johnson A, et al. Antibiotic resistance in sputum isolates of Streptococcus pneumoniae in chronic obstructive pulmonary disease is related to antibiotic exposure. COPD. 2010;7(5):337–44.
28. Herzog R, Cunningham-Rundles S. Immunologic impact of nutrient depletion in chronic obstructive pulmonary disease. Curr Drug Targets. 2011;12(4):489–500.
29. Fletcher C, Peto R. The natural history of chronic airflow obstruction. Br Med J. 1977;1(6077):1645–8.
30. Celli BR. Predictors of mortality in COPD. Respir Med. 2010;104(6):773–9.
31. Celli BR, Cote CG, Marin JM, Casanova C, de Montes OM, Mendez RA, et al. The body-mass index, airflow obstruction, dyspnea, and exercise capacity index in chronic obstructive pulmonary disease. N Engl J Med. 2004;350(10):1005–12.
32. Pinnock H, Kendall M, Murray SA, Worth A, Levack P, Porter M, et al. Living and dying with severe chronic obstructive pulmonary disease: multi-perspective longitudinal qualitative study. BMJ. 2011;342:d142. doi:10.1136/bmj.d142.:d142.
33. O'Neill CL, Williams TL, Peel ET, McDermott CJ, Shaw PJ, Gibson GJ, et al. Non-invasive ventilation in motor neuron disease: an update of current UK practice. J Neurol Neurosurg Psychiatry. 2012;83(4):371–6.
34. Temel JS, Greer JA, Muzikansky A, Gallagher ER, Admane S, Jackson VA, et al. Early palliative care for patients with metastatic non-small-cell lung cancer. N Engl J Med. 2010;363(8):733–42.

Review Questions

1. Treatments of proven benefit in dyspnoea do not include:

   (a) Opioids
   (b) Oxygen for patients with hypoxia
   (c) Benzodiazepines
   (d) Heliox

2. Treatment of symptomatic cough includes:

   (a) Bronchodilator therapy
   (b) Physiotherapy
   (c) Dextromethorphan
   (d) All of the above

3. Patients with hemoptysis:

   (a) Suffer underlying lung conditions
   (b) Need to be managed as inpatients
   (c) Have massive hemoptysis if they exporate > 50 ml of blood over 24 h
   (d) If massive, may have up to 80% mortality

4. For the effective treatment of dyspnoea, opioids may be give

   (a) Orally
   (b) Intravenously
   (c) Transdermally
   (d) All of the above

5. Stridor:

   (a) Is a medical emergency
   (b) Can be alleviated quickly by i.v steroids
   (c) Can only be treated by physical means, e.g. stenting/tracheostomy
   (d) Should be treated by administering back to back salbutamol nebulisers

6. In haemoptysis:

   (a) A CXR is usually sufficient to diagnose cause and aetiology
   (b) Patients should receive high flow oxygen therapy
   (c) "Massive" bleeds are defined as blood loss > 50 ml
   (d) Patients should receive nebulised therapy

7. The treatment of lung infections in immunosuppressed patients should include:

   (a) Broad spectrum antibiotics
   (b) The use of mucolytics
   (c) Physiotherapy
   (d) All of the above

8. Patients with respiratory muscle weakness are most likely to hypoventilate:

   (a) When awake
   (b) In Stage $1+2$ sleep
   (c) In Stage $3+4$ sleep
   (d) In REM sleep

9. Poor prognosis in lung cancer compared to other malignancies is typically due to:

   (a) Late presentation of disease
   (b) Advanced stage of disease at presentation
   (c) Poor performance status of patients due to co-existing medical conditions
   (d) All of the above

Answers

1. (c). While opioids have been shown to be effective in a number of trials, as have oxygen for hypoxic patients or heliox, particularly for patients with large airway obstruction, there is little evidence for the use of benzodiazepines. However, treatment of dyspnoea often includes benzodiazepines such as midazolam, as it is felt that patients may still benefit.

2. (d). Treatment of symptomatic cough is important as it can be a disabling feature of many illnesses. Treatment of cough requires the diagnosis and management of the underlying condition—which may be pulmonary or extra-pulmonary, such as post-nasal drip and gastro-esophageal reflux disease. Cough, particularly caused by airways disease such as asthma or COPD may respond to bronchodilator therapy. Physiotherapy can be important in teaching cough suppression techniques. Dextromethorphan is a pharmacological cough suppressant.

3. (d). In patients presenting with hemoptysis, it is important to rule out bleeding from other sites, such as the oral cavity or nose, which can present as hemoptysis without any overt epistaxis or pooling of blood in the mouth. Not all hemoptysis needs to be managed as an inpatient, and patients with mild hemoptysis who are haemodynamically stable and have little co-morbidities may be managed as outpatients after thorough assessment. Massive hemoptysis is defined as expectoration over 100 ml of blood over 24 h. Massive hemoptysis may be fatal and requires intensive management and resuscitation, if appropriate. However, the mortality of massive hemoptysis may approach 80%.

4. (d). In terms of pharmacological treatment of dyspnoea, opioids are still considered first line. Opioids may be administered in a number of different routes, including orally, subcutaneously, transdermally or intravenously. However, it is important that in the treatment of dyspnoea a patient centred multi-disciplinary team approach is taken. This will include the treatment of patients with non-pharmacological methods such as psychological support, exercise, nutritional advice and other methods, such as cooling fans.

5. (a). Stridor is considered to be a medical emergency which can rapidly progress to death due to complete airway obstruction. Although steroids are beneficial, their mode of action means that they usually take a few hours to work. Treatment of stridor is dependent on the cause, i.e. small cell lung cancer or lymphoma causing airway obstruction due to mediastinal lymphadenopathy may respond to chemotherapy agents. Tracheostomy is only helpful in high tumours, i.e. those above the vocal cords. Nebulised therapy with *epinephrine* has been shown to be beneficial.

6. (b). A CXR is often quick and easy to arrange. However, more detailed radiology such as CT scanning is often necessary in order to determine the cause for haemoptysis. Patients with haemoptysis should be treated with high flow oxygen and cough suppressant medications such as opiates. They should be managed in a calm, relaxed manner, positioned lying on the side of the diseased lung, so protecting the "good" lung. Nebulised therapy can lead to coughing

which can precipitate further bleeding. Massive haemotysis is defined as blood loss of 100–600 ml in a 24-h period.

7. (d). All of the above are suggested. Physiotherapy can help clear secretions. Mucolytics such as carbocysteine and nebulised saline can help loosen secretions to help expectoration. Infections in immunosuppressed patients maybe due to atypical or unusual pathogens, therefore, initial treatment with broad spectrum antibiotics is recommended whilst culture results are awaited.

8. (d). During REM sleep flaccid paralysis occurs meaning breathing is via the diaphragm only. If a patient has a neuromuscular weakness affecting the diaphragms, they will breathe less effectively during this phase of sleep. Stage $1+2$ is defined as light sleep, Stage $3+4$ is defined as deep sleep.

9. (d). Patients with lung cancer often present late and with advanced disease. They often have co-existent COPD and cardiac disease due to their shared aetiology (i.e. smoking).

Chapter 24
Palliative Care in Critical Care Units

Rita Agarwala, Ben Singer, and Sreekumar Kunnumpurath

Introduction

Modern Critical Care Units admit increasingly more complex cases and are able to offer novel, often very invasive, interventions in order to achieve favourable outcomes. Despite this over 20% of deaths in the USA occur in critical care units and over half of those who die in hospital are cared for in critical care units within 3 days of their death [1]. It is, therefore, essential to appreciate the integral role of palliative care within this environment.

The majority of patients admitted to the critical care unit are treated aggressively for acute, potentially reversible diseases [1]. However, palliative care within this group should not be ignored. These patients will still experience pain, discomfort, fear and confusion [2]. Also, a subset of these patients will fail to respond to treatment and further aggressive management will no longer be in their best interests. Palliative care in these patients then becomes the main focus of therapy in the critical care unit.

There is also a group of patients with chronic conditions such as chronic obstructive pulmonary disease or lung fibrosis who are admitted to the critical care unit with the hope of reversing an acute exacerbation or treating a complication of their condition. Palliative care in this group plays a more significant role. Again, a proportion of these patients will continue to deteriorate and symptom control becomes the main goal of treatment.

Many of the principles of palliative care discussed throughout this book, particularly those relating to terminal care, still apply to patients within critical care.

R. Agarwala, B.M., B.Sc. • B. Singer, M.B.B.S., F.R.C.A. (✉)
S. Kunnumpurath, M.B.B.S., M.D.
Department of Anesthetics, Epsom and St Helier University Hospitals NHS Trust,
Carshalton, Surrey, UK
e-mail: b.singer@doctors.org.uk

N. Vadivelu et al. (eds.), *Essentials of Palliative Care*,
DOI 10.1007/978-1-4614-5164-8_24,
© Springer Science+Business Media New York 2013

Maintaining dignity, good communication, ensuring adequate pain management, providing treatment for anxiety, dyspnoea and secretions should not be forgotten. This chapter, however, will focus on palliative care issues and diseases often seen in the critical care unit.

Non-invasive Ventilation

Non-invasive positive pressure ventilation (NIPPV) is one method of assisting ventilation without an endotracheal tube. Pressurised gas is delivered to the airways via a mask, inflating the lungs. Exhalation then occurs by the passive elastic recoil of the lungs and the active contraction of the expiratory muscles [3]. The mask is tight fitting and is applied over the mouth and nose, or in some circumstances, just the nose alone. It is then held in place with elasticated straps (Fig. 24.1). The patient breathes spontaneously and each breath is supported. There are two forms of NIPPV, continuous positive pressure ventilation (CPAP) and bilevel inspiratory positive pressure ventilation (BIPAP).

In CPAP, a constant pressure is delivered during both inspiration and expiration. By doing so, collapsed or underventilated alveoli are opened up, increasing functional residual capacity and improving oxygenation. CPAP also helps improve lung compliance and decreases the work of breathing [4]. In pulmonary oedema, excess alveolar fluid weighs down the closed alveoli. At the end of expiration the energy required to re-open the alveoli for gas exchange is high. This can lead to rapid fatigue and worsening in the patient's condition. The application of CPAP splints the alveoli open and reduces the energy expenditure making breathing much easier for the patient. It also causes a reduction in afterload making CPAP an attractive treatment for pulmonary oedema [3].

In some conditions, CPAP would fail to provide adequate respiratory support and BiPAP may be more appropriate. In BiPAP, two levels of pressure are delivered to the patient. The first, as in CPAP, is a constant pressure delivered throughout the respiratory cycle and is known as expiratory positive airway pressure or EPAP. The second is the inspiratory positive airway pressure, IPAP. When the ventilator detects the negative pressure generated by the patient breathing in it delivers a pre-set pressure (the IPAP) of oxygen/air mix above the pressure already being delivered by the EPAP. This not only reduces the work of breathing but also increases ventilation [3].

NIPPV is now regularly used to reverse and cure acute respiratory failure [3]. Studies have proven its benefit in chronic obstructive airway disease (COAD) [5], respiratory failure in immunocompromised hosts [6] and in cardiogenic pulmonary oedema [7]. A consensus statement in 2001 on non-invasive ventilation for acute respiratory failure also supported the use of palliative NIPPV in selected patients. The consensus suggested palliative NIPPV could be used when endotracheal intubation was inappropriate provided the cause of respiratory failure was known to be reversible and that the NIPPV helped to improve patient comfort [8]. A society for

Fig. 24.1 Examples of masks used for non-invasive ventilation (**a**) oronasal mask. (**b**) Nasal mask

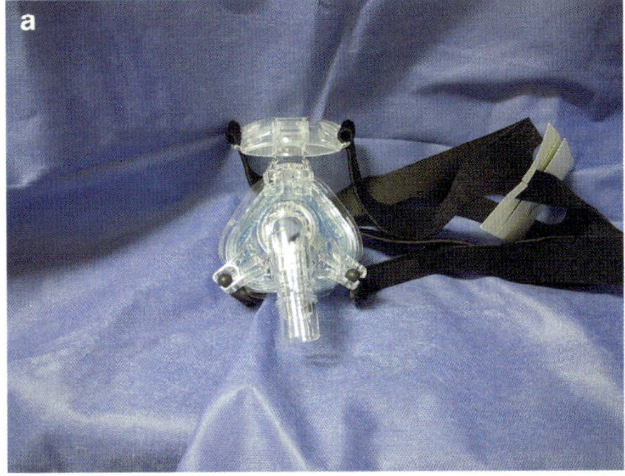

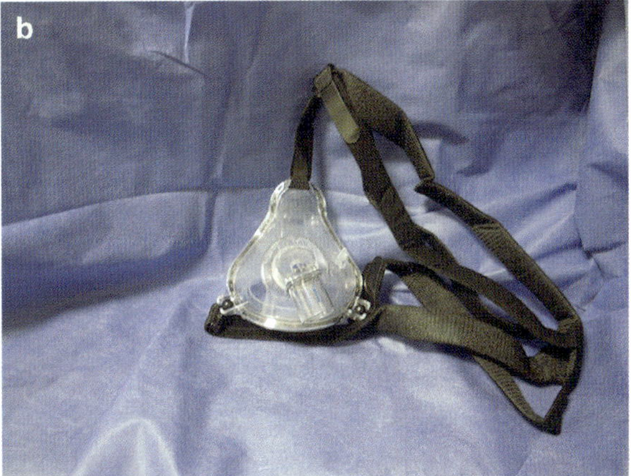

critical care medicine task force built on this and provided one approach to categorise the use of NIPPV [4]: Those without preset limits on the provision of advanced life support; NIPPV for patients who decline endotracheal intubation and invasive mechanical ventilation; NIPPV as a comfort measure for patients who decline endotracheal intubation [4]. The latter two categories describe palliative NIPPV.

In the second category, NIPPV is being used to help support ventilation whilst the underlying cause of acute respiratory failure is treated. It is commonly used in patients with a chronic condition with the hope of reversing an acute exacerbation or treating a complication of their illness. Though the patient should be comfortable on NIPPV, some discomfort may be tolerated if oxygenation or ventilation is improving. If NIPPV, however, is not tolerated or not improving the patient's acute illness, then comfort measures should be adopted after discussion between the patient, family and the healthcare team [4].

Table 24.1 Adverse side effects of NIPPV [3]

Adverse effect	Possible solution
Discomfort from the mask	New type of mask, check fit
Facial skin erythema	Loosen straps
Nasal Bridge ulceration	Loosen straps, artificial skin
Nasal congestion	Nasal decongestant, antihistamine
Eye irritation	Check mask fits
Gastric insufflations	Reduce pressure, Reassure
Air leaks	New mask type, encourage mouth closure
Aspiration pneumonia	Careful patient selection, adequate consciousness
Hypotension	Reduce pressures
Pneumothorax	Stop NIPPV if possible. Chest drain if indicated

NIPPV can be used as a comfort measure. Though limited, evidence suggests that NIPPV can reduce the sensation of dyspnoea [9, 10]. This may allow a reduction in the amount of opiate and anxiolytic required to treat this distressing symptom and thus reduce side effects (such as reduced consciousness) associated with these drugs. Though the mask itself may hinder speech, the relief of dyspnoea and the improved consciousness may help maintain communication for longer.

However, NIPPV is associated with adverse side effects. One side effect is discomfort [3], not only associated with the very tight fitting mask, but also due to the high pressures giving an initial sensation of trying to breathe through a strong wind tunnel. Some strategies exist for circumventing these problems such as using different masks [3] (hood masks, nasal masks), or starting on low pressures and increasing gradually. Another approach is to use light sedation to reduce patient anxiety but this carries significant risks of reducing the patient's respiratory drive and conscious level and may negate the original reasons for using NIPPV. Other adverse effects are listed in Table 24.1 [3].These effects may be unacceptable to the patient and outweigh the relief of dyspnoea NIPPV may provide. For this reason, for patients in the third category in particular, it is vital they are able to communicate the decision to start or continue support as any discomfort is this group should not be tolerated [4].

There are also several relative contraindications for starting NIPPV. These include patients actively or at high risk of vomiting (i.e. bowel obstruction), reduced consciousness, untreated significant pneumothorax and oral–facial abnormalities [11].

The use of palliative NIPPV still remains a controversial issue. The concern is the inadvertent prolongation of the dying process [12]. There is no data currently which supports or refutes this. Also, data proving NIPPV in the dying patient improves the quality of end-of-life care or the family experience does not exist either.

Diabetic Ketoacidosis

A potentially life-threatening complication seen in patients with diabetes is diabetic ketoacidosis (DKA). Mortality rates have improved greatly due to the improved management over the past 20 years and have fallen from close to 8% to now just 0.67% [13]. It remains high in developing countries and those not hospitalised indicating the importance of early diagnosis, prompt treatment and disease prevention [14].

DKA occurs due to absolute or relative insulin deficiency and excessive counter-regulatory hormones such as glucagon, cortisol and growth hormone. This imbalance leads to severe hyperglycaemia, acidosis and ketonaemia [15]. The deficiency of insulin within the body enhances hepatic glucose production causing the hyperglycaemia. The high blood glucose levels trigger an osmotic diuresis resulting in severe dehydration. The dehydration is then exacerbated by the vomiting associated with the disease process and the reduced fluid intake secondary to the decreased level of consciousness. With such severe dehydration, electrolyte shifts occur which can also be life threatening.

Hepatic glucose production is increased by the breakdown of fat and protein. When fat is metabolised like this it produces large amounts of fatty acids. These fatty acids are then converted to ketones (mainly acetone, 3 beta hydroxybutyrate and acetoacetate) resulting in the ketonaemia and acidosis [16].

As soon as a diagnosis of DKA is made a rapid assessment of airway, breathing and circulation should be done. If the dehydration is severe enough to cause a decreased level of consciousness and airway compromise this must be dealt with first, often requiring intubation and ventilation. After this initial assessment, large bore intravenous cannula should be inserted and intravenous fluids commenced. A medical history should be elicited and a clinical examination performed to help identify potential triggers such as infection and non-compliance with medications. Initial investigations, such as those listed in Table 24.2 [15], should also be completed to aid diagnosis and management. Intravenous fluids must also be started promptly to restore the circulating blood volume. Initially, one litre of 0.9% saline is infused over an hour. Subsequent litre bags of 0.9% saline containing potassium chloride are then infused over 2, 4 and 6 h. If a patient is haemodynamically unstable (hypotensive and tachycardic) then these fluids must be given faster without any additional potassium. Due to the greater risk of complications from DKA and its treatment, caution in the rate of fluid resuscitation must be exercised in the elderly, those aged 18–25, in pregnancy and in patients with heart or kidney failure. In these patients fluid should be replaced cautiously and guided by central venous pressure measurements.

Potassium chloride is often added to the second and subsequent bags of fluid because treatment of DKA often drives potassium back into cells causing a hypokalaemia. It is not added to the first litre of fluid in case the DKA has caused a renal failure and an associated hyperkalaemia. In fact, hyperkalaemia is often seen in patients with DKA at presentation due to the acidosis and potassium should not be

Table 24.2 Suggested initial investigations when managing DKA

Blood ketones
Capillary blood glucose
Venous plasma glucose, urea and electrolytes, full blood count
Blood cultures
Venous blood gas
Electrocardiogram
Chest radiograph
Urinalysis and culture

added if the level is greater than 5.5 mmol/l. Once fluid has been initiated a fixed rate intravenous insulin infusion should be commenced at 0.1 unit of fast acting soluble insulin per kilogramme per hour. If there will be a delay in starting the infusion a once only dose of intramuscular fast acting insulin can be given at 0.1 unit/kg. Continue any long acting insulin the patient normally takes at the usual dose and time [15].

Once treatment has been initiated reassessment of the patient and the metabolic parameters is required. A catheter should be considered if the patient is anuric, oliguric or incontinent as this aids assessment of the response to treatment. Also a nasogastric tube may be beneficial in patients who are persistently vomiting and again will help quantify fluid loss. Metabolic parameters should also be reviewed and if a fall in blood ketones by at least 0.5 mmol/l/h or, a fall in blood glucose by 3 mmol/l/h or, a rise in venous bicarbonate of 3 mmol/l/h is not achieved the insulin infusion rate should be increased by 1 unit/h until these rates of improvement are seen. Once the blood glucose is below 14 mmol/l, 10% dextrose fluid infusion at 125 ml/h should be started alongside the 0.9% saline. Again caution in fluid volumes must be taken in high-risk patients and should be adjusted to the patient's clinical condition and the measured variables. The glucose fluid is added to prevent hypoglycaemia as the insulin infusion must continue to suppress the production of ketones. Serum potassium must also be measured frequently and potassium replacement within the fluids continued if the potassium remains between 3.5 and 5.5 mmol/l and the patient continues to pass urine. Again, above this range potassium should not be added and below this further potassium may need to be given. Additional potassium can be given in concentrated volumes via central venous access and in the presence of close cardiac monitoring.

After 24 h the acidosis and ketonaemia is likely to have resolved. Resolution is defined as ketones less than 0.3 mmol/l and pH more than 7.3. The precipitating factor should continue to be treated but if the patient is eating and drinking normally they can be transferred to a subcutaneous insulin regime. A dose of fast acting insulin should be given subcutaneously before a meal and then the intravenous infusion stopped 1 h later. This transfer to subcutaneous insulin is ideally managed by the specialist diabetes team and the team should be involved in the care of DKA patients from a very early stage [15]. Their involvement has been shown to reduce length of hospital stay [17].

The management of DKA involves aggressive fluid management. This has consequences including hyperchloraemic acidosis, due to the large volumes of 0.9% saline used, and more significantly pulmonary and cerebral oedema. The hyperchloraemic acidosis has not been shown to cause significant morbidity or increase length of stay in hospital. However, it is the reason why bicarbonate is not used to define resolution of DKA. Cerebral and pulmonary oedema are uncommon in DKA. They occur within a few hours of treatment and are thought to be iatrogenic though this has been disputed [15]. Cerebral oedema is more likely to occur in the younger population whereas pulmonary oedema is more likely to be seen in the elderly and in those with cardiac and renal dysfunction [15].

The treatment of DKA involves numerous blood tests to assess progress and can be distressing for the patient. Though central venous access will reduce the number of needle pricks, its insertion can be difficult, painful and associated with complications. Response to treatment can be assessed using venous blood and arterial puncture or arterial catheter insertion is not required unless there is any concern regarding oxygenation, ventilation or haemodynamic stability in severe DKA. Arterial puncture is again very painful. Whatever method is used for venesection, the distress it can cause the patient should be considered and local anaesthetic should be thought about with each attempt.

Hyperkalaemia

Potassium is the most abundant cation in the body, the majority of which lies intracellularly. Despite variable daily potassium intake the serum potassium levels remain within a very narrow normal range. This is due to strict regulation of potassium excretion at the kidney, gastrointestinal losses and the transfer between the extracellular and intracellular compartments. Potassium plays a key role in the excitability of cells and therefore, abnormalities in the potassium level can result in life-threatening arrhythmias and cardiac arrest [18].

Causes of hyperkalaemia are listed in Table 24.3 [18]. No exact definition for mild, moderate and severe hyperkalaemia exist, however most authorities advise treatment if the potassium is more than 6 mmol/l. Often multiple factors are involved in causing hyperkalaemia which leads to either decreased excretion of potassium or increased release from cells. Increased potassium intake can also cause hyperkalaemia especially in the presence of renal failure. Intake can be dietary, secondary to a blood transfusion as potassium is released from haemolysis and iatrogenic when too much potassium is given via intravenous fluids or total parenteral nutrition. Spurious results must be excluded first before other causes are searched for. Though over 75% of severe hyperkalaemia cases are due to renal failure, potassium excretion is relatively well preserved in chronic renal disease until the renal dysfunction is advanced. There are a group of patients in whom hyperkalaemia occurs without severe renal failure due to damage of the juxtoglomerulus apparatus in the kidney. The main cause of this is diabetes and it results in a reduced renin production and therefore reduced aldosterone production. Aldosterone is key in regulating

Table 24.3 Causes of hyperkalaemia [18]

Spurious result
Lab error
Excessive tourniquet
Traumatic venipuncture
Ingestion of foods with high potassium content
Figs
Chocolate
Banana/kiwi
Spinach/tomatoes
Tissue breakdown
Rhabdomyolysis
Tumour lysis syndrome
Severe burns
Insulin deficiency
Metabolic acidosis
Renal failure
Addisons disease
Hyporeninaemic hypoaldosteronism
End organ insensitivity to aldosterone
Sickle cell disease
Amyloidosis
Drugs
Beta blockers
Suxamethonium
Potassium supplements
Angiotensin converting enzyme inhibitors
Angiotensin II receptor blockers
Non-steroidal anti-inflammatory drugs
Potassium sparing diuretics

potassium excretion and with reduced aldosterone there is reduced potassium excretion by the kidney. There are also diseases and drugs which can cause an absolute or relative aldosterone deficiency [18].

One of the main contributors to the development of hyperkalaemia is drug therapy. Angiotensin Converting Enzyme Inhibitors and angiotensin receptor blockers are being increasingly used for its reno- and cardioprotective properties in particular groups of patients. Not only do they reduce renal perfusion but they also impair aldosterone release thus reducing potassium excretion by the kidney. In patients with normal renal function, this reduction in potassium excretion is rarely sufficient to cause a hyperkalaemia. However, these drugs are often targeted at those with underlying co-morbidities such as the elderly, those with diabetes, renal disease and cardiovascular dysfunction who are therefore at high risk of developing hyperkalaemia. Drugs like this must be started cautiously in these patients and slowly titrated with potassium being checked within a week of any dose change [18].

In the majority of cases, hyperkalaemia is asymptomatic. Palpitations, lethargy and muscle weakness are often described when symptoms are present due to the

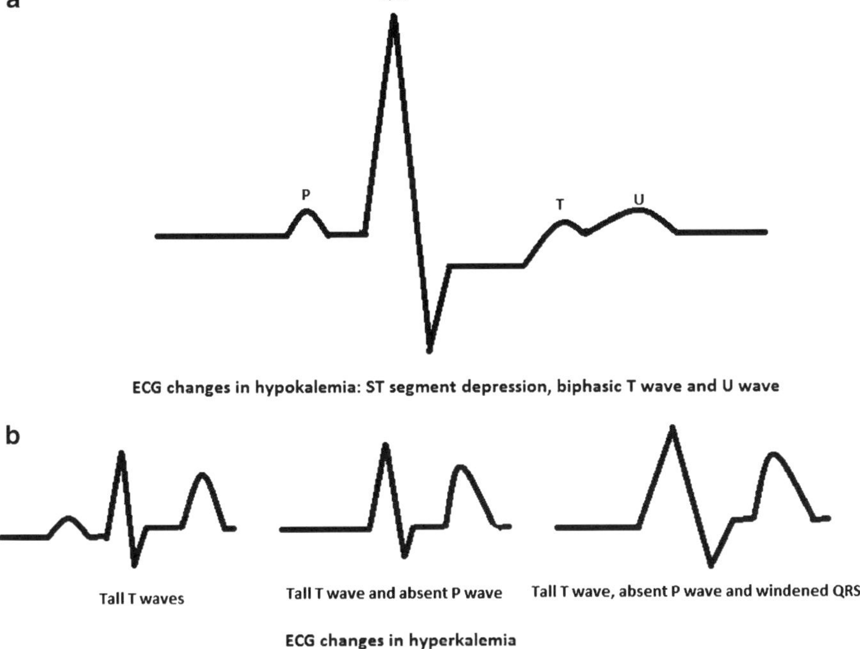

Fig. 24.2 Electrocardiogram changes in (**a**) hyperkalaemia and (**b**) hypokalaemia

cardiac arrhythmias and abnormal muscle function that can occur when high potassium levels exist. When hyperkalaemia is identified on laboratory results an electrocardiogram should be performed as specific changes may be seen as shown in Fig. 24.2a. A medical history and examination must also be performed to help identify potential causes so that further investigations can be directed [18] to pinpointing the disorder.

Mild to moderate hyperkalaemia may be managed by a loop diuretic to increase potassium excretion, though this may be ineffective in patients with renal failure. Dietary potassium should be restricted and contributing drugs should be stopped or reduced where possible [18].

Severe hyperkalaemia is life threatening and requires prompt and aggressive management. Initial treatment involves stabilisation of the myocardium with calcium (10 ml of 10% calcium gluconate infused over 3–5 min). Though this does not reduce the serum potassium level it does protect the heart, reducing the risk of fatal arrhythmias and resolution of electrocardiogram changes can be seen. Once the myocardium has been stabilised, the hyperkalaemia itself must be corrected. This is done by driving potassium from the extracellular compartment, intracellularly. Both insulin and beta-2 agonists activate the sodium–potassium pump, thus shifting potassium into cells [19]. Beta-2 agonists can be given via a nebuliser or intravenously. Both produce a response within 30 min but the intravenous route is thought to achieve a maximal response more rapidly [20]. However, due to the ease to set up, the nebulised route is often used and complements the effect of insulin. Insulin is given as a rapid intravenous infusion with glucose to minimise potential hypoglycaemia. It has been shown to have a more rapid effect on serum potassium levels than beta-2 agonists and sodium bicarbonate though the overall maximal effect is similar [21]. The use of sodium bicarbonate for treatment of hyperkalaemia remains controversial as evidence supporting its use remains inconclusive [18, 21]. It may have a role in the acidotic hyperkalaemic patient or the patient in cardiac arrest. When the above interventions have failed, urgent renal replacement therapy (RRT) is required to remove the potassium from the body. RRT is the process by which blood is removed from the body, filtered via a semipermeable membrane to remove unwanted solutes and then returned back to patient in a continuous cycle. The difficulty is that RRT is time consuming to set up, requires a specialised catheter for intravenous access and can cause haemodynamic instability. Though it is the definitive treatment for hyperkalaemia it is not therefore the first-line management option. Removal of potassium from the body can also be promoted by drug therapy such as diuretics in those with normal renal function or cation exchange resins [18].

Once the acute severe hyperkalaemia has been managed, the cause must be identified and treated to prevent reoccurrence.

Hypokalaemia

The majority of cases of hypokalaemia are mild (between 3.0 and 3.5 mmol/l) and are often iatrogenic as a consequence of prescribed drugs. Though it is mostly asymptomatic, hypokalaemia can cause fatal arrhythmias and cardiac arrest. If symptoms are present, they are often non-specific such as muscle weakness, cramps and palpitations [22]. As with hyperkalaemia, if low potassium is identified on laboratory tests, an electrocardiogram should be performed as characteristic changes of hypokalaemia can be seen and are shown in Fig. 24.2b.

Table 24.4 [22, 23] lists some of the causes of hypokalaemia which can essentially be divided into those that cause potassium to shift into cells and those that increase potassium loss from the body [22]. The cause should be investigated, starting with history and examination followed by laboratory tests.

By establishing the cause the underlying disorder can be treated and the hypokalaemia resolved. In the majority of cases, this approach is adequate at correcting the potassium deficiency. If potassium replacement is required it can be given orally or intravenously. Oral preparations are associated with an increased risk of gastrointestinal ulceration and so should always be given with plenty of fluid. Ingestion of foods with high potassium content such as bananas, pineapples and avocados can also be used to raise the serum potassium. Intravenous potassium is required to treat severe hypokalaemia (serum potassium less than 2.5 mmol/l) but should not be given at a rate greater than 20 mmol/h and should not be concentrated more than 40 mmol in 1 l

Table 24.4 Causes of hypokalaemia

Diuretics
Vomiting and diarrhoea
Pyloric stenosis
Rectal villous adenoma
Intestinal fistula
Hypomagnesaemia
Hyperaldosteronism
Conns syndrome
Cushings disease
Renal tubular acidosis
Excess liquorice ingestion
Transcellular shifts
Alkalosis
Insulin administration
Catecholamines
Phosphodiesterase inhibitors
Activation of the renin–angiotensin pathway
Bartter syndrome
Gitelman syndrome
Malnutrition

as it is irritant to veins [22, 23]. If faster replacement or more concentrated solutions are required, for example in symptomatic severe hypokalaemia or patients with heart failure who cannot tolerate large fluid volumes, then potassium must be given via a central venous catheter with close cardiac monitoring. In all patients having potassium replacement, levels must be frequently checked to avoid the danger of rebound hyperkalaemia. As the risk of hyperkalaemia is so high in oliguric patients, potassium should not be replaced without expert advice [22].

The treatment of acute hypokalaemia is more urgent than the treatment of chronic hypokalaemia which can often be resolved by treating the cause alone. Chronic hypokalaemia may also be treated with potassium sparing diuretics, though again the risk of rebound hyperkalaemia, especially in those with chronic kidney disease, is high [22].

Hyponatremia

Sodium is the primary extracellular cation and it plays a significant role in determining the extracellular fluid volume. Low serum sodium levels can be seen in 15–30% of hospitalised patients [24] and has been shown to be a predictor of mortality in critically unwell patients [25].

If hyponatremia is identified on laboratory tests, a detailed history and examination will help guide the clinician to the most likely cause. By determining the extracellular volume status of the patient, the hyponatremia can be classified into three categories: hypovolemic, euvolemic and hypervolemic hyponatraemia [26].

Table 24.5 Causes and management options of hyponatremia [26]

Hyponatraemia	Causes	Urinary sodium	Treatment
Hypovolemic hyponatra-emia	*Renal losses* Diuretic excess Mineralocorticoid deficiency Polycystic kidney disease Interstial nephritis Renal tubular acidosis Osmotic diuresis	Urinary sodium concentration more than 20 mmol/l	Isotonic saline
	Extrarenal loss Gastrointestinal (vomiting, diarrhoea, peritonitis, pancreatitis, ileus) Burns Haemorrhage	Urinary sodium concentration less than 10 mmol/l	
Euvolaemic hyponatra-emia	Glucocorticoid deficiency Hypothyroidism Hypopituitarism Primary polydipsia Pain Psychiatric disorders SIADH	Urinary sodium concentration more than 20 mmol/l	Water restriction
Hypervolemic hyponatremia	Nephrotic syndrome Cardiac failure Cirrhosis	Urinary sodium concentration less than 10 mmol/l	Sodium and water restriction
	Acute renal failure Chronic renal failure	Urinary sodium concentration more than 20 mmol/l	

In hypovolemic hyponatremia there is a deficit of both total body water and total body sodium. The patient may be hypotensive or complain of orthostatic hypotension, be tachycardic, have a low jugular venous pressure and be peripherally vasoconstricted with increased capillary refill time. The cause can then be further classified into renal losses and extra renal losses which are explored in Table 24.5 [26].

In euvolemic hyponatremia, the total body sodium content is normal but there is a gain of water due to excessive amounts of antidiuretic hormone (ADH) which impairs water excretion. The ADH may be produced in excess from the pituitary itself by inappropriate stimulation or it may come from an ectopic source. This is called SIADH or syndrome of inappropriate ADH secretion, the causes of which are extensive and listed in Table 24.6. Before SIADH is considered however, other causes of euvolemic hyponatremia must be excluded and are listed in Table 24.5 [26].

In hypervolemic hyponatremia, though both are raised, the total body water is increased to a greater extent than the total body sodium causing a relative hyponatremia.

Table 24.6 Causes of SIADH (this list is by no means complete)

Malignant disease
Small cell carcinoma
Pancreatic carcinoma
Bladder cancer
Prostate cancer
Lymphoma
Pulmonary disorders
Pneumonia
Tuberculosis
Cystic fibrosis
Central nervous system
Infection—AIDS, meningitis, abscess
Masses—subdural haematoma, subarachnoid haemorrhage, brain tumour, hydrocephalus
Multiple sclerosis
Guillain–Barre syndrome
Drugs
Tricyclic antidepressants
Serotonin selective receptor inhibitors
Nicotine
Non-steroidal anti-inflammatory drugs
Desmopressin
Vasopressin
Oxytocin
Pain
Stress
General anaesthesia

The patient may present with ascites, peripheral oedema or pulmonary oedema. Again causes and management options are listed in Table 24.5 [26].

Low serum sodium levels can be acute or chronic. When acute it can present as a life-threatening event due to swelling of the brain causing herniation and cardiopulmonary arrest. Other neurological signs may precede this such as acute psychosis, hallucinations, tremor, hemiparesis and seizures. Some patients may present with more non-specific symptoms such as lethargy, agitation, nausea and anorexia. In chronic hyponatremia, the neurological findings tend to be mild as the brain has time to adapt to changes in sodium concentration [26].

The management of hyponatremia is influenced by many factors including, the rate of onset, the severity and the presence of symptoms. In severe, life-threatening acute hyponatremia, presenting with seizures or coma, immediate treatment with 3% hypertonic saline should be started at 100 ml/h. This will increase the serum sodium concentration by 2 mmol/l/h and should be continued until improvement is seen in the patient's signs and symptoms [26]. However, if correction of the hyponatremia is too rapid, especially in those with chronic hyponatremia, damage to the brain will occur, called osmotic demyelination, with pontine and extrapontine sites being most vulnerable. This can present as a delayed onset of neurological signs following treatment [27]. To avoid osmotic demyelination in chronic hyponatremia, correction should be limited to less that 12 mmol in 24 h and less than 18 mmol in 48 h [28]. However in high-risk patients with malnutrition, hypokalaemia, alcoholism and liver disease, correction should be slower than this [26].

The management of hyponatremia is also determined by the category it falls in to. Hypovolemic hyponatremia is treated by volume expansion. The underlying cause must also be addressed such as discontinuation of the offending medication or hormone replacement if hypothyroidism or glucocorticoid deficiency is suspected. In euvolemic and hypervolemic hyponatremia fluid restriction may resolve the low serum sodium concentration. However, fluid intake must be less than daily urine output and insensible losses which many patients find difficult to adhere to. Demeclocycline is another approach which induces a nephrogenic diabetes insipidus so that the kidney can no longer conserve water. It can cause nephrotoxicity and caution must be taken when using in patients with liver disease or congestive cardiac failure. Lithium has also been used to induce a nephrogenic diabetes insipidus but the effect is inconsistent and its narrow therapeutic window makes risk–benefit ratio high [26]. Recently, V2 vasopressin receptor antagonists and dual V1/V2 receptor antagonists have been developed. They are still in the early stages of clinical use but certain types have been approved for use in both America and Europe in specific conditions. Their effect is to increase solute free water excretion and thus they are well suited for the treatment of hypervolemic and euvolemic hyponatremia. At the time of writing this chapter, data supporting their use are promising but studies are small [26, 29].

Hypercalcaemia

The majority of the body's calcium is stored in bone, however only a very small proportion of it is readily exchangeable with extracellular calcium. The extracellular calcium may be either bound (to mostly protein but also to phosphorous and lactate) or free. It is this free calcium that is tightly regulated and when abnormal causes the symptoms of hyper- or hypocalcaemia [30]. Symptoms of hypercalcaemia are non-specific and include muscle weakness, fatigue, confusion, abdominal pain and arrhythmias. A more complete list, as well as a list of causes of hypercalcaemia, is provided in Table 24.7 [31]. Within the outpatient setting, primary hyperparathyroidism is the most common cause of hypercalcaemia; however, this is superseded by malignancy in the inpatient population [31].

Twenty per cent of patients with a malignancy will develop hypercalcaemia at some point during their disease process [32] and the pathological process can be classified into four types. Local osteolytic hypercalcaemia occurs in malignancies with extensive bone involvement such as breast cancer. The tumour cells enter the bone's microenvironment, release factors that stimulate

Table 24.7 Causes and clinical features of hypercalcaemia [31]

Causes	Clinical features
Malignancy associated hypercalcaemia	Muscle weakness
Primary and tertiary hyperparathyroidism	Fatigue and lethargy
	Headache
Parathyroid carcinoma	Confusion and psychosis
Familial benign hypocalciuric hypercalcaemia	Coma
	Abdominal pain
Granulomatous disorders	Constipation
Sarcoidosis	Nausea and vomiting
Crohns disease	Pancreatitis
Tuberculosis	Polyuria and polydipsia
Drugs	Nephrocalcinosis and nephrolithiasis
Thiazides	Arrhythmias
Lithium	Short QT interval
Vitamin D	Cardiac arrest
Thyrotoxicosis	Bone pain
Adrenal insufficiency	
Milk-alkali syndrome	
Renal failure	

osteoclasts and thus increase bone resorption. Humoral hypercalcaemia of malignancy occurs due to the secretion of parathyroid hormone related peptide (PTHrP) by the tumour cells. The PTHrP increases osteoclastic activity in the bone as well as increasing calcium reabsorption by the kidney. Vitamin D mediated hypercalcaemia is rare but it is due to the production of 1,25-dihydroxyvitamin D by the malignant cells. It is also the process by which granulomatous disorders cause hypercalcaemia. The vitamin D increases calcium reabsorption from the gut. The forth pathological process responsible for hypercalcaemia of malignancy is the ectopic production of parathyroid hormone (PTH) by the cancerous cells and is again very rare [30, 31].

Hypercalcaemia has a potent diuretic effect and, therefore, the initial management of hypercalcaemia of malignancy is fluid replacement with 0.9 % saline. Loop diuretics increase renal calcium excretion; however, if they are given to patients who are not volume replete they could worsen the hypercalcaemia. In dehydration the kidney increases tubular absorption to prevent sodium loss but calcium reabsorption is also increased during this process. Bisphosphonates inhibit bone resorption so are frequently used to treat the high calcium in malignancy. The effect on serum calcium concentrations, however, is not seen until 24–48 h later. They also cause an acute phase reaction causing flu-like symptoms, can affect renal function so must be used in caution in patients with renal disease and can cause transient hypocalcaemia and hypophosphataemia [31, 32]. Glucocorticoids are sometimes used to treat vitamin D mediated hypercalcaemia with reductions in serum calcium concentration occurring 3 days later [33]. RRT using a dialysate containing no calcium would also be effective in reducing serum calcium concentrations and may be appropriate in patients with severe hypercalcaemia and renal dysfunction when aggressive fluid replacement and bisphosphonates are contraindicated. All the above management options only have a temporary effect, but they may provide enough time for treatment of the underlying malignancy [31].

Parathyroid hormone secretion is normally stimulated by hyperphosphataemia and hypocalcaemia. It increases bone resorption, enhances renal absorption of calcium and excretion of phosphate and aids the formation of active vitamin D which increases calcium absorption from the gastrointestinal tract. Primary hyperparathyroidism (PHPT) affects 1 in 1,000 people, mostly female and most frequently in the 6th decade of life [30]. If diagnosed at a younger age, multiple endocrine neoplasia (MEN) must be investigated and ruled out. Eighty per cent of PHPT cases are due to a single benign adenoma with the remaining cases due to four gland hyperplasia. Parathyroid cancers are rare, responsible for less than 0.5% of cases [31].

PHPT is a curable disease by excision of the gland and guidelines were developed to direct the timing of surgery. In symptomatic PHPT with overt renal or bone disease and episodes of life-threatening hypercalcaemia, surgical excision of the parathyroid tissue is the appropriate treatment. In asymptomatic PHPT, surgery should be performed when the serum calcium is more than 1 mg/dl above the local reference range; the creatinine clearance is less than 60 ml/min; the patient is under 50 years old and the bone mineral density T-score is less than −2.5 [34]. Those that do not meet the criteria for surgery should be managed medically with yearly bone mineral density scans, blood tests every 6 months and advice including the importance of hydration and the avoidance of drugs that increase serum calcium such as thiazides and lithium [31]. Bisphosphonates are also used in the medical management of PHPT. Alendronate has been the most extensively studied and though it does not reduce serum calcium or PTH concentration, it does reduce bone turnover and improve bone mineral density [35]. Intravenous bisphosphonates should only be used in life-threatening hypercalcaemia.

Cinacalcet is an oral calcimimetic that increases the sensitivity of the calcium sensing receptor found in both the kidney and the parathyroid gland. In PHPT, this receptor fails to respond to the high circulating calcium levels and thus fails to suppress PTH secretion [36]. Initial studies of cinacalcet in the treatment of PHPT are promising achieving normocalcaemia in the majority of patients [36]; however, it is not yet licenced for routine use in these patients. It may be used in patients with parathyroid carcinoma and persistent hypercalcaemia when surgery is not an option [31].

Familial Benign Hypercalcaemia is an autosomal dominant inherited disorder of the calcium sensing receptor. The PTH levels may be inappropriately normal or even raised and therefore this disorder should always be considered as part of the differential diagnosis of PHPT. Surgical excision of the parathyroid gland is reserved for those with severe hypercalcaemia and recurrent pancreatitis as parathyroidectomy is rarely successful with rebound hypercalcaemia occurring within 1 week despite the operation [37].

Hypocalcaemia

Hypocalcaemia can be as high as 85% in the critical care population but can also be seen in the outpatient setting [38]. When it develops gradually it can be completely asymptomatic but those with acute reductions in their serum calcium levels will experience severe symptoms including muscle spasms and cardiac arrhythmias. The extracellular calcium concentration plays an important role in the functioning of nerves and muscles. When hypocalcaemia develops, neuromuscular excitability occurs, causing muscle twitching, tingling sensations, carpopedal spasm, seizures and tetany. The neuromuscular excitability can also be provoked if the above signs are not evident by Chvosteks test (tapping the parotid gland over the facial nerve to cause facial twitch) or Trousseau's test (inducing carpopedal spasm by inflation of a blood pressure cuff) [39].

The causes of hypocalcaemia are listed in Table 24.8 [39]. Vitamin D acts on the gastrointestinal tract to promote calcium absorption. Though a small proportion is taken by diet, the majority of vitamin D is synthesised in the skin and then activated by the liver and finally the kidney. Synthesis in the skin requires exposure to sunlight and this process is reduced by pigmented skin [39].

Hypoparathyroidism, often iatrogenic after thyroid or parathyroid surgery, can also be idiopathic or due to an autoimmune process. With reduced PTH, renal calcium excretion is increased, there is reduced calcium absorption from the gut due to reduced production of active vitamin D and bone resorption slows. Pseudohypoparathyroidism produces a similar picture but occurs due to tissue resistance to the PTH. Though the PTH levels are high, the hypocalcaemia persists. It is a genetic disease often associated with skeletal abnormalities such as shortening of the metacarpal bones. There are a group of patients that exhibit these same skeletal abnormalities but have no biochemical irregularities and they are said to have pseudohypoparathyroidism.

The treatment of hypocalcaemia very much depends on the speed of onset, the signs, symptoms and the severity. In acute hypocalcaemia with neuromuscular excitability, calcium must be replaced intravenously. Even if patients are asymptomatic with a corrected serum calcium concentration of 1.9 mmol/l or less, calcium should be replaced [40]. With electrocardiographic monitoring, 10 ml of 10% calcium gluconate (can be diluted in 5% dextrose to larger volumes) should be infused slowly over 10 min. If correction is too rapid cardiac arrhythmias can occur but as long as done slowly, the treatment can be repeated until symptoms have resolved. Calcium chloride can also be used but is associated with more local irritation. Oral calcium replacement should also be commenced. Occasionally, a continuous infusion of a dilute calcium solution may be required to maintain the serum calcium within the normal range. Calcitriol may also need to be given if the cause of the hypocalcaemia is due to a relative or absolute deficiency in PTH.

When the hypocalcaemia is mild, treatment is directed towards the underlying cause. For example, in vitamin D deficiency, vitamin D can be replaced either

Table 24.8 Causes or hypocalcaemia

Vitamin D deficiency
Hypoparathyroidism
Renal disease
Parathyroid hormone resistance
Hypomagnesaemia
Infusion of phosphate or calcium chelators such as citrate
Critical illness

orally or intramuscularly. In hypoparathyroidism, treatment can either be with active vitamin D (calcitriol or alfacalcidol) or with synthetic parathyroid hormone [39, 40].

Conclusion

The critical care unit can offer respiratory, cardiac and renal support and is also well placed to aid correction of biochemical and metabolic disturbances. The intensive monitoring, organ support and increased nursing care that critical care units provide makes the management of complex chronic diseases possible.

However, investigation and treatment must be directed to the individual patient. There will be circumstances when aggressive management of the disease process is no longer in the patient's best interest. When this occurs comfort becomes the main goal of therapy.

References

1. Angus DC, Barnato AE, Linde-Zwirble WT, Weissfeld LA, Watson RS, Rickert T, et al. Use of intensive care at the end of life in the United States: an epidemiologic study. Crit Care Med. 2004;32(3):638–43.]Multicenter Study Research Support, Non-U.S. Gov't Research Support, U.S. Gov't, P.H.S.].
2. Nelson JE, Puntillo KA, Pronovost PJ, Walker AS, McAdam JL, Ilaoa D, et al. In their own words: patients and families define high-quality palliative care in the intensive care unit. Crit Care Med. 2010;38(3):808–18 [Research Support, N.I.H., Extramural Research Support, U.S. Gov't, Non-P.H.S.].
3. Mehta S, Hill NS. Noninvasive ventilation. Am J Respir Crit Care Med. 2001;163(2):540–77 [Research Support, U.S. Gov't, P.H.S. Review].
4. Curtis JR, Cook DJ, Sinuff T, White DB, Hill N, Keenan SP, et al. Noninvasive positive pressure ventilation in critical and palliative care settings: understanding the goals of therapy. Crit Care Med. 2007;35(3):932–9 [Case Reports Review].
5. Keenan SP, Sinuff T, Cook DJ, Hill NS. Which patients with acute exacerbation of chronic obstructive pulmonary disease benefit from noninvasive positive-pressure ventilation? A systematic review of the literature. Ann Intern Med. 2003;138(11):861–70 [Research Support, Non-U.S. Gov't Review].

6. Hilbert G, Gruson D, Vargas F, Valentino R, Gbikpi-Benissan G, Dupon M, et al. Noninvasive ventilation in immunosuppressed patients with pulmonary infiltrates, fever, and acute respiratory failure. N Engl J Med. 2001;344(7):481–7 [Clinical Trial Comparative Study Randomized Controlled Trial].
7. Masip J, Betbese AJ, Paez J, Vecilla F, Canizares R, Padro J, et al. Non-invasive pressure support ventilation versus conventional oxygen therapy in acute cardiogenic pulmonary oedema: a randomised trial. Lancet. 2000;356(9248):2126–32 [Clinical Trial Comparative Study Randomized Controlled Trial Research Support, Non-U.S. Gov't].
8. International Consensus Conferences in Intensive Care Medicine: noninvasive positive pressure ventilation in acute Respiratory failure. Am J Respir Crit Care Med. 2001;163(1):283–91 [Consensus Development Conference Review].
9. Hilbert G, Gruson D, Vargas F, Valentino R, Chene G, Boiron JM, et al. Noninvasive continuous positive airway pressure in neutropenic patients with acute respiratory failure requiring intensive care unit admission. Crit Care Med. 2000;28(9):3185–90.
10. Cuomo A, Delmastro M, Ceriana P, Nava S, Conti G, Antonelli M, et al. Noninvasive mechanical ventilation as a palliative treatment of acute respiratory failure in patients with end-stage solid cancer. Palliat Med. 2004;18(7):602–10 [Multicenter Study].
11. Brochard L, Mancebo J, Elliott MW. Noninvasive ventilation for acute respiratory failure. Eur Respir J. 2002;19(4):712–21 [Review].
12. Clarke DE, Vaughan L, Raffin TA. Noninvasive positive pressure ventilation for patients with terminal respiratory failure: the ethical and economic costs of delaying the inevitable are too great. Am J Crit Care. 1994;3(1):4–5 [Comment Editorial].
13. Lin SF, Lin JD, Huang YY. Diabetic ketoacidosis: comparisons of patient characteristics, clinical presentations and outcomes today and 20 years ago. Chang Gung Med J. 2005;28(1):24–30 [Comparative Study].
14. Otieno CF, Kayima JK, Omonge EO, Oyoo GO. Diabetic ketoacidosis: risk factors, mechanisms and management strategies in sub-Saharan Africa: a review. East Afr Med J. 2005;82(12 Suppl):S197–203 [Review].
15. Savage AM. The management of diabetic ketoacidosis in adults. 2010. http://www.diabetes.nhs.uk/document.php?o=212.
16. Savage MW. Management of diabetic ketoacidosis. Clin Med. 2011;11(2):154–6 [Review].
17. Cavan DA, Hamilton P, Everett J, Kerr D. Reducing hospital inpatient length of stay for patients with diabetes. Diabet Med. 2001;18(2):162–4 [Comparative Study Research Support, Non-U.S. Gov't].
18. Nyirenda MJ, Tang JI, Padfield PL, Seckl JR. Hyperkalaemia. BMJ. 2009;339:b4114 [Review].
19. Mahoney BA, Smith WA, Lo DS, Tsoi K, Tonelli M, Clase CM. Emergency interventions for hyperkalaemia. Cochrane Database Syst Rev. 2005;(2):CD003235 [Meta-Analysis Review].
20. Elliott MJ, Ronksley PE, Clase CM, Ahmed SB, Hemmelgarn BR. Management of patients with acute hyperkalemia. CMAJ. 2010;182(15):1631–5 [Case Reports Research Support, Non-U.S. Gov't Review].
21. Allon M, Shanklin N. Effect of bicarbonate administration on plasma potassium in dialysis patients: interactions with insulin and albuterol. Am J Kidney Dis. 1996;28(4):508–14 [Clinical Trial Controlled Clinical Trial].
22. Unwin RJ, Luft FC, Shirley DG. Pathophysiology and management of hypokalemia: a clinical perspective. Nat Rev Nephrol. 2011;7(2):75–84 [Review].
23. Longmore JM. Oxford handbook of clinical medicine. 8th ed. Oxford: Oxford University Press; 2010.
24. Upadhyay A, Jaber BL, Madias NE. Incidence and prevalence of hyponatremia. Am J Med. 2006;119(7 Suppl 1):S30–5 [Review].
25. Bennani SL, Abouqal R, Zeggwagh AA, Madani N, Abidi K, Zekraoui A, et al. [Incidence, causes and prognostic factors of hyponatremia in intensive care]. Rev Med Interne. 2003;24(4):224–9.

26. Elhassan EA, Schrier RW. Hyponatremia: diagnosis, complications, and management including V2 receptor antagonists. Curr Opin Nephrol Hypertens. 2011;20(2):161–8 [Review].
27. Sterns RH, Hix JK, Silver S. Treatment of hyponatremia. Curr Opin Nephrol Hypertens. 2010;19(5):493–8 [Review].
28. Verbalis JG, Goldsmith SR, Greenberg A, Schrier RW, Sterns RH. Hyponatremia treatment guidelines 2007: expert panel recommendations. Am J Med. 2007;120(11 Suppl 1):S1–21 [Practice Guideline].
29. Veeraveedu PT, Palaniyandi SS, Yamaguchi K, Komai Y, Thandavarayan RA, Sukumaran V, et al. Arginine vasopressin receptor antagonists (vaptans): pharmacological tools and potential therapeutic agents. Drug Discov Today. 2010;15(19–20):826–41 [Research Support, Non-U.S. Gov't Review].
30. Shepard MM, Smith 3rd JW. Hypercalcemia. Am J Med Sci. 2007;334(5):381–5 [Review].
31. Makras P, Papapoulos SE. Medical treatment of hypercalcaemia. Hormones (Athens). 2009;8(2):83–95 [Review].
32. Stewart AF. Clinical practice. Hypercalcemia associated with cancer. N Engl J Med. 2005;352(4):373–9 [Research Support, U.S. Gov't, P.H.S. Review].
33. Favus MJ. Primer on the metabolic bone diseases and disorders of mineral metabolism. 6th ed. Washington, DC: American Society for Bone and Mineral Research; 2006.
34. Bilezikian JP, Khan AA, Potts Jr JT. Guidelines for the management of asymptomatic primary hyperparathyroidism: summary statement from the third international workshop. J Clin Endocrinol Metab. 2009;94(2):335–9 [Consensus Development Conference].
35. Khan AA, Bilezikian JP, Kung AW, Ahmed MM, Dubois SJ, Ho AY, et al. Alendronate in primary hyperparathyroidism: a double-blind, randomized, placebo-controlled trial. J Clin Endocrinol Metab. 2004;89(7):3319–25 [Clinical Trial Multicenter Study Randomized Controlled Trial Research Support, Non-U.S. Gov't Research Support, U.S. Gov't, P.H.S.].
36. Nemeth EF, Heaton WH, Miller M, Fox J, Balandrin MF, Van Wagenen BC, et al. Pharmacodynamics of the type II calcimimetic compound cinacalcet HCl. J Pharmacol Exp Ther. 2004;308(2):627–35.
37. Egbuna OI, Brown EM. Hypercalcaemic and hypocalcaemic conditions due to calcium-sensing receptor mutations. Best Pract Res Clin Rheumatol. 2008;22(1):129–48 [Review].
38. Hastbacka J, Pettila V. Prevalence and predictive value of ionized hypocalcemia among critically ill patients. Acta Anaesthesiol Scand. 2003;47(10):1264–9.
39. Cooper MS, Gittoes NJ. Diagnosis and management of hypocalcaemia. BMJ. 2008;336(7656):1298–302 [Review].
40. Warrell DA, Cox TM, Firth JD. Oxford textbook of medicine. 4th ed. Oxford: Oxford University Press; 2003.

Review Questions

1. In hyperkalaemia which one of the following ECG changes does not occur?

   (a) Tall tented T waves
   (b) Loss of p wave
   (c) Appearance of u wave
   (d) Widened QRS complexes
   (e) Normal ECG

2. Which one of the following is a cause for hypokalaemia?

   (a) Spironolactone
   (b) Addisons disease
   (c) Conns syndrome
   (d) Rhabdomyolysis
   (e) Metabolic acidosis

3. Which one of the following statements is false?

   (a) Continuous positive pressure ventilation opens up underventilated alveoli
   (b) Continuous positive pressure ventilation delivers two levels of pressure to the patient
   (c) Non-invasive ventilation can be used as a comfort measure
   (d) Non-invasive ventilation should not be used in those at high risk of vomiting
   (e) Non-invasive ventilation can cause hypotension

4. Which one of the following statements about diabetic ketoacidosis is false?

   (a) The breakdown of proteins results in the excessive production of ketones
   (b) Diabetic ketoacidosis causes severe dehydration and requires prompt fluid resuscitation
   (c) Treatment of diabetic ketoacidosis may cause hypokalaemia
   (d) Treatment of diabetic ketoacidosis may cause a hyperchloraemic acidosis
   (e) Resolution of acidosis and ketonaemia usually occurs within 24 h

5. Which one is not a cause of hyponatraemia?

   (a) Pain
   (b) Hyperthyroidism
   (c) Vomiting
   (d) Renal tubular acidosis
   (e) Nephrotic syndrome

6. Which one of the following statements about calcium is false?

   (a) The majority of the bodies calcium is stored in bone
   (b) Vitamin D aids calcium absorption from the gut

(c) It is the amount of bound calcium that causes symptoms of hyper- or hypocalcaemia

(d) Normally, parathyroid hormone increases the renal absorption of calcium

(e) The extracellular calcium concentration plays an important role in the functioning of nerves and muscles

7. Which one of the following causes hypocalcaemia

   (a) Primary hyperparathyroidism
   (b) Sarcoidosis
   (c) Thiazide diuretic drugs
   (d) Pseudohypoparathyroidism
   (e) Lithium therapy

8. Which one of the following regarding treatment of hyponatraemia is false?

   (a) If hyponatraemia is corrected too quickly it may result in osmotic demyelination
   (b) Hypovolaemic hyponatraemia should be treated with water restriction
   (c) Hypertonic Saline should be considered if hyponatraemia presents with seizures
   (d) Vasopressin receptor antagonists have recently been developed for the treatment of hyponatraemia
   (e) Demeclocycline may cause nephrotoxicity

9. Which one of the following is a cause of hyperkalaemia

   (a) Hypomagnesaemia
   (b) Alkalosis
   (c) Gitelman syndrome
   (d) Rhabdomyolysis
   (e) Phosphodiesterase inhibitors

10. Which one of the following is not a sign or symptom of hypercalcaemia

    (a) Short QT interval on electrocardiogram
    (b) Pancreatitis
    (c) Nephrocalcinosis
    (d) Constipation
    (e) Chvosteks test

Answers

1. (c)
2. (c)
3. (b)
4. (a)
5. (b)
6. (c)
7. (d)
8. (b)
9. (d)
10. (e)

Chapter 25
Pediatric Palliative Care

Shu-Ming Wang, Paul B. Yost, and Leonard Sender

Introduction

Many people confuse palliative care with hospice care. However, the two approaches are very different. Hospice care specifically is end-of-life care. The World Health Organization (WHO) defines palliative care and pediatric palliative care in the following way:

Palliative care is an approach that improves the quality of life of patients and their families facing the problems associated with life-threatening illness, through the prevention and relief of suffering by means of early identification and impeccable assessment and treatment of pain and other problems: physical, psychosocial, and spiritual. Palliative care:

- Provides relief from pain and other distressing symptoms
- Affirms life and regards dying as a normal process
- Intends neither to hasten or postpone death
- Integrates the psychological and spiritual aspects of patient care
- Offers a support system to help patients live as actively as possible until death
- Offers a support system to help the family cope during the patient's illness and in their own bereavement

S.-M. Wang, M.D. (✉)
Department of Anesthesiology and Perioperative Care, University of California,
Irvine School of Medicine, Irvine, CA, USA
e-mail: Shuminw1@uci.edu; smwang800@gmail.com

P.B. Yost, M.D., F.A.A.P.
Department of Anesthesiology, St. Joseph's of Orange, Orange, CA, USA

L. Sender, M.D.
Department of Medicine, University of California, Irvine School of Medicine,
Irvine, CA, USA

N. Vadivelu et al. (eds.), *Essentials of Palliative Care*,
DOI 10.1007/978-1-4614-5164-8_25,
© Springer Science+Business Media New York 2013

- Uses a team approach to address the needs of patients and their families, including bereavement counseling, if indicated
- Will enhance quality of life, and may also positively influence the course of illness
- Is applicable early in the course of illness, in conjunction with other therapies that are intended to prolong life, such as chemotherapy or radiation therapy, and includes those investigations needed to better understand and manage distressing clinical complications

WHO Definition of Palliative Care for Children

Palliative care for children represents a special, albeit closely related field to adult palliative care. WHO's definition of palliative care appropriate for children and their families is as follows; the principles apply to other pediatric chronic disorders [1]:

- Palliative care for children is the active total care of the child's body, mind, and spirit, and also involves giving support to the family.
- It begins when illness is diagnosed and continues regardless of whether or not a child receives treatment directed at the disease.
- Health providers must evaluate and alleviate a child's physical, psychological, and social distress.
- Effective palliative care requires a broad multidisciplinary approach that includes the family and makes use of available community resources; it can be successfully implemented even if resources are limited.
- It can be provided in tertiary care facilities, in community health centers, and even in children's homes.

This chapter includes the demographics of children who would benefit from palliative care, description of pediatric palliative care, the barriers why pediatric palliative care has not been fully accepted and implemented, as well as discussion of death with children at various stages of development, issues related to palliative care in special situations such as neonatal ICU, and information regarding the well-being of health care providers and caregivers.

Background and Demographics

Each year in the United States more than 50,000 children die, with around 50% of the deaths occurring in the first year of life. The common causes of death in infants and children are summarized in Table 25.1 [2]. Congenital malformations and chromosome abnormalities are the number one cause of death in infants. For children (age

Table 25.1 Causes of death

Infant
1. Congenital malformations (20.1%)
2. Prematurity/low birth weight (16.9%)
3. Sudden infant death syndrome (8.2%)
4. Maternal complication (6.3%)
5. Unintentional/accidental injury (4.6%)
6. Complications caused by placenta, cord, or membrane (3.8%)
7. Bacterial sepsis (2.5%)
8. Respiratory distress (2.2%)
9. Diseases of circulatory system (2.1%)
10. Neonatal hemorrhage (2.0%)

Infant with chronic complex conditions
1. Cardiovascular (32%)
2. Congenital/genetic (26%)
3. Respiratory (17%)
4. Neuromuscular (14%)

All children (1–19 years)
1. Accident (38.8%)
2. Assault (12.4%)
3. Malignancy (8.6%)
4. Suicide (8.0%)
5. Congenital malformation, deformity, and chromosomal diseases (4.7%)
6. Heart disease (3.4%)
7. Cerebrovascular disease (1.9%)

All children with chronic complex conditions (1–19 years)
1. Malignancy (43%)
2. Neuromuscular (23%)
3. Cardiovascular (17%)

1–19 years) the number one cause of death is accidental/unintentional injury. The second leading cause of death for children for ages 1–4 is congenital malformations, deformities, and chromosomal abnormalities; for ages 5–14: malignancy and for ages 15–19: homicide [3]. Three-fourth of pediatric deaths occur in hospitals each year, mostly in the ICUs where aggressive, life-sustaining, medical therapy is typically provided. Of the deaths that occur in children, around 25% are due to Chronic Complex Conditions [4–7]. Chronic complex conditions (CCC) were defined by Feudtner et al. [4] as "any medical condition that can be reasonably expected to last at least 12 months (unless death intervenes) and to involve either several different organ systems or one organ system severely enough to require specialty pediatric care and probably some period of hospitalization in a tertiary care center." In 2007, the American Academy of Pediatrics issued recommendation for an integrated palliative care model. In this model, the integrated palliative care emphases the provision of curative therapies and comfort measures should be initiated at the time of disease diagnosis [8]. More importantly, a recent study suggests that a high-volume specialist palliative care unit and team may reduce in-hospital end-of-life care cost [9].

Pediatric Palliative Care [10–14], (Himelstein 2005, 2006)

Pediatric palliative care is about helping children and families to live their fullest while facing a life-limiting or complex medical condition. It is an interdisciplinary practice that includes inputs from physicians, social workers, pastoral care providers, and nurses. The principles of palliative care are based on open, honest discussions earlier in the disease trajectory, and allow patients and families participate in decision-making process.

The pediatric palliative care should be:

- Child-focused, family-oriented, and relationship-centered
- Focusing on relief of suffering and enhancing quality of life for the child and family, not to shorten life
- Incorporated into mainstream of medical care regardless of the curative intent of therapy
- Coordinated across all sites of care delivery
- Goal directed and consistent with the beliefs and values of the child and caregivers

All children suffering from chronic, life threatening, and terminal illnesses should be eligible to receive palliative care. Successful pediatric palliative care should give patients and their family the opportunities to express their feelings and concerns as well as actively incorporate their concerns into the care that address the physical, psychological, and spiritual aspects of patients as individuals and family as a unit.

Barriers to Implementation of Pediatric Palliative Care [15, 16]

- Uncertain prognosis
- Communication problems: readiness of the family, cultural differences, religious beliefs, etc.
- False hope for cure
- Inappropriate use of advanced life-saving technology
- Ethical and legal issues
- Inappropriate eligibility criteria
- Inadequate assessment and management of symptoms
- Lack of training and expertise to approach the parents and patient regarding the trajectory of disease process.

- Fragmented care, limited access to specialty care in rural areas
- Lack of adequate data and scientific knowledge to deliver effective care and to design supportive public policies
- Limited financial resources for specialized pediatric care

Clearly, the problem of pediatric palliative care is a multifaceted one that will need to be addressed through multiple reinforcing strategies: medical education, regulatory reform, changes in health care financing, and hospital quality improvement efforts, as well as broad social changes in the ways in which our society views children, families, death, and dying. Lastly, the advances in pediatric medical/surgical care have steadily decreased the overall number of deaths in children with CCC from 1989 to 2003 [17]. In other words, children with CCC are living longer. Therefore, it is important to establish the delivery of comprehensive care early on and find creative ways to provide and coordinate care over a longer period [3]. While previous analysis reveals that most CCC do not lead to death in childhood, the death rate is more than twice that of an age-matched unaffected population and death could potentially occur at any time [5].

Issues Related to the Delivery of Pediatric Palliative Care [18, 19]

Initiation and Formation of Team

Which of the healthcare practitioners is best suited to supervise the medical care of children with CCC and life-threatening illnesses? Pediatricians often have strong relationships with the child and his/her family and they play an important role in influencing the acceptance of palliative care services for the patient and family. The increased awareness of the need of palliative care has reorganized the curriculum during pediatric residency training. However, not every pediatrician feels comfortable in disclosing the potential impending death or shouldering the palliative care alone, and most pediatricians may not be aware of the many services available to alleviate the suffering of a CCC or dying child and their family. A team approach between various specialists, therapists, and religious leaders provides the best comprehensive care of the patient with CCC, with the care coordinator being a practitioner of pediatric palliative care.

Physical and Emotional Suffering

Pain is a common symptom associated with children with life-limiting illness. Pain is unique to an individual. Based on the age and developmental stage of the patient,

Table 25.2 Pain assessment scales

	Child's age
Objective pain assessment scale	
Premature Infant Pain Scale (PIPP)	>36 weeks gestational age
Neonatal Infant Pain Scale (NIPS)	<1 year of age
Face, Leg, Activity, Cary, Consolability Scale (FLACC)	2 months–7 years of age
Children's Hospital Eastern Ontario Pain Scale (CHEOPS)	1–7 years of age
Subjective pain assessment scale	
Wong-Baker FACE Rating Scale	>3 years of age
OUCHER	3–13 years of age
Numerical Rating Scale (NR-22, NRS-101)	>9 years of age
Visual Analog Scale	>7 years of age

the level of pain can be assessed through observation or asking the caregiver and patient using a pain rating scale as listed in Table 25.2. For a nonverbal child, one can evaluate the patient's behavior and physiological signs. Most importantly, family members should be included early on in the treatment process. Various pain medications can be prescribed based on the recommendation of WHO's pain relief. Prior to prescribing the pain medication, several considerations should be taken: (1) Whether the child can and will take medication by mouth. (2) Routes of administering the pain medication. (3) Dose adjustment based on the maturity of organs and co-existing diseases. (4) May consider long-acting analgesics. (5) Consider adding alternative interventions such as acupressure, music, guided imagery, hypnosis, etc. Once the analgesic medications are prescribed, the assessment should be obtained from the child and/or caregivers regularly to assess the effectiveness of therapy.

Other symptoms which may be associated with the last phase of a child with chronic complex condition, e.g., anxiety, dyspnea, nausea, vomiting, etc. Anxiety and dyspnea may be difficult to assess, but once it is identified, the underlying causes should be addressed. If there is no acute process, but is a progression of illness, benzodiazepine and supplemental oxygen should be provided. Similarly, if the child experiences nausea and vomiting, antiemetics should be administered with or without the adjunctive alternative treatments to decrease the frequency and symptoms should be considered. Many children who suffer with CCC also have problems with anxiety and depression; however, the emotional/psychological suffering is an experience that results from a threat to any part of an individual's personhood; however, it is poorly understood especially for those children who are very young and nonverbal. Through the Mandela technique such as drawings, the depth and complexity of cognition and emotion of a very young child might be appreciated, thus the appropriate intervention and guidance can be provided. Having a specialist in child psychology, psychiatry, child life, play therapy, music therapy, pet therapy, and social workers available are important aspects of the team approach to palliative care. Some children may benefit from antidepressant and/or sedative medications as well. Palliative care is not only providing medical support, but also providing the support for the emotional needs of the patient and the emotional support and needs of patient's family members. Team approach and group meetings should be initiated early on to identify specific needs and interventions to prevent emotional fatigue of the family.

Spiritual Care

Last, but certainly not least, spiritual care. Robinson et al. [20] conducted a survey on parents of 56 children who died in three pediatric intensive care units in Boston, Massachusetts. The survey results indicated that 73% of parents reported that prayers, faith, access to and care from clergy, and belief that the parent–child relationship transcends death, help them the most in dealing with their child' last phase of life. Spiritual care should be an integral part of the team approach to palliative care. Clergy and leaders from the faith of the family should be included in the process.

The Understanding and Discussion About Death

Similar to adults, the past experiences with death for the terminally ill child, as well as his/her age, emotional development, and surrounding have significant impact on how he/she perceive death. Every child, at any age, has his/her own unique concept of death. Adult's misconceptions and fear about death are often transferred to his/her children. Treating death as part of life is difficult for children with CCCs or life-threatening illnesses, but treating death in this way may alleviate some of the fear and confusion associated with it. When managing a terminally ill child and his/her siblings, the age and development will be an important factor.

Infant

Death is not a concept but a terminally ill infant will require care and comforting both physically and emotionally to maintain a consistent routine because he/she does react to the separation of parent, painful procedures, and any alteration of his/her routine.

Toddler

Death bears little meaning. Instead he/she may receive the most anxiety from the emotion of those around him/her. The words "death" or "forever" or "permanent" may not have any real value to him/her. Even with previous experiences with death, the toddler may not understand the relationship between life and death.

Preschool Children

Children of the age group may begin to understand that death is something feared by adults but they do not understand that death is permanent and every living thing will eventually die. People around this group of children can influence their experience with death. They may ask questions about "why?" and "how?" death occurs. The preschool children may feel shame and guilt. It is not uncommon for this age group of children to believe that becoming seriously ill is a form of punishment for something they did or thought about. When handling children at this age, death should not be explained as "sleep" to prevent the possible development of a sleep disorder. At times, they do not understand how their parents could not protect them from their illnesses. If siblings of a dying child are at this age group, they may feel as if they are the cause of illness and death. Therefore, a preschool sibling of a dying child also requires reassuring and comforting.

School Age Children

When children reach this stage of development, they may have a more realistic understanding about death and frequently death is personified as an angel, skeleton, or ghost. They may start to understand death as permanent, universal, and inevitable. They may be interested in the physical process of death and what happens after a person dies. They may fear their own death because of uncertainty of what happens to them after they die. Children in the age range tend to mirror the emotions of their parents. When the parents are scared and anxious, the kids may feel similarly.

Adolescent

Adolescents understand the concept that death is permanent. Past experience and emotional development greatly affect the adolescent's concept of death. Similar to adults, adolescents may want to observe their religious or cultural ritual. In spite of the predominant theme in adolescence is a feeling of immortality or being exempt from death. Their realization of their own death threatens all of these objectives. Denial and defiant attitudes may suddenly change the personality of a teenager facing death. An adolescent may feel as if they no longer belong or fit in with their peers or feel an inability to communicate with his/her parents. The adolescent may feel alone in their struggle, scared, and angry.

Issues Related to Palliative Care in the NICU [21, 22]

Few health care environments or patient populations present more challenges than neonates dying in the Neonatal Intensive Care Unit. However, 50% of children die in the first year of life and 25% die in the first month. Palliative care can be very helpful in defining the goals and limits of care, and can help parents and the health care team make good decisions on behalf of the neonate when crises occur. Three unique situations have been identified in newborn ICU in which palliative care team should intervene and offer the support in decision making and comfort for the neonate and parents. These scenarios are described as following [23]:

- When a serious health issue is identified prenatally by ultrasound, amniocentesis, or other prenatal exam.
- When a very premature infant is born or an infant is born with a life-threatening condition diagnosed in the delivery room.
- When a very ill neonate develops multiorgan system failure and care becomes futile.

While supporting neonates through the use of ECMO, high-frequency oscillatory ventilation and other new technologies, one fact is that neonates do feel pain, and every effort should be made to ensure the baby is comfortable and free of physical suffering during painful procedures. Care should be taken to ensure sedative and analgesic agents are given when any paralyzing agents are used. It is always difficult to discuss with parents of infant with terminal illness because of their emotions. Regardless of level of education, religion, socioeconomic, and age factors, it is important for them to understand the issues surrounding the care of their critically ill neonate who cannot speak for him- or herself. It is important to know that palliative care of newborns is holistic and extensive care for an infant who is not going to "get better" or having decent quality of life. The focus of palliative care in NICU is for both the infant and his/her family and may be initially combined with cure-oriented, disease-modifying care; then modify accordingly based on the condition of infant. Its goals are to prevent and relieve infant suffering and to improve the condition of the infant's living or dying and well-being of the family [23].

Issues Related to Health Care Practitioners and Care Givers

Stress and Burnout in Health Care Practitioners

Caring for children with life-limiting conditions is a stressful task not only for patient's family, friends, and siblings, but also for health care providers. Although little is known about how health care professionals cope with the challenges of children with life-threatening and life-limiting disease, studies suggest that they are at risk for developing compassion fatigue and burnout. Difficulties in communications with young patients and parents and inadequate support system were listed as common issues for health care providers in many countries. In addition, the uncertainty of most childhood life-threatening conditions and the continued hope for survival make decisions to shift from cure to palliation difficult and distressing for many health care providers. The emotional impact of the dying process and death of a child and grieving of health care providers are frequently hidden and disenfranchised.

The society expects health care providers remain strong and stoic in the face of death. Papadatou et al. [24] demonstrated that even though health care providers work in different environments and cultures, the grieving process of health care providers has unique characteristics. Some may grieve over the loss of a personal bond they have developed with a child, some over the nonrealization of their efforts to cure or control the disease, and others over unresolved personal loss that surface with the death of a child. Nevertheless, health care professional's grieving process is an ongoing fluctuation between experiencing grief by focusing on the loss, and avoiding or repressing grief by moving away from it. When healthcare providers do not have fluctuating feelings, suppress and deny the feelings, or submerge in their grief, complications occur. Frequently, the health care professionals rely on their colleagues for support, not their family members. Through information exchanges, clinical collaboration, and sharing personal experiences, the healthcare providers try to cope with their loss.

Bereavement

Suffering from CCC and life-threatening illnesses does not end with the wake or funeral. Pediatric palliative care should extend beyond the patient's death. Communication with the family should continue not only to offer support for the family, but to monitor siblings and the parents for signs of difficulty adjusting to life without their son, daughter, sister, or brother. A simple note or phone call may mean a lot to the family, and a referral to a psychologist or therapist may help the grieving process.

Summary

Pediatric Palliative care is systematic coordinated care of patients with CCCs and life-threatening illnesses. Palliative care is not specifically end-of-life care. Pediatric Palliative Care should be initiated early in the disease process and it should extend beyond the patient's death. The goal of pediatric palliative care is to alleviate the physical, emotional, psychosocial, and spiritual suffering of children and their families suffering CCCs and life-threatening illness. The hallmark of successful care of the patient with a CCC is open, straightforward communication with the patient, their families, and amongst those taking care of the patient. Successful palliative care is usually multifaceted and includes the expertise of many specialties including but not limited to social work, psychology, psychiatry, pain and symptom management, child life, play therapy, music therapy, and pet therapy. Care should include clergy and spiritual leaders. Pediatric palliative care is the multidisciplinary approach to the pediatric patient with a CCC and life-threatening illnesses and it can make all the difference in the world.

References

1. http://www.who.int/cancer/palliative/definition/en/.
2. Feudtner CF, DiGiuseppe DL, Neff JM. Hospital care for children and young adults in the last year of the life: a population-base study. BMC Med. 2003;1:3.
3. Friebert S. NHPCO Facts and Figures – pediatric palliative and hospice care in America. 2009. http//www.nhpco.org/files/public/quality/Pediatric_Facts-Figures.pdf.
4. Feudtner C, Silveria MJ, Christakis DA. Where do children with complex chronic conditions die? Patterns in Washington State, 1980–1998. Pediatrics. 2002;109:656–60.
5. US Department of Health and Human Service, Health Resources and Service Administration, Maternal and Child Health Bureau. The National Survey of Children with Special Health Care Needs Chartbook 2005–2006. Rockville, MD: US Department of Health and Human Service; 2007.
6. Simon TD, Feudtner C, Stone BL, Sheng X, Bratton SL, Dean M, Srivastava R. Children with complex chronic conditions in patient hospital settings in the United States. Pediatrics. 2010;126:647–55.
7. Mathews TJ, Miniño AM, Osterman MJK, Strobino DM, Guyer B. Annual summary of vital statistics: 2008. Pediatrics. 2011;127:146–57.
8. American Academy of Pediatrics (Committee on Bioethics and Committee on Hospital Care). Palliative care for children 2007. http://aappolicy.aappublications.org/cgi/reprint/pediatrics;106/2/351.pdf.
9. Smith TJ, Coyne P, Cassel B, Penberthy L, Hopson A, Hager MA. A high-volume specialist palliative care unit and team may reduce in-hospital end-of life care cost. J Palliat Med. 2003;6:699–705.
10. Feudtner CF, Hays RM, Haynes G, Geyer R, Neff J, Koepsell TD. Death attributed to pediatric complex chronic condition: national trends and implications for supportive care services. Pediatrics. 2001;107:e99.
11. Korones DN. Pediatric palliative care. Pediatr Rev. 2007;28:e46.
12. Himelstein BP, Hilden JM, Boldt AM, Weissman D. Pediatric palliative care. N Eng J Med. 2004;350:1752–62.
13. Himelstein BP. Palliative care in pediatrics. Anesthesiol Clin N Am. 2005;23:837–56.
14. Himelstein BP. Palliative care for infants, children, adolescents and their families. J Palliat Med. 2006;9:163–81.
15. Davies B, Sehring SA, Partridge JC, Cooper BA, Hughes A, Philp JC, et al. Barriers to palliative care for children: perceptions of pediatric health care providers. Pediatrics. 2008;121:282–8.
16. Liben S, Papadatou D, Wolfe J. Paediatric palliative care: challenges and emergence ideas. Lancet. 2008;371:852–64.
17. Feudtner CF, Feinstein JA, Satchell M, Zhao H, Kang TI. Shifting place of death among children with complex chronic conditions in the United States, 1989–2003. JAMA. 2007;297:2725–32.
18. Masera G. Who can decide what is in a child's best interest? A problem-solving approach. Med Pediatr Oncol. 2001;36:649–51.
19. Hynson JL, Sawyer SM. Paediatric palliative care: distinctive needs and emerging issues. J Paediatr Child Health. 2001;37:323–5.
20. Robinson MR, Thiel MT, Backus MM, Meyer EC. Matters of spirituality at the end of life in the pediatric intensive care unit. Pediatrics. 2006;118:e719.
21. Rebagliato M, Cuttini M, Broggin L, Berbik I, de Vonderweid U, Hansen G, et al. Neonatal end-of-life decision making: physicians' attitudes and relationship with self-report practice in 10 European Countries. JAMA. 2000;284:2451–9.

22. Dealing with death in the NICU – a conversation with neonatal care expert Anita Catlin. http://www.medscape.com/viewarticle/715963.
23. Carter BS, Levetown M, editors. Palliative care for infants, children, and adolescents – a practical handbook. Baltimore, MD: The Johns Hopkins University Press; 2004.
24. Papadatou D, Martinson IM, Chung P-M. Caring for dying children: a comparative study of nurses' experienced in Greece and Hong Kong. Cancer Nurs. 2001;24:402–12.

Review Questions

1. What is the palliative care?

    (a) Supportive care only
    (b) Only those who is terminally ill can receive it
    (c) Both supportive care and curative care together
    (d) Only being administered in hospice
    (e) The goal is to make patient comfortable

2. Which statement is true?

    (a) Palliative care can only be delivered in hospital
    (b) Hospice care and palliative care are the same
    (c) Palliative care requires multiple disciplinary service
    (d) Palliative care can only be delivered in hospice
    (e) Every case for palliative care should be treated uniformly

3. What are the barriers of pediatric palliative care?

    (a) Inadequate education and exposure
    (b) Uncomfortable in discussing the issue related to death
    (c) Cultural and religious differences
    (d) Uncertainty of disease progression
    (e) All of the above

4. Which one is not included in pediatric palliative care?

    (a) Spiritual consultation
    (b) Social support, family consultation
    (c) Curative treatments
    (d) All services are covered by insurance and Medicaid
    (e) Symptomatic treatments

5. Pediatric palliative care should include the following service

    (a) Religious clergy or cultural leader
    (b) Social worker
    (c) Nursing
    (d) Doctor
    (e) All of the above

6. The similarities between hospice and palliative care are *except*

    (a) Symptomatic treatments
    (b) Curative treatment
    (c) Majority of services are covered by Insurance
    (d) Both types of care can be delivered at home
    (e) Both types of care can be delivered in the hospital

7. The pediatric palliative care is as described below *except*

    (a) Mainly delivered through one person
    (b) Deliver at home, hospital, or nursing facility
    (c) Doctor, nurse, social worker, chaplain, home health aide are included in the team
    (d) Patients with chronic complex illness can benefit from it
    (e) Provide support to the whole family

8. What are symptomatic treatments?

    (a) Pain management
    (b) Anxiety treatment
    (c) Spiritual consultation
    (d) None of the above
    (e) All of the above

9. The barriers to establish neonatal palliative care are all *except*

    (a) The advancement of surgical techniques and life-support technology
    (b) The prognosis of the illness is undetermined
    (c) Social circumstance when the neonate was conceived, e.g., unplanned or IVF
    (d) The decision of palliative care should be made prenatally or immediately when resuscitation is warranted
    (e) None of the above

10. Pediatric palliative care

    (a) The goal of palliative care is to provide most aggressive treatment for pediatric patients
    (b) All neonates need palliative care
    (c) The advancement of technology and surgical interventions warrant excellent overall outcomes
    (d) The person who has the best interest of the child should make the decision regarding the care for the child
    (e) All of the above

Answers

1. (c)
2. (c)
3. (e)
4. (d)
5. (e)
6. (b)
7. (a)
8. (e)
9. (d)
10. (e)

Chapter 26
New Pain Management Vistas in Palliative Care

Christopher K. Merritt, Lien B. Tran, Rinoo V. Shah, and Alan David Kaye

Palliative care medicine is an evolving field, unique with respect to the diverse patients that it treats and drawing from all fields of medicine. Within the field of palliative care, new treatment modalities are continuously under development, and existing modalities are increasingly being applied to ease the suffering patients. This chapter will look toward some of the new treatments under development that may shape the future of palliative care, including new pharmacologic agents, new methods of drug delivery, and the application of regional anesthesia to control pain in palliative care patients.

Novel Agents in Pain Management

Anti-nerve Growth Factor Agents

Nerve growth factor (NGF) is a neurotrophic agent that acts through binding to the tropomyosin-related kinase A receptor (TrkA). Patients with mutations in the gene encoding the TrkA receptor demonstrate congenital analgesia and anhidrosis but few additional adverse effects [1]. Through the interaction with TrkA, NGF functions not only in the growth of nerve fibers, but it also enhances acute nociceptive pain and is also involved in pathologic chronic pain states and hyperalgesia [2]. NGF is released in response to tissue injury by mast cells, eosinophils, macrophages, and others, and in turn stimulates the release of additional inflammatory mediators

C.K. Merritt, M.D. (✉) • L.B. Tran, M.D. • A.D. Kaye, M.D., Ph.D.
Department of Anesthesiology, Louisiana State University School of Medicine,
New Orleans, LA, USA
e-mail: cmerr2@lsuhsc.edu; alankaye44@hotmail.com

R.V. Shah, M.D., M.B.A.
Department of Anesthesiology, Guthrie Clinic-Big Flats,
Horseheads, NY, USA

N. Vadivelu et al. (eds.), *Essentials of Palliative Care*,
DOI 10.1007/978-1-4614-5164-8_26,
© Springer Science+Business Media New York 2013

that enhance the nociceptive response. In addition, the NGF–TrkA complex undergoes retrograde transport to the dorsal root ganglion, where it induces transcriptional changes that increase nociceptive sensitivity and contribute to hyperalgesia [2]. Novel anti-NGF agents have shown significant promise in animal models attenuating both acute inflammatory pain in addition to chronic pain and hyperalgesia. Three monoclonal antibodies are under development by Pfizer (tanezumab), Janssen (fulranumab), and Regeneron (REGN475) with promising analgesic results. Concerns exist about the possibility of rapidly progressive osteoarthritis with at least one of these agents, tanezumab. Nevertheless, the potential benefit of anti-NGF agents for patients suffering with chronic pain led the FDA to endorse the continued development of these drugs [3].

$Na_v1.7$ Blocking Agents

The role of the sodium channel subunit, $Na_v1.7$, has recently come to light as a promising potential analgesic target. In 2006, Cox et al. identified three families with congenital analgesia, mapped the chromosomal location of their mutation, and identified their mutation in the SCN9A gene [4]. This results in loss of function of the $Na_v1.7$ subunit of the voltage-gated sodium channel. Although voltage-gated sodium channels are ubiquitous in neurons, the $Na_v1.7$ subunit is highly expressed in nociceptive fibers. Loss of function of the $Na_v1.7$ subunit results in congenital analgesia but few additional effects [4]. Sodium channel blockade is widely utilized in local anesthetics as well as antiarrhythmic agents such as mexiletine. However, no currently available sodium channel blocking agents are specific to the $Na_v1.7$ subunit [5]. A selective $Na_v1.7$ blocking agent could potentially stop nociceptive pain without otherwise interrupting nerve transmission. Such an agent would present a very attractive analgesic and is the subject of ongoing investigation.

High Dose Topical Capsaicin

Topical capsaicin has long been used as a treatment for neuropathic pain syndromes including painful diabetic neuropathy, HIV-associated peripheral neuropathy, postherpetic neuralgia, as well as in over-the-counter formulations [6]. Capsaicin activates the TRPV1 receptor on nociceptive fibers resulting in calcium influx into cells, depolarization, and the sensation of heat and pain. Repeated applications can cause a decrease in sensitivity to pain and hyperalgesia. It was previously believed that topical capsaicin resulted in analgesia by causing depletion of substance P in the spinal cord. More recent evidence, however, points to "defunctionalization" of nociceptive fibers by topical capsaicin, a multifactorial effect signaling ability of nociceptive pathways [7]. Although successful, the benefits of formulations ranging from 0.025 to 0.075% are limited with respect to the duration of their effect and the ceiling of their benefit [7]. Eight percent capsaicin for topical application (Qutenza™ patch) has recently been FDA approved for the treatment of HIV-associated peripheral neuropathy and postherpetic neuralgia. A single 60-min treatment results in a significant decrease in pain for 12 weeks [8–11]. Temporary pain and local irritation were the most common adverse events and rarely resulted in inability to complete treatment [12, 13].

Voltage-Gated Calcium Channel Blocking Agents

Voltage-gated calcium channels (VGCCs) function in diverse physiologic roles in many neurological systems. Activation of these channels affects the membrane potential of neurons and their depolarization, release of neurotransmitters, as well as affecting the enzymatic activity and genetic transcription of neurons [14]. Through these effects, VGCCs have been implicated in physiologic nociception, as well as pathologic pain conditions. The high voltage activated N-Type calcium channel is highly expressed in dorsal root ganglion cells bodies and at the synapse of afferent nociceptive fibers and dorsal horn neurons. At these sites, N-Type VGCC function in both the transmission and modulation of pain. Currently, one N-Type VGCC blocking agent is available clinically, ziconotide (Prialt™). Ziconotide is a peptide first isolated from the poison of a marine cone snail. The peptide structure of ziconotide necessitates intrathecal administration to reach its site of action in the spinal cord. Ziconotide is indicated for the treatment of patients with severe chronic pain of various etiologies in those who are refractory to or unable to take first-line systemic analgesics, adjunctive therapies, or IT morphine. Studies of intrathecal ziconotide infusion reduced pain scores in chronic pain patients approximately 30–50% including those with HIV-associated chronic pain, cancer-related pain, as well as patients with nonmalignant chronic pain. Although generally well tolerated, ziconotide can cause neuropsychiatric side effects including confusion, dizziness, and somnolence. Despite ziconotide's significant benefit, its clinical utility remains limited by cost and the need for delivery by intrathecal microinfusion catheters.

Cannabinoids

Smoked or ingested cannabis has long been used both recreationally, as well as for medical purposes to treat symptoms such as pain, nausea, cachexia, and glaucoma. As a pharmacologic agent, however, the potential benefit of cannabis has been complicated by psychotropic side effects, legal restrictions, inconsistency in regulation and potency, and risks of smoke inhalation [15–17]. Currently, the US Drug Enforcement Agency classifies cannabis as a Schedule I agent with high potential for abuse, no currently accepted medical use, and a lack of accepted safety for use even under medical supervision [18]. Despite this, 14 states have enacted laws allowing the use of cannabis for medical purposes under physician supervision [16].

The primary active agent in cannabis, delta-9-tetrahydrocannabinol, acts via the cannabinoid receptors CB_1 and CB_2 to produce its varied psychotropic and therapeutic effects, with the majority of psychotropic effects occurring via CB_1 signaling [15]. Synthetic preparations of delta-9-tetrahydrocannabinol or dronabinol (Marinol™) have been classified by the DEA as a Schedule III agent and are FDA approved for the treatment of anorexia in patients with AIDS-associated wasting as well as nausea associated with cancer chemotherapy that has failed conventional treatment [19]. Small studies have also suggested that dronabinol also significantly reduces pain scores in patients with central pain due to multiple sclerosis as well as in patients with chronic pain syndromes using opioids [20, 21].

Recently, improved understanding of cannabinoid pharmacology has created the potential for new pharmacologic agents for symptom management. The CB_2 receptor is primarily expressed in peripheral immune and inflammatory cells, though it may also be expressed in the central nervous system, particularly in pathologic pain states [15]. In these two locations, the CB_2 receptor is thought to modulate nociception in both inflammatory as well as neuropathic and central pain states [15, 22]. In animal models selective CB_2 receptor agonists attenuated both acute and chronic pain. In addition, rats subjected to painful nerve injury self-administered the CB_2 receptor agonist more than control rats [15]. This may suggest that action at the CB_2 receptor possesses more analgesic effects than psychotropic effects, and therefore future selective CB_2 receptor agonists may provide analgesia with limited abuse potential [15].

Fatty-Acid Amide Hydrolase Inhibitors

In addition to these exogenous cannabinoids, endogenous cannabinoids exert effects via the CB_1 and CB_2 receptors, and modulation of these endogenous cannabinoids presents an attractive target for future analgesics. The two best-characterized cannabinoids are anandamide (AEA) and 2-arachidonoylglycerol (2-AG), and these are thought to be the primary endogenous ligands of the CB_1 and CB_2 receptors, respectively [22]. AEA and 2-AG are hydrolyzed and inactivated via the intracellular enzyme fatty-acid amide hydrolase (FAAH) [22, 23]. FAAH knockout mice demonstrate reduced sensitivity to painful stimuli and increased levels of endogenous cannabinoids presumably due to decreased endocannabinoid hydrolysis [24]. This suggests that inhibition of FAAH could be a viable strategy to therapeutically increase endogenous cannabinoids, and preliminary data supports this. URB597 is an experimental specific FAAH inhibitor that enters the CNS, and in animal models results in anxiolysis, reduced sensitivity to pain and antidepressant activity [23, 25–27]. URB937 is another specific FAAH inhibitor; however, it only functions in peripheral tissues since it is actively transported out of the CNS [23]. Interestingly, in animal models, this purely peripheral FAAH inhibition results in significant reduction in inflammatory mediated as well as neuropathic pain [23]. FAAH inhibition, particularly if limited to peripheral tissues, holds significant promise to maximize the analgesic benefits of the cannabinoid system while minimizing psychotropic side effects and potential for abuse.

AMPA and Kainate Ionotropic Glutamate Receptor Antagonists

Glutamate is the primary excitatory neurotransmitter, and glutamate signaling has been indicated in a wide variety of disease states including neuronal injury after cerebral ischemia, epilepsy, Parkinson's disease, Alzheimer's disease, chronic pain, and hyperalgesia [28, 29]. Excessive glutamate signaling can damage neurons through elevated intracellular calcium release, although enhancing glutamate excitation may have benefits in promoting synaptic connections in learning disorders or neurodegenerative conditions. AMPA and Kainate subclasses of ionotropic glutamate receptors (iGluRs) serve different functions in the CNS and may be expressed peripherally; AMPA iGluRs are responsible for the majority of glutamate signaling, where Kainate iGluRs perform more modulatory functions [28, 29]. AMPA agonists such as CX717 increase excitatory transmission and may encourage synaptic connections and learning. CX717 has shown success for the treatment of ADHD, though it did not receive FDA approval. AMPA agonists continue to be investigated to enhance learning in Alzheimer's disease as well as prevention of opiate-induced respiratory depression, both with preliminary evidence of promise in animal studies [30, 31].

In contrast, AMPA and AMPA/Kainate antagonists such as talampanel, perampanel, and tezampanel decrease excitatory glutamate signaling and have been investigated for prevention of neurodegeneration in Alzheimer's, as adjunctive antiepileptic medications, and may decrease pain in patients with painful diabetic neuropathy [29]. In addition, AMPA/Kainate receptor antagonists have shown preliminary benefit in the treatment of migraines and postoperative pain in animal studies [32–34]. Excitatory glutamate serves myriad and complex roles in normal physiology and both excessive and inadequate glutamate signaling function in pathological conditions and have the potential to be modulated for therapeutic benefit.

Human Chorionic Gonadotropin

Human chorionic gonadotropin (hCG) is an endogenous hormone which stimulates the production of testosterone, thyroid hormones, estradiol, and progesterone [35]. Exogenous subcutaneous recombinant hCG (Ovidrel™/Novarel™) is currently indicated for the treatment of prepubertal cryptorchidism, hypogonadotropinism and hypogonadism, and for the induction of ovulation and pregnancy in anovulatory women [36]. Emerging case reports suggest that hCG may have analgesic benefits to patients with chronic pain particularly those on chronic opioid therapy [37]. Opioids can cause suppression of pituitary gonadotropin release and produce a state of relative hypogonadotropinism and hypogonadism [38–40]. Androgen replacement in male patients with testosterone deficiency improves mood, sleep, and energy, though without consistent improvement in pain scores [39]. However, in patients with hypogonadotropinism, subcutaneous injection of hCG 500–1,000 units one to three times per week has been reported to significantly improve pain control in addition to energy, mood, and libido [37].

Somatropin/Human Growth Hormone

Somatotropin [human growth hormone (hGH)] is another endogenous anabolic hormone that promotes muscle and bone growth, lipolysis, gluconeogenesis, and organ growth [35]. Exogenous recombinant hGH (somatropin) has been widely reported in the popular media due to its frequent abuse by athletes and celebrities for its anabolic properties. Nevertheless, FDA indicated for the treatment of documented hGH deficiency, pediatric chronic kidney disease, and pediatric disorders associated with significant short stature [35, 41]. More recently and relevant to palliative care, rhGH has been indicated for the treatment of HIV-associated wasting syndrome and parenteral nutrition-dependent short bowel syndrome. In these situations, rhGH has been shown to increase body weight, muscle mass, and improve physical endurance. Research is ongoing into the use of rhGH in the treatment of cachexia related to other syndromes such as CHF, COPD, and cancer-related wasting with some evidence of benefit [42–51].

In addition to rhGH, the peptide hormone ghrelin, a hGH secretagogue released by the stomach in response to fasting, has shown promise for patients with wasting disorders. Ghrelin stimulates the release of hGH and other orexigenic hormones. Exogenous administration of ghrelin increases appetite and food intake, and preliminary studies have examined ghrelin administration to patients with cancer cachexia or protein malnutrition related to dialysis-dependent kidney disease. These data suggests that ghrelin may increase food intake and lean body mass in [41, 47, 52–57]. Concerns exist, however, with both ghrelin and rhGH that these agents could potentially stimulate tumor growth in patients with malignancy. In addition, a randomized controlled trial of hGH administration to acutely and critically ill patients demonstrated a significantly increased mortality rate in those patients who received hGH [58].

New Directions in Drug Delivery

Advances in the delivery of medications have allowed for improvements in the pharmacokinetic profile of medications and the minimization of unwanted side effects. These advances have been particularly important in expanding the utility of existing medications to better serve a variety of patients.

Extended Release Enteral Formulations

Extended release formulations of medications allow for simpler dosing regimens, improved patient satisfaction, and improved patient compliance [59, 60]. In addition, they can provide more stable blood concentrations of therapeutic agents and may avoid the peaks and troughs of immediate release drugs. This may result in fewer adverse effects that occur at high peak concentrations and fewer periods of inadequate treatment due to low drug concentrations at trough points.

Extended release medications use a variety of drug delivery strategies. Early extended release formulations mixed the active agent within an insoluble matrix that slowed the dissolution of the drug. Newer formulations, for example Exalgo™ (hydromorphone extended release), is based on the osmotic-controlled release oral delivery system (OROS). In OROS delivery systems, the active agent is encapsulated in an insoluble shell with a laser-drilled hole. The osmotic pressure of gastrointestinal fluids dissolving into the tablet generates the driving force for a slow, predictable release of active medication.

Some newer extended release formulations use a polymer matrix to both delay release of agent and slow gastric transit. Gralise™ (gabapentin extended-release) represents a newer class of extended release formulations that uses a polymeric system to delay transit of the tablet from the stomach [61]. Gabapentin has been successfully used to treat a variety of neuropathic pain states including diabetic neuropathy and postherpetic neuralgia with few adverse effects [62–64]. In contrast to traditional immediate release formulations of gabapentin, Gralise™ tablets expand in the stomach when taken with food. Gabapentin is slowly released from a polymeric matrix where it is subsequently absorbed in the small intestine. This allows not only for more convenient once-daily dosing, but it also decreases the peaks and troughs of thrice-daily gabapentin dosing. Furthermore, Gralise™ allows for a peak plasma gabapentin concentration at night when the undesired side effect of somnolence is unnoticed.

Parenteral Formulations

Transdermal and transmucosal delivery systems present attractive options for palliative care patients in whom enteral delivery may be limited by nausea, malabsorption, or dysphagia, as well for drugs with poor oral bioavailability in which enteral formulations are unavailable. The potent opioid fentanyl is a prototypical example of a medication with poor oral bioavailability whose utility has been greatly enhanced by the development of transmucosal (Actiq™, Fentora™) and transdermal formulations (Duragesic™). Transmucosal fentanyl allows for rapid treatment of breakthrough pain, while Duragesic™ patches deliver a basal rate of fentanyl to the patient to treat chronic pain, but cannot be used to treat breakthrough pain. In contrast, Ionsys is an iontophoretic transdermal fentanyl delivery system under

Fig. 26.1 The Sufentanil
NanoTab® PCA System (with
permission from AcelRx
Pharmaceuticals, Inc.)

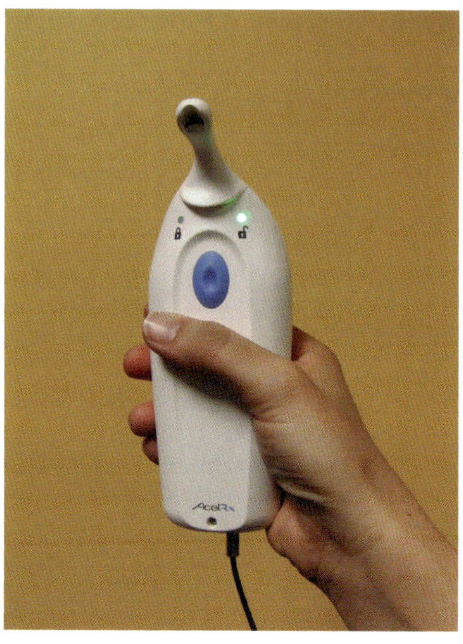

development that would allow patient controlled analgesia (PCA) through the active delivery of transdermal fentanyl on patient demand with the added safety of timing lockouts [65].

Newer transmucosal formulations of the opioid sufentanil may be able to provide rapid and enduring pain control through dosing as a sublingual patient controlled analgesia (PCA) system, the Sufentanil NanoTab® PCA System [66]. The system is shown in Fig. 26.1. Sufentanil is an analog of fentanyl that is approximately 10 times more potent than fentanyl and 1,000 times more potent than morphine [67]. Sufentanil provides superior analgesia with lower rates of respiratory depression than fentanyl or morphine after intravenous administration [67]. However, it is extremely lipophilic resulting in a short duration of action due to rapid redistribution into lipid-rich tissues in the body. Transmucosal absorption of sufentanil results in a longer plasma half-life, which may expand its clinical utility [66–72]. The Sufentanil NanoTab® PCA System delivers a 3-mm tablet on demand under the patient's tongue with programmed timing lockouts [72]. The advantage of this technology is that there is no need for the placement of an iv or classic PCA equipment for the system to be effective. Clinical data, thus far, has been quite positive with this innovative system that has been developed through AcelRx Pharmaceuticals, Inc.

In addition to opioids, transdermal delivery systems of NSAIDs such as diclofenac are being prescribed to treat localized pain and inflammation. Delivery systems such as the Flector™ patch and Voltaren™ gel allow targeted application of anti-inflammatory agents. Systemic absorption of diclofenac gel is approximately 94% less than an equivalent oral dose of diclofenac [73]. This decreased systemic absorption may result in an improved safety profile with fewer side effects. Transdermal lidocaine (Lidoderm™) has been previously discussed in this text and represents an additional safe localized analgesic adjunct. In addition to these transdermal and sublingual delivery systems, intranasal delivery systems of morphine (Rylomine™) and fentanyl are being investigated, as are intranasal, oral, and sublingual formulations of medications such as ketamine, which are currently commercially available only for intravenous administration [74]. The ever-expanding complement of new drug delivery systems promises to greatly improve the safety and utility of medications available for symptom management in palliative care.

Regional Anesthesia and Palliative Care

Introduction to Regional Anesthesia

Regional anesthesia consists of the application of local anesthetic agents to nerve roots or peripheral nerves to provide anesthesia or analgesia to a portion of the body. Regional anesthesia provides targeted analgesia while not affecting a person's consciousness or resulting in physiologic impairment of vital organ systems. Local and regional anesthesia has long been used within the fields of obstetrics, dentistry, and anesthesiology to provide pain control during and after surgical procedures. In addition to perioperative pain control, neuraxial (intrathecal and epidural) blockade and peripheral nerve blockade have proven useful in the treatment of diverse pain conditions. These include cancer pain, complex regional pain syndromes, radicular pain from herniated vertebral discs, ischemic pain, sickle-cell crises, posttraumatic pain, neuropathy, and/or the complications of treatments such as postradiation pain and lymphedema.

Regional blockade can provide rapid and complete control of existing pain but can also form a component of preemptive analgesia to ameliorate anticipated acute pain. Regional anesthesia may have benefits in interrupting the neurophysiological and psychophysiological response to pain thereby improve control chronic pain through psychological relief [75]. As these benefits have become apparent, the safety of regional anesthesia has also improved through newer medications and ultrasound-guided nerve localization. The utility of regional anesthesia has expanded from single injections lasting hours to indwelling peripheral nerve catheters that can provide analgesia for many days.

The increasing utility and safety of regional anesthesia make it an attractive future tool for palliative care medicine. However, patients with advanced systemic disease may present challenges for the use of regional anesthesia, particularly with the insertion of indwelling catheters. Patients receiving palliative care often have pain in multiple portions of their body, may have coagulopathies, or may present anatomical challenges due to the presence of edema, contractures, scar tissue, or absence of peripheral pulses and normal anatomic landmarks [76].

Local Anesthetic Agents

Local anesthetics (LAs) are the key agents used to achieve neural blockade in regional anesthesia. The basic structure of LAs consists of an aromatic end and an amine end connected to each other through an ester or and amide chain [77]. These molecules act primarily via targets on neuronal sodium channels thereby blocking the conduction of action potentials along the course of nerves.

Na Channel Blockade

The susceptibility of a nerve to blockade by LAs depends on characteristics of the individual drug (e.g., potency, pKa, buffering), characteristics of the tissue (e.g., presence of local inflammation and acidosis), and characteristics of individual nerve fibers (e.g., diameter, myelination, activity). LAs tend to block small nerve fibers both earlier and at lower concentrations than large nerve fibers, and blockade resolves in the reverse order. For example, blockade of 0.15-μm C-fibers (postganglionic autonomic, pressure, dull pain, and temperature) occurs before 1.5-μm Aδ fibers (sharp pain), and blockade of 15-μm Aα (motor) is the last to occur [77]. In addition to blocking Na channels on sensory and motor fibers, at high doses or after inadvertent intravascular injection, LAs can block Na channels in the brain and heart potentially resulting in loss of consciousness, seizures, myocardial depression, and even cardiac arrest.

Ester and Amide LAs

LAs can be broadly divided into two categories: those with an amide linking chain and those with an ester linking chain. Ester LAs can generally be identified as those with only one "i" in their names, and they include the first clinically utilized LA, cocaine, as well as procaine, chloroprocaine, and tetracaine. Amide LAs can generally be identified as those with two "i's." Amides are more commonly available, and include lidocaine, mepivacaine, bupivacaine, and ropivacaine. Allergy to ester LAs is much more common than amide LAs, due to the metabolism of ester LAs to the common allergen para-aminobenzoicacid (PABA). Amide LAs can generally be safely used in patients with a history of allergy to ester LAs. Ester LAs are primarily metabolized by pseudocholinesterase, whereas amide LAs undergo hepatic metabolism.

Lidocaine is an intermediate-duration amide local anesthetic with significant potency, fast onset, good tissue penetration, and low cardiac toxicity. The concentration of lidocaine used for regional anesthesia ranges from 1 to 2%, and a single injection can provide up to approximately 6 h of analgesia. Lidocaine is often used in combination with a long-acting local anesthetic, such as bupivacaine or ropivacaine in order to achieve both rapid and enduring analgesia. The duration of analgesia with this technique may be less compared to a long-acting local anesthetic such as ropivacaine or bupivacaine used alone [78].

Bupivacaine was the first long-acting amide local anesthetic created. The concentration of bupivacaine used for peripheral nerve blockade ranges from 0.25 to 0.5%, and a single injection can provide up to approximately 16–24 h of analgesia. It is more hydrophobic than lidocaine and has a slower onset. Bupivacaine is highly protein bound which allows for a longer duration; however, this also contributes to the potential for cardiotoxicity. Due to its narrow therapeutic index, bupivacaine has greatly been replaced by ropivacaine.

Levobupivacaine is the levorotatory enantiomer of bupivacaine. Commercial bupivacaine is a racemic mixture of both enantiomers (R and S). Levobupivacaine is approximately equivalent to its racemic bupivacaine with respect to onset, duration, and dosing in regional anesthesia. However, cardiac and CNS toxicity of levobupivacaine is approximately 35% less than racemic bupivacaine.

Exparel™ is a bupivacaine liposome injectable suspension (1.3% 266 mg/20 ml or 13.3 mg/ml). DepoFoam, which is a multivesicular liposome, consists of tiny 10–30 μm in diameter lipid-based particles which contain discrete water-filled chambers of bupivacaine dispersed through a lipid matrix. This novel preparation allows for increased duration of efficacy and pain relief up to 72 h after injection. This drug preparation recently came to market in early 2012.

Ropivacaine is a long-acting amide local anesthetic derived from mepivacaine and is a structural analog of bupivacaine. Ropivacaine differs from bupivacaine in that it exists as a pure S enantiomer, and it demonstrates reduced cardiac and CNS toxicity and may result in reduced motor blockade [79]. Concentrations of ropivacaine ranging from 0.2 to 1% are used for regional anesthesia, and a single injection can provide up to approximately 16 h of analgesia.

Mixtures of lidocaine with a long-acting local anesthetic such as bupivacaine or ropivacaine are commonly used for peripheral nerve blocks. This combination does achieve a quicker onset of analgesia; however, the plasma levels of the long-acting local anesthetics are lower than when using only long-acting local anesthetics.

Additives to LAs

Vasoconstrictors such as epinephrine or phenylephrine are often added to LAs to improve the duration and quality of neural blockade. Vasoconstriction slows the rate of systemic absorption, which can allow for the administration of higher doses of LAs before encountering toxicity. The addition of epinephrine to LAs can also serve as a marker of intravascular injection. If LA with epinephrine is injected intravascularly, the patient will demonstrate signs of tachycardia, hypertension, or T-wave peaking on EKG. Epinephrine may also improve the quality of neuraxial LA blockade independent of vasoconstriction through α-2 adrenergic activity [80].

Sodium bicarbonate is frequently added to LAs to increase the speed of onset of some LAs. LAs are weak bases and are often packaged as their water-soluble salt forms at an acidic pH. The addition of sodium bicarbonate raises the pH of the solution and increases the fraction of LA that exists in its unionized form. LAs must cross the cell membrane in this unionized form to gain access to the intracellular receptor site of the Na channel. By favoring this unionized state, sodium bicarbonate can hasten onset of blockade. The correct ratio is 1 ml of sodium bicarbonate per 10 ml of lidocaine or 30 ml of bupivacaine.

Additional adjuncts are occasionally added to LA solutions in certain clinical scenarios. Opioids such as fentanyl, morphine, or hydromorphone are commonly added to solutions of neuraxial LAs in epidural infusions or spinals. They improve pain control while minimizing the systemic side effects of opioids and decrease the necessary concentration of LA to achieve similar pain control. This decreased concentration of LA may allow for decreased motor block; however, risks of respiratory depression must be considered when administering neuraxial narcotics. α-2 adrenergic agonists such as clonidine or dexmedetomidine can also be added to mixtures of LAs for neuraxial administration. They improve pain control, but may result in hypotension and bradycardia. The NMDA-antagonist ketamine has also been added to mixtures of LAs for neuraxial administration with improved analgesia, but this is uncommonly used in the USA [81]. Steroids such as dexamethasone have been added to LAs for peripheral nerve blockade with reports of improved duration and quality of blockade. Any medication administered perineurally should be preservative free, as some preservative preparations contain the neurotoxic agent phenol. This is particularly critical for neuraxial administration where neurotoxicity could result in devastating cauda equina syndrome or paraplegia.

Toxicity of LAs

The primary concern in the administration of LAs is the risk of systemic LA absorption resulting in CNS and cardiac toxicity. This can occur from inadvertent intravascular injection of LA or from systemic absorption of LA. The risk of systemic toxicity depends on the LA agent and the site of administration. For example, even a very small dose of lidocaine can rapidly cause unconsciousness and seizure if inadvertently injected into the vertebral artery. Even without intravascular injection, rates of absorption and risk of systemic toxicity vary by location of administration. For example, rates of systemic absorption are highest with interpleural or intercostal injection, lowest with subcutaneous infiltration, and lower still with the addition of vasoconstrictors. Toxicity also varies with specific LA agents. The potent, lipophilic, long-acting amide agent bupivacaine presents much higher risk of cardiotoxicity than the less potent, rapidly metabolized ester agent chloroprocaine.

CNS Toxicity

At sufficient doses or after intravascular injection, LAs cause CNS stimulation. Early symptoms can include lightheadedness, metallic taste, tinnitus, and circumoral numbness. This can progress to restlessness, unconsciousness, and tonic–clonic seizures. At higher doses, CNS depression occurs which can result in respiratory failure and death.

Cardiovascular Toxicity

LAs can additionally cause cardiovascular toxicity, though this generally occurs at doses higher than those causing CNS symptoms. LAs act on the myocardium, decreasing electrical excitability, conduction rate, and contractile force. On rare occasions LAs have caused cardiovascular collapse and death without preceding CNS symptoms. This may be due to either an action on the pacemaker or the sudden onset of ventricular fibrillation. Ventricular tachycardia and fibrillation are relatively uncommon consequences of local anesthetics but can occur, particularly with bupivacaine. Bupivacaine-associated cardiotoxicity is very resistant to resuscitation and defibrillation. In addition to ACLS, treatment should include rapid administration of lipid emulsion bolus and infusion [82].

Methemoglobinemia

Clinically significant methemoglobinemia may occur with the local anesthetics benzocaine and priolocaine [83]. Benzocaine is commonly available in a spray form for topical anesthesia to mucous membranes (Hurricaine™ Spray), and prilocaine is a component in eutectic mixture of local anesthetic (EMLA) cream often used to provide topical anesthesia prior to intravenous line placement in children.

Performing Regional Nerve Blocks

Any patient considering regional anesthesia should be advised of the risks of the procedure (infection, bleeding, damage to nerves, damage to adjacent structures, local anesthetic toxicity, etc.). They should also be forewarned of side effects of nerve blockade such as motor block that may present a risk of falls and care of the numb limb. In addition, patients with continuous catheters should be evaluated in person or via telephone to assess for any signs or symptoms of infection or local anesthetic toxicity.

Strict sterile technique including antibiotic skin preparation, sterile gloves, hat, and mask should be used for all peripheral nerve blocks, and asepsis is especially critical with peripheral nerve catheters. Monitoring patients for regional anesthesia is additionally important, as patients may require procedural sedation, and complications such as local anesthetic toxicity, pneumothorax, nerve injury, vascular puncture, and bleeding can occur. Standard monitoring should include pulse oximetry, electrocardiography, and blood pressure monitoring. Some centers use capnography to ensure adequate ventilation, but pulse oximetry and frequent verbal communication with the patient are often sufficient [84].

Resuscitation equipment should also be available, including a self-inflating bag-valve-mask, oxygen source with face-mask, suction, intravenous access, laryngoscope, and endotracheal tubes. Resuscitation medications such as vasopressors and lipid emulsion should also be readily available.

Single-Shot Peripheral Nerve Blocks and Peripheral Nerve Catheters

Single shot peripheral nerve blocks are intended for the treatment of acute pain. They provide rapid analgesia, but even with long-acting local anesthetics, single shot blockade can provide analgesia for only up to 24 h. In order to provide more enduring analgesia, continuous peripheral nerve catheters can be placed near the target nerve to deliver a continuous infusion of local anesthetic and extend the duration of analgesia for days. Initial use of continuous peripheral nerve blockade was limited to the inpatient population, but increasingly patients are being sent home with peripheral nerve catheters. Despite the benefits and widespread use of continuous peripheral nerve catheters, few studies exist regarding the prevention of complications during peripheral nerve catheter placement, management, and removal. In a series of 620 outpatients treated with continuous peripheral nerve blocks, there were surprisingly few interventions requiring an anesthesiologist. Patients were able to manage and remove their catheters at home without additional follow-up. This suggests that with adequate instruction and telephone access to health care providers, patients are comfortable with managing and removing continuous peripheral nerve catheters at home [85].

The duration of continuous peripheral nerve blocks is limited primarily by the risk of infection, which increases with the duration of infusion. Most clinicians remove catheters after approximately 3–7 days, though case series have been published with duration greater than 2 weeks [86, 87]. Additional challenges with peripheral nerve catheters include more difficult placement, possibility of malpositioning resulting in failure or complication.

Specific Regional Techniques

Common blocks for the upper and lower extremities will be discussed, with ultrasound-guided techniques described when possible. Although far from exhaustive, these techniques allow for analgesia to all or part of the upper and lower extremities with either single shot or continuous catheter techniques. All regional anesthesia techniques carry risks of vascular injury and bleeding, local anesthetic toxicity, and

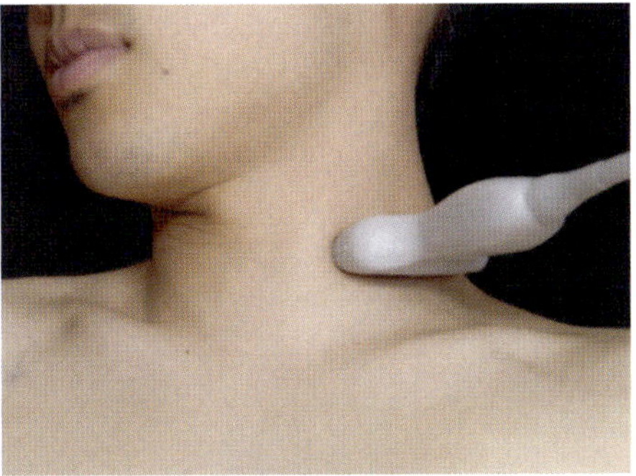

Fig. 26.2 Position of an ultrasound probe for interscalene brachial plexus block, obtained with permission from Essentials of Regional Anesthesia, Tran De QH, Dugani S, Asenjo J. Kaye AD, Urman R, Vadivelu N (editors), Springer, Chap. 13, p. 345

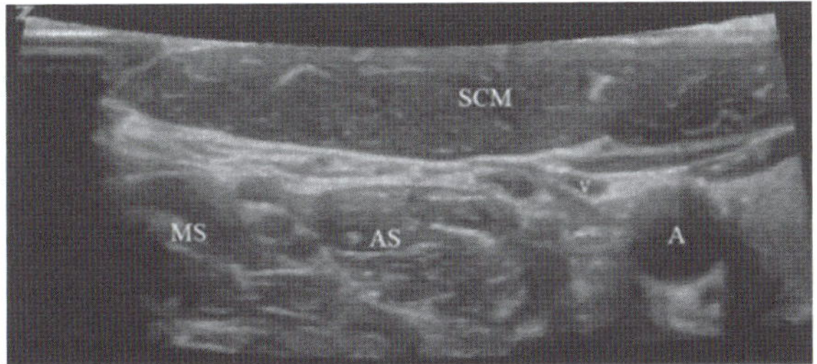

Fig. 26.3 Ultrasonographic appearance of the interscalene and cervical paravertebral brachial plexus (*A* carotid artery, *AS* anterior scalene muscle, *MS* middle scalene muscle, *SCM* sterno-cleidomastoid muscle, *V* internal jugular vein, obtained with permission from Essentials of Regional Anesthesia, Tran De QH, Dugani S, Asenjo J. Kaye AD, Urman R, Vadivelu N (editors), Springer, Chap. 13, p. 346

nerve injury from intraneural injection or neurotoxicity of local anesthetics and additives. Upper extremity nerve blocks carry additional risks, such as pneumothorax, injury or blockade of the recurrent laryngeal and phrenic nerves, and inadvertent intrathecal or epidural injections. Among others, relative contraindications to all peripheral nerve blocks include pathologic coagulopathy, blood thinning agents, infection at the site, systemic infection, and preexisting nerve damage. Figure 26.2 shows a typical probe utilized for ultrasound guided regional techniques. Figure 26.3 demonstrates imaging from an ultrasound guided regional block.

Peripheral Nerve Blocks of the Upper Extremity

Interscalene Brachial Plexus Block

The interscalene nerve block is the most proximal approach to the brachial plexus, anesthetizing the shoulder, clavicle, and proximal humerus innervated by roots and trunks. This block typically spares the C8-T1 nerve roots (ulnar nerve.) Using the in-plane ultrasound approach, the subclavian artery is first identified. The brachial plexus should appear as a cluster of hypoechoic circles superior and posterolateral to the artery. When it is followed in the cephalad direction, the cluster takes on a stacked "stop-light" appearance between the anterior and middle scalene muscles. Approximately 30 ml of local anesthetic is typically deposited between the first and second or second and third nodules, which are likely the nerve roots of C5, C6, and C7 [84].

Interscalene brachial plexus blockade can cause recurrent laryngeal nerve injury, pneumothorax, vertebral artery injury or injection, neuraxial injection, and Horner's syndrome by injuring the cervical sympathetic chain. Interscalene brachial plexus blockade results in nearly universal blockade of the ipsilateral phrenic nerve. Therefore, interscalene block may be contraindicated in patients with significant respiratory insufficiency, contralateral hemidiaphragmatic paralysis, contralateral pneumonectomy, etc.

Supraclavicular Brachial Plexus Block

The supraclavicular block anesthetizes the distal clavicle, humerus, forearm, and hand through blockade at the trunks and divisions of the brachial plexus. It is identified by ultrasound as the hypoechoic cluster that appears superior and postero-lateral to the subclavian artery as described in the interscalene brachial plexus block above. Local anesthetic is injected toward the "corner pocket," i.e., the intersection between the subclavian artery and the first rib.

As with the interscalene nerve block, Horner's syndrome, recurrent laryngeal nerve injury can occur. Phrenic nerve blockade occurs approximately 30% of the time with the supraclavicular nerve block due to cephalad spread of local anesthetic. The close proximity of the brachial plexus to the subclavian artery and the apex of the lung make pneumothorax, intravascular injection, and vascular injury the most common complications of supraclavicular blockade.

Infraclavicular Brachial Plexus Block

The infraclavicular approach blocks the brachial plexus at the level of the lateral, medial, and posterior cords, providing anesthesia to the humerus, forearm, and hand. Placing the ultrasound probe sagitally in the infraclavicular fossa, medial to the coracoid process will obtain a short-axis view of the axillary vessels. Using an in-plane technique and a cephalad to caudad direction, a 10-cm block needle is advanced until the tip lies just deep to the artery, where local anesthetics can be injected.

Vascular puncture is the primary concern during an infraclavicular block. External compression can be difficult to achieve due to the depth of the vessels. Caution should be taken in coagulopathic patients, and perhaps a different approach should be considered. There have also been anecdotal reports of Horner's syndrome, phrenic nerve paralysis, and pneumothorax associated with infraclavicular blocks.

Axillary Brachial Plexus Block

The axillary brachial plexus block anesthetizes the terminal branches of the brachial plexus (musculocutaneous, median, radial, and ulnar nerves.) The musculocutaneous and median nerves are situated ventral relative to the artery. The musculocutaneous nerve has generally split away from the rest of the branches and may need to be individually targeted a few centimeters ventrolateral to the artery. The radial and ulnar nerves are located dorsal relative to the artery. Using an in-plane technique and puncture sites above or below the artery, a 5-cm block needle is directed toward each of the four neural structures. Care must be taken to visualize the entire length of the needle during the advancement process. Local anesthetic is injected until circumferential spread is achieved for each nerve.

The overall safety margin for this block is extremely high. The biggest risk is vascular puncture. Continuous block catheters in the axilla are generally avoided due to higher rates of infection.

Peripheral Nerve Blocks of the Lower Extremity

Sciatic Nerve Block

The sciatic nerve is the largest nerve in the human body and provides sensory and motor innervation to the posterior thigh and lower leg. It arises from the lumbosacral plexus (ventral rami of L4–5 and S1–3). There are many approaches to the sciatic nerve block. Here, the classic approach and an ultrasound-guided approach will be discussed [84].

The classic or Labat approach utilizes the nerve stimulator to verify plantar flexion at the ankle, which is the desired response. The patient is placed in the lateral position with the targeted side up, slightly flexed at the hip and knee. This position will bring the sciatic nerve into a more superficial position. The unaffected or dependent leg is positioned down and straightened. The landmarks include the posterior superior iliac spine (PSIS), greater trochanter, and sacral hiatus. A first line is drawn between the greater trochanter and PSIS. A second line is drawn from the sacral hiatus to the greater trochanter. A third line is drawn perpendicular to the first at its midpoint and will intersect the second line. The needle insertion point is where lines two and three intersect. Insert the needle perpendicular to all planes. Stimulation of the gluteus maximus muscle is often encountered just before the sciatic nerve stimulation which is seen as plantar or dorsiflexion at the ankle or toes. Plantar flexion indicates stimulation of the tibial component of the nerve and is associated with greater block success.

The subgluteal approach is one of several ways to block the sciatic nerve under ultrasound guidance. The patient is again placed in the lateral position with the targeted leg up. The landmarks are the greater trochanter and ischial tuberosity. A line is drawn between these two structures, and a low frequency ultrasound probe is placed at the midpoint of the line. The sciatic nerve can be identified as a hyperechoic structure (wide, flat, or triangular) beneath the gluteus maximus muscle and between the greater trochanter and ischial tuberosity. Using an in-plane technique, 20–30 ml of local anesthetic can be injected around the nerve.

Sciatic blockade is fairly safe with complications including intravascular injection and damage to the sciatic nerve.

Popliteal Sciatic Nerve Block

The sciatic nerve can be blocked lower in the leg as it splits into the common peroneal and tibial nerves for anesthesia of the entire lower leg, foot, and ankle with the exception of the medial saphenous distribution. The patient can be either in the supine or lateral position. If in the supine position, the leg will need to be elevated so that the ultrasound probe can be placed under the leg. The ultrasound probe is first placed in the popliteal crease to identify the popliteal artery (deep) and tibial nerve (superficial). Once these structures have been identified, follow the tibial nerve cephalad until the common peroneal nerve can be seen coming in laterally to join the tibial nerve forming the sciatic nerve. This junction usually occurs approximately eight centimeters cephalad from the popliteal crease but may vary among patients. Using an in-plane technique from a lateral direction, inject local anesthetic around the nerve. The proximity of the sciatic nerve to the popliteal artery and vein makes intravascular injection the primary concern.

Femoral Nerve Block

The femoral nerve is derived from the L2–L4 nerve roots in the lumbar plexus. It provides sensory innervation to the anterior thigh, anterior knee, and medial lower leg, as well as motor innervation to the quadriceps. This nerve can be easily blocked using a nerve stimulator or by ultrasound. The patient is placed in the supine position. The inguinal ligament is identified by drawing a line from the pubic tubercle to the anterior superior iliac spine. The femoral artery can be palpated just distal to the ligament, and the femoral nerve should be about 1–1.5 cm lateral to the femoral artery. With a nerve stimulator technique, insert the needle in a cephalad direction at a 45–60° angle to the skin and monitor for contraction of the rectus femoris (patellar snap). Under ultrasound, locate the femoral artery and vein. The femoral nerve is the hyperechoic bundle about 1 cm lateral to the femoral artery. Using an in-plane technique, approach the nerve from a lateral direction, carefully visualizing the needle tip to avoid puncture and injection into the femoral artery. The proximity of the femoral nerve to the femoral artery and vein makes intravascular injection the primary concern.

Saphenous Nerve Block

The saphenous nerve is a terminal branch of the posterior division of the femoral nerve (L3–L4). It provides sensory innervation to the medial aspect of the upper thigh, lower leg, ankle, and foot. It is the only nerve that innervates the lower leg that is not derived from the sciatic nerve, and below the knee it has no motor component. The patient is placed in the supine position, and the ultrasound probe is placed in the transverse fashion on the anterior thigh. The sartorius muscle will be most superficial and medial, and the vastus medialus laterally and deeper. The saphenous nerve can be found deep to the sartorius muscle and travelling with the deep genicular artery, a branch of the superficial femoral artery. An in-plane approach is used from the lateral edge of the ultrasound probe. Inject 8–15 ml of local anesthetic with intermittent aspiration to exclude vascular injection.

In summary, drug development and technology advances have given the practitioner additional tools to manage pain. This is particularly good news in palliative care. Though the drugs and technologies are not perfect, it is an exciting time and the future appears quite exciting in that our patients should be afforded greater opportunity for excellent patient care and comfort.

References

1. Indo Y. Nerve growth factor, pain, itch and inflammation: lessons from congenital insensitivity to pain with anhidrosis. Expert Rev Neurother. 2010;10(11):1707–24.
2. Mantyh PW, et al. Antagonism of nerve growth factor-TrkA signaling and the relief of pain. Anesthesiology. 2011;115(1):189–204.
3. FDA. FDA Arthritis Advisory Committee Meeting to Discuss Safety Issues Related to the Anti-Nerve Growth Factor Agents. http://www.fda.gov/downloads/AdvisoryCommittees/CommitteesMeetingMaterials/Drugs/ArthritisDrugsAdvisoryCommittee/UCM295202.pdf 2012; FDA.gov.
4. Cox JJ, et al. An SCN9A channelopathy causes congenital inability to experience pain. Nature. 2006;444(7121):894–8.
5. Heinzmann S, McMahon SB. New molecules for the treatment of pain. Curr Opin Support Palliat Care. 2011;5(2):111–5.
6. Derry S, et al. Topical capsaicin for chronic neuropathic pain in adults. Cochrane Database Syst Rev. 2009;(4):CD007393.
7. Anand P, Bley K. Topical capsaicin for pain management: therapeutic potential and mechanisms of action of the new high-concentration capsaicin 8% patch. Br J Anaesth. 2011;107(4):490–502.
8. Backonja MM, et al. NGX-4010, a high-concentration capsaicin patch, for the treatment of postherpetic neuralgia: a randomized, double-blind, controlled study with an open-label extension. Pain Med. 2010;11(4):600–8.
9. Clifford DB, et al. A randomized, double-blind, controlled study of NGX-4010, a capsaicin 8% dermal patch, for the treatment of painful HIV-associated distal sensory polyneuropathy. J Acquir Immune Defic Syndr. 2012;59(2):126–33.
10. Irving GA, et al. NGX-4010, a capsaicin 8% dermal patch, administered alone or in combination with systemic neuropathic pain medications, reduces pain in patients with postherpetic neuralgia. Clin J Pain. 2012;28(2):101–7.
11. Irving GA, et al. A multicenter, randomized, double-blind, controlled study of NGX-4010, a high-concentration capsaicin patch, for the treatment of postherpetic neuralgia. Pain Med. 2011;12(1):99–109.
12. Peppin JF, et al. Tolerability of NGX-4010, a capsaicin 8% patch for peripheral neuropathic pain. J Pain Res. 2011;4:385–92.

13. Simpson DM, et al. Long-term safety of NGX-4010, a high-concentration capsaicin patch, in patients with peripheral neuropathic pain. J Pain Symptom Manage. 2010;39(6):1053–64.
14. Perret D, Luo ZD. Targeting voltage-gated calcium channels for neuropathic pain management. Neurotherapeutics. 2009;6(4):679–92.
15. Li JX, Zhang Y. Emerging drug targets for pain treatment. Eur J Pharmacol. 2012;681(1–3):1–5.
16. Leung L. Cannabis and its derivatives: review of medical use. J Am Board Fam Med. 2011;24(4):452–62.
17. Lynch ME, Campbell F. Cannabinoids for treatment of chronic non-cancer pain; a systematic review of randomized trials. Br J Clin Pharmacol. 2011;72(5):735–44.
18. DEA. Drug Enforcement Agency Definition of Controlled Substances. 2012. http://www.deadiversion.usdoj.gov/schedules/index.html.
19. FDA. Marinol (dronabinol) FDA approved label. 2006. http://www.accessdata.fda.gov/drugsatfda_docs/label/2006/018651s025s026lbl.pdf.
20. Svendsen KB, Jensen TS, Bach FW. Does the cannabinoid dronabinol reduce central pain in multiple sclerosis? Randomised double blind placebo controlled crossover trial. BMJ. 2004;329(7460):253.
21. Narang S, et al. Efficacy of dronabinol as an adjuvant treatment for chronic pain patients on opioid therapy. J Pain. 2008;9(3):254–64.
22. Rice AS, Farquhar-Smith WP, Nagy I. Endocannabinoids and pain: spinal and peripheral analgesia in inflammation and neuropathy. Prostaglandins Leukot Essent Fatty Acids. 2002;66(2–3):243–56.
23. Sasso O, et al. Peripheral FAAH inhibition causes profound antinociception and protects against indomethacin-induced gastric lesions. Pharmacol Res. 2012;65(5):553–63.
24. Cravatt BF, et al. Supersensitivity to anandamide and enhanced endogenous cannabinoid signaling in mice lacking fatty acid amide hydrolase. Proc Natl Acad Sci USA. 2001;98(16):9371–6.
25. Kathuria S, et al. Modulation of anxiety through blockade of anandamide hydrolysis. Nat Med. 2003;9(1):76–81.
26. Gobbi G, et al. Antidepressant-like activity and modulation of brain monoaminergic transmission by blockade of anandamide hydrolysis. Proc Natl Acad Sci USA. 2005;102(51):18620–5.
27. Russo R, et al. Synergistic antinociception by the cannabinoid receptor agonist anandamide and the PPAR-alpha receptor agonist GW7647. Eur J Pharmacol. 2007;566(1–3):117–9.
28. Catarzi D, Colotta V, Varano F. Competitive AMPA receptor antagonists. Med Res Rev. 2007;27(2):239–78.
29. Swanson GT. Targeting AMPA and kainate receptors in neurological disease: therapies on the horizon? Neuropsychopharmacology. 2009;34(1):249–50.
30. Zheng Y, et al. Effects of the Putative Cognitive-Enhancing Ampakine, CX717, on Attention and Object Recognition Memory. Curr Alzheimer Res. 2011;8(8):876–82.
31. Ren J, et al. Ampakine CX717 protects against fentanyl-induced respiratory depression and lethal apnea in rats. Anesthesiology. 2009;110(6):1364–70.
32. Lee HJ, Pogatzki-Zahn EM, Brennan TJ. The effect of the AMPA/kainate receptor antagonist LY293558 in a rat model of postoperative pain. J Pain. 2006;7(10):768–77.
33. Jin HC, et al. Epidural tezampanel, an AMPA/kainate receptor antagonist, produces postoperative analgesia in rats. Anesth Analg. 2007;105(4):1152–9. Table of contents.
34. Sang CN, et al. LY293558, a novel AMPA/GluR5 antagonist, is efficacious and well-tolerated in acute migraine. Cephalalgia. 2004;24(7):596–602.
35. Melmed S, Williams RH. Williams textbook of endocrinology. 12th ed. Philadelphia: Elsevier/Saunders; 2011. xviii, 1897 p.
36. FDA. FDA approved label: chorionic gonadotropin. http://www.accessdata.fda.gov/drugsatfda_docs/label/2011/017067s057lbl.pdf 2011.
37. Tennant FS. Hormone Treatments in Chronic and Intractable Pain. Pract Pain Manag. 2005;5(3):57–67.

38. Elliott JA, Horton E, Fibuch EE. The endocrine effects of long-term oral opioid therapy: a case report and review of the literature. J Opioid Manag. 2011;7(2):145–54.
39. Aloisi AM, et al. Hormone replacement therapy in morphine-induced hypogonadic male chronic pain patients. Reprod Biol Endocrinol. 2011;9:26.
40. Reddy RG, et al. Opioid induced hypogonadism. BMJ. 2010;341:c4462.
41. Gullett NP, Hebbar G, Ziegler TR. Update on clinical trials of growth factors and anabolic steroids in cachexia and wasting. Am J Clin Nutr. 2010;91(4):1143S–7.
42. Anker SD, et al. Wasting as independent risk factor for mortality in chronic heart failure. Lancet. 1997;349(9058):1050–3.
43. Burdet L, et al. Administration of growth hormone to underweight patients with chronic obstructive pulmonary disease. A prospective, randomized, controlled study. Am J Respir Crit Care Med. 1997;156(6):1800–6.
44. Cittadini A, et al. Growth hormone deficiency in patients with chronic heart failure and beneficial effects of its correction. J Clin Endocrinol Metab. 2009;94(9):3329–36.
45. Frustaci A, Gentiloni N, Russo MA. Growth hormone in the treatment of dilated cardiomyopathy. N Engl J Med. 1996;335(9):672–3. Author reply 673–4.
46. Isgaard J, et al. A placebo-controlled study of growth hormone in patients with congestive heart failure. Eur Heart J. 1998;19(11):1704–11.
47. Mijan-de-la-Torre A. Recent insights on chronic heart failure, cachexia and nutrition. Curr Opin Clin Nutr Metab Care. 2009;12(3):251–7.
48. Neary NM, Goldstone AP, Bloom SR. Appetite regulation: from the gut to the hypothalamus. Clin Endocrinol (Oxf). 2004;60(2):153–60.
49. Osterziel KJ, et al. Randomised, double-blind, placebo-controlled trial of human recombinant growth hormone in patients with chronic heart failure due to dilated cardiomyopathy. Lancet. 1998;351(9111):1233–7.
50. Pape GS, et al. The effect of growth hormone on weight gain and pulmonary function in patients with chronic obstructive lung disease. Chest. 1991;99(6):1495–500.
51. Pupim LB, et al. Recombinant human growth hormone improves muscle amino acid uptake and whole-body protein metabolism in chronic hemodialysis patients. Am J Clin Nutr. 2005;82(6):1235–43.
52. Garcia JM, Polvino WJ. Effect on body weight and safety of RC-1291, a novel, orally available ghrelin mimetic and growth hormone secretagogue: results of a phase I, randomized, placebo-controlled, multiple-dose study in healthy volunteers. Oncologist. 2007;12(5):594–600.
53. Nagaya N, et al. Treatment of cachexia with ghrelin in patients with COPD. Chest. 2005;128(3):1187–93.
54. Nagaya N, et al. Effects of ghrelin administration on left ventricular function, exercise capacity, and muscle wasting in patients with chronic heart failure. Circulation. 2004;110(24):3674–9.
55. Neary NM, et al. Ghrelin increases energy intake in cancer patients with impaired appetite: acute, randomized, placebo-controlled trial. J Clin Endocrinol Metab. 2004;89(6):2832–6.
56. Strasser F, et al. Safety, tolerability and pharmacokinetics of intravenous ghrelin for cancer-related anorexia/cachexia: a randomised, placebo-controlled, double-blind, double-crossover study. Br J Cancer. 2008;98(2):300–8.
57. Wynne K, et al. Subcutaneous ghrelin enhances acute food intake in malnourished patients who receive maintenance peritoneal dialysis: a randomized, placebo-controlled trial. J Am Soc Nephrol. 2005;16(7):2111–8.
58. Takala J, et al. Increased mortality associated with growth hormone treatment in critically ill adults. N Engl J Med. 1999;341(11):785–92.
59. Corsonello A, et al. Regimen complexity and medication nonadherence in elderly patients. Ther Clin Risk Manag. 2009;5(1):209–16.
60. Claxton AJ, Cramer J, Pierce C. A systematic review of the associations between dose regimens and medication compliance. Clin Ther. 2001;23(8):1296–310.

61. Chen C, Cowles VE, Hou E. Pharmacokinetics of gabapentin in a novel gastric-retentive extended-release formulation: comparison with an immediate-release formulation and effect of dose escalation and food. J Clin Pharmacol. 2011;51(3):346–58.
62. Sampathkumar P, Drage LA, Martin DP. Herpes zoster (shingles) and postherpetic neuralgia. Mayo Clin Proc. 2009;84(3):274–80.
63. Rowbotham M, et al. Gabapentin for the treatment of postherpetic neuralgia: a randomized controlled trial. JAMA. 1998;280(21):1837–42.
64. Irving G, et al. Efficacy and tolerability of gastric-retentive gabapentin for the treatment of postherpetic neuralgia: results of a double-blind, randomized, placebo-controlled clinical trial. Clin J Pain. 2009;25(3):185–92.
65. FDA. FDA approved label: IONSYS™ (fentanyl iontophoretic trandermal system). http://www.accessdata.fda.gov/drugsatfda_docs/label/2006/021338lbl.pdf 2006.
66. Griffin DW, Skowronski RJ, Dasu BN, Palmer PP. A phase 2 open-label functionality, safety, and efficacy study of the sufentanil NanoTab™ PCA System in patients following elective unilateral knee replacement surgery. In: American Society of Regional Anesthesia and Pain Medicine: Poster Presentation, 35th annual spring meeting and workshops; 2010.
67. Monk JP, Beresford R, Ward A. Sufentanil. A review of its pharmacological properties and therapeutic use. Drugs. 1988;36(3):286–313.
68. Dale O, Hjortkjaer R, Kharasch ED. Nasal administration of opioids for pain management in adults. Acta Anaesthesiol Scand. 2002;46(7):759–70.
69. Kunz KM, Theisen JA, Schroeder ME. Severe episodic pain: management with sublingual sufentanil. J Pain Symptom Manage. 1993;8(4):189–90.
70. Palmer PP, Hamel LG, Skowronski RJ. Single- and repeat-dose pharmacokinetics of sublingual sufentanil NanoTab in healthy volunteers [abstract A1222]. In: Proceedings of the annual meeting of the American Society of Anesthesiologists; 2009.
71. Passmore MJ. Sublingual sufentanil for incident pain and dementia-related response agitation. Int Psychogeriatr. 2011; Feb 25:1–3.
72. Singla NK, Skowronski R, Palmer PP. A phase 2 multicenter, randomized, placebo-controlled study to evaluate the clinical efficacy, safety, and tolerability of sublingual sufentanil NanoTab™ in patients following major abdominal surgery. In: American Society of Regional Anesthesia and Pain Medicine: Poster Presentation, 35th annual spring meeting and workshops; 2010.
73. Information, V.G.P. 2009. http://www.voltarengel.com/common/pdf/Voltaren-PI-10-19.pdf. Cited March 2012.
74. Blonk MI, et al. Use of oral ketamine in chronic pain management: a review. Eur J Pain. 2010;14(5):466–72.
75. Pogatzki-Zahn EM, Englbrecht JS, Schug SA. Acute pain management in patients with fibromyalgia and other diffuse chronic pain syndromes. Curr Opin Anaesthesiol. 2009;22(5):627–33.
76. Chambers WA. Nerve blocks in palliative care. Br J Anaesth. 2008;101(1):95–100.
77. Miller RD. Miller's anesthesia. 7th ed. Philadelphia, PA: Churchill Livingstone/Elsevier; 2010.
78. Cuvillon P, et al. A comparison of the pharmacodynamics and pharmacokinetics of bupivacaine, ropivacaine (with epinephrine) and their equal volume mixtures with lidocaine used for femoral and sciatic nerve blocks: a double-blind randomized study. Anesth Analg. 2009;108(2):641–9.
79. Casati A, Baciarello M. Enantiomeric local anesthetics: can ropivacaine and levobupivacaine improve our practice? Curr Drug Ther. 2006;1:85–9.
80. Niemi G, Breivik H. Epinephrine markedly improves thoracic epidural analgesia produced by a small-dose infusion of ropivacaine, fentanyl, and epinephrine after major thoracic or abdominal surgery: a randomized, double-blinded crossover study with and without epinephrine. Anesth Analg. 2002;94(6):1598–605. Table of contents.
81. Congedo E, Sgreccia M, De Cosmo G. New drugs for epidural analgesia. Curr Drug Targets. 2009;10(8):696–706.

82. Corman SL, Skledar SJ. Use of lipid emulsion to reverse local anesthetic-induced toxicity. Ann Pharmacother. 2007;41(11):1873–7.
83. Guay J. Methemoglobinemia related to local anesthetics: a summary of 242 episodes. Anesth Analg. 2009;108(3):837–45.
84. Kaye A, Urman R, Vadivelu N, editors. Essentials of regional anesthesia. New York: Springer; 2011.
85. Swenson JD, et al. Outpatient management of continuous peripheral nerve catheters placed using ultrasound guidance: an experience in 620 patients. Anesth Analg. 2006;103(6):1436–43.
86. Lai TT, et al. Continuous peripheral nerve block catheter infections in combat-related injuries: a case report of five soldiers from Operation Enduring Freedom/Operation Iraqi Freedom. Pain Med. 2011;12(11):1676–81.
87. Head S, Enneking FK. Infusate contamination in regional anesthesia: what every anesthesiologist should know. Anesth Analg. 2008;107(4):1412–8.

Review Questions

1. Members of which of the following classes of agents are currently available for clinical use (select all that apply):

   (a) Anti-NGF agents
   (b) VGCC blocking agents
   (c) High-dose topical capsaicin
   (d) FAAH inhibitors

2. Extended release enteral formulations may allow for all of the following except:

   (a) Improved compliance
   (b) Reduced adverse effects
   (c) Improved rapidity of effect onset
   (d) Simpler dosing regimen

3. Which of the following parenteral analgesics would be least suited to rapid control of breakthrough pain?

   (a) Sufentanil NanoTab® PCA System
   (b) Transdermal fentanyl patch
   (c) Buccal fentanyl lozenge
   (d) Ionsys® iontophoretic transdermal fentanyl

4. Monitoring for regional anesthesia under moderate sedation include all of the following except:

   (a) Electrocardiography
   (b) Pulse oximetry
   (c) Neurological checks every 1 h
   (d) End-tidal CO_2 monitoring

5. Regional anesthesia:

   (a) May not be feasible in patients with severe edema or contractures
   (b) Can be used in any patient suffering from chronic pain
   (c) Is more effective than opioids and should be the first-line treatment for chronic pain
   (d) Is not recommended for patients experiencing a sickle cell crisis

6. Risks of continuous catheter regional nerve blocks include which of the following?

   (a) Infection at the site of catheter insertion
   (b) Cardiovascular collapse from local anesthetic toxicity
   (c) Falls from lower extremity nerve blocks
   (d) All of the above

Answers

1. (b, c)
2. (c)
3. (b)
4. (c)
5. (a)
6. (d)

Chapter 27
Ethics in Palliative and End-of-Life Care

Jack M. Berger

Introduction

"Do the kind thing, and do it first," said William Osler as advice to physicians (circa 1904) [1]. But in 1904 there were limited things that physicians could do for their patients with chronic pain or who were in need of care at the end of life. **William Osler in his Ingersoll Lecture 1904 entitled Science and Immortality (Houghton, Mifflin and Comp., Riverside Press, Cambridge 1904) stated**: "I have careful records of about five hundred death-beds, studied particularly with reference to the modes of death and the sensations of the dying…" "Ninety suffered bodily pain or distress of one sort or another…" (This is about 20%) [1].

Osler continued, "…eleven showed mental apprehension, two showed positive terror, while one expressed spiritual exaltation, and one expressed bitter remorse. The great majority gave no sign one way or the other; like their births, their deaths were as a sleep and a forgetting…." "As a rule, man dies as he has lived, uninfluenced practically by the thought of a future life…wondering but uncertain, generally unconscious and unconcerned" [1].

In Osler's time, that's how people died… a doctor could visit a patient and could tell the patient's family that death was imminent. The doctor's duty was then to provide comfort to the patient and the family, and to diminish suffering. The patient got plenty of Laudanum® and humane care.

J.M. Berger, M.S., M.D., Ph.D. (✉)
Department of Anesthesiology, Keck School of Medicine,
University of Southern California,
Los Angeles, CA, USA
e-mail: jmberger@usc.edu

N. Vadivelu et al. (eds.), *Essentials of Palliative Care*,
DOI 10.1007/978-1-4614-5164-8_27,
© Springer Science+Business Media New York 2013

Extent of the Problem

Weiss et al. report that the number of seriously ill patients who experience *"substantial"* pain ranges from 36 to 75% [2]. And according to Jennings and his associates *"…too many Americans die unnecessarily bad deaths—deaths with inadequate palliative support, inadequate compassion, and inadequate human presence and witness. These deaths are preceded by a dying marked by fear, anxiety, loneliness, and isolation; deaths that efface dignity and deny individual self-control and choice"* [3]. So, we are not even doing as well as Osler over 100 years ago.

Defining Death

With advances in life support, the line between who is alive and who is dead has become blurred [4]. Thus, we need to define death in order to be able to declare a person physically and legally dead. In the first edition of *Encyclopaedia Britannica* "DEATH" was defined as the separation of the soul and body; in this sense death stood opposed to life, which consisted in the union of the soul and body [5].

The **Uniform Determination of Death Act (UDDA)**, written by the President's Commission on Bioethics in 1981, confronts the complexities concerning the declaration of death [6]. The UDDA wording specifically states: "An individual who has sustained either (1) irreversible cessation of circulatory and respiratory functions, or (2) irreversible cessation of all the functions of the entire brain, including the brain stem, is dead." In other words, the UDDA states that a person can be declared dead when *either* the heart and lungs *or* the brain and brain stem stop functioning permanently [7].

The problem today is not so much determining death but rather with our modern interventions, we can *prolong the dying process* (dialysis, ventilators, intravenous fluids, antibiotics, furosemide, etc.) and therefore, we are *unable to recognize when death will occur*. It appears that we health care providers and physicians suffer from "Mural Dyslexia" defined as the inability to read the handwriting on the wall [8].

In their article, "Care of the dying: An ethical and historical perspective" published in Critical Care Medicine in 1992, Cowley, Young, and Raffin conclude that: "Despite the miraculous advances in medical theory and medical practice, *the ethics* surrounding medical care for the dying are more troubling today than they were in ancient Athens at the time of Plato [9]. In classical antiquity, the primary concerns were for health and living well. The 'Middle Ages' saw the emergence of the principle of sanctity of life. To these basic ideals, the 'Renaissance' and the 'Enlightenment' added the aspiration to prolong life. Finally, in the twentieth century, modern science has rendered this aspiration a reality of unclear merit" [9]. And we can expand that to include the twenty-first century now.

In making end-of-life decisions regarding symptom management and palliative care, one must have the ability to estimate accurately a patient's length of survival

(**LOS**) and improved quality of life. In 1994, Daas wrote that "we do not have the ability to accurately estimate LOS and that we have little knowledge or understanding of the end-stage illness experience" [10]. It is known that anorexia/cachexia in association with increased heart rate does correlate with the terminal cancer syndrome. Dysphagia, cognitive failure, and weight loss are highly correlated with shorter LOS, <4 weeks. The presence of *pain*, although producing poor quality of life, does not contribute to decreased LOS in terminal illness [10].

According to Spiegel, Stroud, and Fyfe, here at the end of the twentieth century, the old adage, to *"cure rarely, relieve suffering often, and comfort always,"* **(Hippocrates) has been rewritten**: The doctor's job has become *to "cure always, relieve suffering if one has the time, and leave the comforting to someone else"* [11]. They further state that the acute disease model, which emphasizes diagnosis, definitive treatment, and cure, works in many situations, but the leading killers of Americans—heart disease, stroke, and cancer—are by and large chronic and progressive rather than acute and curable [11]. Western Medicine's success is also its weakness. The application of a curative model when disease management is all that can be given leaves doctors and patients dissatisfied [11].

Ethical Principles

In providing palliative and end-of-life care, one must consider Medical Ethics and Ethical Conduct, Moral Obligations, and Legal Responsibilities.

In end-of-life care, there are four guiding ethical principles which govern our decision making and care of patients. These are the same principles that guide us in the conduct of medicine in general.

- **Nonmaleficence** [11] (minimize harm) (Hippocratic oath)
- **Beneficence** [12] (do good if you can) (St. Thomas Aquinas thirteenth century)
- **Patient autonomy** [13] (respect for the patient as a person, informed consent) (Nuremberg trial of Nazis physicians who performed experiments on humans without consent)
- **Justice** [14] (fair distribution of available resources) (not everyone is entitled to everything that medicine has to offer when resources are limited)

In implementing the above principles the physician has to balance "Three Dichotomies."

- The potential benefits of treatment must be balanced against the potential burdens.
- Striving to preserve life but, when biologically futile, providing comfort in dying.
- Individual needs are balanced against those of society.

Eric J. Casssel, in his article the "Nature of suffering and the goals of medicine," stated "…The relief of suffering and the cure of disease must be seen as twin obligations of a medical profession that is truly dedicated to care of the sick. Physicians' failure to understand the nature of suffering can result in medical intervention that (though technically adequate) not only fails to relieve suffering, but becomes a source of suffering itself" [15].

Rule of Double Effect

At the end of life, providing pain relief can present a dilemma for physicians who operate under misconceptions of both the law and ethics. The "Rule of Double Effect" which is the moral doctrine taken from the teachings of St. Thomas Aquinas of the thirteenth century gives physicians the ethical duty and moral obligation to relieve pain and suffering [12]. Yet these philosophical arguments do not provide insight into the ambivalence that practitioners feel when they legitimately engage in these practices. Why should a physician feel ambivalence about doing the "*right thing?*"

With regard to palliation and comfort care, many clinicians are unaware of the current ethical and legal consensus regarding palliative care at the end of life. This consensus is built around **the principle of the double effect**. The thrust of the principle is to **focus on the intention** of the caregiver in seeking to provide comfort to terminally ill patients, even if the clinician realizes that a side effect of the therapy could be an earlier death [14].

The principle of double effect continues to be an area of lively debate in bioethics, in part because of the ambiguous intentions of caregivers in treating patients at the end of life. For example, even when a physician has no desire to hasten the patient's death, the death of the patient may nevertheless be seen as a good or desirable outcome. Despite these ambiguities, however, the principle remains an ethical and legal touchstone around treatment of the terminally ill [14].

The US Supreme Court in **Vacco v. Quill**, validated the rule of double effect when Justice Rehnquist stated that "It is widely recognized that the provision of pain medication is ethically and professionally acceptable even when the treatment may hasten the patient's death if the medication is intended to alleviate pain and severe discomfort, and not to cause death" [16].

In the **Vacco v. Quill** case, a landmark decision was reached by the Supreme Court of the United States regarding the right to die [16]. It ruled that a New York ban on physician-assisted suicide was constitutional and preventing doctors from assisting their patients in bringing about death, even those terminally ill and/or in great pain, was a legitimate State interest that was well within the authority of the State to regulate [16]. In brief, this decision established that, as a matter of law, there was no constitutional guarantee of a "right to die" [16]. But it also affirmed that a patient retains the **Right** to choose not to continue treatment, even life sustaining treatment, and that choosing to discontinue treatment or declining treatment is not equivalent in the eyes of the law to requesting a treatment to end life [16].

Not only is the rule of Double Effect well ensconced in the law, but also all of the major religions have doctrines that support this approach. The principle of double effect was initially developed in the Catholic tradition, from the teachings of St. Thomas

Aquinas in the thirteenth century [12]. Clinicians should, therefore, never withhold needed pain medications from terminally ill patients for fear of hastening their death through respiratory depression or other complications [12, 15].

The "Rule of Double Effect" states that an action having two effects, one good and one bad is permissible if five conditions are fulfilled:

1. The act itself is good or at least morally neutral, e.g., giving morphine to relieve pain.
2. Only the good effect is **intended** (relieving pain) and not the bad effect (ending the patient's life).
3. The good effect is not achieved through the bad effect (pain relief does not depend on hastening death).
4. There is no alternative way to attain the good effect (pain relief).
5. There is a proportionately grave reason for running the risk, e.g., relief of intolerable pain and suffering.

Clearly, to justify use of this rule, the patient or surrogate decision maker would need to be informed of the risks and give valid consent (***Principle of Autonomy***). It is clear that any patient coming for surgery is expecting that his/her physician will attend to the pain which results from the surgery including the use of opioids. If other forms of pain relief are to be used, such as epidural analgesia or peripheral nerve blockade, then additional consent discussions should be undertaken so that patients can make informed decisions about their pain management care.

According to the Rule of Double Effect, it is clear in end-of-life care that there are ethical and legal sanctions for the use of whatever doses of opioids that are necessary so long as death is not directly intended. If the doses of the opioids necessary to relieve pain are large enough to produce deep sedation, this too would be permissible, if suffering can be relieved in no other way.

Thorn and Sykes studied 238 consecutive dying patients [17]. In a retrospective study they found that there was no difference in survival between those patients requiring escalating doses of opioids versus those patients that were on stable doses of opioids [17]. Because of this finding, they concluded that the rule of double effect was not even needed to justify the use of opioids for the control of pain at the end of life, and this could be that the first two principles of ethical conduct, nonmaleficence and beneficence, are maintained [17].

Ethics and the Use of Opioids

Much of inadequate pain management, particularly in end-of-life care can be traced to lack of knowledge on the part of physicians. In a typical example, a physician was managing an end-stage AIDS patient who had a DNR status and a documented pain scores of 6/10 (10/10 on the verbal analogue scale is the worst possible pain imaginable). The patient was receiving 3 mg/h IV morphine infusion from which the physician stated, "***We must wean off the morphine. We're killing him.***" The physician wanted to give naloxone to reverse the effects of the morphine and then remedicate the patient with 25 mg Meperidine IV q4 h PRN for pain control. What's wrong with this scenario?

- **3 mg/h of IV Morphine = 72 mg/day**
- **1 mg Morphine IV = 10 mg Meperidine IV**
- **72 mg Morphine = 720 mg Meperidine**
- **25 mg Meperidine q4 h = 150 mg/day**
- **The patient was already in moderate to severe pain at the current dosage which was already inadequate, and the Physician was reducing the dose by 80%. Further, by writing a PRN order, the physician was insuring that the patient would not even receive the 25 mg of Meperidine q4 h**

This is a classic case of *"Opiophobia"*—*"the unreasonable fear of opioid use, based on an inaccurate assessment of its dangers."* It affects patients as well as physicians and may be one of the greatest barriers to the provision of effective pain medication [18]. The 1993 California Medical Board Statement on the Prescribing of Controlled Substances stated that…Concerns about regulatory scrutiny should not make *physicians who follow appropriate guidelines* reluctant to prescribe or administer controlled substances, including Schedule II drugs, for patients with a legitimate medical need for them [19].

Likewise, the Federal Controlled Substances Act (**CSA**) does *NOT* address medical treatment issues such as the selection or quantity of prescribed drugs [20]. The US Supreme Court addressed these issues in the 1990s [21]. While the Court did not support either using drugs to terminate life or the legalization of drugs and controlled substances, it fully encouraged and supported adequate pain and symptom management, as reported in the New England Journal of Medicine in 1997: *A [United States Supreme] Court majority effectively required all states to ensure that their laws do not obstruct the provision of adequate palliative care, especially for the alleviation of pain and other physical symptoms of people facing death* [21].

The CSA regulates drugs, not the practice of medicine. **The practitioner's judgment, based upon training, medical specialty, and practice guidelines determines what may be considered** *legitimate medical purpose, (DEA Policy Statement)* [22]. According to the federal CSA, in order for a prescription to be valid, it must be issued for a legitimate medical purpose by an individual practitioner acting in the usual course of professional practice. A dentist, for example, cannot prescribe opioids for gynecological pain even though he/she has a DEA number.

Model guidelines for the use of controlled substances for the treatment of pain were developed jointly by the DEA and Federation of State Medical Boards of the United States and adopted May 2, 1998 [23, 24]. The purpose was: *(to) protect legitimate medical uses of controlled substances while preventing drug diversion and eliminating inappropriate prescribing practices. Simply put, you have a license to drive your car but you have to recognize stop signs and traffic lights.*

Good faith prescribing requires an equally good faith history, physical examination and documentation {of benefit}. One can always be sued by a patient or the family claiming injury or the patient becoming addicted to opioids. One can always be manipulated or deceived by individual patients seeking to abuse opioid medications. But careful monitoring and particularly ***documentation of benefit*** will reduce these risks to both the physician and patient to a minimum.

Ethics in Decision Making

In providing symptom management and palliative care at the end of life, difficult decisions have to be made with respect to initiating therapeutic interventions or discontinuing interventions. There appears to be a great deal of discrepancy between what physicians state as to their biases for withdrawing life support measures and what they actually practice in real life. Asthenia, malnutrition, and cachexia are common in dying patients with advanced cancer. They may in fact be adaptive mechanisms which do not require intervention [25].

Enteral feedings can lead to pneumonia from aspiration or diarrhea from poor absorption. Parenteral feeding requires intravenous access, and there is no evidence for improved survival, no evidence for improved tumor response to chemotherapy, and no evidence of decreased chemotherapy toxicity. Decreased surgical complications with the use of total parenteral nutrition are debatable. In animal studies, there is evidence of actual enhanced tumor growth, and there is no evidence for enhanced quality of life or satisfaction of hunger [26].

Withdrawing Supportive Measures

In their study on "Biases in how physicians choose to withdraw life support," Christakis et al. reported that in order of preference, physicians find it easier to withdraw or withhold treatments in the following order: blood products, hemodialysis, intravenous vasopressors, total parenteral nutrition, antibiotics, mechanical ventilation, tube feedings, and finally intravenous fluids [27].

These therapies correlate with the preferences to withdraw forms of therapy supporting organs that failed for natural rather than iatrogenic reasons, to withdraw recently instituted rather than long-standing interventions, to withdraw forms of therapy resulting in immediate death rather than delayed death, and to withdraw forms of therapy resulting in delayed death when confronted with diagnostic uncertainty [27].

In their report entitled Outcome of Cancer Patients Receiving Home Parenteral Nutrition, Cozzaglio et al. retrospectively studied patients with metastatic cancer who were treated with home parenteral nutrition [28]. They note that the use of parenteral nutrition in end-stage cancer patients varies from country to country [28]. In the USA, Japan, and Italy, 40–60% of all patients getting home parenteral nutrition have cancer while only 18% in France and 5% in the UK [8]. Cozzaglio et al. state that "the variance reflects a difference in cultural, ethical, social, and economic approaches to the problem, with a lack of a scientific basis resulting from the scarcity of specific literature" [28]. Cozzaglio et al. conclude that home parenteral nutrition does not benefit cancer patients with a Karnofsky score of <50 [28]. In those patients who were treated less than 3 months (Karnofsky <50) there was no benefit in quality of life improvement [28].

Since dyspnea is a subjective experience like pain, it has a complicated pathophysiology that is affected by physical, psychological, social, and spiritual factors. The involvement of the entire interdisciplinary team is essential for treating dyspnea effectively, particularly in the terminal stages of disease.

Hydration is another area that presents ethical problems for physicians in the dying patient. Too much hydration in a patient who is unable to eliminate the fluid can lead to pulmonary congestion and dyspnea, edema around encapsulated tumors leading to pain. Yet withholding fluids may make the family members uncomfortable or suspicious. One must explain to the family about the harmful effects of excess fluid and that if the patient is thirsty, he/she will tell the doctor or nurse. In dealing with pain or end-of-life care, we must make every effort to control pain, being mindful of the risks of our interventions, but at the same time not be afraid to take action.

Futility

Luce [29] discussed in detail the Consensus report on the "Ethics of Foregoing Life-Sustaining Treatments in the Critically Ill" prepared by the Task Force on Ethics of the Society of Critical Care Medicine and published in 1990 [30]. Much of Luce's discussion centers on the definition of futility of care. This term generally conveys the idea that a patient cannot benefit from treatment, that the patient's acute disorder is not reversible, that the patient will not survive the current hospital stay, or that the quality of the patient's life following discharge will be poor [31].

Many barriers to decision making center on misunderstandings of the legal aspects of withholding and withdrawing life support measures. As a result (according to Luce) the courts in recent years have underscored the right of patients to refuse treatment, affirmed the concept that human life is more than a biologic process that must be continued in all circumstances, defined how therapeutics may or may not benefit patients, argued against a distinction between the withholding and withdrawing of life support, established guidelines for limiting life-sustaining treatments, and approached the resolution of disagreements among physicians and patients or their surrogates [16, 31].

Generally the courts have ruled that most patients would accept or refuse medical therapy based on the ability of the therapy to support sentient life over mere biologic existence. Of course, it is always best if the patient is able to participate directly in informed decision making, but baring this the concept of "substituted judgement" is employed where family or surrogate decision makers speak for the patient, based on their intimate knowledge of what the patient would have wanted.

In *Barber V Superior Court of California*, 1983, the court did not distinguish between removing mechanical ventilation or removing fluids or nutrition because all were interventions that could either benefit or burden [32]. ***But the issue of futility of care was entered into court proceedings***. In a case in Boston at Massachusetts General Hospital, the Suffolk Superior Court decided that physicians and the hospital could discontinue life-sustaining therapy despite the objections of a patient or surrogate if further care was deemed futile [33]. This decision has not been tested in the appellate courts. But among ethicists and intensivists a consensus is evolving for physicians to have the medical responsibility and privilege to decide to limit care, even against the wishes of the patient or the patient's legal representative [34, 35].

An illness may well be incurable, but not necessarily terminal. *Terminal* is used herein to mean a condition that will directly and inexorably result in death within the foreseeable future. If the condition is also *incurable*, then death will result regardless of whether medical treatment is undertaken or not [36]. And thus would be considered *futile*.

Surveys from ICU's in 1994–1995 involving 71,513 admissions indicate that 75% of the deaths involved patients in whom some form of limitation of treatment took place [37]. Therapies commonly withheld or withdrawn were cardiopulmonary resuscitation (CPR), mechanical ventilation, vasoactive drugs, antibiotics, renal dialysis, blood and blood products. Decisions to recommend withholding or withdrawal of therapies deemed futile depend often on the presence or absence of the "persistent vegetative state," as discussed by Waisel and Truog [37].

A presumptively terminally ill patient may request a therapy the clinician does not believe will be successful. Some hospitals have incorporated policies that permit physicians to unilaterally withhold treatments with a low likelihood of success [12]. Others recognize the inherent problems in determining qualitative and quantitative thresholds for futility judgments. For example, how low does the probability of success have to be for a therapy to be considered futile? How great a benefit must a patient receive from a therapy for that therapy not to be considered futile? How certain must physicians be of their predictions? [38]. How do the patient's values play into these determinations? [38]. Because these questions are difficult to answer, a growing trend is to step away from defining a specific policy to limit futile care and instead focus on individual benefits and burdens in the particular situations [39].

Principle of Double Effect

With regards to palliation and comfort care, many clinicians are unaware of the current ethical and legal consensus regarding palliative care at the end of life. As stated earlier, this consensus is built around the ***Principle of the Double Effect***. The thrust of the principle is to focus on the intention of the caregiver in seeking to provide comfort to terminally ill patients, even if the clinician realizes that a side effect of the medications or treatments could be respiratory depression and earlier death.

Comatose patients on ventilatory support look the same to family members as other patients, even though they may be in a persistent vegetative state or even brain dead. These patients may even be theoretically capable of reproduction which biologists sometimes cite as the ***sine qua non* of life**. Using a phrase such as "withdrawing life support" is not only incorrect but is also misleading, and potentially harmful to family members struggling with the diagnosis of brain death or persistent vegetative state. Life support cannot be withdrawn from a patient who is already dead, and such linguistic imprecision can confuse an already shaken family as to the meaning of the diagnosis. At this point, the only purpose of "life" support is to maintain homeostasis. (This section was taken out of context from Waisel and Truog but it fits with the concept of futility of care) [37].

Although individual convictions and religious beliefs should be respected and supported, maintenance of prolonged intensive care is expensive and State Laws differ in the degree to which they require clinical diagnosis to defer to religious conviction.

Palliative

As stated earlier, the goals of end-of-life care encompass symptom management for comfort. Palliative interventions may be necessary for improved comfort. Palliative care is defined as care that recognizes the inevitability of the patient's death and therefore whose goal is to lessen, ease, and make less severe the patient's suffering, without curing the disease. Symptom control of such things as pain, nausea/vomiting, constipation, dyspnea, etc., should be the goal [38].

A multidisciplinary or interdisciplinary team approach to end-of-life care is the most successful. Medical decision making such as withdrawal of treatments, total parental nutrition, ventilator support, and DNR discussions should be part of the duties of this palliative care team. In providing palliative care one must maintain a respect for life, while at the same time be able to accept the ultimate inevitability of death. The potential benefits of treatment must be balanced against the potential burdens of such treatment. The physician must strive to preserve life but, when biologically futile, provide comfort in dying. At the same time the physician must recognize that individual needs must be balanced against those of society [39].

Luce and Rubenfeld considered the question of whether costs could be reduced by limiting futile care [40]. The public must define futility if they are to accept limits on such care! But it is unrealistic to expect the lay public to accept this responsibility. Therefore, the healthcare profession must take the lead. Borrowing from the nursing profession *"**Compassionate Stewardship**"* is also part of physician behavior [41]. During 1993, an estimated 118 attempts at CPR were reported for 172 facilities with a total of 19,596 licensed beds, for a frequency of one CPR attempt per 166 beds per year in one survey [42].

Reductio ad Absurdum, having a 108-year-old man make a decision about CPR suggests the unreal and macabre. The level of competence to which patients should be held varies with the expected harms or benefits of acting in accordance with the patient's choice. A minimal level of decision making competence should be applied to a patient who consents to a lumbar-puncture for presumed meningitis. A maximum standard should be applied for a patient who refuses surgery for a simple appendectomy. CPR discussions held at the time of acute illness may lead patients and their families to believe erroneously that any last hope is being withheld.

Decisions About Cardiopulmonary Resuscitation and Do Not Resuscitate Orders

When patients were educated about CPR, 87% chose to forego CPR or allow the physician to decide if it was appropriate. When surveyed, patients consistently over-estimated their chances of surviving CPR and survival to discharge. The physician must initiate discussion of CPR since no patients reported initiating the discussion themselves although most desired to have this type of conversation [43]. The general public has an inflated perception of CPR success. While most people believe that CPR works 60–85% of the time, in fact the actual survival to hospital discharge is more like 10–15% for all patients and less than 5% for the elderly and those with serious illnesses [44].

DNR Discussion

Although the techniques of CPR were originally intended only for use after acute, reversible cardiac arrests, the current practice is to use CPR in all situations unless there is a direct order to the contrary [45]. Since cardiac arrest is the final event in all terminal illness, everyone is eventually a candidate for this medical procedure [45]. DNR orders were developed to spare patients from aggressive attempts at revival when imminent death is anticipated and inevitable [45]. Nevertheless, patients or families sometimes request CPR even when care givers believe such attempts would be futile [45]. Some have argued that in these circumstances a physician should be able to enact a DNR order without consent of the patient or family [45, 46].

Many physicians feel "uncomfortable" about discussing DNR status with their patients. Regardless of this when a physician initiates such a discussion, the manner in which the discussion takes place could lead to a medical dilemma if not done appropriately. A proper discussion consists of two questions.

Question 1

"Would you want to be resuscitated in the event of cardiopulmonary arrest?"

This question needs to be asked in lay terms that the patient can understand. This question needs to be presented in the manner of informed consent with a presentation of the true risks and realistic chances of successful outcome. If the patient chooses to have full resuscitation, then a second question must be asked.

Question 2

"Let us assume you were resuscitated. If the critical care team, despite doing everything they can to save your life, determine after 72 h that you have no chance to regain a reasonable quality of life, would you agree to let them withdraw support and allow natural death to occur with peace and dignity?" It is believed that most patients who choose to be resuscitated will choose to not have their death prolonged if there is no reasonable chance to recapture a meaningful life. The earlier these questions are discussed in the course of a terminal illness, the more likely that a prolonged course of suffering in dying can be avoided.

If one only asks a patient with a terminal disease "if your heart stops, would you want us to start it again," the implication is that the resuscitation will be successful and all will be well. This of course is untrue. By simply changing a few words, "if your heart stops beating, would you want us to **try** to start it again," immediately places doubt that the resuscitation will be successful and can then lead to further inquire by the patient about "odds" "consequences," etc. If the patient still wants an attempt at resuscitation, the second question must be asked. There is of course the possibility that a patient with capacity to make his/her own decisions about care will still want everything done. Then an ethics consult should be obtained if the physician feels that the act of CPR would be futile and potentially lead to more harm and suffering for the patient.

DNR Status and Palliative Surgical Procedure

A final issue that must be addressed is whether do-not-resuscitate (DNR) orders should be routinely rescinded when terminally ill patients undergo palliative surgery? If so, patients will be forced to balance the benefits of palliative surgery against the risks of unwanted resuscitation. On the other hand, if physicians are required to honor intraoperative DNR orders, they may feel unacceptably restrained from correcting adverse effects for which they feel responsible [47]. Walker argued for the permissibility of honoring intraoperative DNR orders [47]. Walker maintains that the patient's right to refuse treatment outweighs physicians' concerns about professional scrutiny over intraoperative deaths [47]. Physicians' moral concerns about hastening patient death are important but may be assuaged by (1) emphasizing patients' acceptance of operative mortality risk; (2) viewing matters as analogous to surgery on Jehovah's Witnesses who refuse lifesaving transfusion; (3)

viewing the patient's intraoperative death as a double effect, that is, an unintended negative effect that is linked to the performance of a good act (palliation); and (4) distinguishing this from assisted suicide [47].

In 1992, Franklin and Rothenberg reported on a survey of 156 accredited hospitals in the USA as to their policies for suspending do not resuscitate (DNR) orders when patients went to surgery even for palliative procedures [48]. One hundred twelve hospitals responded. The majority (81%) noted that they suspended the DNR order when patients went to surgery [48].

Today it is customary to engage in an informed discussion with all concerned parties about the consequences of performing CPR, a chemical code only, or withholding resuscitative efforts should a code occur during palliative surgery and anesthesia. More recently it has been recommended by the American Society of Anesthesiology, multiple Surgical Societies, as well as the AMA that the DNR order could be maintained in force even during surgery [49].

Now it is obvious that the induction of general anesthesia including endotracheal intubation incorporate life sustaining measures and it may not be possible to immediately extubated patients at the end of surgery. These acts alone do not constitute cardiopulmonary resuscitation. It therefore requires full discussion with the patient, family, or surrogate decision makers and the surgeon about informed consent.

Next, resuscitative efforts can be expressly limited to chemical resuscitation without chest compressions if full CPR would result in more harm to the patient than good. Again this is a joint decision made by the patient and the entire care team.

Concluding Remarks

Neville Goodman stated that "Words are all we have to describe what we do, the way we do it, and what we infer from clinical research [50]. We must use them carefully and properly" [50].

The late Primo Levi, an Italian journalist said "If we know that pain and suffering can be alleviated, and we do nothing about it, then we ourselves become the tormentors" [51]. *But "when men lack goals, they tend to engage in activity," (unknown author)* [52]. It is our job as compassionate and professional physicians to "Do the right thing, and do it first" as William Osler told us so many years ago [1].

References

1. Osler W. Science and Immortality. Boston/Cambridge: Houghton, Mifflin/Riverside; 1904.
2. Weiss SC, Emanuel LL, Fairclough DL, Emanuel EJ. Understanding the experience of pain in terminally ill patients. Lancet. 2001;357:1311–5.
3. Jennings B, Rundes T, D'Onofrio C, et al. Access to hospice care: expanding boundaries, overcoming barriers. Hastings Cent Rep. 2003;33(2):S3–4.

4. Capron AM. Definition and determination of death: II. Legal issues in pronouncing death. In: Reich WT, editor. Encyclopedia of bioethics. New York: Simon & Schuster MacMillan; 1995. p. 536.
5. Encyclopaedia Brittanica 1st edition 1768, Encyclopaedia Brittanica Inc., Edinburgh, United Kingdom. Vol. 2. 1768. p. 309.
6. Defining death: a report on the medical, legal and ethical issues in the determination of death: review of the Uniform Determination of Death Act (UDDA), written by the President's Commission on Bioethics in 1981. http://hdl.handle.net/1805/707.
7. Guidelines for the determination of death: report of the medical consultants on the diagnosis of death to the President's Commission for the Study of Ethical Problems in Medicine and Biomedical and Behavioral Research. J Am Med Assoc. 1981;246(19):2184–6.
8. Scherger J. Overcoming 'Mural dyslexia,' or not reading the writing on the wall. In: Crosson FJ, Tollen LA, editors. Partners in health: how physician practices and hospitals can be accountable together. San Francisco, CA: Jossey-Bass; 2010.
9. Cowley LT, Young E, Raffin T. Care of the dying: an ethical and historical perspective. Crit Care Med. 1992;20(10):1473–82.
10. den Daas N. Estimating length of survival in end-stage cancer: a review of the literature. J Pain Symptom Manage. 1995;10(7):548–55.
11. Spiegel D, Stroud P, Fyfe A. Complementary medicine. West J Med. 1998;168(4):241–7.
12. Waisel DB, Truog RD. The cardiopulmonary resuscitation not indicated order: futility revisited. Ann Intern Med. 1995;122:304–8.
13. Weindling P. Nazi medicine and the Nuremberg Trials: from medical war crimes to informed consent. New York: MacMillan; 2004.
14. Gillon R. Medical ethics: four principles plus attention to scope. BMJ. 1994;309:184.
15. Casssel EJ. Nature of suffering and the goals of medicine. N Engl J Med. 1982;306:639–45.
16. *Vacco v. Quill*, 521 U.S. 793. 1997.
17. Thorns A, Sykes N. Opioid use in last week of life and implications for end-of-life decision-making. Lancet. 2000;356:398–9.
18. Joranson DE, Ryan KM, Gilson AM, Dahl JL. Trends in medical use and abuse of opioid analgesics. JAMA. 2000;283(13):1710–4.
19. Clark HW, Sees KL. Opioids, chronic pain, and the law. J Pain Symptom Manage. 1993;8(5):297–305 (1993 California Medical Board Statement on the Prescribing of Controlled Substances).
20. Miller NS. Failure of enforcement controlled substance laws in health policy for prescribing opiate medications: a painful assessment of morbidity and mortality. Am J Ther. 2006;13(6):527–33 (Federal Controlled Substances Act).
21. Burt RA. The Supreme Court speaks: not assisted suicide but a constitutional right to palliative care. N Engl J Med. 1997;337:1234–6.
22. DEA Policy Statement.
23. Joranson DE. Medical board guidelines for intractable pain treatment. APS Bull. 1995;5(3):1–5.
24. Federation of State Medical Boards of the United States. Model guidelines for the use of controlled substances for the treatment of pain. Fed Bull. 1998;85:84–9.
25. Baracos VE. Cancer-associated cachexia and underlying biological mechanisms. Annu Rev Nutr. 2006;26:435–61.
26. Torosian M, Daly J. Nutritional support in the cancer-bearing host. Cancer. 1986;58:1915–29.
27. Christakis NA NA, Asch DA, Christakis NA, Asch DA. Biases in how physicians choose to withdraw life support. Lancet. 1993;342:642–6.
28. Cozzaglio L, et al. Outcome of cancer patients receiving home parenteral nutrition. J Parenter Enteral Nutr. 1997;21(6):339–42.
29. Luce JM. Withholding and withdrawal of life support from critically ill patients. West J Med. 1997;167:411–6.
30. Task Force on Ethics of the Society of Critical Care Medicine. Crit Care Med. 1990;18:1435–9.

31. Luce J. Physicians do not have a responsibility to provide futile or unreasonable care if a patient or family insists. Crit Care Med. 1995;23:760–6.
32. Barber V Superior Court of California. 1983.
33. Boston at Massachusetts General Hospital, the Suffolk Superior Court.
34. Raffin TA. Withdrawing life support: how is the decision made? JAMA. 1995;273(9):738–9.
35. Asch DA, Hansen-Flaschen J, Lanken PN. Decisions to limit or continue life-sustaining treatment by critical care physicians in the United States: conflicts between physicians' practices and patients' wishes. Am J Respir Crit Care Med. 1995;151:288–92.
36. Meyers DW. Legal aspects of withdrawing nourishment from an incurably ill patient. Arch Intern Med. 1985;145(1):125–8.
37. Waisel DB, Truog RD. The end-of-life sequence. Anesthesiology. 1997;87(3):676–86.
38. Brody BA, Halevy A. Is futility a futile concept? J Med Philos. 1995;20:123–44.
39. Tomlinson T, Czlonka D. Futility and Hospital Policy. Hastings Cent Rep. 1995;25(3):28–35.
40. Luce J, Rubenfeld G. Can health care costs be reduced by limiting intensive care at the end of life? Am J Respir Crit Care Med. 2002;165(6):750–4.
41. Dorn K. Caring-healing inquiry for holistic nursing practice. Top Adv Pract Nurs. 2004;4(4):1.
42. Kane RS, Burns EA. Cardiopulmonary resuscitation policies in long-term care facilities. J Am Geriatr Soc. 1997;45(2):154–7.
43. Von Gunten C. Discussing do-not-resuscitate status. J Clin Oncol. 2001;19(5):1576–81.
44. Von Gunten CF, Weissman DE. Fast facts and concepts #24. July 2005; 24.024 Discussing DNR Orders-Part 2. 2nd ed. http://www.eperc.mcw.edu/fastfact/ff_024.htm.
45. Truog RD, Brett AS, Frader J. Sounding board: the problem with futility. N Engl J Med. 1992;326(23):1560–4.
46. Hackler JC, Hiller C. Family consent to orders not to resuscitate. JAMA. 1990;264:1281–3.
47. Walker R. DNR in the OR: resuscitation as an operative risk. JAMA. 1991;266:2407–12.
48. Franklin CM, Rotherberg DM. Do-not-resuscitate orders in the presurgical patient. J Clin Anesth. 1992;4:181–4.
49. Tungpalan L, Tan SY. DNR orders in the OR. Hawaii Med J. 2001;60(3):64–8.
50. Goodman N. Neither obsession nor distraction: words must be chosen well. Anesth Analg. 1998;87:742–3.
51. Primo Levi, an Italian journalist.
52. But "when men lack goals, they tend to engage in activity" (unknown author).

Review Questions

1. The number of seriously ill patients who experience "*substantial*" pain ranges from…

   (a) 36–75%
   (b) 5–10%
   (c) 75–90%
   (d) 25–30%

2. The Uniform Determination of Death Act (UDDA) defined death as a state of…

   (a) Irreversible cessation of circulatory and respiratory functions
   (b) Irreversible cessation of all the functions of the entire brain including the brain stem
   (c) Irreversible cessation of both cardio-respiratory function and brain functions
   (d) Either irreversible cessation of circulatory and respiratory functions or irreversible cessation of all levels of brain function including the brain stem
   (e) Any of the above

3. Symptoms that correlate with the terminal cancer syndrome are except…

   (a) Anorexia/cachexia in association with increased heart rate
   (b) Dysphasia
   (c) Cognitive failure
   (d) Weight loss
   (e) The presence of pain

4. Which of the following acts is not protected by the rule of double effect?

   (a) Do good if you can
   (b) Do no harm
   (c) Rationing of health care
   (d) Physician-assisted suicide

5. Appropriate prescribing of opioids requires all of the following except…

   (a) Complete medical history
   (b) Diagnosis of pain generator
   (c) Documentation of physical examination
   (d) Documentation of benefit
   (e) Treatment of side effects
   (f) Increasing dosing of opioids for terminal sedation is not sanctioned by the rule of double effect

6. Which of the following is not true with respect to do not resuscitate (DNR) orders?

   (a) DNR orders must be suspended when patients go to have palliative surgery
   (b) DNR orders are written by physicians after obtaining consent from the patient or assigned patient decision maker
   (c) DNR orders obtained in the appropriate manner may not be over turned by physicians or family members
   (d) DNR does not mean "do not treat" or "do nothing"

7. Which of the following is a true statement about CPR?

   (a) CPR is meant to be used in all circumstances of cardio-pulmonary arrest
   (b) CPR is successful in more than 70% of cases
   (c) Patients with end-stage disease who undergo CPR after cardiac arrest have virtually no chance of leaving the hospital and returning home
   (d) Most patients in long-term nursing care facilities do receive CPR when they have a cardio-pulmonary arrest

8. Which statement is not true relative to the rule of double effect?

   (a) Providing opioids for pain relief or terminal sedation is permissible as long as the intent is not to hasten death
   (b) Providing opioids and other sedatives for relief of suffering is permissible even if there is a risk of hastening death as long as death is not the intent of the treatment
   (c) Providing treatments that can have a bad outcome are permissible as long as the intent of the treatment is to provide the good effect and the patient or authorized designee has consented to undergo the treatment and is aware of the risks
   (d) Physician-assisted suicide is protected by the rule of double effect

Answers

1. (a)
2. (e)
3. (e)
4. (d)
5. (f)
6. (a)
7. (d)
8. (d)

Chapter 28
Physician Coding, Billing, and Reimbursement for Palliative Care

Rene R. Rigal

The advances of medical care as well as the social advances in our societies have transformed the outcomes of many disease processes. Fatal conditions such as cancer, coronary artery disease, AIDS, and CNS diseases are now conditions with which patients live for many years (living with disease) [1]. This has been compounded by the increasingly graying of the population, particularly in the most economically advanced countries. Thus, we find ourselves as physicians not "curing" disease processes, but providing respite from symptoms such as shortness of breath, nausea, fatigue, or chronic pain.

Palliative care has evolved as an interdisciplinary medical activity focused on providing quality of life instead of curing diseases. Palliative care physicians and their care teams strive to decrease pain and other symptoms associated with serious illnesses and enhance the remaining quality of life to the patients and their families [2].

Proper coding and billing for palliative care services provided is a core competency for palliative care physicians. Only then can we insure the continued services that are provided to patients. Physicians practicing palliative medicine should obtain fair reimbursement for their services and valuable skills. Intimate knowledge of billing and coding rules and resources is imperative.

Physicians and their practice staff report the provision of medical procedures and services through the current procedural terminology (CPT), commonly referred as the CPT codebook [3]. CPT is a listing of descriptive terms and identification codes for reporting medical services and procedures performed by physicians and other qualified health care professionals. The purpose of the terminology is to provide uniform language that accurately describes medical, surgical, and diagnostic services. It also provides an effective means for reliable nationwide communications between physicians, Medicare, and third-party payers.

R.R. Rigal, M.D. (✉)
Pain Management Center, Divine Providence Hospital,
Williamsport, PA, USA
e-mail: tainomd@hotmail.com

N. Vadivelu et al. (eds.), *Essentials of Palliative Care*,
DOI 10.1007/978-1-4614-5164-8_28,
© Springer Science+Business Media New York 2013

Physician palliative care services are coded for billing using the same CPT that other physicians use to bill Medicare or other insurance payers for any type of patient care service they provide. There are, nevertheless, several "quirks" that are innate to palliative medicine practice [4].

As in all areas of medicine, physicians must document the services provided to patients and submit for billing (usually using form HC 1500) of that care to the appropriate payer. Palliative medicine physician services, whether for hospice or non-hospice care patients, whether provided in the home, in the office, or in the hospital setting, are reimbursed using the *same* billing and coding guidelines that apply throughout the healthcare system.

Two sets of codes are used to describe physician services to payers [4]:

- **Current Procedural Terminology (CPT) Codes**, which describe the type and extent of services provided, the location of the service, and the relationship of the physician to the patient [5].
- **The International Classification of Diseases, 9th Revision (soon 10th), and Clinical Modification** codes define the medical diagnosis for which the physician service was required [6].

For physicians involved in the provision of palliative care services, the most frequently used codes are for **Evaluation and Management (E/M)**. The Center for Medicare and Medicaid Services (CMS), has as of January 2010, eliminated Medicare payment for consultations [7], thus most of the CPT coding will involve E/M codes 99201-99349. These groups include evaluation and management codes in the usual settings such as ambulatory outpatient, acute impatient hospital, extended care institutions, or in patients' homes.

Since palliative care physicians provide care in which there are extensive amounts of information and counseling given to the patient, family, nursing staff, and requesting physicians, the time component in the physician–patient visit becomes an important aspect in coding. "When more than 50 % of a patient/physician interaction is comprised of counseling and/or information giving, then the TIME becomes the factor that determines which E/M code to use" [3].

Time is defined differently depending on the setting [4, 8]:

- **In the hospital**: the time used to determine which E/M code to use is defined as the **total time** that the physician is present in the hospital unit.
- **In the nonhospital setting**: total time is the time that the physician spends in actual **face to face** with the patient.

When time is taken into account, we have the choice of either using an E/M codes that incorporates the time spent providing the service, or independently bill for the time (using codes 99354-99357) [8]. Local issues must be taken into account when making this decision.

An ICD-9 (soon to be ICD-10) code must also be selected and must reflect the reason for the services provided [4, 6]. A decision must be made between coding for a symptom vs. a diagnosis. For example, it is probably safer to bill for a symptom (back pain 724.2) instead of spinal stenosis, and thus avoid concurrent care issues with the patient's primary care physician or other consultants [9].

In addition, if the palliative care physician provides other than E/M (procedural) services, then these procedures can be billed using the appropriate procedural codes for the specific procedures performed, such as pain management blocks, paracentesis, thoracentesis, etc. The time required to perform the procedure is not counted, as it is included in the "global payment" for the particular procedure code submitted [8].

All the Federal and State agencies (CMS, HCFA) require extensive documentation prior to payment (and must be present to survive an audit). The documentation should include the domains of quality palliative care [10] and should include the following:

- Structure and process of care
- Physical aspect of care
- Psychological and psychiatric aspects of care
- Social aspects of care
- Spiritual, religious, and existential aspects of care
- Cultural aspects of care
- Care of the imminently dying patient
- Ethical and legal aspects of care
- Clarify the patient's definition of quality of life and advance directives
- Detailed physical exam
- Development of an assessment and plan of care
- Communication of all of the above to primary care physician

The billing and coding guidelines previously described are common in many billing situations by all physicians. However, there are some issues that are unique to palliative care physicians, particularly those employed by Hospice Agencies [4, 8, 9]:

- **Attending Physician—Hospice Employee**: Care plan oversight, supervisory activities, establishment of eligibility and of governing policies for the Hospice is covered as part of the administrative duties and is included in the per diem reimbursement that the Hospice receives. Patient care services for direct patient care are not included in the per diem payment provided to the hospice agency and these services should be submitted for payment to the hospice.
- **Attending Physician not employed with the Hospice**: can submit bills for direct patient services using the CPT and ICD-9 codes as previously described and submits these claims directly to Medicare Part B.

Most commercial insurance companies follow the CMS billing guidelines and thus require physicians to code for direct patient services using the CPT and ICD-9 codes. Nevertheless, it is always prudent to verify with the commercial insurance company and follow their proprietary processes.

Reimbursement for palliative care services provided to patients follows the usual guidelines used for reimbursement in the USA. When these are followed, and the care is properly documented, then the usual and customary payment (as established by CMS or commercial insurance companies) can be expected. The most important thing to do is to document what you do and how long it takes to do it.

References

1. Cassell EJ. The nature of suffering and the goals of medicine. N Engl J Med. 1982;306:639–45.
2. Morrison RS, Meier DE. The national palliative care research center and the center to advance palliative care: a partnership to improve care for persons with serious illness and their families. J Pediatr Hematol Oncol. 2011;33:S126–31.
3. American Medical Association. Current procedural terminology. Chicago, IL: American Medical Association; 1999.
4. Von Gunten CF, Ferris FD, Kirschner C, Emanuel LL. Coding and reimbursement mechanisms for physician services in hospice and palliative care. J Palliat Med. 2000;3(2):157–64.
5. Standardizing CPT codes, guidelines and conventions; Administrative simplification White Paper, May 19, 2009.
6. American Medical Association. International classification of diseases. 9th revision, clinical modification. Chicago, IL: American Medical Association; 1997.
7. American Medical Association. Consultation services and transfer of care. 2010.
8. American Academy of Hospice and Palliative Medicine. AAHPM Coding & Billing task force: Quick reference guide for physicians coding, billing and reimbursement for hospice and palliative medicine services. 2006.
9. Ely JC, Twaddle ML. Essentials of coding and billing in palliative care. Paper presented in annual assembly of AAHPN and HPNA. 2006.
10. National Consensus Project for Quality Palliative Care. Clinical practice guidelines for quality palliative care. 2nd ed. 2006. http://www.nationalconsensusproject.org.

Index

A

Accumulation of respiratory tract secretions (ARTS), 62

Acetaminophen, 110

Activities of daily living (ADLs), 182

Adjustment disorders, 30–32, 47

Adjuvants, 108, 114

Advanced certified hospice and palliative social worker (ACHP-SW), 4

Advanced heart failure (HF) patients
communication, 379–380
dyspnea
benzodiazepines, 377
nonpharmacological approach, 378
opioids, 377, 383, 384
hospice care reimbursement, 380
implantable cardioverter defibrillator, 378–379
incidence, 375
left ventricular assist device, 379
pacemakers, 378
palliative care and hospice, 376
pharmacological treatment, 377
prognosis, 375, 376, 383, 384
symptoms, management of, 378

Aloysi, A.S., 111

American Board of Medical Specialties, 2

AMPA ionotropic glutamate receptor antagonists, 461

Analgesics, 108

Angiography
catheter insertion, 255, 256
contraindications, 254
guide wire passage, 255, 256
indications, 254
vessel puncture, 255, 256

Angioplasty
balloon catheter, 255
complications, 256–257
interventional options, 255
stent insertion, 256

Anorexia, 218. *See* Cachexia syndrome

Anticonvulsants, 115

Antidepressants, 115

Anti-nerve growth factor agents, 457–458

Anxiety disorder
benzodiazepines, 36–37
clinical interview based on DSM criteria, 47
patient-physician relationship, 35
relaxation training and deep breathing exercises, 37
screening, 36

Arrhythmias
bradyarrhythmias, 389
tachyarrhythmias, 387–389

Artiticial nutrition (AN)
clinical indications, 148
complications of, 148–149
enteral nutrition, 146
immunonutrition, 148
parenteral nutrition, 146–148

Asenjo, J., 471

Atrial fibrillation
case study, 391–393
embolic stroke risk, 388
palliative care goals, 388
rhythm control strategies, 387
symptoms, 387
treatment, 387

Aura, 316, 346, 347

Axillary brachial plexus block, 473

Axillary lymph node resection (ALND), 183

N. Vadivelu et al. (eds.), *Essentials of Palliative Care*,
DOI 10.1007/978-1-4614-5164-8,
© Springer Science+Business Media New York 2013

B

Bilevel inspiratory positive pressure
    ventilation (BIPAP), 418
Biliary catheter insertion, 270–271
Blalock, A., 370
Blalock–Taussig shunt, 370
Blind loop syndromes, 140
Boyle, G., 202
Bradyarrhythmias, 389
Brain aneurysms
    coils for, 260
    contraindications, 260
    indications, 259–260
    Seldinger percutaneous catheter insertion,
        260
    triple-H therapy, 260
Breaking bad news
    assess patient readiness, 77
    availabilities and resources, 79
    body language, 80
    briefly assess patient, 77
    cultural and spiritual issues, 80–81
    delivery news, 77–78
    delivery requirements, 75
    determining presence, 76–77
    elements for meeting, 76
    over-optimism, 79
    patient remembering, 80
    planning, 78
    recommendation, 74–75
    respond to emotion, 78
    team members limits, 79
    touching patients, 80
Breast cancer, 183
Breathlessness. *See* Dyspnea
Bryson E.O., 111
Bupivacaine, 467

C

Cachexia syndrome, 218
    agent, 122
    causes of, 120–121
    definition, 120
    melatonin, 122
    nutritional care, 159
        anorexia and decreased food intake,
            138–139
        counseling, 143–144
        definitions, 138
        energy expenditure, 159
        inflammatory and humoral activities, 141
        metabolic perturbations, 139–140
        oral nutritive supplements, 144–146
    systemic inflammatory response, 120

Cannabinoids, 459–460
Cardiac electrophysiology
    cardiac pacing, 386
    catheter ablation, 387
    implantable cardioverter-defibrillators,
        386–387, 391, 393
Cardiac pacing, 386
Cardiac surgical procedures, 370–371
Cardiopulmonary resuscitation (CPR), 493,
    499, 500
Cardiothoracic surgery, 369–371
Casssel, E.J., 485
Catheter ablation, 387
Celiac plexus neurolysis, 303–304
Cement, 307, 308, 311, 312, 314
Central venous catheters (CVCs), 266–267
Cerebral angiography, 259–260
Certified Hospice and Palliative Care
        Administrator (CHPCA), 4
Certified Hospice and Palliative Licensed
        Nurse (CHPLN), 3
Certified Hospice and Palliative Nursing
        Assistant (CHPNA), 4
Chest pain, 398
Christakis, N.A., 489
Christopher, K., 1, 50
Chronic migraine, 328–329
Chronic obstructive pulmonary disease
        (COPD), 405–406
Cluster headaches
    abortive treatment, 335, 338
    criteria, 332–333
    definition, 332
    diagnosis, 334–335
    etiology, 333–334
    features, 333
    hallmark of, 332
    medications for, 335–337
    pathophysiology, 333, 334
    prevalence, 332
    preventive treatment
        antiepileptic drugs, 340
        civamide, 341
        lithium carbonate, 340
        melatonin, 340–341
        polypharmacy, 339
        verapamil, 340
    prognosis, 342
    surgical treatment, 341–342
    transitional treatment, 339
Coeliac plexus blocks
    anterior and posterior approaches, 269
    biliary interventions, 270
    complications for, 269
    contraindications, 269

indication, 268
procedural method, 270
Colostomy, 220–221
Communication among physicians, 84
Communication skills
breaking bad news, 86
assess patient readiness, 77
availabilities and resources, 79
body language, 80
briefly assess patient, 77
cultural and spiritual issues, 80–81
deliver news, 77–78
delivery requirements, 75
determining presence, 76–77
elements for meeting, 76
over-optimism, 79
patient remembering, 80
planning, 78
recommendation, 74–75
respond to emotion, 78
team members limits, 79
touching patients, 80
coordinated team work, 74
distressed families, 81–83
formal training, 86
health professionals, 83–84
physician interrupting patient, 86
recognising diagnosis, 86
training models, 74
Community palliative care programs, 10
Comprehensive health enhancement support
system, lung cancer module
(CHESS-LC), 98
Confusion assessment method (CAM), 38
Connor, S.R., 376
Constipation, 134
bowel regimen, 119, 120
management of
laxatives, 150–151
opioid antagonists, 151
rectally administered medications, 151
Continuous catheter techniques, 469, 470,
480, 481
Continuous positive pressure ventilation
(CPAP), 418
Cooley, D., 370
Coordination of care, 16–17, 20
Cortical spreading depression (CSD), 317–318
Corticosteroids, 116–117, 145
Cough, 124–125, 399–400, 414
Covered self-expanding metal stents
(CSEMS), 352, 357–358, 365, 367
Cowley, L.T., 484
Cox, J.J., 458
Cozzaglio, L., 489, 490

Critical care units
diabetic ketoacidosis, 437, 439
aggressive fluid management, 423
complications, 421
initial investigations, 421, 422
metabolic parameters, 422
mortality rates, 421
occurence, 421
potassium chloride, 421
treatment, 422, 423
hypercalcaemia, 430–432
hyperkalaemia
aldosterone, 423, 424
beta-2 agonists, 425, 426
causes of, 423, 424, 438, 439
drug therapy, 424
electrocardiogram, 425, 437, 439
insulin, 425, 426
myocardium stabilisation, 425
renal replacement therapy, 426
hypocalcaemia, 433–434, 438, 439
hypokalaemia, 426–427, 437, 439
hyponatremia
causes and management options,
428
classification, 427
management, 429–430
SIADH, 428, 429
NIPPV
acute respiratory failure, 418
adverse side effects, 420
comfort measures, 419, 420
contraindications, 420
nasal mask, 418, 419
oronasal mask, 418, 419
Cruzan, N., 153
Current procedural terminology (CPT) codes,
501, 502

D
Decision conflict, 94, 95
Decision making process
guidance with end-of-life decisions
clinical decisions, 99
decision for specific situations,
100–101
initiating process, 99–100
patient's needs/values and goal, 100
providing information to patient and
family, 100
specific areas, 99, 104
time-limited trial, 101
models, 90–91
support, 94–99

Decision support
    aids
        definition, 95–96
        online resource guidance, 97
        standards, 96
    clinical encounter, 96
    coaching, 104
        CHESS-LC, 98
        definition, 95
        health professionals, 97–98
        randomized controlled trials, 98–99
    definition, 94–95
    interventions, 95, 104
Dehydration management, 149
Delirium, 47, 134
    agents, 126–127
    causes of, 125–126
    confusion assessment method, 38
    environmental and psychosocial
            interventions, 40
    MDAS, 38
    medication, 39
    perceptual disturbances, 37
    pharmacologic treatment, 126
    subtypes, 125
    tripartite approach, 38
den Daas, N., 485
DepoFoam, 467
Depression disorder
    antidepressants, 34–35
    cognitive-behavioral therapy, 35
    HADS, 33
    hastened death, 32
    medical conditions and medication use, 34
    prevalence rates, 32
    suicidal ideas, 32–33
Diabetic ketoacidosis (DKA), 437, 439
    aggressive fluid management, 423
    complications, 421
    initial investigations, 421, 422
    metabolic parameters, 422
    mortality rates, 421
    occurence, 421
    potassium chloride, 421
    treatment, 422, 423
Do-not-resuscitate (DNR) orders, 493–495,
            499, 500
Drug delivery
    extended release enteral formulations,
            463, 480, 481
    parenteral formulations, 463–465
Drug formulary
    codeine
        administration, 236

        amitriptyline, 236–237
        benzodiazepines, 240
        candida albicans, 241
        carbamazepine, 237
        clonazepam, 241
        CYP2D6 function, 236
        dexamethasone, 239–240
        gabapentin, 237
        glycopyrrolate, 238–239
        haloperidol, 238
        lactulose, 239
        megestrol acetate, 239
        metaclopramide, 238
        midazolam, 240
        nystatin, 241
        senna, 239
    diclofenac
        COX enzyme inhibition, 235
        tapentadol, 236
        topical preparations, 235–236
        tramadol, 236
    dosing, PRN, 245
    levorphanol
        buprenorphine, 243
        modafinil, 243–244
        octreotide, 244
    mirtazepine, 242
    pain
        acetaminophen, 231
        fentanyl, 233
        methadone, 233–235
        morphine, 231–233
    routes, 245–246
    symptoms, 229, 230
Dugani, S., 471
Duragesic™, 463
Dyspnea
    benzodiazepines, 377
    BORG score, 396
    definition, 122–123, 396
    medical management, 397
    non-invasive ventilation, 397
    nonpharmacological approach, 378
    opioids, 123–124, 377
    pschological components, 124
    reversible causes, treatment of, 123
    treatment, 396, 412, 414

E
Elwyn, G., 96
Embolisation
    chemoembolisation, 259
    contraindications, 257–258

indications, 257
radioembolisation, 259
End-of-life care
cardiopulmonary resuscitation,
493, 499, 500
death, definition of, 484–485
do-not-resuscitate orders, 493–495
ethics
decision making, 489
and opioids use, 487–489
principles of, 485–486
futility of care, definition of, 490–491
length of survival, 484–485
and palliative care, 492–493
principle of double effect, 491–492
rule of double effect, 486–487, 498, 500
substantial pain, 484, 498, 500
supportive measures, withdrawal of,
489–490
Enteral nutrition (EN), 146, 160
Enteral tube feeding, dementia patients,
153, 159
Epilepsy
drug-resistant epilepsy, 285
palliative treatment
hemispherectomy, 285–286
ketogenic diet, 286
multiple subpial transection, 286
sudden unexpected death, 285
Euvolemic hyponatremia, 428, 430
Exercise, 179
Exparel™, 467
Extended release enteral formulations, drug
delivery, 463, 480, 481

F
Fainsinger, R., 289
Fatty-acid amide hydrolase (FAAH) inhibitors,
460–461
Femoral nerve block, 474
Figley, C.R., 201
Franklin, C.M., 495
Fyfe, A., 485

G
Gastroduodenal obstruction, 353, 365, 367
Gastrointestinal malignancies, endoscopic
therapies
endoscopic retrograde
cholangiopancreatography, 356, 359
esophagus
argon plasma coagulation, 349, 350
esophageal dilation, 350, 351
laser photoablation, 349, 350
photodynamic therapy, 349, 350
self-expanding metal stents,
351–353
nutrition, 360–361
pain management, 360
pancreas and biliary tract, 356–360
small and large intestines
biliary stent, 353
complications, 354–356
enteral/duodenal stent insertion,
353, 354
gastrojejunostomy, 353, 354
self-expanding metal stents, 354–355
stent occlusion, 356, 357
Gastrointestinal symptoms
cachexia syndrome and fatigue,
120–122
constipation, 119–120
cough, 124–125
delirium, 125–127
dyspnea, 122–124
insomnia, 127–128
nausea and vomiting, 117–119
xerostoma, 117
Gastrostomy
complications, 272
contraindications, 271
procedural method, 272
Gastrostomy tube, 220
Glenn shunt, 370, 373, 374
Glenn, W., 370
Goodman, N., 495
Groshong, 266

H
Headaches
cluster
abortive treatment, 335, 338
criteria, 332–333
definition, 332
diagnosis, 334–335
etiology, 333–334
features, 333
hallmark of, 332
medications for, 335–337
pathophysiology, 333, 334
prevalence, 332
preventive treatment, 339–341
prognosis, 342
surgical treatment, 341–342
transitional treatment, 339

Headaches (*cont.*)
  migraine
    chronic, 328–329
    definition, 316
    diagnosis, 318–320
    etiology and pathophysiology, 317–318
    gender difference, 316
    International Headache Classification,
      316–317
    pediatric populations, 331
    phases, 316
    pregnancy and lactation, 330–331
    prevalence, 316
    prognosis, 331–332
    refractory, 329–330
    status migrainosus, 316
    treatment options, 302–328
Head and neck cancer, 183
Healthcare system
  access
    doctors appointment, 213
    hospice experience, 213
    information, 211–212
    insurance, 212–213
    resources, 212–213
  communication, 209–211
Hemispherectomy, 285–286
Hemoptysis
  blood screening, 403, 412, 414
  bronchial artery embolisation, 403
  causes for, 403
  chest X-ray, 403, 412, 414
  computer tomography, 403, 412, 414
  description, 402
  massive, 404, 412, 415
Hickman, S., 266
High dose topical capsaicin, 458–459, 480, 481
Himelstein, B.P., 444
Home palliative care, 57
Hopkins, J., 370
Hospice
  average length of stay, 68
  benefits and coverage, 51–52
  complication of immobility, 68
  continuous care, 52
  definition, 50–51
  discharge patient and re-enroll, 67
  functional decline, 58–59
  funding and eligibility
    life-prolonging therapy, 57
    medicare guidelines, 53–57
    reasonable likelihood, 52
  general inpatient care, 52
  history, 50
  home palliative care, 57

    hospital bed, oxygen, and commode
      for home use, 67
  impending death, 68
  length of stay, 68
  nurse, role of, 166
  open access hospice, 58
  oral intake reduction, 59, 67–68
  physiology of death, 63
  primary caregiver, 67–68
  routes of medication administration, 68
    pharmacotherapy, 59
    rectal route, 61
    subcutaneous route, 61
    transdermal route, 60, 68
    transmucosal route, 61
  routine home care, 52
  statements, 67
  symptom management, 67
    death rattle, 62
    terminal agitated delirium, 62–63
  terminal phase of illness, 58, 69
  time of symptoms, 63
  treatment, 67–68
  type of sedation, 68
Hospice and Palliative Medicine (HPM), 1
Hospice medicare benefit, 51–52
Hospital anxiety and depression scale
    (HADS), 33
Human chorionic gonadotropin (hCG),
    461–462
Hypercalcaemia
  causes and clinical features, 430, 431,
    438, 439
  diuretic effect, 431
  familial benign, 432
  parathyroid hormone related peptide, 431
  primary hyperparathyroidism, 432
  vitamin D, 431
Hyperkalaemia
  aldosterone, 423, 424
  beta-2 agonists, 425, 426
  causes of, 423, 424, 438, 439
  drug therapy, 424
  electrocardiogram, 425, 437, 439
  insulin, 425, 426
  myocardium stabilisation, 425
  renal replacement therapy, 426
Hypervolemic hyponatremia, 428, 430
Hypocalcaemia, 433–434, 438, 439
Hypokalaemia, 426–427, 437, 439
Hyponatremia, 437–439
  causes and management options, 428
  classification, 427
  management, 429–430
  SIADH, 428, 429

Hypothalamic stimulation, cluster headaches,
       342
Hypovolemic hyponatremia, 428, 430

I
Ileostomy, 220–221
Implantable cardioverter defibrillators (ICDs)
       advanced HF patients, 378–379
       implantation, 386
       non-invasive strategy, 387
       reprogramming, 386
Inferior vena cava (IVC) filters, 265–266
Informed choice model, 90–91, 103
Infraclavicular brachial plexus block, 472
Insomnia
       causes, 127
       definition, 127
       melatonin, 128
       sedating antidepressants, 128
Institutional palliative care programs, 11
Interactive health communication systems
       (IHCS), 98
Intercostal neurolysis, 307
Interdisciplinary team communication, 84
International Association of Hospice and
       Palliative Care (IAHPC), 229, 230
International Classification of Diseases
       (ICD-9) codes, 502
International Patient Decision Aids Standards
       (IPDAS), 96, 104
Interscalene brachial plexus block, 471–472
Interventional pain blocks, 313, 314
Interventional techniques
       neurolysis
              alcohol, 300, 311, 314
              celiac plexus, 303–304
              complications, 302
              cryoablation, 301–302
              equipments, 302
              glycerol, 301, 311, 314
              informed consent, 302
              intercostal, 307
              intrathecal, 303
              peripheral nerve, 303
              phenol, 300–301, 311, 314
              radiofrequency thermocoagulation, 301
              sympathetic, 304–306
       noncancer palliative care, 309–310
       skeletal metastases (*see* Skeletal
              metastases)
       trigeminal ganglion, 306–307,
              313, 314
Intra-arterial thrombolysis (IAT)
       contraindications, 263

indications, 262–264
       procedural method, 263
Intrathecal neurolysis, 303
Intrathecal opioid pumps, 308–309
Ionsys, 463–464
Ischaemic stroke
       monitoring and reimaging, 262
       tissue plasminogen activator
              contraindications, 261–262
              dosage, 262
              indications, 261

J
Joint commission on Accreditation of
       Healthcare Organizations, 4

K
Kainate ionotropic glutamate receptor
       antagonists, 461
Kaye, A.D., 471
Klinner, W., 370

L
Leao, A., 317
Left ventricular assist device (LVAD),
       379, 383, 384
Lema, M., 5
Length of survival (LOS),
       484–485
Levobupivacaine, 467
Lidocaine, 466–467
Local anesthetics (LAs)
       dexamethasone, 468
       epinephrine addition, 467
       ester and amide, 466–467
       methemoglobinemia, 469
       Na channel blockade, 466
       opioids, 468
       sodium bicarbonate addition,
              467–468
       structure of, 466
       toxicity, 468–469
       vasoconstrictors, 467
Luce, J., 490, 492
Lumbar sympathetic neurolysis, 304–305
Lung cancer, 413, 415
       incidence, 408
       mortality rates, 408
       superior vena caval obstruction, 409
       ventilatory failure risk, 408, 409
Lung infections, 404–405, 412, 415
Lymphedema, 183–184

M
Mandela technique, 446
McCarthy, M., 380
Memorial delirium assessment scale
   (MDAS), 38
Migraine
   chronic, 328–329
   definition, 316
   diagnosis, 318–320
   etiology and pathophysiology, 317–318
   gender difference, 316
   International Headache Classification,
      316–317
   nonpharmocologic treatment, 321
   pediatric populations, 331
   phases, 316
   pregnancy and lactation, 330–331
   prevalence, 316
   prognosis, 331–332
   prophylaxis
      abortive medications, 325–328
      goals, 321
      indications for, 321
      nonprescription prophylactic
         medications, 322–325
   refractory, 329–330
   status migrainosus, 316
Miner, P.M., 317
Mirtazepine, 242
Multidisciplinary team (MDT)
   advantages and effectiveness, 14
   barriers, 14–15
   benefits, 20
   continuity of care, 20
   coordination of care, 16–17, 20
   interdisciplinary team, 9–10
   models, 10–11
   overlapping dimensions, 9
   roles of, 11–13
Multiple subpial transection, 286

N
National Board for Certification of Hospice
      and Palliative Nurses (NBCHPN),
      3–4
Nausea and vomiting, 117–119
Na$_v$ 1.7 blocking agents, 458
Navigante, A.H., 377
Neonatal Intensive Care Unit (NICU),
      pediatric palliative care, 448–449
Neurological cases, respiratory disease
   bulbar weakness, 406
      diaphragmatic weakness, 407

   mortality, 406
   rapid eye movement, 407, 413, 415
   treatment options, 407–408
Neurological disease
   advance care planning, 287
   communication, 287
   drug administration routes, 288
   symptom management
      death rattle, 288
      delirium, 289
      depression, 291–292
      drowsiness, 289–290
      dyspnea, 288
      epileptic seizures, 290
      myoclonus, 290
      nausea and vomiting, 291
      pain, 290–291
      terminal restlessness, 288–289
   at terminal stage, 286–287
Neurolysis
   alcohol, 300
   celiac plexus, 303–304
   complications, 302
   cryoablation, 301–302
   equipments, 302
   glycerol, 301
   informed consent, 302
   intercostal, 307
   intrathecal, 303
   peripheral nerve, 303, 313, 314
   phenol, 300–301
   radiofrequency thermocoagulation, 301
   sympathetic, 304–306
NIPPV. *See* Non-invasive positive pressure
      ventilation (NIPPV)
N-methyl-d-aspartate (NMDA) antagonists,
      116
Non-cardiac thoracic surgery, 371
Non-invasive positive pressure ventilation
      (NIPPV)
   acute respiratory failure, 418
   adverse side effects, 420
   comfort measures, 419, 420
   contraindications, 420
   nasal mask, 418, 419
   oronasal mask, 418, 419
Nonopioids, 109–110
Nonsteroidal anti-inflmatory drugs (NSAIDs),
      109–110, 235, 326, 464
Norwood, W.I., 370
Numeric Pain Intensity Instrument/Scale, 170
Nursing perspective and considerations
   coaching, 164
      cultural and spiritual considerations, 172

Index   513

hospice care, 166
interdisciplinary care team
    design and composition, 165
    meetings, 165–166
nurse's role, 164
nursing pain management
    education, 170, 171
    family caregivers, 167
    nursing assessment, 166–167
    terminology, 168–169
pain assessment ways, 165
patient controlled analgesia (PCA)
    intravenous and subcutaneous routes, 172
    pain team, 172
    parameters, 171
    patient and family education, 171–172
    symptoms, 172
Nutritional care
appetite and rehabilitation clinic teams, 143
artiticial
    clinical indications, 148
    complications of, 148–149
    enteral nutrition, 146
    immunonutrition, 148
    parenteral nutrition, 146–148
assessment, 141–142, 159
cachexia
    anorexia and decreased food intake, 138–139
    counseling, 143–144
    definitions, 138
    inflammatory and humoral activities, 141
    metabolic perturbations, 139–140
    oral nutritive supplements, 144–146
ethical decision making, 153–155, 160
maintain weight, 159
with noncancer chronic illnesses, 152–153
prevalence of malnutrition, 160
score, 142
support on tumor, 141
weight change, 142

O
Occipital nerve stimulation, cluster headaches, 342
Olanzepine, 242
Olsen, J., 317
Olson, D.P., 80
Opioids, 134
atute monitoring, 112
conversion table, 111
dyspnoea, 397
nalbuphine, 110
systematic titration, 111–112
toxicities, 110
Orexigens, 145
Osler, W., 483, 484, 495
Osmotic-controlled release oral delivery system, 463
Ostomy, 221
Outpatient Palliative Care Programs, 10
Overall, Y., 144

P
Pacemakers
advance HF patients, 378
bradyarrhythmias, 389, 391, 393
Pain
antineuropathic benefit, 134
distress, 107
emergencies and emergency departments, 113
pharmacologic tools, 108
WHO analgesic ladder, 108–109
Pain Assessment Tool/Scale, 170
Pain management
AMPA and kainate ionotropic glutamate receptor antagonists, 461
anti-nerve growth factor agents, 457–458
cannabinoids, 459–460
drug delivery
    extended release enteral formulations, 463
    parenteral formulations, 463–465
fatty-acid amide hydrolase inhibitors, 460–461
high dose topical capsaicin, 458–459
human chorionic gonadotropin, 461–462
Na_v 1.7 blocking agents, 458
regional anesthesia (*see* Regional anesthesia)
somatotropin, 462
voltage-gated calcium channel blocking agents, 459
Palliative care
decision making (*see* Decision making process)
definition of, 453, 455
    by NCP, 8–9
    by NQF, 9
    by WHO, 8, 19
and education
    HPM, 1
    nursing, 3–4
    physicians, 2
    program certification, 4–5
    social work, 4
    symptoms, 1–2

Palliative care (*cont.*)
  facilities, 151–152
  goals of, 93
  guidance with complex treatment choices,
      93–94, 103
  hospice based, 20
  level of, 19
  MDT (*see* Multidisciplinary team (MDT))
  medical specialty risk, 86
  number of domains, 19
  nutrition (*see* Nutritional care)
  patient-and family centered, 19
  preference-sensitive decisions, 92–93, 103
  professionals, 19
  requirements, 19
Palliative care physician services
  coding and billing, 501, 502
  documentation, 502, 503
  employed by Hospice Agencies, 503
  global payment, 503
  to payers
      clinical modification codes, 502
      current procedural terminology codes,
          501, 502
      evaluation and management, 502
      ICD-9 codes, 502
  reimbursement, 503
  time component, physician–patient visit, 502
Papadatou, D., 449
Parenteral nutrition, 146–148, 160
Paternalistic model, 90–91, 103
Patient controlled analgesia (PCA)
  intravenous and subcutaneous routes, 172
  pain team, 172
  parameters, 171
  patient and family education, 171–172
  symptoms, 172
Pediatric palliative care, 453–455
  causes of death, 442, 443
  chronic complex conditions, 443
  deaths in
      adolescents, 448
      infant, 447
      preschool children, 447–448
      school age children, 448
      toddler, 447
  health care practitioners, stress and
          burnout, 449–450
  implementation barriers, 444–445
  initiation and team formation, 445
  integrated palliative care model, 443
  NICU, 448–449
  pain assessment scales, 445, 446
  physical and emotional suffering, 445–446

  principles of, 444
  spiritual care, 447
  WHO definition, 441–442
Percutaneous endoscopic gastrostomy (PEG),
    220, 360, 361
Percutaneous transhepatic cholangiography
    (PTC)
  contraindications, 270–271
  procedural method, 271
Percutaneous vertebroplasty and kyphoplasty,
    267–268
Peripheral nerve blocks, regional anesthesia
  contraindications, 471
  of lower extremity
      femoral nerve block, 474
      popliteal sciatic nerve block, 474
      saphenous nerve block, 474–475
      sciatic nerve block, 473–474
  single shot, 470
  of upper extremity
      axillary brachial plexus block, 473
      infraclavicular brachial plexus block,
          472
      interscalene brachial plexus block,
          471–472
      supraclavicular brachial plexus block,
          472
Peripheral nerve neurolysis, 303, 313, 314
Photodynamic therapy (PDT), 365, 367
  cholestasis, 359
  esophageal cancer, 349, 350
  photosensitizing agent usage, 350
Physical and occupational therapy
  anorexia, 178
  cachexia, 178
  muscle wasting, 178
  primary fatigue, 178
  rehabilitation strategies
      breast cancer, 183
      exercise, 179
      head and neck cancer, 183
      hospice and palliative care patient,
          180–181
      lymphedema, 183–184
      occupational therapy, 182
      physical modalities, 182
      pulmonary rehabilitation, 182
  rehab team and setting, 179
Pleurx catheters, 221
Popliteal sciatic nerve block, 474
Postdrome, 316, 317
Potts shunt, 370
Preference-sensitive decisions, 92–93, 103
Prodrome, 316

Protein metabolism abnormalities, 141
Psychiatric disorders
  adjustment, 30–32, 47
  anxiety
    benzodiazepines, 36–37
    clinical interview based on DSM
      criteria, 47
    patient-physician relationship, 35
    relaxation training and deep breathing
      exercises, 37
    screening, 36
  assessment types, 28
  delirium, 47
    confusion assessment method, 38
    environmental and psychosocial
      interventions, 40
    MDAS, 38
    medication, 39
    perceptual disturbances, 37
    tripartite approach, 38
  depression
    antidepressants, 34–35
    cognitive-behavioral therapy, 35
    hastened death, 32
    Hospital Anxiety and Depression Scale,
      33
    medical conditions and medication use,
      34
    prevalence rates, 32
    suicidal ideas, 32–33
  phases of illness, 27
  prognostic factors, 30
  psychopharmacologic agents, 28, 30
  psychotherapeutic interventions, 28–29
  symptoms, 28, 47
Psychological distress and psychiatric
      comorbidities
  adjustment disorder, 30–32, 47
  anxiety disorder
    benzodiazepines, 36–37
    clinical interview based on DSM
      criteria, 47
    patient-physician relationship, 35
    relaxation training and deep breathing
      exercises, 37
    screening, 36
  delirium, 47
    confusion assessment method, 38
    environmental and psychosocial
      interventions, 40
    MDAS, 38
    medication, 39
    perceptual disturbances, 37
    tripartite approach, 38

depression disorder
    antidepressants, 34–35
    cognitive-behavioral therapy, 35
    HADS, 33
    hastened death, 32
    medical conditions and medication use,
      34
    prevalence rates, 32
    suicidal ideas, 32–33
  end of life, psychosocial demands, 23–24
  grief, 24
  life meaning, 24–25
  patient-provider communication
    factors, 26–27
    guidelines, 27
    ineffective coping strategies and
      beliefs, 25
    primary medical caregiver, 26
    resources, 25
  phases of illness, 27
  prognostic factors, 30
  psychopharmacologic agents, 28, 30
  psychotherapeutic interventions, 28–29
  repertoire of skills, 47
  spiritual distress, 25
  symptoms, 28, 47
  types of assessments, 28
Psychopharmacology, 28, 30
Psychotherapy, 28–32, 35, 37
Pulmonary artery banding, 370–371
Pulmonary rehabilitation, 182
Pyenson, B., 376

Q
Quinlan, 154

R
Radiofrequency thermocoagulation, 311, 314
  cluster headaches, 341
  lumbar sympathetic neurolysis, 305
  thoracic sympathetic neurolysis, 306
  trigeminal ganglion, 307
Radiology
  angiography
    catheter insertion, 255, 256
    contraindications, 254
    guide wire passage, 255, 256
    indications, 254
    vessel puncture, 255, 256
  angioplasty
    balloon catheter, 255
    complications, 256–257

Radiology (*cont.*)
    interventional options, 255
    stent insertion, 256
  brain aneurysms
    coils for, 260
    contraindications, 260
    indications, 259–260
    Seldinger percutaneous catheter
      insertion, 260
    triple-H therapy, 260
  central venous catheters (CVCs), 266–267
  cerebral angiography, 259–260
  coeliac plexus blocks
    anterior and posterior approaches, 269
    biliary interventions, 270
    complications for, 269
    contraindications, 269
    indication, 268
    procedural method, 270
  embolisation
    chemoembolisation, 259
    contraindications, 257–258
    indications, 257
    radioembolisation, 259
  gastrostomy
    complications, 272
    contraindications, 271
    procedural method, 272
  intra-arterial thrombolysis
    contraindications, 263
    indications, 262–264
    procedural method, 263
  ischaemic stroke, 261–262
  percutaneous transhepatic
    cholangiography, 270–271
  percutaneous vertebroplasty and
    kyphoplasty, 267–268
  transjugular intrahepatic portosystemic
    shunt
    complications, 273
    contraindications, 272
    procedural method, 273
  venous thromboembolism
    indications, 265
    inferior vena cava filters, 265–266
Raffin, T., 484
Ravasco, P., 143
Refeeding syndrome, 148–149
Refractory migraine, 329–330
Refractory status epilepticus (RSE), 290
Regional anesthesia, 480, 481
  benefits, 465
  local anesthetics
    dexamethasone, 468
    epinephrine addition, 467
    ester and amide, 466–467
    methemoglobinemia, 469
    Na channel blockade, 466
    opioids, 468
    sodium bicarbonate addition, 467–468
    structure of, 466
    toxicity, 468–469
    vasoconstrictors, 467
  peripheral nerve blocks, 470–475
  regional nerve blocks, 469–470
  utility and safety, 465
Regional nerve blocks, 469–470
Respiratory disease
  American Thoracic Society, 395
  symptoms, management of
    chest pain, 398
    chronic obstructive pulmonary disease,
      405–406
    cough, 399–400
    dyspnoea, 396–397
    hemoptysis, 402–404
    lung cancer, 408–409
    lung infections, 404–405
    neurological cases, 406–408
    stridor, 400–401
    wheeze, 400
Robinson, M.R., 447
Ropivacaine, 467
Rotherberg, D.M., 495
Rubenfeld, G., 492
Rule of double effect, 486–487, 498–500

S
Sano shunt, 370
Saphenous nerve block, 474–475
Saunders, C., 1, 50
Schiavo, T., 153
Sciatic nerve block, 473–474
Self-expanding metal stents (SEMS)
  cost of, 358
  esophageal, 352–353
  malignant biliary obstruction, endoscopic
    relief of, 356
  nitinol composition, 351
  outcomes, 359
  proximal colon cancers, 354
  types, 352
Seven "Cs" planning model, 193–194
Shang, E., 146
Shared decision model, 91, 95, 103
Shoulder-hand syndrome, 282
Single shot peripheral nerve blocks, 470
Skeletal metastases
  cement, 307, 308, 311, 312, 314

complications, 308
intrathecal opioid pumps, 308–309
kyphoplasty, 307, 308
morbidity, 307
neurosurgical ablative approaches, 308
vertebroplasty, 307, 308
Social work
care planning
communication and, 196–197
family members, 197–198
model, 195
and patient–family meeting, 193–194
core therapeutic interventions, 199
Dr. L's view, 200–201
Marcia R's view, 200
patient and family, 199
cultural awareness, 195–196
emotional support, 203
family meeting
bedside care, 198
Mary G's view, 198
Ramona F's view, 198–199
stories sharing, 197
limitations of, 202
National Association of Social Workers, 190
palliative care social worker
compassion fatigue, 201–202
consult, 192–193
psychosocial and spiritual aspects, 202–203
role of, 190–191
social work assessment, 192–193
team configurations, 191
team evolution, 191–192
supervision, 203
Somatotropin, 462
Spiegel, D., 485
Spinal cord
modulation, 312–314
stimulation, 308, 309, 312, 314
Status migrainosus, 316
Stent occlusion, 356, 357
Stridor, 412, 414
description, 400
emergency management, 400–401
long-term management, 401
Stroke
incidence, 280
medical care, 280
nutritional needs and access, 280–281
pressure sores, 281–282
shoulder-hand syndrome, 282
venous thrombosis, 281
reduce disability and impairment
depression, 284
language and perceptual impairment, 283
rehabilitation practice, 282
sensorimotor training, 283
spasticity, 284
Stroud, P., 485
Stuppy D.J., 170
Sufentanil NanoTab® patient controlled analgesia system, 464
Superior hypogastric plexus, 268–270
Supraclavicular brachial plexus block, 472
Supraventricular tachycardia (SVT), 388, 392, 393
Sykes, N., 487
Sympathetic neurolysis
lumbar, 304–305
thoracic, 305–306
Symptom management
adjuvants, 114
anticonvulsants, 115
antidepressants, 115
breakthrough pain, 112–113
corticosteroids, 116–117
gastrointestinal system
cachexia syndrome and fatigue, 120–122
constipation, 119–120, 134
cough, 124–125
delirium, 125–127, 134
dyspnea, 122–124, 134
insomnia, 127–128
nausea and vomiting, 117–119
xerostoma, 117
hospice, 67
death rattle, 62
terminal agitated delirium, 62–63
NMDA antagonists, 116
nonopioids, 109–110
opioids, 134
atute monitoring, 112
conversion table, 111
nalbuphine, 110
systematic titration, 111–112
toxicities, 110
pain
antineuropathic benefit, 134
distress, 107
emergencies and emergency departments, 113
pharmacologic tools, 108
WHO analgesic ladder, 108–109
side effects, 113–114
Systemic-to-pulmonary arterial shunt, 370, 373, 374

T
Tachyarrhythmias
  supraventricular, 387–388
  supraventricular tachycardia, 388
  ventricular tachycardia, 388–389
Taussig, H.B., 370
Terminal phase of illness, 58, 69
Thomas, V., 370
Thoracic sympathetic neurolysis, 305–306
Thorns, A., 487
Time-limited trial (TLT), 101
Total parenteral nutrition (TPN), 146–148, 160
Tracheotomy, 218–219
Tramadol, 236
Tran De, Q.H., 471
Transformed migraine. *See* Chronic migraine
Transjugular intrahepatic portosystemic shunt
    (TIPS)
  complications, 273
  contraindications, 272
  procedural method, 273
Trigeminal-autonomic cephalgias (TAC), 332
Trigeminal ganglion, 306–307, 313, 314
Triple-H therapy, 260
Truog, R.D., 491, 492
Tuckman, B.W., 191
Tunnelled central venous access, 266–267
Type I cyclo-oxygenase (COX-I), 109–110
Type II cyclo-oxygenase (COX-II), 109–110

U
Uncovered self-expanding metal stents, 352,
    354, 356, 358
Uniform Determination of Death Act
    (UDDA), 484, 498, 500
Urinary diversion, 221
Urman, R., 471

V
Vadivelu, N., 471
Vascular access
  adjuvant or supplementary analgesic
    agents, 218

  anorexia and cachexia syndrome,
    218
  autonomy assessment, 223
  delirium, 218
  end-of-life assistance, 223–224
  gastrointestinal or urinary tract
    obstructions, 220–221
  heart failure patients, 222
  hospice movement, 217
  interstitial lung disease,
    218–219
  nutritional evaluation,
    219–220
  opioids, 218, 219
  pain evaluation, 218
  patient's comfort, 217
  pleural effusion, 221
  psychological problems, 218
  tracheotomy, 218–219
Veldink, J.H., 287
Venous thromboembolism
  indications, 265
  inferior vena cava filters,
    265–266
Ventricular tachycardia, 388–389
Voltage-gated calcium channel
    (VGCC) blocking agents,
    459, 480, 481

W
Waisel, D.B., 491, 492
Walker, R., 494
Waterston shunt, 370
Weiss, S.C., 484
Wheeze, 400
Wolffe, H., 317

X
Xerostoma, 117

Y
Young, E., 484

Printed by Printforce, the Netherlands